MANUAL OF CLINICAL PROBLEMS IN INFECTIOUS DISEASE

Fifth Edition

MANUAL OF CLINICAL PROBLEMS IN INFECTIOUS DISEASE
Fifth Edition

Nelson M. Gantz, MD, FACP
Chief of Infectious Disease
Boulder Community Hospital
Boulder, Colorado
Former Clinical Professor of Medicine
Penn State College of Medicine
Hershey, Pennsylvania

Richard B. Brown, MD, FACP, FCCP
Professor of Medicine
Tufts University School of Medicine
Chief, Division of Infectious Disease
Baystate Medical Center
Springfield, Massachusetts
Professor of Medicine
Tufts University School of Medicine
Boston, Massachusetts

Steven L. Berk, MD
Regional Dean
Professor of Medicine and Family Medicine
Mirick-Myers Endowed Chair in Geriatric Medicine
Texas Tech University Health Science Center
School of Medicine at Amarillo
Amarillo, Texas

James W. Myers, MD
Associate Professor of Medicine
Division of Infectious Disease
East Tennessee State University
Johnson City, Tennessee

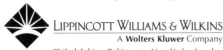
LIPPINCOTT WILLIAMS & WILKINS
A **Wolters Kluwer** Company
Philadelphia • Baltimore • New York • London
Buenos Aires • Hong Kong • Sydney • Tokyo

Acquisitions Editor: Frances R. DeStefano
Managing Editor: Joanne Bersin
Project Manager: Fran Gunning
Manufacturing Manager: Ben Rivera
Marketing Manager: Kathy Neely
Design Coordinator: Teresa Mallon
Production Services: TechBooks
Printer: RR Donnelley-Crawfordsville

Library of Congress Cataloging-in-Publication Data

Manual of clinical problems in infectious disease / Nelson M. Gantz . . .
   [et al.].— 5th ed.
      p. ; cm.
   Includes bibliographical references and index.
   ISBN 0-7817-5929-3 (alk. paper)
   1. Communicable diseases—Handbooks, manuals, etc.   I. Gantz, Nelson
Murray, 1941-
   [DNLM: 1. Communicable Diseases—Handbooks.   WC 39 M294 2006]
   RC112.M368 2006
   616.9—dc22   2005019158

Care has been taken to confirm the accuracy of the information presented and to describe generally accepted practices. However, the authors, editors, and publisher are not responsible for errors or omissions or for any consequences from application of the information in this book and make no warranty, expressed or implied, with respect to the currency, completeness, or accuracy of the contents of the publication. Application of this information in a particular situation remains the professional responsibility of the practitioner.

The authors, editors, and publisher have exerted every effort to ensure that drug selection and dosage set forth in this text are in accordance with current recommendations and practice at the time of publication. However, in view of ongoing research, changes in government regulations, and the constant flow of information relating to drug therapy and drug reactions, the reader is urged to check the package insert for each drug for any change in indications and dosage and for added warnings and precautions. This is particularly important when the recommended agent is a new or infrequently employed drug.

Some drugs and medical devices presented in this publication have Food and Drug Administration (FDA) clearance for limited use in restricted research settings. It is the responsibility of the health care provider to ascertain the FDA status of each drug or device planned for use in their clinical practice.

10 9 8 7 6 5 4 3 2

To purchase additional copies of this book, call our customer service department at (800) 638-3030 or fax orders to (301) 824-7390. International customers should call (301) 714-2324.

Visit Lippincott Williams & Wilkins on the Internet: http://www.LWW.com. Lippincott Williams & Wilkins customer service representatives are available from 8:30 am to 6:00 pm, EST.

CONTENTS

VIII: BONES AND JOINTS

IX: SKIN AND SOFT TISSUE

X: BACTEREMIA

XI: FEVER

XII: IMMUNITY

XIII: NOSOCOMIAL INFECTIONS

XIV: ZOONOSES

XV: NEWLY APPRECIATED INFECTIONS

XVI: PROPHYLAXIS OF INFECTION IN TRAVELERS

XVII: TUBERCULOSIS

XVIII: SELECTED LABORATORY PROCEDURES

XIX: ANTIMICROBIAL, ANTIVIRAL, ANTIPARASITIC, ANTIFUNGAL AGENTS

*W*e would like to express appreciation for those who have assisted us in the preparation of this book. We thank Ellen Teig and Peg Fletcher at the Boulder Community Hospital library for their invaluable assistance in searching the literature. We are grateful to Kimberly Decker, Alicia Maltzman, Darcy Perez, and Christina Ells, who did an excellent job typing the manuscript.

*I*n 1979, at the request of our students and house officers, Drs. Richard Gleckman and Nelson Gantz prepared the first edition of *Manual of Clinical Problems in Infectious Disease*. At the time, our aim was to provide medical students, house officers, and practitioners with a contemporary approach to selected problems in infectious disease; key annotated references supported in the text.

In 1986, with the help of two additional authors, Drs. Richard Brown and Anthony Esposito, the second edition of *Manual of Clinical Problems in Infectious Disease* was published and covered a list of new subjects.

Since that time, numerous infectious agents have been recognized, new concepts have evolved, and new treatments have emerged. For the third edition, to satisfy the contemporary text addressing this information, we prepared a new list of subjects and added Dr. Steven Berk to our team.

The fifth edition of *Manual of Clinical Problems in Infectious Disease* is not simply an updated version of the four earlier books: it re-examines some older material and explores new subjects such as West Nile virus, SARS, and Parvovirus. For this edition, we are pleased to add Dr. James Myers to the team. Every effort has been made to add contemporary references to the text to enhance the accuracy of the manual and to provide a springboard for further reading; many references are annotated.

Like the four previous editions, this manual is not meant to be all-inclusive. Numerous major texts that fulfill this mission have already been published. The fifth edition of *Manual of Clinical Problems in Infectious Disease* represents an attempt to provide contemporary, scientifically accurate, and readable material on selected topics of concern to the practicing physician, house officer, and medical student. All of the editors are clinicians who see patients on a regular basis and have written chapters based on a "real world" approach to patient care while keeping with a scientific basis of management. Chapters have been added, removed, or revised in keeping with changes in infectious disease over the past 6 years. We are proud of our effort and feel that this book will prove valuable to the clinician in the day-to-day management of patients with infectious disease.

NMG
RBB
SLB
JWM

Javed Ashfraf, MD
Fellow in Geriatrics
Baystate Medical Center
Springfield, Massachusetts
Instructor in Medicine
Tufts University School of Medicine
Boston, Massachusetts
(Chapter 77)

Stewart F. Babbott, MD
Associate Director, Medicine Residency
  Program
Baystate Medical Center
Assistant Professor of Medicine
Tufts University School of Medicine
Boston, Massachusetts
(Chapter 47)

Andrew Balder, MD
Member, Division of General
  Medicine
Baystate Medical Center
Assistant Professor of Medicine
Tufts University School of Medicine
Boston, Massachusetts
(Chapter 6)

Sandra Bellantonio, MD
Director Geriatric Fellowship Program
Baystate Medical Center
Assistant Professor of Medicine
Tufts University School of Medicine
Boston, Massachusetts
(Chapter 77)

Kurt A. Diebold, MD, MPH
Director, Academic Hospital Medicine
  Program Track
Baystate Medical Center
Springfield, Massachusetts
Assistant Professor of Medicine
Tufts University School of Medicine
Boston, Massachusetts
(Chapters 15 and 33)

Marjorie Jenkins, MD
Associate Professor of Medicine
Department of Obstetrics and
  Gynecology and Internal Medicine
Texas Tech University Health
  Science Center
School of Medicine at Amarillo
Amarillo, Texas
(Chapter 26)

Brendan P. Kelly, MD
Associate Director, Medicine-Pediatrics
  Residency Program
Baystate Medical Center
Assistant Professor of Medicine
Tufts University School of Medicine
Boston, Massachusetts
(Chapter 32)

Kenda L. Kroodsma, MD
Member, Division of General Medicine
Baystate Medical Center
Assistant Clinical Professor of Medicine
Tufts University School of Medicine
Boston, Massachusetts
(Chapter 85)

Donna Leco Mercado, MD
Director, Medical Consultation
  Program
Baystate Medical Center
Assistant Professor of Medicine
Tufts University School of Medicine
Boston, Massachusetts
(Chapter 74)

James L. Mugford, MD
Member, Division of General Medicine
Baystate Medical Center
Assistant Professor of Medicine
Tufts University School of Medicine
Boston, Massachusetts
(Chapter 3)

Sivakumar Natanasabapathy, MD
Fellow in Geriatrics
Baystate Medical Center
Springfield, Massachusetts
Instructor in Medicine
Tufts University School of
    Medicine
Boston, Massachusetts
(Chapter 77)

Michael S. Picchioni, MD
Associate Director, Internal Medicine
    Residency Program
Baystate Medical Center
Assistant Professor of Medicine
Tufts University School of
    Medicine
Boston, Massachusetts
(Chapter 37)

David N. Rose, MD
Chief, General Medicine and
    Geriatrics
Baystate Medical Center
Springfield, Massachusetts
Professor of Medicine
Tufts University School of
    Medicine
Boston, Massachusetts
(Chapters 67 and 78)

Michael Rothberg, MD, MPH
Member, Division of General Medicine
Baystate Medical Center
Assistant Professor of Medicine
Tufts University School of Medicine
Boston, Massachusetts
(Chapter 1)

Stephen J. Ryzewicz, MD
Member, Division of Internal Medicine
Baystate Medical Center
Assistant Professor of Medicine
Tufts University School of Medicine
Boston, Massachusetts
(Chapter 31)

Irina Schiopescu, MD
Fellow in Infectious Diseases
Baystate Medical Center
Springfield, Massachusetts
Instructor in Medicine
Tufts University School of Medicine
Boston, Massachusetts
(Chapter 54)

Afzal Siddiqui, MD
Associate Professor of Medicine
Texas Tech University Health
    Science Center
School of Medicine at Amarillo
Amarillo, Texas
(Chapter 70)

Upper Respiratory Tract

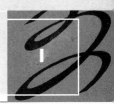

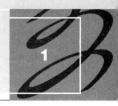

*S*ore throat is the third most common complaint in office-based practice, accounting for up to 40 million outpatient visits each year and resulting in as many as 100 million days lost from work annually. Pharyngitis, the cause of most sore throats, is characterized by the presence of inflammation in the mucous membranes of the throat and can be caused by a variety of pathogens, including viruses and bacteria. Of these, group A β-hemolytic streptococcal (GAS) infection has received the most attention because of its potential for suppurative complications and its association with both acute rheumatic fever and post-streptococcal glomerulonephritis.

Timely antibiotic therapy can shorten the course of GAS infection by approximately 1 day, decrease spread, and prevent the development of suppurative complications and rheumatic fever, but not glomerulonephritis. Most sore throats, however, are not strepto-coccal. With the exception of other bacterial causes of pharyngitis such as *Corynebacterium diphtheriae* or *Neisseria gonorrhoeae*, antibiotics are generally not indicated. Thus, distin-guishing between streptococcal pharyngitis and other causes of sore throat is important to minimize both bacterial complications and antibiotic side effects and costs. Clinical presen-tation, rapid testing, and traditional throat culture can all be used for this purpose. This chapter will focus on strategies for diagnosing and treating sore throats.

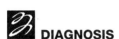 **DIAGNOSIS**

Clinical Presentation

The clinical presentation of pharyngitis is similar regardless of the causative organism. Patients usually complain of soreness in the throat, sometimes accompanied by dysphagia, and if the uvula is involved, the feeling of a "lump" upon swallowing. Associated symptoms may include headache, fever, nausea, vomiting, or abdominal pain. Any inability to manage secretions or the presence of severe dysphagia should alert the clinician to the possibility of epiglottitis or abscess.

Physical examination reveals pharyngeal erythema, while frank exudate is noted in at least 50% of cases, regardless of etiology. The presence of this is definitive of neither streptococcal pharyngitis nor bacterial infection, as it also is regularly noted with infectious mononucleosis and adenoviral pharyngitis, among others. Anterior or posterior adenopathy may be present. With streptococcal infection, there may be a beefy red tongue, swollen uvula, palatal petechiae, and a scarlatiniform rash, but none of these findings is specific. The presence of trismus or deviation of the uvula should alert the examiner to the possibility of tonsillopharyngeal cellulitis or abscess.

Although GAS is responsible for up to 30% of pharyngitis in children, among adults, only 10% of pharyngitis is caused by GAS. Certain clinical predictors, specifically the Cen-tor Criteria, have been shown in combination to differentiate between streptococcal and nonstreptococcal pharyngitis. These criteria include:

> Measured temperature >37.8°C
> Tonsillar or pharyngeal exudates
> Tender anterior cervical adenopathy
> Absence of cough

Adults meeting at least three of these criteria have a 30 to 50% chance of having streptococcal infection, whereas those meeting 0 or 1 criterion have a <7% probability of infection. McIsaac further adapted this score by adding one point for patients younger than age 15, and subtracting one point for patients older than age 45. Patients with definite exposure to *Streptococcus pyogenes* within 2 weeks are twice as likely as others to have GAS pharyngitis. Alternatively, finding vesicles or ulceration is common with viral infections and makes GAS less likely. Other viral manifestations such as conjunctivitis, coryza, hoarseness, or diarrhea also make GAS infection unlikely.

Rapid Antigen Testing

A number of commercial products are available that can detect GAS carbohydrate antigen directly from a throat swab. The major advantage of these "rapid tests" is that results are available at the point-of-care, usually within 10 minutes, and can be incorporated into clinical decision making. Compared with conventional cultures, specificity of the tests is generally 90 to 95%; thus, false positive tests are uncommon, and a positive test may be acted upon with confidence. Sensitivity of the rapid tests is more variable, with rates no greater than 80 to 90%. As a result, negative tests may require confirmation with conventional culture, especially when clinical suspicion is high. The sensitivity of these tests depends greatly on the adequacy of the sample. This requires vigorous swabbing of both tonsils and the posterior pharynx.

Throat Culture

Conventional culture from a throat swab plated on sheep's blood agar remains the gold standard for diagnosing GAS infection. A single swab has a sensitivity of 90 to 95%, assuming an adequate sample. Specimens obtained from sites other than the tonsils or posterior pharynx, as well as any recent antibiotic use, can cause a false-negative result. The culture is read after overnight incubation. Negative cultures should be reexamined 24 hours later to increase the yield. Throat culture cannot reliably distinguish between GAS pharyngitis and asymptomatic colonization with this organism. Therefore cultures generally should only be obtained from truly symptomatic persons and should not be used as "test of cure" or other considerations. Other bacterial causes of pharyngitis, such as *N. gonorrhoeae*, require special media for growth and will not be diagnosed by strep culture. If one of these other causes is suspected, specific instructions to look for the pathogen in question should be communicated to the laboratory.

Diagnostic Strategies

The goals of treatment for streptococcal pharyngitis include shortening the course of illness, avoiding suppurative complications and rheumatic fever, minimizing contagiousness, and limiting use of unnecessary antibiotics. This is best achieved by risk stratifying patients based on clinical grounds. Two different approaches have been advocated: the Infectious Disease Society of America recommends no treatment of patients with Centor scores of 0 or 1, with rapid testing or culture of all other individuals. Negative rapid tests should also be confirmed by throat culture. This strategy tends to minimize the number of unnecessary antibiotic prescriptions but will miss selected cases with few clinical signs. It may also result in delayed diagnosis for patients with negative rapid tests, who must wait overnight before receiving treatment. The American College of Physicians and the Centers for Disease Control and Prevention endorse a similar guideline, but allow for immediate treatment without testing for adults with Centor scores of 4 and rapid testing for patients with scores of 2 to 3, without confirmation of negative tests. This strategy maximizes the number of patients who are treated immediately at a cost of some unnecessary prescriptions and some missed cases. A prospective trial comparing these two guidelines confirmed these trade-offs. Neither strategy is clearly superior because the value of the outcomes is similar. Unnecessary courses of penicillin very rarely result in anaphylaxis or other severe reactions. Alternatively, missed cases of GAS cause rheumatic fever in adults so rarely today that it may almost be removed from consideration. Both approaches also appear to have similar cost effectiveness. For patients who are extremely uncomfortable and fulfill all four Centor criteria, empirical therapy can be recommended, whereas patients in less distress can be treated symptomatically while awaiting results of rapid testing, and if necessary, traditional culture.

TREATMENT

The major goals of treatment are to decrease duration of illness, prevent suppurative complications and rheumatic fever, and contain spread. Therapy begun within the first 48 hours of illness leads to a prompt resolution of fever and shortens overall illness by 1 to 2 days. Failure to respond clinically should cast doubt on the correctness of the diagnosis. Other complications are rare in clinical practice. Studies from the 1950s confirmed the ability of penicillin to prevent acute rheumatic fever if initiated up to 9 days after onset of symptoms. However, the incidence of acute rheumatic fever today in the United States is less than 1/million population. In contrast, transmission of GAS to close contacts occurs in about 35% of cases. Treatment is effective in reducing the spread of GAS after 24 hours of therapy.

Penicillin V remains the treatment of choice for GAS. It is both inexpensive and effective; to date, resistance has not been demonstrated. The traditional dose is 250 mg t.i.d. to q.i.d. for 10 days. Twice-daily dosing has been shown to be effective in children, and 500 mg b.i.d. may be effective in adults as well, though evidence is lacking. Even once-daily amoxicillin 750 mg may be effective, but more studies are needed. Shorter courses of penicillin have been associated with relapse, but 5-day courses of amoxicillin, amoxicillin-clavulanate, and several cephalosporins, including cefadroxil, cefuroxime, and cefpodoxime have eradication rates similar to those obtained with 10 days of penicillin V. For patients who are unreliable, benzathine penicillin G, a single dose of 1.2 million units intramuscularly, is an acceptable alternative. For those allergic to penicillin, treatment should be with either erythromycin or a first-generation cephalosporin (assuming there is no history of immediate-type hypersensitivity to beta-lactams). Newer macrolides, although effective and convenient, should be avoided to prevent induction of resistance and to minimize costs. Routine culturing of asymptomatic household contacts is not indicated.

OTHER CAUSES OF PHARYNGITIS

GAS is responsible for only 10% of pharyngitis in adults (Table 1-1). Most cases are due to viruses and are not treatable. However, a number of diagnoses are important for either treatment or prognostic purposes.

Infectious Mononucleosis

Infectious mononucleosis is a systemic disease characterized by lymphadenopathy and fatigue. Splenomegaly, weight loss, and hepatitis may also be present. Epstein-Barr virus (EBV) is responsible for 80% of disease, with most of the remainder being caused by cytomegalovirus (CMV). Both viruses are associated with pharyngeal exudate and can mimic bacterial disease. A complete blood count can also provide useful information. In up to 50% of cases, EBV pharyngitis can be complicated by infection with *S. pyogenes*, and in the presence of EBV infection, many clinicians associate severe pharyngitis with the presence of both pathogens. Gram's stain and culture of pharyngeal exudate often can clarify the situation. When EBV or CMV is considered, neither ampicillin nor amoxicillin (with or without beta-lactamase inhibitors) should be used because of risk of severe dermatitis. This feature is the result of a toxic rather than allergic reaction. Thus, reuse of these products after clinical recovery can be safely performed. Rapid test kits (e.g., Monospot) detect heterophile antibodies specific to EBV and are positive in up to 95% of cases. Specific EBV serologies are rarely indicated. Treatment is supportive.

| TABLE 1-1 | Notable Causes of Pharyngitis in Adults and Percentages of Cases |

Bacterial/treatable	Viral/untreatable
Streptococcus pyogenes (5–20)	Rhinovirus (42)
Other "groupable" streptococci (6)	Adenovirus (19)
Haemophilus influenzae	Epstein-Barr Virus (7–15)
Arcanobacterium hemolyticum (0.4–2)	Cytomegalovirus
Corynebacterium diphtheriae (rare)	Respiratory syncytial virus (2)
Neisseria gonorrhoeae (rare)	Myxovirus (10)
Mycoplasma pneumoniae (10–13)	
Chlamydia pneumoniae	

(Adapted from Carroll K, Reimer L. Microbiology and laboratory diagnosis of upper respiratory tract infections. *Clin Infect Dis* 1996;23:442–448.)

Primary HIV

When assessing acute pharyngitis, careful attention should be paid to HIV risk factors, because the acute retroviral syndrome can mimic infectious mononucleosis, including fever, lymphadenopathy, weight loss, and splenomegaly. The examiner should specifically address high-risk behaviors in the preceding several weeks. Diagnosis can be made by measuring HIV viral load, which should be >10,000 copies. Routine HIV testing may be falsely negative during the acute phase of illness.

Viral Influenza

Influenza occurs in winter epidemics and generally presents with fever, cough, and myalgia. Pharyngitis, however, may be a prominent symptom. When influenza is known to be in the community, diagnosis may be made solely on clinical grounds. At other times, rapid testing should be used and, if positive, treatment with one of four antiviral drugs—amantadine, rimantadine, oseltamivir, or zanamivir—can be initiated. If begun within 48 hours of onset, therapy shortens duration of illness and may decrease secondary bacterial complications.

Neisseria gonorrhoeae

Gonococcal pharyngitis is a rare but an important consideration in all persons who are sexually active, and is statistically correlated with oral sex. It has been best described in prostitutes, servicemen, and male homosexuals. In high-risk populations, positive cultures (requiring special media) may be noted in up to 6% of patients. Infection is usually asymptomatic but may be associated with erythema or exudate. Lymphadenitis and constitutional symptoms are uncommon. However, the pharynx may still serve as a nidus for disseminated disease. Therapy with ceftriaxone, 250 mg IM as a single dose, is effective, and should usually be accompanied by therapy for chlamydial infection.

Corynebacterium diphtheriae

Currently, fewer than five cases of diphtheria are reported in the United States annually. In several outbreaks noted in the 1970s, disease occurred almost entirely in nonimmunized populations. The organism is noninvasive, and most morbidity and mortality is associated with complications resulting from elaboration of toxin. This disease should be suspected in patients representing populations unlikely to have been immunized: selected religious sects, immigrants from Third World countries, and people of lower socioeconomic status. Pharyngitis is associated with exudative or membranous changes that involve the soft palate and uvula. Onset is often rapid and in the early stage resembles other forms of exudative pharyngitis. Within days, a membrane forms, then turns from white to dark. Extent of membrane correlates with severity of disease and may involve the larynx and trachea. Treatment includes antimicrobial therapy with penicillin or erythromycin at standard doses for 14 days, diphtheria antitoxin, in doses of 20,000 to 100,000 units IM or IV, and strict isolation until cultures are proved negative on several occasions. Patients identified as carriers also should be treated, although eradication may prove difficult.

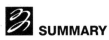 **SUMMARY**

Streptococcal infection is the most common treatable cause of pharyngitis, but still represents only 10% of pharyngitis in adults in clinical practice. Clinical predictors of this infection can be used to risk stratify patients better. Those with very low probability of infection can be managed with observation and symptomatic therapy. Patients at higher risk should have rapid testing or throat culture to confirm the diagnosis before treatment is started. Those at highest risk can either be tested or treated empirically. Penicillin remains the agent of choice for shortening illness and preventing complications, though many alternative regimens are acceptable. In specific populations, other causes of pharyngitis should also be considered. (RBB)

Bibliography

Adam D, Scholz H, Helmerking M. Short-course antibiotic treatment of 4782 culture-proven cases of group A streptococcal tonsillopharyngitis and incidence of poststreptococcal sequelae. *J Infect Dis* 2000;182:509–516.
Large, randomized trial of short-course antibiotic therapy in children. A 5-day course of six different drugs was found to be at least as effective as 10 days of penicillin V.

Bisno AI, et al. Practice guidelines for the diagnosis and management of group A streptococcal pharyngitis. *Clin Infect Dis* 2002;5:113–125.
Infectious Diseases Society of America guideline. Well-written summary of evidence for diagnosis and treatment of GAS pharyngitis. Addresses clinical presentation, rapid testing, culture and treatment options with graded evidence and specific recommendations.

Carroll K, Reimer L. Microbiology and laboratory diagnosis of upper respiratory tract infections. *Clin Infect Dis* 1996;23:442–448.

Ebell MH, et al. The rational clinical examination. Does this patient have strep throat? *JAMA* 2000;284:2912–2918.
Clinician-oriented review of the evidence for history and physical examination in determination of GAS pharyngitis. Includes sensitivity, specificity, and likelihood ratios for 22 signs and symptoms from 9 different trials. Also reviews several clinical prediction rules with easy-to-apply tables.

McIsaac WJ, et al. Empirical validation of guidelines for the management of pharyngitis in children and adults. *JAMA* 2004;291:1587–1595.
Comparison of ISDA and ACP/CDC guidelines in 787 children and adults in Canada. Highlights the tradeoffs inherent in adopting either of the guidelines. Outcomes are expressed in sensitivity and specificity for detecting GAS pharyngitis, total antibiotic prescriptions, and unnecessary antibiotic prescriptions.

Neuner JM, et al. Diagnosis and management of adults with pharyngitis. A cost-effectiveness analysis. *Ann Intern Med* 2003;139:113–122.
Cost-effectiveness analysis comparing different strategies for diagnosing and treating GAS pharyngitis, including one using a decision rule. Introduces another dimension—cost—into the tradeoffs addressed in other studies.

2 SINUSITIS

$\mathcal{S}$inusitis presents a number of diagnostic and therapeutic problems to the clinician. The classic features of the disease—fever, purulent nasal discharge, facial pain, and tenderness—may be absent. It is often difficult to differentiate a viral upper respiratory infection from a superimposed bacterial sinusitis requiring antimicrobial therapy. No simple diagnostic tests are available to establish the diagnosis, and the sinus radiographs may be confusing at times. Laboratory confirmation of the etiologic agent is also difficult to obtain without an invasive procedure. Because the throat or nasal swab cultures are generally misleading in a patient with sinusitis (sinus aspirations are not routinely performed), empiric antimicrobial therapy is usually initiated.

Sinusitis is a common disorder, occurring from the first year of life. About 11.6 million office visits are made for sinusitis yearly in the United States. Infection occurs most often in the maxillary sinus and rarely in the sphenoid sinus. The opening of the maxillary sinus is located on the upper part of the medial wall of the sinus, and as a result, the maxillary sinus does not drain by gravity in the upright position. The close relationship of the sinuses to the orbits, frontal and maxillary bones, and intracranial structures easily explains the potentially life-threatening complications that can result from either contiguous spread or hematogenous dissemination of infection from the sinuses. Complications of sinusitis include orbital cellulitis, subperiosteal abscess, orbital abscess, frontal (Pott's puffy tumor) and maxillary osteomyelitis, subdural abscess, cavernous sinus thrombosis, meningitis, and brain abscess. The most common complication is periorbital swelling resulting from impaired venous drainage, which can occur with maxillary or ethmoid sinusitis.

Obstruction of the sinus ostia by anatomic causes, such as a nasal foreign body or vascular congestion secondary to a viral upper respiratory infection, or by allergic rhinitis can result in an alteration of the local flora and sinusitis. Sinusitis also can occur when local host defenses are impaired, as in patients with the immotile cilia syndrome. About 10% of adult patients have maxillary sinusitis with a dental source—the extension of a periapical abscess of an upper tooth directly to the maxillary sinus. Sinusitis can be caused by diving into a pool or by barotrauma. In a hospitalized patient with a nasotracheal or nasogastric tube, sinusitis should be considered as a possible occult source of unexplained fever. In the majority of patients in whom sinusitis develops, however, a preceding viral upper respiratory infection or, less often, a history of allergic rhinitis can be elicited.

The etiologic agents involved in acute sinusitis are similar to those in acute otitis media. Aspiration of the maxillary sinuses has shown that *Streptococcus pneumoniae* and *Haemophilus influenzae* are responsible for just over half the cases. The *H. influenzae* strains are usually nontypeable, and 17 to 68% produce β-lactamase. About 20% or more of the cases in children, depending on the cultural methods, are caused by *Moraxella (Branhamella) catarrhalis*, an organism that is almost always β–lactamase-positive. Other organisms recovered from the sinuses of patients with acute infection include anaerobes, *Staphylococcus aureus*, and *Streptococcus pyogenes* (group A). Viruses account for about 10 to 20% of the cases. Gram-negative rods, such as *Pseudomonas* species, are the most frequent cause of nosocomial sinusitis. Anaerobes are isolated more often in patients with associated dental disease and in those with chronic sinusitis. A variety of anaerobes, such as anaerobic streptococci and *Bacteroides* species, can be found in half the patients with chronic sinusitis. *Pseudomonas aeruginosa* and *H. influenzae* are the predominant organisms found in patients with acute maxillary sinusitis and cystic fibrosis. The possibility of fungal infection caused by *Mucor* species, *Aspergillus* species, or Scedosporium apiospermum (*Pseudoallescheria boydii*) should be considered when a diabetic patient, a renal transplant recipient, or patient with acute leukemia presents with acute illness, usually maxillary or ethmoid sinusitis. Rhinocerebral mucormycosis results from extension of the fungi from the sinuses to the orbit, meninges, and frontal lobes of the brain.

The presenting features of maxillary sinusitis can include nasal discharge, which is usually purulent; facial pain; impaired sense of smell; and sense of fullness of the sinus. Only half of children and adults with maxillary sinusitis will be febrile, but a nasal discharge is generally present. In children, a cough, nasal discharge, and fetid breath are frequently present. Facial pain and headache are major complaints in older children. Patients can have pus in the sinuses and still be asymptomatic. A clue to the diagnosis of acute sinusitis is an unusually severe or protracted "cold" (persisting beyond 10 days). Sphenoid sinusitis is frequently misdiagnosed and should be considered in patients with a severe headache, fever, purulent nasal discharge, and paresthesias of cranial nerve V. Facial tenderness, periorbital swelling, and pus on rhinoscopy may be present, but in the majority of patients, the physical examination is not helpful in establishing the diagnosis of acute sinusitis.

A variety of diagnostic tests are available to help confirm the diagnosis of sinusitis: transillumination, radiography, ultrasonography, computed axial tomography (CAT), magnetic resonance imaging (MRI), and sinus endoscopy. Routine sinus radiographs may reveal the presence of an air-fluid level, complete opacification, or 4 mm or more of mucosal thickening correlates with a positive sinus aspirate in 75% of patients. Sinus radiographic studies are of value in persons older than age 1, but findings are often abnormal in those younger than age 1 without a history to suggest acute sinusitis. CT is the noninvasive modality of choice to evaluate the sinuses. Sinus endoscopy is recommended for patients with recurrent acute and chronic sinusitis. Determination of the bacteriology of sinusitis requires that sinus secretions be obtained directly from the sinus by needle aspiration. Unfortunately, nose, throat, and nasopharyngeal cultures do not predict the etiology of the sinusitis well in comparison with sinus aspiration cultures. Indications for sinus aspiration are (a) nosocomial sinusitis, (b) sinusitis in an immunocompromised host, (c) sinusitis in a severely ill patient, and (d) failure of the sinus infection to respond to several courses of antimicrobial therapy. Aspiration of the maxillary sinus can be performed safely in patients age 2 or older.

Sinusitis should be considered as a cause of unexplained fever in patients with acute leukemia or HIV. The clinical presentation is often subtle. *Aspergillus* is a frequent pathogen in patients with acute leukemia. Approximately 75% of patients with HIV have a diffuse sinus infection. The etiology of the sinus disease in patients with HIV infection remains unclear. For patients with a presumed sinus infection who fail to respond to conventional antimicrobial therapy, consideration should be given to aspirating the sinus. If the aspirate is nondiagnostic, a mucosal biopsy is indicated.

Because sinus aspirates are not routinely performed, antimicrobial therapy of this disease is usually empirically based on the bacteriology from previous studies. The antimicrobial agents selected should be at least adequate for *S. pneumoniae* and *H. influenzae*. *M. catarrhalis* appears to have an increasing role in this disease.

There is no antimicrobial agent of choice for the therapy of acute sinusitis (Table 2-1). The presence of a penicillin allergy, the prevalence of penicillin-resistant *H. influenzae* and *M. catarrhalis*, the frequency and nature of adverse effects, and drug cost are important factors to consider. Amoxicillin appears to be the preferred drug to initiate treatment of a patient with acute sinusitis. Amoxicillin-clavulanic acid, azithromycin, cefaclor, cefprozil, cefuroxime axetil, a fluoroquinolone, clarithromycin, doxycycline, telithromycin, loracarbef, and trimethoprim-sulfamethoxazole (TMP-SMX) are suitable alternative therapeutic agents (Table 2-2). TMP-SMX is ineffective in patients with group A streptococcal infections. The optimal duration of therapy is unknown, but 10 to 14 days is conventional for acute disease.

Although controlled studies are lacking, establishing drainage with topical or oral decongestants is important. The best decongestant is steam. Decongestants, however, inhibit ciliary motion, an important local defense mechanism. Antihistamines should be avoided;

TABLE 2-1	Principles of Management of a Patient with Sinusitis

1. Most cases of sinusitis in the outpatient setting are caused by viruses.
2. Acute bacterial sinusitis is suggested by the presence of severe symptoms (unilateral maxillary pain, facial swelling, and high fever) or for symptoms which persist for seven days.
3. Most patients with sinusitis do not require an imaging study unless patients have severe symptoms or fail to respond to antibiotic therapy.
4. Select a first-line agent for initial therapy. Direct therapy against *H. influenzae* and *S. pneumoniae*.
5. Select a second-line agent for patients who fail therapy or if a resistant pathogen is suspected.
6. Surgical drainage is often required for patients with chronic sinusitis. Therapy should be guided by the results of sinus cultures. Clindamycin should be added for anaerobes.

they tend to thicken sinus secretions and impair drainage. Topical corticosteroids help reduce edema and are useful for patients with allergic rhinitis and chronic sinusitis. Guaifenesin has a limited role in thinning secretions. Analgesics are indicated, and any underlying predisposing factors should be corrected. Irrigation and surgical drainage are usually reserved for patients who fail to respond to conventional therapy. It is reasonable to try an alternative antimicrobial agent, such as amoxicillin-clavulanic acid, azithromycin, cefaclor, cefuroxime axetil, clarithromycin, cefprozil, ciprofloxacin, doxycycline, levofloxacin, or loracarbef if a patient fails to respond to a course of amoxicillin.

TABLE 2-2	Common Antimicrobial Agents for the Treatment of Sinusitis

First line

Drug	Adult dose	Duration/days
Amoxicillin	500 mg three times daily	10
Amoxicillin	875 mg twice daily	10
Doxycycline	100 mg twice daily	10
Trimethoprim- Sulfamethoxazole	160 mg/800 mg 1 tab DS twice daily	10

Second line

Drug	Adult dose	Duration/days
Amoxicillin-clavulanic acid (Augmentin)	875 mg/125 mg twice daily	10
Amoxicillin-clavulanic acid (Augmentin XR)	2000 mg/125 mg twice daily	10
Azithromycin (Zithromax)	500 mg daily	3
Clarithromycin (Biaxin)	500 mg twice daily	14
Telithromycin (Ketek)	800 mg daily	5
Cefprozil (Cefzil)	500 mg twice daily	10
Loracarbef (Lorabid)	400 mg twice daily	10
Ciprofloxacin (Cipro)	500 mg twice daily	10
Gatifloxacin (Tequin)	400 mg daily	10
Levofloxacin (Levaquin)	500 mg daily	10
Moxifloxacin (Avelox)	400 mg daily	10

The optimal therapy for chronic sinusitis is unknown, but amoxicillin and clindamycin are reasonable drugs with which to initiate therapy. If the patient fails to respond to therapy, then other disorders, such as Wegener's granulomatosis or neoplastic disease, should be investigated. (NMG)

Bibliography

Axelsson A, Runze U. Comparison of subjective and radiological findings during the course of acute maxillary sinusitis. *Ann Otol Rhinol Laryngol* 1983;92:75.
Radiographic improvement lags the clinical course.
Bluestone CD, Steiner RE. Intracranial complications of acute frontal sinusitis. *South Med J* 1965;58:1.
Classic description of neurologic complications of acute frontal sinusitis.
Brook I. Bacteriology of chronic maxillary sinusitis in adults. *Ann Otol Rhinol Laryngol* 1989;98:426.
Anaerobes were isolated in 88% of adults with chronic sinusitis.
Chandler JR, Langenbrunner DJ, Stevens ER. The pathogenesis of orbital complications in acute sinusitis. *Laryngoscope* 1970;80:1414.
Orbital complications with vision loss may result from sinusitis.
Chow AW. Acute sinusitis: Current states of etiologies, diagnosis and treatment. *Current Clin Top Infect Dis* 2001;21:31–63.
Review.
DeShazo RD, Chapin K, Swain RE. Fungal sinusitis. *N Engl J Med* 1997;337:254.
Aspergillus is the most common cause of fungal sinusitis. Noninvasive disease (e.g., allergy or mycetoma) must be distinguished from invasive disease.
Evans FO Jr, et al. Sinusitis of the maxillary antrum. *N Engl J Med* 1975;293:735.
Results of nasal swab cultures correlated poorly with those of direct sinus aspirate cultures.
Frederick J, Braude AI. Anaerobic infection of the paranasal sinuses. *N Engl J Med* 1974;290:135.
Classic article. Anaerobes are an important cause of chronic sinusitis.
Gurney TA, Lee KC, Murr AH. Contemporary issues in rhinosinusitis and HIV infection. *Curr Opin Otolaryngol Head Neck Surg* 2003;11:45–48.
Gwaltney JM Jr. Acute community-acquired sinusitis. *Clin Infect Dis* 1996;23:1209–1225.
Review. About 60% of cases of acute sinusitis are caused by bacteria; in 15% of cases, viruses are isolated.
Gwaltney JM, Wiesinger BA, Patrie JT. Acute community-acquired bacterial sinusitis: the value of antimicrobial treatment and the natural history. *Clin Infect Dis* 2004;38:227–233.
Review. Treatment for 7–10 days is recommended.
Hamory BH, et al. Etiology and antimicrobial therapy of acute maxillary sinusitis. *J Infect Dis* 1979;139:197.
S. pneumoniae and H. influenzae accounted for 64% of the isolates.
Kuhn FA, Susin R Jr. Allergic fungal sinusitis: diagnosis and treatment. *Curr Opin Otolaryngol Head Neck Surg* 2003;11:1–5.
Criteria for diagnosis include (1) guidance of type I hypersensitivity (immunoglobulin E [IgE] mediated), (2) nasal polyposis, (3) characteristic computed tomography findings, (4) eosinophilic mucus, and (5) positive fungal smear.
Lawson W, Reino A. Isolated sphenoid sinus disease: an analysis of 132 cases. *Laryngoscope* 1997;107:1590–1595.
Isolated sphenoid sinus disease had an infectious etiology in 61% and was caused by a benign or malignant tumor in 29%. Cranial nerve defects were noted in 12% of infectious cases and 60% of neoplasms.
Lew D, et al. Sphenoid sinusitis. *N Engl J Med* 1983;309:1149.
Often unsuspected. An intense unilateral, frontal, or occipital headache occurs. Neurologic complications such as cavernous sinus thrombosis and meningitis can be life-threatening.
McAlister WH, Lusk R, Muntz HR. Comparison of plain radiographs and coronal CT scans in infants and children with recurrent sinusitis. *AJR Am J Roentgenol* 1989;153:1259.

CT scans are superior to plain radiographs in establishing the diagnosis.

Mofenson LM, et al. Sinusitis in children infected with human immunodeficiency virus: clinical characteristics, risk factors, and prophylaxis. *Clin Infect Dis* 1995;21:1175–1181.

Sinusitis in HIV-infected children is most often subacute and recurrent, with nasal discharge and cough common. Fever is usually absent.

Mondy KE, et al. Rhinocerebral mucormycosis in the era of lipid-based amphotericin B: case report and literature review. *Pharmacotherapy* 2002;22:519–526.

A cure using amphotericin B lipid complex without surgery.

Piccirillo, JF. Acute bacterial sinusitis. *New Engl J Med* 2004;351:902–910.

Review. Treat with antibiotics if symptoms persist for more than 10 days or begin worsening after 5 to 7 days.

Remmler D, Boles R. Intracranial complications of frontal sinusitis. *Laryngoscope* 1980; 90:1814.

Subdural empyema is the most frequent complication of frontal sinusitis.

Senior BA, et al. Long-term results of functional endoscopic sinus surgery. *Laryngoscope* 1998;108:151–157.

At the 7-year follow-up, most (98%) patients after endoscopic sinus surgery were improved and did not require further surgery.

Shapiro ED, et al. Bacteriology of the maxillary sinuses in patients with cystic fibrosis. *J Infect Dis* 1982;146:589.

P. aeruginosa was isolated most commonly.

Snow V, Mottur-Pilson C, Hickner JM. Principles of appropriate antibiotic use for acute sinusitis in adults. *Ann Intern Med* 2001;134:495–497.

Treatment guidelines. See also Ann Intern Med 2001;134:498–505.

Talmor M, Li P, Barie PS. Acute paranasal sinusitis in critically ill patients: guidelines for prevention, diagnosis, and treatment. *Clin Infect Dis* 1997;25:1441–1446.

Nosocomial sinusitis occurs in 18 to 32% of endotracheally intubated patients and is usually caused by gram-negative bacilli or is polymicrobial.

VanBuchem FL, et al. Primary-care-based randomised placebo-controlled trial of antibiotic treatment in acute maxillary sinusitis. *Lancet* 1997;349:683–687.

In patients with mild acute maxillary sinusitis, amoxicillin was not better than placebo in improving the outcome of the disease.

Wald ER. Chronic sinusitis in children. *J Pediatr* 1995;127:339–347.

Chronic sinusitis caused by infection is uncommon in children; persistent nasal symptoms are often caused by allergy.

Wald ER, et al. Acute maxillary sinusitis in children. *N Engl J Med* 1981;304:749.

Classic study in children. Cough and nasal symptoms occur most often. Only half of children had fever initially.

Williams JW Jr, et al. Antibiotics for acute maxillary sinusitis. *Cochrane Database Syst Rev* 2003;3:1–82.

A review of treatment. Amoxicillin should be given for 7 to 14 days.

Williams JW Jr, et al. Clinical evaluation for sinusitis. *Ann Intern Med* 1992;117:105.

Best predictors of sinusitis include maxillary toothache, abnormal transillumination, poor response to nasal decongestants, colored nasal discharge, and mucopurulence on examination.

Williams JW Jr, Holleman DR Jr, Samsa GP. Randomized controlled trial of 3 vs 10 days of trimethoprim/sulfamethoxazole for acute maxillary sinusitis. *JAMA* 1995;273:1015–1021.

A 3-day course of TMP-SMX plus oxymetazoline was as effective as a 10-day course of the same drug in patients with mild sinusitis.

INFECTIOUS MONONUCLEOSIS— MANY FACES OF A COMMON DISEASE

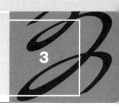

$\mathscr{T}$he Epstein-Barr Virus (EBV), a member of the herpesvirus family, is the etiologic agent of infectious mononucleosis (IM). Disease can occur in all age groups, with presenting symptomatology generally being age dependent. Infections in adolescents and young adults frequently result in classic IM, manifested by the triad of fever, lymphadenopathy, and pharyngitis. Most EBV infections in infants and children are asymptomatic. With advances in serologic testing for IM, a spectrum of disease caused by this virus has been increasingly recognized. The varied and often unusual presentations of EBV-related disease may produce diagnostic challenges. The following discussion will focus on atypical manifestations of EBV-related disease; these are summarized in Table 3-1. An awareness of these syndromes can lead to prompt diagnosis and avoid unnecessary testing and treatment.

HEMATOLOGIC

Up to 3% of patients with IM manifest hematologic abnormalities that can involve any primary marrow component. In most instances, problems arise during the first 2 to 4 weeks of illness, and thus complicate a more classic presentation. Some patients may present with primarily hematologic symptoms. Hemolytic anemia is the most commonly recognized of these abnormalities. Hemolysis may be severe and life threatening and may require administration of corticosteroids. Thrombocytopenia, primarily owing to peripheral destruction rather than primary marrow suppression, with platelet counts below 1,000/mm^3, has been

TABLE 3-1	Unusual Manifestations of Infectious Mononucleosis

Hematologic	Neurologic
Hemolytic anemia	Guillain-Barré syndrome
Neutropenia	Cranial nerve palsy
Thrombocytopenia	Radiculopathy
	Encephalitis
	Aseptic meningitis

Gastrointestinal	Cardiopulmonary
Hepatitis	Interstitial pneumonitis
Jaundice	Myo/pericarditis
Splenic rupture	

Dermatologic	Renal
Maculopapular rash	Oliguric renal failure
Petechiae	Interstitial nephritis

reported. Fortunately, such critically low levels, along with the subsequent risk for major bleeding, are extremely rare. Neutropenia and absolute granulocytopenia secondary to maturation arrest, as well as aplastic anemia also have been reported. These are also rare, though fatalities have been documented.

 ## GASTROINTESTINAL

Hepatomegaly, splenomegaly, or both, and their complications are examples of gastrointestinal complications of IM. In patients diagnosed with "typical" IM, approximately 50% will experience subclinical elevations in hepatic enzymes. Rarely, the degree of hepatitis can become severe, with jaundice and fulminant hepatic failure reported. More commonly, acute hepatitis caused by EBV is associated with complete recovery.

Although splenomegaly is often noted in IM, splenic rupture may make accurate diagnosis of IM difficult. This complication represents the most common cause of death from EBV infection, and most commonly occurs during weeks 2 to 3 of illness. Given this risk, all patients with IM should be cautioned of the risk of rupture and counseled to avoid contact sports and other risks of trauma.

 ## CARDIOPULMONARY

Myocarditis, pericarditis, atypical pneumonia, pleural effusions, hilar adenopathy, and pulmonary hypertension are all reported complications of IM. Electrocardiographic (ECG) changes are noted in up to 6% of patients and include nonspecific ST-T wave changes, likely resulting from myocardial inflammation. Resolution is the rule, and deaths are rare. Atypical pneumonia, characterized by mild respiratory symptoms (e.g., nonproductive cough) has been described in 3 to 5% of patients with IM, whereas pulmonary infiltrates are seen in 3 to 10% of individuals. Other observations include hilar adenopathy (1.5–13.6%), and pulmonary venous hypertension (2%). Pulmonary involvement leading to significant hypoxemia has been described on only six occasions, and respiratory failure requiring mechanical ventilation on only three.

 ## OTORHINOLARYNGOLIC

Pharyngitis, which may include exudative tonsillitis, is part of classic IM. Some of the complications noted occur when bacterial infection (typically *Streptococcus pyogenes*) occurs. Up to 50% of severe exudative tonsillitis ("kissing tonsils") is thought to be IM complicated by streptococcal pharyngitis. Atypical presentations include upper airway obstruction and peritonsillar abscess; neither of these need be associated with bacterial secondary infection. However, when primary infection is complicated by secondary bacterial infection, sinusitis and periorbital cellulitis may also be documented. In a retrospective investigation of IM in children, 50 to 60% of patients with IM complicated by tonsillopharyngitis developed severe airway obstruction. Most responded to systemic corticosteroids, whereas three individuals required surgery. Obstruction is due to EBV-induced hypertrophy of the tissue comprising Waldeyer's ring. Whenever patients present with dysphagia and significant tonsillar hypertrophy, care must be taken to investigate and rule out the possibility of a bacterial secondary infection.

 ## NEUROLOGIC

Epstein-Barr virus is a well-described independent cause of neurologic disease, but such complications may also be regularly noted in classic IM. In up to 7% of cases, a neurologic syndrome may either herald or be the sole manifestation of IM. Aseptic meningitis, the most common central nervous system (CNS) abnormality associated with IM, is reported in up to 25% of cases. Cerebrospinal fluid analysis frequently reveals lymphocytic pleocytosis, normal glucose, and minimal protein abnormalities. The presence of atypical lymphocytes can facilitate diagnosis of EBV infection.

Guillain-Barré syndrome, typically characterized by areflexia, ascending paresis, paresthesia, and risk for respiratory compromise, is a well-documented complication of IM. In a prospective investigation of the role of EBV in neurologic disease, more than 25% of persons with Guillain-Barré syndrome demonstrated serologic evidence of acute EBV infection, despite having negative heterophile antibody testing and no other clinical symptoms of IM.

Meningoencephalitis, with symptoms of fever, headache, photophobia, and behavioral changes (especially in children), has been reported. Other presenting symptoms may include memory loss, personality changes, reduced level of consciousness, and brainstem disorders. The ability of EBV to cause acute cerebellitis has been documented, although more global forms of encephalitis are possible. In rare cases, seizures complicate the clinical course. Death from CNS complications may occur rarely and substantial neurologic residuae may complicate survival. Facial paralysis or other focal cranial nerve palsies and headache are other presentations of IM. Most commonly, complete neurologic recovery is anticipated. However, long-term complications may be noted, especially in children where global developmental delay, autistic behavior, and limb paresis have been ascribed to this condition.

 DERMATOLOGIC

Skin disorders in IM are noted in less than 5% of patients. Some of these may be the result of therapy of presumed streptococcal infection, however. Skin rashes that may be erythematous, pruritic, or maculopapular complicate up to 95% of patients with IM treated with amoxicillin or ampicillin. Reasons for this are undefined, but are not truly allergic. Other rashes include petechiae (often related to thrombocytopenia), and periorbital edema. Immune-suppressed patients with IM appear particularly susceptible to atypical dermatologic manifestations. Reactivation of varicella-zoster virus associated with IM has been described. Other dermatologic manifestations include exacerbation of preexisting mild acne vulgaris; erythema nodosum; oral, nasal, and genital ulcers; and cutaneous lymphomas. The exact relationship to IM is uncertain.

 RENAL

Renal involvement associated with IM is unusual. However, oliguric renal failure requiring hemodialysis and immune complex-mediated glomerulonephritis have been reported.

 ONCOLOGIC

The oncogenic potential of EBV is well known, and rarely, families may develop these after typical IM. Examples include Burkitt's lymphoma, nasopharyngeal carcinoma, Hodgkin's disease, and other lymphoproliferative diseases. Regarding nasopharyngeal carcinoma, virtually 100% of anaplastic or poorly differentiated nasopharyngeal carcinomas contain EBV genomes and express EBV proteins. Similarly, in Burkitt's lymphoma, more than 90% of cases are associated with EBV. Patients with congenital or acquired immunodeficiency states who develop Hodgkin's lymphoma and lymphoproliferative diseases are more likely to have EBV presence in tumor cells when compared with healthy individuals with the same processes.

 EPSTEIN-BARR VIRUS IN THE ELDERLY

Although IM in adults older than age 30 has historically been thought to comprise less than 3% of cases, this is likely an underestimation. Disease in older persons is well described and may present only with fever and fatigability. Typical symptoms and signs of splenomegaly, lymphadenopathy, and pharyngitis are often not noted. Disease course, particularly fever, may be substantially more prolonged (13 days vs. 7 days in adolescents), and peak white blood cell counts may be lower (6,600/mm^3 in adults vs. 11,000/mm^3 in adolescents). As a consequence of these observations, EBV infection should be considered in the differential diagnosis of fever in the older individual.

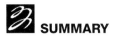

SUMMARY

EBV represents the etiologic agent of IM and typically is associated with a syndrome that is easily identified in adolescents and young adults. However clinical presentation is variable in some age groups, and atypical manifestations of IM can result in delayed diagnosis, extensive testing, and unnecessary treatment. This may be particularly true in immunocompromised persons, who are at highest risk for the most severe complications of EBV and IM. (RBB)

Bibliography

Andersson J, et al. Effect of acyclovir on infectious mononucleosis: a double-blind placebo-controlled study. *J Infect Dis* 1986;153:283–290.
> *Thirty-one patients with recent-onset IM received either acyclovir or placebo. No important clinical parameters were impacted upon by use of acyclovir. There is no role for acyclovir in the routine management of this disease.*

Carter J, Edson RC, Kennedy CC. Infectious mononucleosis in the older patient. *Mayo Clin Proc* 1978;53:146–150; also Halevy J, Ash S. Infectious mononucleosis in hospitalized patients over forty years of age. *Am J Med Sci* 1988;295:122.
> *These reports focus on older persons serologically diagnosed with IM. Both studies demonstrate that clinical presentation is often different from that seen in younger individuals and may consist primarily of prolonged fever. This should allow for earlier diagnosis, potentially avoiding unnecessary testing and treatment.*

Cohen J. Epstein-Barr virus infection. *N Engl J Med* 2000;343:481–492.
> *A contemporary review of EBV infection and clinical manifestations, it is also an excellent single source for information about pathogenesis and immunity. Limited information about "classic" IM is provided, but other syndromes, including cancers and x-linked immunoproliferative disease, are explored. Additionally, a section on EBV in HIV is presented. Regarding therapy of IM, the author provides a potential justification for corticosteroids in selected patients with severe complications, but does not feel that they are justified for most individuals.*

Ghosh A, et al. Infectious mononucleosis hepatitis: report of two patients. *Indian J Gastroenterol* 1997;16:133–114.
> *The authors describe two patients with hepatitis with jaundice. Fulminant hepatic failure with death ensued in one. IM as a cause of clinical hepatitis, even severe, should be considered if others are ruled out.*

Ikediobi N, Tyring S. Cutaneous manifestations of Epstein-Barr virus infection. *Dermatol Clin* 2002;20:283–289.
> *The authors present a review of typical features of IM, the unusual dermatologic manifestations, and other EBV-related skin conditions.*

Okano M, Gross T. A review of Epstein-Barr infection in patients with immunodeficiency disorders. *Am J Med Sci* 2000;319:392–396.
> *This review article discusses the biology and immunopathology of EBV and its clinical correlations in a variety or immunodeficiency states.*

Strauss SE, et al. Epstein-Barr virus infections: biology, pathogenesis, and management. *Ann Intern Med* 1993;118:45–58.
> *This National Institutes of Health conference remains an excellent overview of the many issues related to infection with EBV. Areas covered include the biology of EBV, serodiagnosis, and clinical manifestations. The authors reinforce the need for supportive care and underplay the role of corticosteroids in management.*

Lower Respiratory Tract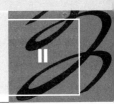

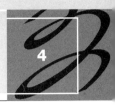

$\mathcal{A}$ cute bronchitis, an inflammatory condition of the bronchi, refers to a clinical syndrome whose most distinctive hallmark is the recent onset of cough, which is usually productive. Diverse viruses such as rhinovirus, coronavirus, adenovirus, and influenza virus presumably cause most acute bronchitis. Less often bacterial pathogens such as *Mycoplasma pneumoniae, Chlamydia pneumoniae, Bordetella pertussis, Bordetella parapertussis, Legionella* species, *Streptococcus pneumoniae,* and *Haemophilus influenzae* cause the syndrome. *M. pneumoniae* and *C. pneumoniae* are each present in about 5% of cases.

No criteria for sputum culture findings distinguish innocent airway colonization from invasiveness. As a result, we are uncertain how often these pathogens really cause bronchitis. Furthermore, neither the appearance of the sputum (purulence) nor the measurement of the white cell count is a reliable indicator of the cause of the acute bronchitis (viral vs. bacterial). Neither blood nor sputum analyses appear to be indicated for the management of immunocompetent patients.

When wheezing, shortness of breath, and tightness of the chest occur, the disease can resemble an acute attack of asthma. The symptoms of acute infectious bronchitis can imitate those of infectious pneumonia, and chest radiography would then be required to distinguish precisely between acute bronchitis and pneumonia. The absence of focal crackles or consolidation suggests bronchitis rather than pneumonia.

The preponderance of evidence indicates that most healthy persons experience spontaneous resolution of bronchitis and do not sustain any sequelae. Many patients, with or without antimicrobial therapy, will cough for weeks. Clinically, acute bronchitis is a recent, commonly productive cough without evident pneumonia. It lasts approximately 2 weeks in 20% of patients, 3 weeks in 30%, 4 weeks in 30%, and longer in 20%. Typically, 3 to 4 weeks elapse from its onset until patients resume all usual daily activities.

With rare exceptions (such as disease caused by influenza virus), the disease in these patients does not progress to pneumonia or cause irreversible anatomic abnormalities of the respiratory tract. Despite these observations, nearly half of prescriptions for adults are for common respiratory tract infections such as bronchitis, pharyngitis, sinusitis, and upper respiratory tract infections. When seeking medical care for conditions labeled as upper respiratory tract infections, bronchitis, and even the common cold, 50 to 70% of adults receive an antibiotic prescription, especially if the clinician believes that the patient expects it. Patients should be reassured that most infections are viral and will not respond to an antibiotic. If a patient fails to improve with 4 to 5 days, efforts should be made to confirm the diagnosis, exclude alternative disorders, including pneumonia, and attempt to identify specific offending pathogens, such as *B. pertussis.*

Pertussis is characterized by a paroxysmal, nonproductive cough that worsens at night. In contrast to children, adults with pertussis do not have absolute lymphocytosis. Several reports of pertussis outbreaks have been documented recently among older children and young adults who were previously immunized by vaccination. Neither immunization against pertussis nor natural disease provides lifelong protection. In the case of immunization, an attack rate greater than 50% has been reported when the interval after immunization exceeds 12 years. Adolescents and adults represent a large reservoir of susceptibles who can transmit the disease to unimmunized infants, and pertussis is an important cause of persistent cough in adults. The period of immunity induced by the pertussis vaccine tends to wane within 5 to 10 years and is shorter than that induced by the disease itself.

Although the number of susceptible adults is increasing, it is difficult to determine the true incidence of pertussis in adults. A characteristic feature suggesting pertussis is a prolonged and disturbing cough that lasts from several weeks to several months. Only 5% have a whoop. Cough is found in more than 85% of immunized adults with pertussis. It is estimated that 20 to 25% of adults with persistent cough might have pertussis. Cultures are difficult to obtain and need to be taken early in the course of the disease. Specimens for culture are best obtained by nasal swab rather than by the cough plate method. A sterile cotton swab wrapped about a flexible copper wire is passed through the nares, and mucus is obtained from the posterior pharynx. The percentage of positive cultures changes precipitously from 67 to 81% shortly after exposure to 25%, 14%, and 0% during the third, fourth, and fifth weeks, respectively.

Compared with cultures, direct fluorescent antigen detection is not more sensitive and is much less specific. Polymerase chain reaction, using a specific probe for *B. pertussis*, may offer an early diagnosis of pertussis with high specificity and sensitivity. In the established paroxysmal stage, the organisms can be readily eliminated by antimicrobial agents, but the course of the illness is unaltered. Antibiotics may be justified to render the patient noninfectious. A macrolide (traditionally erythromycin) is the drug of choice. The organism is eliminated after a few days of therapy, but because bacteriologic relapse may occur, treatment should be continued for 14 days.

Trimethoprim/sulfamethoxazole (8 mg/kg and 40 mg/kg per day in two doses) is a possible alternative for patients who do not tolerate erythromycin. Exposed susceptibles should receive erythromycin prophylaxis for 14 days, and close (household, day care, classroom) contacts younger than age 7 who have been previously immunized should receive a booster dose of vaccine in addition to erythromycin. Booster doses of vaccine or erythromycin chemoprophylaxis have been used to protect adults, such as hospital staff. Precautions to prevent respiratory droplet transmission or spread by close or direct contact should be used in the care of patients admitted to the hospital with suspected or confirmed pertussis. These precautions should remain in effect until patients are clinically improved and have completed at least 5 days of appropriate antimicrobial therapy.

Healthcare workers in whom symptoms (i.e., unexplained rhinitis or acute cough) develop after known pertussis exposure may be at risk for transmitting pertussis and should be excluded from work. Vaccination of adolescents and adults with whole-cell *B. pertussis* vaccine is not recommended because local and systemic reactions have been observed more frequently in these groups than in children. Acellular pertussis vaccine is immunogenic in adults and carries a lower risk of adverse events than does whole-cell vaccine. However, the acellular vaccine has not been licensed for use in persons age 7 or older. Postexposure prophylaxis is indicated for personnel exposed to pertussis; a 14-day course of either erythromycin (500 mg orally four times daily) or trimethoprim-sulfamethoxazole (1 tablet twice daily) has been used for this purpose. The efficacy of such prophylaxis has not been well documented, but studies suggest that it may minimize transmission.

There are no data on the efficacy of newer macrolides (clarithromycin or azithromycin) for prophylaxis in persons exposed to pertussis. Restriction from duty is indicated for personnel with pertussis from the beginning of the catarrhal stage through the third week after onset of paroxysms, or until 5 days after the start of effective antimicrobial therapy. Exposed personnel do not need to be excluded from duty. (An excellent Centers for Disease Control and Prevention [CDC] publication regarding pertussis can be found at http://www.cdc.gov/nip/publications/pink/pert.pdf.)

A systematic review performed by the Cochrane Collaboration in 1998 evaluated trials in which patients with the diagnosis of upper respiratory tract infection or the common cold were treated with antibiotics or placebo. Trials in which 5% or more of participants had group A beta-hemolytic streptococci on throat swab, those in which bronchitis was diagnosed, those in which patients had purulent sputum or purulent nasal discharge, and those in which symptoms lasted for more than 6 days were excluded. Analysis of seven trials including patients of all ages revealed that antibiotic treatment did not affect resolution of illness (summary odds ratio, 0.95 [95% CI, 0.70 to 1.28]) or loss of work time (measured in only one study). The three trials that enrolled adults only also showed no benefit of treating routine upper respiratory tract infections with antibiotics.

Instead of prescribing antibiotics, clinicians should explain that cough persists for 2 to 4 weeks, occasionally longer, and that sputum purulence is unimportant unless other features, such as high fever and chills, suggest pneumonia, which is a rare complication. An antitussive agent, such as dextromethorphan, may relieve symptoms, and inhaled bronchodilators help some patients, especially those with dyspnea, wheezing, or severe cough.

 ## ACUTE EXACERBATION OF CHRONIC BRONCHITIS

Clinically defined, chronic bronchitis is sputum production on most days for at least 3 months annually for 2 consecutive years. Patients are usually current or prior cigarette smokers. Most studies characterize exacerbations by one or more of these features: purulent phlegm or increased dyspnea, cough, or sputum volume.

Probably viruses cause 20 to 50% of attacks. *C. pneumoniae* is implicated in about 5% and *M. pneumoniae* in less than 1%. In most investigations, sputum cultures yield *S. pneumoniae* and *H. influenzae* from about 30 to 50% of patients during purulent exacerbations. *M. catarrhalis* is present in about 5 to 15% of exacerbations, but usually with *S. pneumoniae* and *H. influenzae*, not as a pure isolate.

Do antibiotics help these exacerbations? A meta-analysis found six trials, two favoring antimicrobials that used peak expiratory flow rate as an objective end point and discovered a 10.75 L/min greater improvement in the antibiotic group. Because the patients' average peak expiratory flow rate was approximately 200 L/min, this result represents about a 5% difference, a finding that is clinically and physiologically inconsequential.

The best study supporting antibiotic therapy investigated 173 patients with 362 exacerbations defined by increased dyspnea, sputum volume, or sputum purulence. Overall, success was significantly greater in those receiving antibiotics (68%) than placebo (55%), and failures were fewer (10% vs. 19%). For exacerbations with only 1 feature, antibiotics conferred no clinical advantage, and, with two features, it was marginal. With all three criteria present—about 40% of exacerbations—antibiotics recipients had greater success (63% vs. 43%) and less deterioration (14% vs. 30%), although whether these differences were statistically significant is unstated.

If antibiotics are used, the quinolones are not necessarily indicated. Less expensive agents like doxycycline and amoxicillin are still useful agents but have adverse reaction rates that are higher than placebo.

In conclusion, microbiologic studies provide no conclusive evidence that bacteria cause exacerbations, and in most investigations, antibiotics provide no significant benefit. Overall, the preponderance of information indicates that obtaining sputum cultures and prescribing antimicrobials are unnecessary, both in mild exacerbations and in the more severe episodes, which should be treated with systemic corticosteroids. (JWM)

Bibliography

Anthonisen NR, et al. Antibiotic therapy in exacerbations of chronic obstructive pulmonary disease. *Ann Intern Med* 1987;106:196–204.
Best study supporting the use of antibiotics.

Arroll B, Kenealy T. Antibiotics for the common cold. Cochrane Database Syst Rev. 2002;(3): CD000247.
There is not enough evidence of important benefits from the treatment of upper respiratory tract infections with antibiotics and there is a significant increase in adverse effects associated with antibiotic use.

Ball P, et al. Acute infective exacerbations of chronic bronchitis. *Q J Med* 1995;88;61–68.
Fever is not a common manifestation of the exacerbation.

Cherry JD. Pertussis in adults. *Ann Intern Med* 1998;128:64–66.
Pertussis as a cause of chronic nonproductive cough in adults who do not demonstrate absolute lymphocytosis.

Crimin N, Mastruzzo C, Vancheri C. The long-term antimicrobial prophylaxis of chronic bronchitis exacerbations. *J Chemother* 1995;7:307–310.

Use of oral administration of bacterial extracts to stimulate immune defenses and reduce recurrent respiratory infections.

Gonzales R, et al. Principles of appropriate antibiotic use for treatment of acute respiratory tract infections in adults: background, specific aims, and methods. *Ann Emerg Med* 2001;37:690–697.
A review article discusses the pitfalls of inappropriate antibiotic therapy for some respiratory infections.

Gonzales R, Steiner JF, Sande MA. Antibiotic prescribing for adults with colds, upper respiratory tract infections, and bronchitis by ambulatory care physicians. *JAMA* 1997;278:901–4.
Although antibiotics have little or no benefit for colds, upper respiratory tract infections, or bronchitis, these conditions account for a sizable proportion of total antibiotic prescriptions for adults by office-based physicians in the United States. Overuse of antibiotics is widespread across geographic areas, medical specialties, and payment sources. Therefore, effective strategies for changing prescribing behavior for these conditions will need to be broad based.

Grant CC, Cherry JD. Keeping pace with the elusive Bordetella pertussis. *J Infect* 2002;44: 7–12.
The persistent circulation of B. pertussis in these older age groups provides a source for epidemics in susceptible infants and young children.

Gump DW. Chronic bronchitis: common and controversial. *Infect Dis Clin Pract* 1996; 5:227–321.
A review of chronic bronchitis.

Hirschmann JV. Do bacteria cause exacerbations of COPD? *Chest* 2000;118:193–203.
The randomized, placebo-controlled trials generally show no benefit for antibiotics, but most have studied few patients. A meta-analysis of these demonstrated no clinically significant advantage to antimicrobial therapy. The largest trials suggest that antibiotics confer no advantage for mild episodes; with more severe attacks, in which patients should receive systemic corticosteroids, the addition of antimicrobial therapy is probably not helpful.

Isada CM. Pro: antibiotics for chronic bronchitis with exacerbations. *Semin Respir Infect* 1993;8:243–253.
An attempt to make the case for the use of an antibiotic to manage the exacerbation.

MacKay DN. Treatment of acute bronchitis without underlying lung disease. *J Gen Intern Med* 1996;11:557–562.
Antibiotics should not be routinely prescribed to healthy adults who experience acute bronchitis.

Roessingh PH, et al. Viral and atypical pathogens causes type 1 acute exacerbation of chronic bronchitis. *Clin Microb Infect* 1997;3:513–514.
An attempt to identify the infectious causes of the exacerbation of chronic bronchitis.

Saint S, et al. Antibiotics in chronic obstructive pulmonary disease exacerbations. A meta-analysis. *JAMA* 1995;273:957–960.
A meta-analysis of randomized trials was performed to estimate the effectiveness of antibiotics in treating exacerbations of chronic obstructive pulmonary disease (COPD).

Senzilet LD, et al. Pertussis is a frequent cause of prolonged cough illness in adults and adolescents. *Clin Infect Dis* 2001;32:1691–1697.
These patients had significantly longer duration of cough than did patients without laboratory evidence of pertussis (56 days vs. 46 days), and more of them had vomiting with cough (45.5% vs. 28.5%, respectively). Pertussis is a common cause of prolonged cough illness in adolescents and adults and is frequently associated with other symptoms of whooping cough.

Weber DJ, Rutala WA. Management of healthcare workers exposed to pertussis. *Infect Control Hosp Epidemiol* 1994;15:411–415.
Guidelines for management in the hospital setting.

ANTIBIOTIC-RESISTANT PNEUMOCOCCI

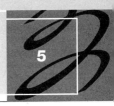

*S*treptococcus pneumoniae causes more cases of community-acquired pneumonia than any other pathogen. The pneumococcus is responsible for more than half of all community-acquired pneumonia deaths. Particular populations are very vulnerable to pneumococcal pneumonia, including older patients, those with chronic obstructive lung disease and congestive heart failure, and patients with asplenia, sickle cell anemia, and multiple myeloma. It is estimated that 500,000 cases of pneumococcal pneumonia occur annually in the United States.

Within the past decade, some strains of pneumococci have developed resistance to penicillin and other antibiotics. The first reports of penicillin resistance occurred in the 1960s, 20 years after the introduction of penicillin. Resistance became a clinically relevant problem in South Africa in the 1970s and in Europe and Asia in the 1980s. Penicillin-resistant strains of the pneumococcus (PRSP) appeared in the United States in the early 1990s and its prevalence has increased rapidly. Antimicrobial resistance among clinical isolates of *S. pneumoniae* have gone from 18% in 1990–1991 to 25% by 1995. At present about 30 to 40% of isolates are not susceptible to penicillin. These percentages can vary dramatically from one region to another and from one patient group to another. Factors that influence the emergence of resistant strains are listed in Table 5-1.

Of particular concern is the increasing incidence of high-level penicillin resistance (MIC greater than 2.0 μg/mL) and of multiresistant species to other classes of antibiotics including macrolides, trimethoprim-sulfamethoxazole, and fluoroquinolones.

In the United States, *S. pneumoniae* resistance to macrolides has risen to about 25% and clinical reports of failure in treatment with azithromycin and clarithromycin are well documented. Of *S. pneumoniae* isolates that are resistant to penicillin or intermediately resistant (minimal inhibitory concentrations [MIC] of .12 to 1.0 μg/mL), 50 to 75% are macrolide or azalide resistant. Hence, penicillin resistance serves as a marker for resistance to the macrolides. The mechanism of resistance is, of course, different, involving the efflux mechanism with respect to macrolides and not the penicillin-binding proteins that determine penicillin resistance.

Fluoroquinolone resistance has also increased particularly where the usage of quinolones is high. In Canada, resistance of more than 4.0% to levofloxacin has been reported in a group of older patients. Clinical failures have correlated with antibiotic-resistant strains in the United States and Canada. There will be some differences in susceptibility among the newer fluoroquinolones.

Until recently, penicillin was the antibiotic of choice for *S. pneumoniae* pneumonia. Now the management of pneumococcal infection is much more complex. The problem is exacerbated by the common practice of using empiric antibiotic therapy for the treatment of

 Factors That Influence Penicillin Resistance

Antimicrobial use over 3-month period
Inappropriate use of antibiotics including dosage
Clonal spread of drug-resistant strains
Presence of comorbidities

community-acquired pneumonia without efforts to determine a particular etiologic agent. This type of empiric therapy is much more difficult in areas where resistant pneumococci have emerged.

The majority of penicillin-resistant pneumococci are of a few specific serotypes, and these serotypes are included in the 23-valent pneumococcal vaccine. Penicillin resistance has developed through chromosomally mediated genetic mutations that have caused changes in penicillin-binding proteins. The affinity of penicillin for these binding proteins is weakened, resulting in less antibiotic activity.

Classification of penicillin activity in regard to pneumococci can be confusing, as different authors have set up somewhat different categories. *S. pneumoniae* with MIC of less than 0.06 μg/mL are always considered penicillin susceptible. Penicillin resistance is defined as intermediate when the MIC falls between 0.1 and 1 μg/mL. High-level resistance is usually defined as greater than 1 μm/mL, but sometimes is greater than 2 μm/mL. These breakpoints are most useful in understanding the treatment of meningitis, in that the breakpoints were determined based on antibiotic levels in cerebrospinal fluid.

Because alterations in penicillin-binding proteins will influence the binding of other β-lactam antibiotics, some pneumococci have developed multiple drug resistance. Resistance to cephalosporins generally develops in association with penicillin resistance, particularly when penicillin-binding proteins 2× and 1a are affected. However, different β-lactams bind to different proteins, and some antibiotics may retain their activity even when penicillin-binding protein changes have occurred. Hence, some β-lactams, such as ceftriaxone and cefotaxime, may be active against penicillin-intermediate and even penicillin-resistant strains.

Antibiotic susceptibility studies should be performed on all isolates of pneumococci that have been obtained from patients who are suspected of having pneumococcal disease. For patients at high risk for penicillin-resistant organisms, these studies must be carried out as quickly as possible. High-risk patients include those who are at the extremes of age, have previously received antibiotic therapy, have been recently hospitalized or institutionalized, or are attending day care or respite care centers.

The 1-μg oxacillin disk is used for screening of nonsusceptible strains. The disk will detect more than 99% of nonsusceptible strains with 80% specificity. These nonsusceptible strains should then be tested for susceptibility to vancomycin, ceftriaxone, fluoroquinolones, and other agents, depending perhaps on local susceptibility data.

The E test is a new, simpler method for MIC determination. A calibrated, antibiotic-impregnated strip is applied to the surface of an inoculated plate. An antibiotic gradient is produced that results in an elliptic zone of inhibition. The test correlates well with microdilution methods for determining MICs to the pneumococcus.

Even if adequate sputum samples and blood cultures are obtained from all patients with pneumococcal pneumonia, culture results will not be available for several days, and initial antibiotic regimens must be chosen without the benefit of this information. In addition, clinical studies are not yet available to settle fully controversy about the importance of in vitro sensitivity testing in treating penicillin-resistant pneumococci. At least one study could not show any difference in mortality among patients with sensitive versus resistant pneumococci as long as meningitis was not present and corrections were made for other predictors of mortality. Another study found that success of treatment was no different for penicillin-sensitive and penicillin-intermediate strains. For treatment of pneumococcal pneumonia when the organism has been isolated and susceptibility tests have been performed, the following recommendations appear appropriate.

1. For penicillin-susceptible strains of pneumococci: Penicillin or ampicillin is recommended (as always in the past before the emergence of resistant pneumococci).
2. For isolates that are intermediately resistant to penicillin (MICs between 0.1 and 1 μg/mL): Parenteral penicillin, ceftriaxone or cefotaxime, amoxicillin, or fluoroquinolones are recommended.
3. For highly resistant strains of pneumococci (MIC >2 μg/mL): Fluoroquinolones or vancomycin is recommended. Other agents can then be chosen based on results of susceptibility tests.

The American Thoracic Society, Infectious Disease Society of America (IDSA), and other groups have proposed guidelines for the empirical treatment of community-acquired pneumonia. These recommendations take into account that the pneumococci is the most likely cause of community-acquired pneumonia, but that other organisms such as mycoplasma, chlamydia, *Haemophilus influenza*, *Moraxella catarrhalis*, are also potential pathogens. Treatment should be based on severity of illness, comorbidities, and previous antibiotic therapy. Both the IDSA and the American Thoracic Society recommend the use of a macrolide or doxycycline in a patient who does not appear ill and is not suspected of having a resistant pneumococcus. If the patient requires hospital admission, has received recent antibiotic therapy, or has comorbidity such as cardiopulmonary disease, then the use of a respiratory fluoroquinolone might be recommended. (SLB)

Bibliography

Anderson KB, et al. Emergence of levofloxacin-resistant pneumococci in immunocompromised adults after therapy for community acquired pneumonia. *Clin Infect Dis* 2003;37:376.
Pneumococci with in vitro resistance to levofloxacin are likely to result in treatment failure.

Aubier M, et al. Once-daily sparfloxacin versus high-dosage amoxicillin in the treatment of community-acquired, suspected pneumococcal pneumonia in adults. *Clin Infect Dis* 1998;26:1312.
Sparfloxacin treatment was successful in patients with pneumococcal pneumonia, including 20 of 24 patients with bacteremia.

Austrian R. The enduring pneumococcus: unfinished business and opportunities for the future. *Microb Drug Resist* 1997;3:111.
Essay puts penicillin resistance in historical perspective and emphasizes the value of the pneumococcal vaccine.

Bartlett JG, et al. Community-acquired pneumonia in adults: guidelines for management. *Clin Infect Dis* 1998;26:811.
Practice guidelines for pneumonia developed by the IDSA. The article emphasizes the importance of specific diagnosis and provides antibiotic recommendations for pneumococcal pneumonia based on whether organism is susceptible to penicillin, intermediately resistant, or completely resistant. The use of fluoroquinolones is recommended for penicillin-resistant pneumococci.

Breiman RF, et al. Emergence of drug-resistant pneumococcal infections in the United States. *JAMA* 1994;271:1831.
Surveillance study found that 6.6% of all pneumococcal isolates from 13 hospitals in 12 states were penicillin-resistant. Most of the resistant isolates were serotypes present in the 23-valent pneumococcal vaccine.

Campbell GD, Silberman R. Drug-resistant *Streptococcus pneumoniae*. *Clin Infect Dis* 1998;26:1188.
Includes discussion of risk factors for antibiotic-resistant pneumococci. These include extremes of age, recent antimicrobial therapy, coexisting illness, HIV infection, attendance at day care centers, and recent hospitalization or institutionalization.

Doern GV, et al. Antimicrobial resistance among clinical isolates of Streptococcus pneumoniae in the United States during 1999–2000 including a comparison of resistance rates since 1994–1995. *Antimicrob Agents Chemother* 2001;45:1721.
One of the best articles to document the increasing resistance of the pneumococcus to penicillin.

Guillemot D, et al. Low-dosage and long-term treatment duration of β-lactam. Risk factors for carriage of penicillin-resistant *Streptococcus pneumoniae*. *JAMA* 1998;279:365.
Low-dose and long-duration therapy with β-lactam antibiotics promotes pharyngeal carriage of penicillin-resistant pneumococci.

File TM. Streptococcus pneumoniae and community-acquired pneumonia: A cause for concern. *Am J Med* 2004;117:39S.
Updates the increasing resistance of the pneumococcus to penicillin, macrolides, and fluoroquinolones. Reviews guidelines for the treatment of community-acquired pneumonia.

Klugman KP. Pneumococcal resistance to antibiotics. *Clin Microbiol Rev* 1990;3:171.
Detailed review of the prevalence and mechanism of resistance of pneumococci to peni-cillin, erythromycin, tetracycline, chloramphenicol, and other agents.

Mandel LA, et al. Update of practice guidelines for the management of community-acquired pneumonia in immunocompetent adults. *Clin Infect Dis* 2003;37:1405.
Recommendations are based on estimating the likelihood of penicillin-resistant and macrolide-resistant pneumococci. If patient is not ill, has no underlying comorbidity, and has not been on antibiotics, then a macrolide or doxycycline is recommended. Flu-oroquinolones are held for those with comorbidity, those requiring hospitalization, and those previously taking antibiotics.

Musher DM. Infections caused by Streptococcus pneumoniae: clinical spectrum, pathogen-esis, immunity, and treatment. *Clin Infect Dis* 1992;14:801.
Summarizes data on the clinical features of pneumococcal pneumonia and approach to diagnosis. Predicted the increasing use of quinolones in the treatment of penicillin-resistant pneumococci.

Nuorti JP, et al. An outbreak of multidrug-resistant pneumococcal pneumonia and bac-teremia among unvaccinated nursing home residents. *N Engl J Med* 1998;338:1861.
A multidrug-resistant (type 23F) pneumococcus caused an outbreak of pneumonia in a nursing home. None of the patients had received the pneumococcal vaccine. After vaccination, there were no additional cases and the colonization rate decreased.

Pallares R, et al. Risk factors and response to antibiotic therapy in adults with bac-teremic pneumonia caused by penicillin-resistant pneumococci. *N Engl J Med* 1987; 317:18.
Patients with penicillin-resistant pneumococci had a higher mortality rate than patients with penicillin-sensitive organisms. Sixty-five percent of patients with resistant pneumo-cocci had previously received β-lactam antibiotics.

Yu VL, et, al. An international prospective study of pneumococcal bacteremia: correlation with in vitro resistance antibiotics administered and clinical outcome. *Clin Infect Dis* 2003;37:230.
Antibiotic resistance correlated with underlying illnesses and previous antibiotic therapy.

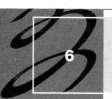

6   FEVER AND PLEURAL EFFUSIONS

leural effusions associated with fever constitute a common medical problem. The clinician must have a thorough understanding of the pathophysiology of pleural effusions and a realistic approach to diagnosis and treatment if optimal treatment is to be provided.

ANATOMY AND PATHOPHYSIOLOGY OF THE PLEURAL SPACE

The pleural space, truly a "potential space," formed at the interface of the parietal and visceral pleura acts as a lubricant, and normally contains only 7 to 14 cc of fluid. The area becomes a bone fide space in diseases in which it may fill with air or fluid. Blood supply to the parietal pleura comes primarily from branches of the intercostal and superior phrenic arteries, whereas the visceral pleura is supplied by both pulmonary and pericardiophrenic arteries. Venous drainage of the parietal pleura is through the intercostal veins; the visceral pleura is drained primarily by pulmonary veins.

Pleural lymphatics, located in the connective tissues that underlie the mesothelial cells of the pleural surfaces, freely interconnect with those below the diaphragm. Materials placed in subdiaphragmatic lymphatics drain into the intercostal and mediastinal nodes, respectively. Drainage is extremely important for removal of erythrocytes and proteins from the pleural space. Gases and liquids are rapidly cleared. In normal individuals, the origin of most pleural fluid is the capillaries of the parietal pleura by a pressure gradient effect. As the pleural space is under relative negative pressure, there is no corresponding effect favoring removal by the visceral pleura. Most pleural fluid is removed via lymphatic vessel stomas in the parietal pleura. Normally 250 to 500 mL/day of fluids and contained materials, including particulate matter and proteins, can be removed in this fashion. A small amount of pleural fluid is removed by a mesothelial cellular mechanism. Pleural effusions develop when there are discrepancies between rates of production and absorption of fluid. Causes include changes in transpleural pressure balance (disturbed hydrostatic or colloid oncotic pressure), impaired lymphatic drainage, or altered capillary permeability.

Pleural fluid is normally sterile, but easily supports microbial growth. This is in part related to the fluid basis of effusion, which allows extreme mobility of bacteria relative to white blood cells, and thus impairs early phagocytosis prior to the presence of opsonins. Empyema formation is divided into an exudative phase, during which pus accumulates; a fibrinopurulent phase, with fibrin deposition and loculation of fluid; and an organizing phase, with fibroblast proliferation and scar formation that may result in lung entrapment. The presence of microbes within pleural effusions initiates a variety of host responses that involve cytokines. If the response fails to inhibit bacterial growth, opsonins and complement become deficient, and the fluid becomes hypoxic and acidic. The inflammatory process typical of empyema releases components capable of bacterial inhibition. In such a state, bacterial reproduction slows and may be reduced to every 24 hours. This may explain in part why antibiotics need to be administered for prolonged periods in patients treated for undrained empyema.

 EVALUATION OF PLEURAL EFFUSIONS

History and Physical Examination

History and physical examination provide important clues for both presence and etiology of effusions. Questions regarding pneumonia, subdiaphragmatic illness, medication use, malignancy, and epidemiology (e.g., travel and tuberculosis exposure) are indicated. Specific risks for human immunodeficiency virus should be assessed. Physical examination should be comprehensive.

Radiography

The chest radiograph is often insensitive, requiring 200 mL of fluid to show blunting of the posterior costophrenic sulcus and often up to 500 mL for obscuring of the hemidiaphragm. Ultrasonography may reveal as little as 5 to 50 cc; lack of echogenicity may indicate a transudate. Computerized tomography (CT) has the advantage of revealing additional details of pulmonary parenchyma and mediastinum and is better at differentiating pleural thickening from fluid. Either ultrasound or CT may be used to guide thoracentesis in selected cases.

Obtaining Pleural Fluid

Thoracentesis is indicated to assess the cause of most effusions and provides a diagnosis in about 75% of cases. There are no absolute contraindications, although bleeding potential and poor patient cooperation are considered relative contraindications. Well-documented congestive heart failure or generalized anasarca may be managed without this study. Occasionally, because of small size or difficult location, thoracentesis using either ultrasound or CT guidance may be indicated. Recent prospective studies demonstrate that this procedure

TABLE 6-1	Tests for Evaluation of Thoracentesis Fluid
Microbiologic	Gram's stain
	Aerobic/anaerobic culture
	Acid fast smear/culture*
	Fungal smear/culture*
	Legionella culture*
Hematologic	Cell count/differential
	Cytology*
Biochemical	pH
	Glucose
	LDH
	Protein
	Amylase
Tests of Occasional Value	Counterimmunoelectrophoresis
	Rheumatoid factor, antinuclear antibody
	Adenosine deaminase
	Gamma interferon
	Polymerase chain reaction for *M. tuberculosis*
	Neutrophil elastase, alpha-1 proteinase inhibitor
	Flow cytometry with immunochemistry

*Performed on stored fluid aliquots or unstained slides if initial assessment is nondiagnostic.

provides useful information in >90% of instances, but may be associated with both technical problems and adverse reactions. Table 6-1 lists studies to be performed once fluid is obtained.

Biochemical Tests

Pleural effusions may be exudative or transudative. The latter are more likely benign and occur when mechanical factors alter pleural fluid formation or resorption. Thus, diagnosing fluid as transudative generally truncates the evaluation. Exudates result from inflammation or malignancy that interfere with pleural surfaces or lymphatic drainage. Differentiation is important because of the broad types of illness that fall into the two categories. Some diagnoses may result in either; for example, significant diuresis may alter pleural fluid protein and lactate dehydrogenase (LDH) so that fluid mimics exudate. Simultaneous measurements of serum and pleural fluid LDH and protein content allow for more accurate assessment. A pleural fluid-serum ratio of LDH >0.6, or protein >0.5, or a pleural fluid LDH more than two thirds the upper limit of normal for the serum LDH generally documents an exudate (Light's criteria). Virtually all exudates exhibit at least one of these characteristics; transudates typically lack all three. When a transudative effusion is strongly suspected by clinical criteria, but Light's criteria are consistent with an exudate, a serum-effusion albumin gradient of >1.2 mg/dL makes a transudate highly likely. Pleural fluid cholesterol >60 mg/dL appears specific for exudative effusion but may not be as sensitive as the prior criteria.

Pleural fluid glucose levels <40 mg/100 mL are generally seen in effusions caused by bacterial infection, tuberculosis, malignancy, or rheumatoid arthritis. The value of a low glucose level lies more in documenting the need for further evaluation than in providing a specific diagnosis. Pleural fluid amylase levels are elevated in pancreatitis, esophageal rupture, and with amylase-producing tumors. Amylase may be further divided into that of salivary or pancreatic origin. Markedly elevated levels almost always result from pancreatitis and are usually associated with pleural fluid-serum amylase levels >1.0. Esophageal rupture may be suspected by the presence of amylase of salivary origin.

Pleural fluid pH is useful in defining parapneumonic effusions that require tube thoracostomy. Low pleural fluid pH values occur primarily in malignancy, tuberculosis, and bacterial infections. Pleural fluid acidosis is defined by a pH <7.3 or, if acidemia is present, by a value >0.15 below blood pH. Some authors now recommend immediate chest tube drainage for parapneumonic effusions associated with pH <7.10, glucose <40 mg/dL, LDH >1,000, or evidence of loculation. Parapneumonic effusions with pH values >7.10, especially if accompanied by glucose levels >40 mg/100 mL, may be successfully treated without tube placement. Repeat thoracentesis to document trends is recommended.

Cell Type

Exudates often contain >1000 cells/mL, but this is not as useful as LDH and protein ratios for distinguishing between exudate and transudate. An elevated percentage of polymorphonuclear leukocytes, seen primarily in bacterial infections, is also noted in pancreatitis, connective tissue disease, and pulmonary infarction. Tuberculosis of short duration has been associated with this cell type as well. Predominance of lymphocytes is seen in >80% of tuberculous and malignant pleural effusions. Tuberculosis is also associated with a relative absence of mesothelial cells in the differential count. Newer tests to define lymphocyte type further may be important in defining etiology of pleural effusions. As an example, recent studies have demonstrated elevated levels of helper T cells in a patient with pleural effusion due to sarcoidosis.

Eosinophilic pleural effusions contain >10% eosinophils and may account for 2 to 9% of all pleural effusions. A recent investigation documented "idiopathic" and postthoracic surgery as statistically correlated with eosinophilia, and survivorship was longer in those with eosinophilic effusions. Such effusions have also been reported with malignancies, tuberculosis, parasitic infection, and drug-related hypersensitivity reactions.

Erythrocytes are common but of uncertain importance. Historically, the presence of blood-tinged fluid was considered indicative of tuberculosis, pulmonary infarction, or malignancy. However, <2 mL/1,000 mL of blood in an effusion creates this appearance. Greater than 100,000 red blood cells (RBCs)/mL is generally associated with malignancy, trauma, and pulmonary infarction.

Malignant cells should be sought in exudative effusions not otherwise diagnosed. Cytologic examination establishes a diagnosis in about 50% of malignant pleural effusions. Fresh samples must be used, and several techniques may be necessary to demonstrate malignant cells.

Bacteriologic Studies

All pleural effusions should be analyzed by Gram's stain and aerobic and anaerobic culture. Although only 5% of bacterial pneumonias are complicated by infected pleural fluid, laboratory information is valuable. Not all effusions need to be evaluated for tuberculosis or fungal infection. Acid-fast bacilli (AFB) and fungal smears and cultures should be obtained with lymphocytic exudative effusions or when diagnosis of an exudate is elusive. Smears for AFB are positive in <25% of cases and increase both patient and laboratory costs.

Tests of Occasional Value

Pleural effusions in systemic lupus erythematosus (SLE) may be associated with antinuclear antibody (ANA) titers >1:160 and pleural fluid-serum ANA ratios >1. Determination of levels of both complement and rheumatoid factor in pleural fluid may help diagnose rheumatoid arthritis. Measurement of adenine deaminase and other studies of potential value in diagnosing pleural tuberculosis are discussed below.

Tests for detection of bacterial antigens may document a bacterial etiology in the absence of viable organisms. Thus, partially treated infections may be diagnosed despite negative cultures. Organisms detectable include *Haemophilus influenzae* type b (rarely noted any longer), *Streptococcus pneumoniae*, and several types of *Neisseria meningitidis*. Results with these techniques have been comparable to routine cultures. Other studies of occasional value include neutrophil elastase and alpha-1 proteinase inhibitor (malignancy), and flow cytometry with immunochemistry (malignancy).

Pleural Biopsy and/or Thoracoscopy

Thoracoscopy, often video assisted, which can include pleural biopsy, should be performed in difficult cases of exudative pleural effusion. Current data demonstrate that >90% of cases of elusive exudative effusions can be diagnosed by use of this procedure. It is especially useful for finding nodular pleural lesions that could then be sampled. Biopsy specimens should be submitted for bacteriology (aerobic/anaerobic, mycobacteriology, and mycology) and histopathology. Despite best efforts, some patients remain undiagnosed. Most turn out to be benign and resolve in 5 to 6 months. Etiologies eventually discovered in a minority of these patients include asbestosis, rheumatoid arthritis, congestive heart failure, cirrhosis, and adenocarcinoma.

Pleural Effusion in the Intensive Care Unit

Patients in adult critical care units often develop pleural effusions. Up to 9% have larger effusions discovered by physical examination, but up 60% are found by ultrasound screening (often transudates). Causes of large effusions are similar to patients not in the intensive care unit (ICU), but likely weighted more to transudates from fluid overload and myocardial dysfunction. However, the relatively compromised state of ICU patients and incidence of pneumonia in this population makes thoracentesis a valuable tool. The more common small effusions do not require sampling unless suspicion for infection or other specific diagnosis is high.

Pleural Disease and AIDS

Pleural effusion is seen in 2 to 27% of hospitalized patients with HIV. Most effusions are small. Three leading causes are parapneumonic effusions, tuberculosis, and Kaposi's sarcoma. *Pneumocystis carinii* pneumonia is found in 4% of pleural effusions and is much more commonly associated with spontaneous pneumothorax than pleural effusion.

 TYPES OF PLEURAL EFFUSIONS

Table 6-2 lists some of the common causes of fever and pleural effusions. Selected ones are discussed below.

TABLE 6-2   **Common Pleural Effusions Associated with Fever**

Condition	Effusion type	Cells	Glucose (mg/dL)	pH
Empyema	Exudate	PMNs*>50,000	<30	<7.0
Parapneumonic effusion	Exudate	PMNs often <50,000	>30	>7.2
Tuberculosis	Exudate	Lymphocytes	30–60	7.0–7.3
Systemic lupus erythematosus	Exudate	PMNs, lymphocytes	Variable	Variable
Malignancy	Exudate	Generally lymphocytes	Variable	Variable, generally >7.2
Pulmonary infarction	Variable (usually exudate)	Variable; RBCs >100,000	Variable, generally >30	Variable

*PMNs, Polymorphonuclear leukocytes.

Parapneumonic Effusions

Parapneumonic effusion is associated with pneumonia, lung abscess, or bronchiectasis. Between 30 and 70% are associated with positive pleural fluid cultures, reflecting the progression from effusion to infected pleural space to empyema. the likelihood of encountering parapneumonic effusions with different pathogens is as follows: *Staphylococcus aureus*, 75%; *Streptococcus pneumoniae*, 57%; viruses, 15 to 25%; *Haemophilus influenzae*, 50 to 75%; and *Streptococcus pyogenes*, 90%. Yield may be related to duration of effusion, as organisms such as *S. pneumoniae* may undergo autolysis. *Mycoplasma pneumoniae* has been associated with parapneumonic effusions in up to 20% of cases. Relative frequency with *Legionella* species or gram-negative enteric bacilli is uncertain.

Management of parapneumonic effusions includes thoracentesis and antimicrobials. β-lactams penetrate the pleural space well and achieve therapeutic levels early in therapy. Concentrations of parenteral aminoglycosides are decreased in the presence of empyema. Although empyema (pus) is the only absolute indication for drainage, other features that suggest the need for drainage to hasten resolution and/or avoid complications include a positive pleural fluid Gram's stain or culture, size and number of loculations, virulence of the pathogen (*Str. pyogenes, Sta. aureus, Klebsiella* sp., anaerobes), low pH, and other features (see Table 6-3). The method of drainage (video-assisted thoracoscopic surgery, tube thoracoscopy, intrapleural fibrinolysis, repeated thoracentesis) should be determined in collaboration with appropriate consultants.

Pleural Empyema

Pleural empyema is pus in the pleural space, and can be demonstrated only by direct sampling. Often, pH values <7.0 and glucose levels <40 mg/100 mL are observed. The most common conditions associated with nontuberculous bacterial empyema include pulmonary infection (56%), surgery (22%), trauma (4%), and esophageal perforation (4%). Presence of pleural empyema requires parenteral antimicrobials and definitive drainage. Although tube thoracostomy has been traditionally used, some persons may now benefit from thoracoscopy with repeated irrigations. Gram's stain, culture, and other standard tests usually provide information sufficient to initiate therapy. Antimicrobial doses higher than those commonly

 TABLE 6-3   **Parapneumonic Effusions Requiring Drainage**

Clinical
Likelihood of anaerobic pneumonia: alcoholic or other cause of aspiration
Prolonged infection by history or presence of anemia and hypoalbuminemia
Failure to respond to antibiotic therapy
Virulent bacterial pathogen

Imaging
Increased size
Intrapleural air-fuid level
Intrapleural loculations
Multiloculations
Size of loculations
Marked thickening of the pleural membranes

Pleural Fluid Characteristics
Gross pus (empyema) (absolute indication)
Positive Gram's stain for bacteria (strong indication)
Positive culture for bacteria (strong indication)
Low pH (<7.1)
Low glucose (<40)
High LDH (>1,000)

used for uncomplicated pneumonia are necessary to ensure adequate drug concentrations within the pleural space. Duration of treatment is variable but generally should be continued until the patient is afebrile, peripheral white blood cell (WBC) count approaches normal, and tube thoracostomy drainage is meager. This is often approximately 3 weeks. If complicated pneumonia or lung abscess is simultaneously present, longer treatment may be needed. Patients who fail to defervesce with appropriate antimicrobials and closed tube thoracostomy should be evaluated for loculated pus. Either ultrasound or CT scanning can be used, and open surgical drainage or thoracoscopy may be necessary.

Tuberculous Pleurisy

Involvement of the pleural space occurs in about 4% of patients diagnosed with tuberculosis, and most commonly is noted as an early complication of primary disease. Presentation may be acute and may mimic bacterial pneumonia, or more chronic and characterized by weight loss and anorexia. Approximately 75 to 80% of patients with tuberculous pleurisy are febrile; 30% have simultaneous pulmonary parenchymal involvement. Pleural effusions most commonly involve the right hemithorax and are unilateral. Lymphocytes predominate; however, early in the course of disease, polymorphonuclear leukocytes may be noted. Glucose levels may be normal or low, and AFB smears are generally negative. Cultures of pleural effusion are positive in about 50% of cases. Diagnosis should be suspected in lymphocyte-predominant exudative effusions, and pleural biopsy represents the procedure of choice if AFB smear of fluid is initially negative. Recommendations are for submission of three biopsy specimens, as yield increases from about 70 to >90% with additional specimens. Adenosine deaminase (ADA) has been recommended as a test for tuberculous pleurisy. In some hands, levels of >50 U/L were >90% sensitive and specific for tuberculosis, whereas levels <45 U/L were 100% specific and sensitive for alternative diagnoses. Pleural interferon (IFN)-γ level >3.7 U/mL is more specific for tuberculosis than ADA activity. In regions of high tuberculous pleuritis prevalence, high pleural fluid ADA or IFN-γ levels with a lymphocytic effusion may obviate the need for pleural biopsy.

Pulmonary Infarction

Fever occurs in up to 68% of angiographically-documented cases of pulmonary thromboembolic disease, may reach levels of 39°C, and can last for many days. Observations suggesting pulmonary thromboembolic disease include (1) history of embolic events, (2) fever, and (3) phlebitis. Pleural fluid evaluation is often nondiagnostic. In 33% of cases, fluid is transudative and contains <10,000 RBCs/mL. RBC counts >100,000/mL suggest this diagnosis if trauma and malignancy are excluded. WBC counts can reach 70,000/mL. Early, polymorphonuclear leukocytes predominate, and lymphocytes are noted after several days.

Iatrogenic Pleural Effusions

Causes of iatrogenic pleural effusions include drugs (heparin, hydralazine, sulfas, nitrofurantoin, albumin, ionic contrast dye, etc.) and procedures (e.g., sclerotherapy, surgery, misadventures with central intravascular lines, and peritoneal dialysis). All can be associated with fever. The diagnostic approach is similar to other effusions, and discontinuation of an offending medication results in clinical improvement.

Rheumatologic and Other Causes

Although detailed discussion is beyond the scope of this chapter, there are multiple other causes of fever and pleural effusion. Rheumatoid arthritis-associated effusions are usually small and unilateral and develop after the onset of rheumatoid synovitis (80%). It is generally exudative, with low pH and glucose. Pleural effusion in systemic SLE is seen as part of the systemic illness. Other rheumatologic causes include polymyositis, dermatomyositis, temporal arteritis, and other vasculitides.

Pleural effusion and fever have also been reported in primary amyloidosis, drug hypersensitivity, fungal infection, parasitic infection, and pulmonary malignancies.

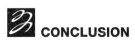 **CONCLUSION**

Pleural effusions associated with fever are common and have many causes. The physician should have a working knowledge of the mechanisms involved in the formation of fluid and be comfortable using tests available for diagnosis. In selected situations, small effusions that have been incidentally identified may be observed. When pleural fluid has been sampled, hematologic, chemical, and microbiologic studies generally provide a diagnosis. Occasionally, cases prove more frustrating, and biopsy or other analyses may be indicated. The cause of an effusion may occasionally remain elusive, and repeat assessments may be necessary. Fortunately, many cases of chronic exudative undiagnosed effusion appear to be benign. (RBB)

Bibliography

Azoulay E. Pleural Effusions in the intensive care unit. *Curr Opin Pulm Med* 2003;9:291–297.
> *A synthesis of data with a discussion of screening ICU patients for pleural effusions, safety of thoracentesis in ventilator patients, and diagnosis and management of effusions in critically ill patients.*

Bartter T, et al. The evaluation of pleural effusion. *Chest* 1994;106:1209–1214.
> *The authors present an excellent review of the roles for imaging, thoracentesis, and other studies in the evaluation of pleural effusions. They also provide a good framework for differentiating exudates from transudates and for the management of exudative pleural effusions.*

Black LF. The pleural space and pleural fluid. *Mayo Clin Proc* 1972;47:493–506.
> *This paper, now more than 3 decades old, remains a superb review of the anatomy and physiology of the pleural space. Although somewhat technical, it provides an excellent basis for the understanding of pleural disease.*

Bryant RE, Salmon CJ. Pleural empyema. *Clin Infect Dis* 1996;22:747–764.
> *This manuscript is an excellent in-depth review of the history, pathophysiology, anatomy, diagnosis, and management of pleural empyema. It contains contemporary information about the role of intrapleural thrombolysis and video-assisted thoracoscopy. Recommendations regarding antibiotic therapy are basic and do not really address the role of newer agents that may have a role for prolonged oral therapy in selected cases.*

Colice GL, et al. Medical and surgical treatment of parapneumonic effusions. *Chest* 2000;118:1158–1171.
> *An American College of Chest Physicians (ACCP) consensus panel statement covering therapy of parapneumonic effusions. Twenty-four articles were eligible for review, although few were randomized, controlled trials. They cover criteria for and methods of drainage. Intrapleural fibrinolysis, video-assisted thoracoscopic surgery and other surgical management appear preferable to tube thoracostomy and therapeutic thoracentesis in high-risk effusions (loculated; low pH; positive culture).*

Cohen M, Sahn SA. Resolution of pleural effusions. *Chest* 2001;119:1547–1562.
> *A review of the literature documenting rates of resolution of pleural effusions. Most treated effusions of infectious origin resolve within 2 months—longer for tuberculosis and shorter for Mycoplasma. Rheumatoid effusions may take months or years to resolve, even with corticosteroid treatment.*

Collins TR, Sahn SA. Thoracentesis: clinical value, complications, technical problems, and patient experience. *Chest* 1987;91:817–822.
> *Eighty-nine patients undergoing 129 consecutive thoracenteses were evaluated. Ninety-two percent of procedures provided useful information. Twenty percent of procedures were associated with complications that included pneumothorax and cough. Subjective patient discomfort was seen in more than 20% of cases, and technical problems were encountered in more than 20% of cases.*

Ferrer Sancho J. Pleural tuberculosis: incidence, pathogenesis, diagnosis and treatment. *Curr Opin Pulm Med* 1996;2:327–334.

The author presents an excellent overview of issues related to pleural tuberculosis and deals with the issue in patients with HIV/AIDS as well. Therapy is primarily with antituberculous agents, with very limited roles for either corticosteroids or repeated thoracenteses.

Ferrer JS, et al. Evolution of idiopathic pleural effusion. *Chest* 1996;109:1508–1513.

This report of 40 patients followed up for as long as 10 years demonstrates that many patients with exudative pleural effusions without a specific diagnosis did well. Mean time to resolution was less than 6 months, and most patients followed benign courses. Part of the entry criteria for this study was adenosine deaminase levels <43 IU/L, which in the opinion of the authors was valuable for ruling out pleural tuberculosis. Despite long-term follow-up, 80% never had a diagnosis, whereas most of the remainder had nonmalignant conditions.

Harris RJ, et al. The diagnostic and therapeutic utility of thoracoscopy. *Chest* 1995;108:828–841.

An excellent review of the historic and current uses of thoracoscopy as a modality for diagnosing and treating pleural disease. This technique is actually not new, but has had a renaissance, in part because of the addition of video assistance, which allows easier imaging of the pleural space. The use of this technique needs to be studied better in controlled trials to avoid overuse. However, it does appear to be extremely valuable as a tool to recognize specific intrapleural lesions.

Heffner JE. Indications for draining a parapneumonic effusion: an evidence-based approach. *Semin Respir Infect* 1999;14:48–58.

A thoughtful assessment of the utility of radiographic and thoracentesis-derived data in assessing the need for drainage of a parapneumonic effusion. The paper includes an algorithm for applying these data in the clinical setting.

Leslie WK, Kinasewitz GT. Clinical characteristics of the patient with nonspecific pleuritis. *Chest* 1988;94:603–608.

This retrospective analysis of 119 patients who underwent pleural biopsy identified variables associated with malignant or granulomatous disease. Patients with a diagnosis of nonspecific pleuritis can be managed conservatively if weight loss, positive tuberculin test, lymphocytosis above 95%, and fluid above half the hemithorax are not demonstrated.

Light RW. Pleural Diseases. 3rd ed. Baltimore: Williams and Wilkins; 1995.

A comprehensive text covering the full range of pleural disease by one of the most experienced physicians in the field.

Mattison LE, et al. Pleural effusions in the medical ICU: prevalence, causes, and clinical implications. *Chest* 1997;111:1018–1023.

The investigators assessed 100 patients admitted to a medical ICU. Of these, 62% were documented to have pleural effusions; about two thirds of these were present upon admission. Most were small and of no clinical significance. Most were present on chest roentgenograms. If patients are not clinically suspected to have infection, the authors feel that most can be observed prospectively without thoracentesis.

Rubins JB, Rubins HB. Etiology and prognostic significance of eosinophilic pleural effusions. *Chest* 1996;110:1271–1274.

This is an interesting brief report of more than 470 patients with pleural effusions, of which almost 10% were eosinophilic. The authors conclude that the only statistical significance of eosinophilia in pleural effusions was with either after postthoracic surgery or in idiopathic cases. No correlations with malignancy were noted, and generally eosinophilic effusions resulted in more prolonged survival than others.

Sahn SA. The differential diagnosis of pleural effusions. *West J Med* 1982;13:99–108.

This excellent basic article by one of the giants in the field of pleural effusion reviews physiology, thoracentesis, and analysis of pleural effusion. Charts are provided to distinguish causes of pleural effusion based on laboratory characteristics. It remains accurate in 2004.

Trejo O, et al. Pleural effusion in patients infected with the human immunodeficiency virus. *Eur J Clin Microbiol* 1997;16:807–815.

A cohort of HIV (+) patients with pleural effusions was compared with a similar number of those without HIV infection but with documented pleural effusion due either to parapneumonic effusion or tuberculosis. Most HIV (+) persons were intravenous drug users, and this population had a high incidence of infection as a cause of the effusion. Tests demonstrated similar results between the two groups for a given diagnosis.

Zocchi L. Physiology and pathophysiology of pleural fluid turnover. *Eur Respir J* 2002; 20:1545–1558.

This paper discusses control of pleural liquid in depth and expands somewhat on the above reference. It clarifies the relationship between the mechanisms of production and characteristics of pleural effusions.

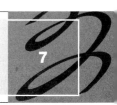

COMMUNITY-ACQUIRED PNEUMONIA IN THE ELDERLY   7

neumonia and influenza are the leading infectious causes of death in the elderly and the fifth most common cause of death overall. Age-specific incidence of pneumonia increases from 15.4 per thousand for those aged 60 to 74 to 34.2 per thousand for those older than age 75. Table 7-1 includes predisposing factors for pneumonia in the older patient.

Mortality from pneumonia also increases with age. In the preantibiotic era, Osler found that 22% of pneumonia patients in the third decade died from pneumonia, 30% in the fourth decade, 47% in the fifth, and 51% in the sixth. Osler stated, "Pneumonia is the special enemy of old age. In the aged, chances are against recovery. So fatal is it in this group, it has been called the natural enemy of the old man." Age is still the most important single factor in predicting the outcome of pneumonia, as evidenced in data developed by the Pneumonia Patient Outcome Research Team. Hence, pneumonia in the aged is an extremely important public health problem.

The management of pneumonia in older patients is based on an evaluation of prognosis. Most older patients will require hospitalization as age, per se, is an important, poor prognostic sign. Table 7-2 describes poor prognostic signs in older patients with pneumonia.

The clinical picture of pneumonia in older patients may be classic, with fever, chills, pleuritic chest pain, shortness of breath, and purulent sputum. However, the onset may be insidious, fever may be absent, and cough less prominent. This more subtle picture of

 TABLE 7-1   **Predisposing Factors for Pneumonia in the Elderly**

Swallowing disorder or aspiration
Low serum albumin level
Comorbid illness: heart failure, asthma, chronic lung disease
Alcoholism
Status of daily living
Advancing age (up to age 90)
Nursing home residence
Immunosuppression

TABLE 7-2	Predictors of Fatal Outcome in Pneumonia in the Elderly

Patient is bedridden
Swallowing disorder
Respiratory rate greater than 30/min
Underlying illnesses such as heart failure, renal failure, and chronic lung disease
Status of activities associated with daily living
Bacteremia
Multilobe involvement
Organism is *S. pneumoniae*
Elevated blood urea nitrogen and creatinine

pneumonia in old age has been described since Osler's time but is also documented in prospective studies. In one recent large study of very elderly patients with pneumonia, older than 80, there was less pleuritic chest pain, less fever, and fewer physical findings on chest examination than in a younger population. Older patients with pneumonia are more likely to have the complications of bacteremia, empyema, and meningitis than younger patients. The higher mortality and increased complication rate are the result, in part, of the increased number of underlying diseases that the older patient with pneumonia is likely to have. However, suboptimal antibody production, particularly in pneumococcal pneumonia, may also explain the worse prognosis.

The etiologic agents that are responsible for pneumonia in this group have not been completely elucidated. Many older patients are unable to cough, so expectorated sputum cannot be obtained for culture. The value of expectorated sputum in determining an etiologic agent is debated and may vary from laboratory to laboratory. Some microbiology laboratories will be more adept at isolating such organisms *as Moraxella catarrhalis, Haemophilus influenzae,* and *Legionella* sp., for example. Nevertheless almost all studies find that *Streptococcus pneumoniae* is the most common cause of pneumonia in the elderly. The more severe the pneumonia, the more likely the pneumococcus is the etiologic agent. In the large study by Fernandez-Sabe, the pneumococcus was isolated from 23% of all patients. Jokinen and colleagues found that 48% of older patients with pneumonia had pneumococcal infection. Other organisms found to be important in pneumonia of old age include *H. influenzae* (nontypeable), *Staphylococcus aureus,* influenza virus, gram-negative bacilli, *M. catarrhalis,* and *Legionella* sp. *Chlamydia pneumoniae* and *Mycoplasma pneumoniae* are probably more common in the young than the elderly. Gram-negative bacilli are more common in the nursing home setting, especially when broad-spectrum antibiotics are used extensively. The gram-negative bacillary pneumonias occur when older patients become colonized by these bacilli and then aspirate them.

Empirical therapy for pneumonia in the older patient is based on covering the following major pathogens.

1. *S. pneumoniae*
2. *H. influenzae*
3. *M. catarrhalis*
4. *Legionella* sp.
5. *M. pneumoniae*
6. *C. pneumoniae*

The importance of covering these atypical organisms (*Mycoplasma, Chlamydia,* and *Legionella*) is controversial, particularly in the elderly. Recommendations for the treatment of pneumonia in Europe generally do not include antibiotics that cover these atypical organisms. In the United States, however, concern for these organisms resulted in guidelines for empiric therapy that do include either a macrolide or fluoroquinolone. Of the atypicals, *Legionella* is of greatest concern, as it is more likely to result in a rapidly downhill course.

In the elderly, additional etiologic agents become of concern under specific circumstances. Intensification or expansion of antibiotic coverage occurs when:

1. The patient is particularly frail, has severe comorbid disease, or is older than age 85.
2. Pneumonia occurs in a nursing home.
3. The presence of aspiration suggests anaerobic or gram-negative infection.
4. Chronic alcoholism increases the likelihood of *Klebsiella pneumoniae* or other gram-negative bacillus.
5. History of infection with a gram-negative bacillus or with resistant *S. pneumoniae.*
6. History of treatment failure.
7. Previous hospitalizations for pneumonia.
8. Other epidemiologic factors suggesting resistant pneumococci, such as a particular community with high resistance or previous treatment with a third-generation cephalosporin.
9. Immunodeficiency disease.

Risk stratification schemes have been increasingly used to decide whether a patient should be admitted to the hospital for pneumonia. Outpatient management is recommended for Class 1 and Class 2 risks, brief inpatient observation for Class 3, and hospitalization for Class 4 and Class 5. Men older than age 70 and women older than age 80 would be in Class 3, based on risk for age alone. Hence it would be the rule to admit the great majority of elderly patients for pneumonia. Although underlying illnesses add significantly to risk, not all comorbid diseases will be appreciated in every elderly patient.

Most guidelines for the treatment of pneumonia in adults differentiate between inpatient and outpatient therapy. A macrolide antibiotic alone may be recommended for outpatient therapy, but not for inpatient treatment. Therefore, most elderly patients will be admitted to the hospital for pneumonia and be treated with both a macrolide and β-lactam antibiotic or with a fluoroquinolone. This empiric regimen provides some assurance that resistant pneumococci, still almost always sensitive to the fluoroquinolones and β-lactams, will be covered.

Empiric regimens have been helpful in guiding appropriate antibiotic therapy in the elderly. Some clinical data are also useful. In one national study, a nonpseudomonal third-generation cephalosporin alone, a second- or third-generation cephalosporin with a macrolide, and a fluoroquinolone alone, showed a reduced mortality rate of 26%, 29%, and 36%, respectively, as compared to a reference group.

Some elderly patients may be treated specifically for an etiologic agent based on some clue in the history, physical examination, or laboratory data. Sputum Gram's stain and culture are still recommended as part of optimal therapy. It is recognized that at times, sputum may not be obtainable or Gram's stain may be difficult to interpret. Nevertheless, cases, for example, of older patients with influenza and staphylococcal pneumonia or β-hemolytic streptococcal pneumonia, can be suspected on Gram's stain. Similarly, foul-smelling sputum, poor dentition, or cavitary lesion on chest radiograph may suggest anaerobic infection, and a better antibiotic regimen for anaerobes will be chosen.

 PREVENTION OF PNEUMONIA IN THE ELDERLY

Annual vaccination against influenza is crucial in preventing influenza and secondary bacterial pneumonia in patients older than age 65. It is now recommended that even patients older than age 50 be immunized, as some will have underlying cardiopulmonary disease that is unrecognized and might predispose to serious illness. Efficacy data on the currently available 23-valent pneumococcal vaccine are somewhat controversial, but most studies do suggest a 60 to 70% protection rate. This vaccine becomes increasingly attractive in the era of antibiotic resistance.

Other measures that may help in the prevention of pneumonia include maintenance of good nutrition and prevention of zinc deficiency. Good oral hygiene may be helpful in preventing aspiration pneumonia. Hand washing will help prevent viral infections, particularly in the institutional setting. To avoid infection by resistant organism, antibiotics should be used only when necessary. (SLB)

Bibliography

Berk SL. Bacterial pneumonia in the elderly: The observations of Sir William Osler in retrospect. *J Am Geriatr Soc* 1984;32:683.
The clinical descriptions of pneumonia in elderly patients from Osler's studies. Pneumonia often presented without fever or chills. It carried a higher mortality rate in the preantibiotic era.

Bosker G. Community-acquired pneumonia (CAP) in the geriatric patient: evaluation, risk-stratification, and antimicrobial treatment guidelines for inpatient and outpatient management. Clinical Consensus Reports 2003. Available at: http://www.ahc. pub.com/ahc_root_html/ccr/geriatric_cap.html
Detailed clinical consensus report on the treatment of community-acquired pneumonia in elderly patients. Includes a review of guidelines as well as available clinical data.

Feldman C. Pneumonia in the elderly. *Clin Chest Med* 1999;20:563.
Includes summary of etiologic agents, diagnostic workup and data to support prevention with influenza and pneumococcal vaccine.

Fernandez-Sabe N, et al. Community-acquired pneumonia in very elderly patients, causative organisms, clinical characteristics, and outcomes. *Medicine* 2003;82:159.
Prospective observational analysis of 1,474 elderly patients with pneumonia. Compares characteristics of the elderly with the very elderly (older than age 80). Very elderly have more subtle clinical findings.

File TM, et al. Guidelines for empiric antimicrobial prescribing in community-acquired pneumonia. *Chest* 2004;125:1888.
This review compares the North American, European, and Canadian guidelines for the empiric treatment of community acquired pneumonia. The reasons for the differences in recommendations are explained.

Koivula I, Sten M, Makela PH. Prognosis after community-acquired pneumonia in the elderly: a population-based 12-year follow-up study. *Arch Intern Med* 1999;159:1550.
The overall mortality rate for pneumonia in the elderly was found to be 8.7 per 1,000 person-years. This was higher than previous studies. Elderly patients who develop pneumonia are at risk for subsequent mortality over several years.

Loeb M. Pneumonia in older persons. *Clin Infect Dis* 2003;37:1335.
Summarizes the best evidence on risk factors, etiologic agents, and prevention.

Marrie TJ. Community-acquired pneumonia in the elderly. *Clin Infect Dis* 2000;37:1335.
Details of epidemiology and risk factors for pneumonia in the elderly.

Verghese A, Berk SL. Bacterial pneumonia in the elderly. *Medicine* 1983;62:271.
This early study details transtracheal aspirate data to define the spectrum of etiologic agents.

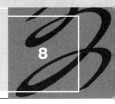

NEW PATHOGENS CAUSING PNEUMONIA— SEVERE ACUTE RESPIRATORY SYNDROME

*S*evere acute respiratory syndrome (SARS) is a respiratory infection now known to be caused by a coronavirus (SARS-CoV). The syndrome was first recognized in the Guangdong Province of mainland China in November 2002. It spread rapidly to Hong Kong, Vietnam, Singapore, and Canada. The pandemic eventually involved 26 countries on five continents. It affected 8,000 patients and caused 774 deaths.

 ## EPIDEMIOLOGY

The epidemiology of the outbreak has provided important public health lessons. The disease does not appear to have been endemic to human populations previously as determined by serologic methods. The initial outbreak involved occupational exposure to live animals being caged and sold, particularly the Himalayan palm civet. Hence, the view was that this pathogenic coronavirus was an animal virus that adapted to humans. Asymptomatic infection seems to be rare. Infection is spread by patients who are very ill and usually 5 to 10 days into their illness. This correlates well with the finding that peak viral load occurs at 10 days. Spread of disease has usually occurred in hospitals and has affected physicians and healthcare workers. Infection, however, has also been spread in the workplace, taxis, and airplanes. The potential spread from country to country by travel has been documented and can be dramatic.

Respiratory droplets are most likely to spread infection, but the fecal–oral route, particularly in those with severe watery diarrhea, is a less common mode of spread.

Food- and water-borne disease have not been documented, but spread through an apartment complex's sewage system is suspected.

 ## CLINICAL SIGNS AND SYMPTOMS

SARS presents with fever, chills, myalgias, and malaise. Upper respiratory symptoms, such as sore throat and rhinorrhea are not characteristic. Some cases of more severe disease include nonproductive cough . Shortness of breath, tachypnea, and pleurisy occur with severe disease. Twenty to thirty percent of infected patients require intensive care and mechanical ventilation.

The clinical presentation in the elderly, as with other respiratory infections, may be more subtle and more severe. Many older patients are afebrile. They may present with poor appetite, malaise, delirium, or falls. They are more likely to die of the disease. Table 8-1 summarizes the frequency of clinical findings.

A three-phase clinical course has been described in one prospective study. Phase 1 includes high fever and myalgias of several days' duration. Phase 2 begins 8 days after the onset of fever and includes recurrence of fever and spread of infiltrate. Arterial oxygen desaturation occurs in about half of all patients. Phase 3 is described as deterioration with evidence of severe lung disease characterized by adult respiratory distress syndrome (ARDS)-like elements.

TABLE 8-1	Clinical Features of SARS
Fever	94–100%
Chills	55–74%
Rigors	43–56%
Myalgias	51–68%
Malaise	50–64%
Loss of appetite	10–54%

 LABORATORY FEATURES

Laboratory abnormalities often include lymphocytopenia, low platelet count, increased lactate dehydrogenase (LDH), and increased alanine aminotransferase. Prolonged prothrombin time (PTT) and increased D-dimer is described in some studies.

The chest radiograph is abnormal in 60 to 100% of patients. Airspace consolidation is a characteristic feature. Ground-glass opacification and focal consolidation are usual findings. Opacity occurs, on average, 8 to 10 days after symptoms. The chest radiograph does not show cavity formation or mediastinal lymphadenopathy. Pleural effusions are described but are not common. Spontaneous pneumomediastinum is commonly reported in some series.

High-resolution computed tomographic (CT) scans have been shown to identify abnormalities several days before appearance on chest radiograph.

 VIROLOGIC DIAGNOSIS

Reverse-transcriptase polymerase chain reaction (RT-PCR) was developed in 2003 to detect the presence of SARS-CoV, the pathogenic agent of SARS. The virus also has been isolated from respiratory secretions, feces, urine, and lung biopsy material. Because most patients do not bring up sputum, throat and nose swabs have been most practical in making a virologic diagnosis. Second-generation PCR has been used to detect disease using these sources, even in the first few days of the illness. Urine and blood specimens can also be used. Eighty percent of patients had positive SARS CoV real time RT-PCR on day 1 but drop to 42% on day 14. In one series of patients studied on day 14, urine cultures were positive in 42% of cases, nasopharyngeal swabs positive in 68%, and stools positive in 97%. Seroconversion by whole virus antibody can be detected after 1 week. There is no IgM antibody test at present.

 PROGNOSTIC FACTORS

The overall fatality rate from all countries was about 11%. Death rarely occurs in children. Age and coexisting disease are the most important prognostic factors, as with other respiratory infections. Fifty percent of patients older than age 65 die of the disease. Diabetes mellitus and coronary artery disease may be the most serious comorbid conditions. An elevated LDH and elevated white blood cell count are reported to be poor prognostic laboratory findings. Other poor prognostic indicators have included lymphopenia, elevated creatine kinase, and recurrence of fever (Table 8-2).

The treatment of SARS will need further clinical study. No antiviral agents have yet been shown to be effective. Ribavirin has been extensively used, but there is no direct clinical evidence to show its efficacy. Interferon-β is also considered as a potential therapy. High-dose steroids have been used but have not been shown to be effective. Many other attempts at therapy, including immunoglobulin and Chinese traditional medicine, are unproven. Patients will often receive broad-spectrum antibiotics until bacterial infection is ruled out.

TABLE 8-2	Poor Prognostic Factors in SARS

Age
Underlying disease, particularly diabetes mellitus
Elevated LDH
Elevated creatine kinase
Recurrent fever
Management

PREVENTION AND PUBLIC HEALTH MEASURES

Patients with SARS need to be identified and isolated early in the course of the disease. Contact and travel history will be most important in suspecting the disease. Patients should be on respiratory precautions, and visitors should be discouraged. SARS patients at home should wear surgical masks and wash their hands frequently. Healthcare workers in facilities that have known patients with SARS should be carefully monitored. Public health recommendations are beyond the scope of this chapter; however, international cooperation, travel advice, and international health regulations will be important in containing pandemics. (SLB)

Bibliography

Antonio GE, et al. Imaging of severe acute respiratory syndrome in Hong Kong. *Am J Radiol* 2003,181:11–17.
The radiologic picture of SARS, its pattern of progression, and the value of high-resolution CT.
Booth CM, et al. Clinical features and short-term outcomes of 144 patients with SARS in the greater Toronto area. *JAMA* 2003;289:2801–2809.
Outcomes of the 144 patients treated in Toronto.
Hui DS, Wong PC, Wang C. SARS: clinical features and diagnosis. *Respirology* 2003;8:S20.
Includes description of clinical features of elderly patients with SARS. Delirium, falls, and atypical febrile response are likely to occur in the elderly.
Naylor CD, Chantler C, Griffiths S. Learning from SARS in Hong Kong and Toronto. *JAMA* 2004;291:2483.
Summary of public health lessons from SARS outbreak.
Olsen SJ, et. al. Transmission of the severe acute respiratory syndrome on aircraft. *N Engl J Med* 2003;349:2416.
One commercial aircraft flight, carrying a single symptomatic person, caused disease in 22 passengers.
Peiris JSM, et al. Coronavirus as a possible cause of severe acute respiratory syndrome. *Lancet* 2003;361:1319.
Describes characteristics of coronavirus that explains pattern of disease.
Peiris JSM, et al. The severe acute respiratory syndrome.*New Engl J Med* 2003;349:2431–2441.
Very comprehensive review article including the epidemiology, clinical features, prognostic factors, management, and prevention of SARS.
Poon L, et al. Early diagnosis of SARS coronavirus infection by real time RT-PCR. *J Clin Virol* 2003;28:233–238.
RT-PCR able to make early diagnosis of SARS.
Poutanen SM, et. al. Identification of severe acute respiratory syndrome in Canada. *N Engl J Med* 2003;348:1995.
Detailed clinical description of the cases of SARS from Canada.
Rainer TH. Severe acute respiratory syndrome: clinical features, diagnosis, and management. *Curr Opin Pulm Med* 2004;10:159.
Review article including summary of clinical, laboratory, and radiologic features of the disease.

Rota PA, et al. Characterization of a novel coronavirus associated with severe acute respiratory syndrome. *Science* 2003;30:1394.
  Describes DNA sequencing of the SARS virus and differences from other coronaviruses.
Update: Outbreak of severe acute respiratory syndrome-worldwide. *Morbid Mortal Wkly Rep* 2003;52:1779.
  Important account of the epidemiology of the SARS outbreak
Wang J, Chang S. Severe acute respiratory syndrome *Curr Opin Infect Dis* 2004;17:143.
  Summary of therapeutic experience with SARS.

Cardiovascular System

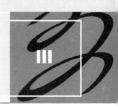

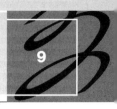

$\mathcal{T}$he diagnosis of bacterial endocarditis has long been based on a constellation of history; physical examination findings; laboratory data, including blood cultures; and an assessment of the patient's risk factors and underlying diseases. Many patients complain only of fever and fatigue and are found to have a new cardiac murmur. The disease, however, presents in many ways. Friable vegetations may result in embolic features, such as stroke, meningitis, blindness, myocardial infarction, or arterial occlusion. Some patients will initially appear septic, whereas some will present with autoimmune disease and others with congestive heart failure secondary to rapid destruction of a heart valve. Embolic signs on physical examination, such as Osler's nodes, Janeway lesions, Roth's spots, and splinter hemorrhages are seen less often today because of the rapid institution of antibiotic therapy in most patients. Although positive results on blood cultures are very helpful in diagnosis, some patients with endocarditis will have persistently negative cultures. Other patients with positive blood cultures may appear to have endocarditis, but are found to have some other focus of infection instead. For these reasons, standardized diagnostic criteria for endocarditis have long been sought.

In 1981, von Reyn et al. published criteria for the diagnosis of endocarditis based on clinical–pathologic criteria. These criteria were helpful, particularly because of the wider spectrum of presentation of the disease in recent decades, including the more subtle presentation that often occurs in the elderly. The von Reyn criteria are listed in Table 9-1.

Endocarditis is categorized as definite only when the characteristic histology is demonstrated on a surgical specimen or at autopsy, or when bacteria are cultured from a heart valve or peripheral embolus. Cases are further categorized as probable endocarditis, possible endocarditis, or diagnosis rejected.

During the past several years, the von Reyn classification of diagnosis has become less useful for several reasons. Most importantly, the use of transthoracic echocardiography has become a major tool in the diagnosis of endocarditis, and results of this test need to be included in the overall assessment of the likelihood of endocarditis. Echocardiography is not part of the von Reyn diagnostic criteria. The von Reyn criteria were not studied prospectively, but recent reports suggest that some patients in whom the diagnosis is rejected by these criteria do in fact have the disease. The von Reyn criteria do not emphasize the importance of intravenous drug abuse as an extremely important predisposing factor.

In 1992, Lukes et al. proposed an endocarditis classification system that has come to be known as the Duke criteria. This classification system was published in 1994 and included an analysis of 67 patients with pathologically proven endocarditis, in whom the system proved to be very sensitive. The original article did not study the specificity of the classification method. Prospective studies have come to prove that this system is more sensitive and specific than the von Reyn system. The Duke approach classifies cases as definite, possible, or rejected on the basis of a scoring system of major and minor criteria (Table 9-2).

For endocarditis to be diagnosed definitively by the system, a patient must show either histologic or pathologic evidence of the disease or exhibit definitive clinical criteria. Two major criteria, one major and three minor criteria, or five minor criteria provide sufficient evidence for a definitive diagnosis. Table 9-3 delineates the definitions of major and minor criteria.

Much like the von Reyn system, the Duke system classifies as definite any case of endocarditis for which there is evidence based on histology from surgery or autopsy or on direct culture from a vegetation or peripheral embolus. Unlike the von Reyn system, the

TABLE 9-1　　The von Reyn Criteria for Diagnosis of Infective Endocarditis

Definite
　Direct evidence of infective endocarditis based on histology from surgery or autopsy or on bacteriology (Gram's stain or culture) of valvular vegetation or peripheral embolus
Probable
　(A) Persistently positive blood culture* plus one of the following:
　　(1) New regurgitant murmur
　　(2) Predisposing heart disease** *and vascular phenomena*‡
　(B) Negative or intermittently positive blood cultures§ plus three of the following:
　　(1) Fever
　　(2) New regurgitant murmur, and
　　(3) Vascular phenomena
Possible
　(A) Persistently positive blood cultures plus one of the following:
　　(1) Predisposing heart disease, or
　　(2) Vascular phenomena
　(B) Negative or intermittently positive blood cultures with all three of the following:
　　(1) Fever
　　(2) Predisposing heart disease, and
　　(3) Vascular phenomena
　(C) For *viridans* streptococcal cases only: at least two positive blood cultures without an extracardiac source, and fever
Rejected
　(A) Endocarditis unlikely, alternative diagnosis generally apparent
　(B) Endocarditis likely, empiric antibiotic therapy warranted
　(C) Culture-negative endocarditis diagnosed clinically, but excluded by postmortem

*At least two blood cultures were obtained, with two of two or three of three positive, or at least 70% of cultures positive if four or more cultures obtained.
**Definite valvular or congenital heart disease or a cardiac prosthesis (excluding permanent pacemakers).
‡Petechiae, splinter hemorrhages, conjunctival hemorrhages, Roth's spots, Osler's nodes, Janeway lesions, aseptic meningitis, glomerulonephritis, and pulmonary, central nervous system, coronary, or peripheral emboli.
§Any rate of blood culture positivity that does not meet the definition of persistently positive.

Duke system can be used to make a definite diagnosis of endocarditis even without direct histologic or culture evidence. This definitive diagnosis requires either two major criteria, one major and three minor criteria, or five minor criteria. It should be noted that major criteria are related either to blood culture data or echocardiographic data. Positive results on blood cultures are not considered major criteria per se. Typical microorganisms, such as α-hemolytic streptococci, isolated from two separate cultures stand as a major criterion. Persistently positive blood cultures with an organism that can cause endocarditis would also count as a major criterion. Three other major criteria are based on data available from echocardiography. They are (a) an oscillating intracardiac mass in the absence of an alternative anatomic explanation (i.e., other than endocarditis); (b) abscess; and (c) a new partial dehiscence of a prosthetic valve or new valvular regurgitation. Hence, the definitive diagnosis of endocarditis is more easily made in the Duke system than in the von Reyn system because of the use of echocardiographic data.

　　The sensitivity and specificity of transesophageal echocardiography for the diagnosis of endocarditis was established between 1981 and 1994, when the two classification schemes were established. The Duke system, unlike the von Reyn, can accept a definitive diagnosis based on clinical criteria as long as enough clinical criteria are available. Five minor criteria establish the diagnosis as definitive, whereas the same clinical data would result only in a classification of possible endocarditis by the von Reyn system. Hence, according to the Duke system, a patient having blood cultures positive for a characteristic organism and

TABLE 9-2   **Proposed New Criteria for Diagnosis of Infective Endocarditis (Duke University)**

Definite infective endocarditis
  Pathologic criteria
    Microorganism: demonstrated by culture or histology in a vegetation, or in a vegetation
      that has embolized, or in an intracardiac abscess, or
    Pathologic lesions: vegetation or intracardiac abscess present and confirmed by
      histology showing active endocarditis
  Clinical criteria, as specifically defined in Table 9-3
    Two major criteria or
    One major criterion and three minor criteria, or
    Five minor criteria
Possible infective endocarditis
  Findings consistent with infective endocarditis that fall short of "Definite," but not
    "Rejected"
Rejected
  Firm alternate diagnosis explaining evidence of infective endocarditis, or
  Resolution of infective endocarditis syndrome, with antibiotic therapy for 4 days or less, or
  No pathologic evidence of infective endocarditis at surgery or autopsy, with antibiotic
    therapy for 4 days or less

TABLE 9-3   **Definition of Terms Used in the Proposed Diagnostic Criteria (Duke University)**

Major criteria
  (A) Positive blood culture for infective endocarditis: typical microorganisms for infective
     endocarditis from two separate blood cultures
    (1) *Streptococcus viridans, Streptococcus bovis,* HACEK* group, or
    (2) Community-acquired *Staphylococcus aureus* or enterococci, in absence of a primary
       focus, or
  (B) Persistently positive blood culture, defined as a microorganism consistent with infective
     endocarditis, from
    (1) Blood cultures drawn more than 12 hours apart, or
    (2) All of three, or a majority of four or more separate blood cultures, with first and last drawn
       at least 1 hour apart
  (C) Evidence of endocardial involvement: positive echocardiogram for infective endocarditis
    (1) Oscillating intracardiac mass, on valve or supporting structure, or in the path of
       regurgitant jets, or on iatrogenic devices, in the absence of an alternative anatomic
       explanation, or
    (2) Abscess, or
    (3) New partial dehiscence of prosthetic valve, or new valvular regurgitation (worsening or
       changing or preexisting murmur not sufficient)
Minor criteria
  (A) Predisposing heart condition or intravenous drug use
  (B) Fever: 38°C or higher
  (C) Vascular phenomena: arterial embolism, septic pulmonary infarcts, mycotic aneurysm,
     intracranial hemorrhage, Janeway lesions
  (D) Immunologic phenomena: glomerulonephritis, Osler's nodes, Roth's spots
  (E) Echocardiogram consistent with infective endocarditis but not meeting major criterion as
     noted previously, or serologic evidence of active infection with organism consistent with
     infective endocarditis

*HACEK, *Haemophilus, Actinobacillus, Cardiobacterium, Eikenella, Kingella* species.

positive findings on echocardiogram would fulfill two major criteria and be given a definitive diagnosis. Similarly, a patient with *Staphylococcus aureus* in the bloodstream (with no other focus of infection) and new valvular regurgitation by echocardiography would also fulfill two major criteria and be given a definitive diagnosis. Five minor criteria, such as fever, Janeway lesion, intravenous drug abuse, Osler node, and glomerulonephritis, would also be a basis for a definitive diagnosis.

Because at least some patients will be available for study who have definitive evidence for infective endocarditis by surgical or autopsy material, the sensitivity of the von Reyn and Duke criteria can be assessed in these cases. At least six studies have compared the Duke criteria with the von Reyn criteria prospectively. By the Duke criteria, 83% of the confirmed cases were considered definitive. None of the confirmed cases was rejected. By the von Reyn methodology, 48% of the confirmed cases were classified only as probable. Twenty-one percent of the confirmed cases would have been rejected by this system.

The usefulness of the Duke criteria was evaluated by reviewing cases during a 3-year period at 54 hospitals in the Philadelphia area. The clinical judgment of three infectious disease experts who reviewed the records of 410 patients was compared with classification that would be generated by the Duke system. There was excellent agreement (91%) for possible and probable cases. However, the experts found 36 cases that they did not feel were likely to be endocarditis, but that would have been classified as definite or probable by the Duke criteria. The authors warn that although the Duke criteria are very sensitive, they may result in overdiagnosis of infective endocarditis.

In general, when the Duke criteria are tested against pathologically confirmed cases, sensitivity is greater than 80%. A high specificity and negative predictive value have also been confirmed.

Nevertheless, a variety of additional modifications have been suggested, including a study based on the Duke University endocarditis database. Li et al. have suggested that the category of "possible IE" that is generated from criteria is too broad. The group recommends that "possible IE" should be redefined as having one major criterion and one minor or three minor criteria. They also recommend that the criterion "echocardiogram consistent with IE but not meeting major criteria" be eliminated. The authors believe that bacteremia due to *Staphylococcus aureus* should always be considered a major criterion—to improve sensitivity. Positive Q fever serology should also be considered a major criterion.

Lamas and Eykyn have suggested the same modifications to the Duke criteria, but they also recommend the addition of some additional minor criteria. These include splenomegaly, splinter hemorrhages, petechiae, newly diagnosed clubbing, elevated erythrocyte sedimentation rate, and the presence of intravascular lines and peripheral intravascular devices. These additions would obviously increase sensitivity and decrease specificity to some extent.

Modifications to the Duke criteria will continue to be made to improve sensitivity, particularly in cases of culture-negative endocarditis. In these cases, additional methods, such as newer histologic and molecular techniques as well as meticulous culture methods for difficult organisms, will become increasingly important. Newer molecular or serologic methods for organisms such as *Bartonella quintana* or *Tropheryma whippelii*, or *Chlamydia* species may become included as major criteria.

Regardless of the modifications to improve sensitivity and specificity, diagnosis and treatment of this heterogeneous disease will continue to be based on the judgment of the individual clinician, on a case-by-case basis, with the modified Duke criteria serving as useful guidelines. (SLB)

Bibliography

Bayer AS, et al. Evaluation of new clinical criteria for the diagnosis of infective endocarditis. *Am J Med* 1994;96:211.
Sixty-three febrile patients with suspected infective endocarditis who had open heart surgery were evaluated, and the von Reyn and Duke criteria for endocarditis were compared. The Duke criteria were superior predominantly because of the use of transthoracic echocardiographic data.
Cecchi E, et al. New diagnostic criteria for infective endocarditis. A study of sensitivity and specificity. *Eur Heart J* 1997;18:1149.

Italian study in which 143 patients with suspected endocarditis had long-term follow-up. The sensitivity and specificity of the von Reyn and Duke criteria were compared. The Duke criteria were more sensitive and specific than the von Reyn criteria.

Durack DT, et al. New criteria for the diagnosis of infectious endocarditis: utilization of specific echocardiographic findings. *Am J Med* 1994;96:200.

Establishes the Duke criteria and uses the system to classify 400 patients as definite, possible, or rejected. The system was 80% sensitive in classifying 69 proven cases. No attempt to determine specificity was made.

Hoen B, et al. The Duke criteria for diagnosing endocarditis are specific: analysis of 100 patients with acute fever or fever of unknown origin. *Clin Infect Dis* 1996;23: 298.

In a study of patients with acute fever admitted to medical wards, the Duke criteria were 99% specific (i.e., cases of acute fever were not misdiagnosed as endocarditis when the Duke criteria were used).

Lamas CC, Eyken SJ. Suggested modifications to the Duke criteria for the clinical diagnosis of native valve and prosthetic valve endocarditis: analysis of 118 pathologically proven cases. *Clin Infect Dis* 1997;25:713.

Shows improved diagnostic sensitivity by adding some minor criteria including splenomegaly, petechiae, splinter hemorrhages, clubbing, elevated erythrocyte sedimentation rate, and presence of central lines.

Li JS, et al. Proposed modifications to the Duke criteria for the diagnosis of endocarditis. *Clin Infect Dis* 2000;30:633.

Recommends including all S. aureus positive blood cultures and Q fever serology as major criteria. Also recommends that the category "possible IE" require one major and one minor, or three minor criteria.

Lisby G, Gitschik E, Durack DT. Molecular methods for the diagnosis of infective endocarditis. *Infect Dis Clin North Am* 2002;16:393.

Polymerase chain reaction is being used to help identify pathogens such as Bartonella, Brucella, Chlamydia, *and* Legionella *species.*

Nettles RE, et al. An evaluation of the Duke criteria in 25 pathologically confirmed cases of prosthetic valve endocarditis. *Clin Infect Dis* 1997;25:1401.

The authors used 25 cases of pathologically confirmed prosthetic valve endocarditis to compare the von Reyn and Duke criteria for diagnosis. When the Duke method was used, 76% of confirmed cases were considered definite. No cases were rejected. The von Reyn method would have rejected five cases, or 20% of the total.

Prendergast BD. Diagnostic criteria and problems in infective endocarditis. *Heart* 2004; 90:611.

The author reviews modifications of the Duke criteria and includes some of the newer techniques useful in the diagnosis of endocarditis.

Sekeres MA, et al. An assessment of the usefulness of the Duke criteria for diagnosing active infective endocarditis. *Clin Infect Dis* 1997;24:1185.

Infectious disease experts reviewed the charts of 410 patients with suspected endocarditis for 3 years at 54 hospitals in Philadelphia. Cases were classified as definite, probable, or possible, and then results were compared with the Duke method of classification. The sensitivity of the Duke method was good to excellent, but some concern about specificity is expressed by the authors.

Tissieres P, et al. Value and limitations of the von Reyn, Duke, and modified Duke criteria for the diagnosis of endocarditis in children. *Pediatrics* 2003;112:647.

Modified Duke criteria were most sensitive in diagnosing children with endocarditis. Positive blood cultures were the most important IE criterion.

von Reyn, et al. Infective endocarditis: an analysis based on strict case definitions. *Ann Intern Med* 1981;94:505.

Established case definitions for endocarditis that have been widely used, especially for clinical studies. The system was not tested prospectively and was developed before breakthroughs in diagnosis by transesophageal echocardiography.

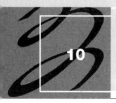

10 CULTURE-NEGATIVE ENDOCARDITIS

*B*lood cultures are the critical element in the diagnosis of bacterial endocarditis. Endocardial vegetations exude bacteria into the bloodstream, causing continuous bacteremia and positive results on blood cultures in most patients. However, in all endocarditis series, some patients are found to have the disease despite negative cultures. The percentage of negative blood cultures varies among studies from 2 to 30%. The mean percentage appears to be about 10%, but with developing methods, probably fewer than 5% of cases of endocarditis will be culture negative. High rates of culture-negative endocarditis from early studies probably resulted from suboptimal technique, less rigorous criteria for diagnosis, and lack of appreciation for certain recently recognized etiologic agents.

The most common cause of culture-negative endocarditis is prior antimicrobial therapy. In one large study, antimicrobial therapy reduced the incidence of positive blood cultures from 97 to 91%. Duration of antimicrobial therapy correlates with the likelihood of negative cultures. When antimicrobial therapy has been continued for several days, blood cultures usually remain negative for weeks or longer.

Several laboratory methods may be helpful when endocarditis is suspected in a patient already on antimicrobial therapy. Antimicrobial removal devices that bind antimicrobials in the serum to a resin have been described but are rarely helpful.

Some studies have suggested that in patients already treated with antimicrobials, more frequent cultures should be taken. One recommendation is to obtain blood cultures every 8 to 12 hours for 3 days. Using 10 to 30 mL of blood (rather than the usual 5 mL) has also been recommended to increase culture positivity. If endocarditis is suspected in a patient who has received antimicrobial therapy, the microbiology laboratory should be asked to incubate blood cultures for at least 2 weeks.

Newer molecular methods appear to have increased the yield in some cases of bacterial infection. Polymerase chain reaction (PCR) amplification of gene targets and rNA loci have been performed on valves themselves and on blood, resulting in positive identification of organisms even though blood cultures are negative. In a study by Millar et al., PCR amplification and subsequent sequencing were done on all blood cultures and valve materials. All patients classified as definite or possible by Duke's criteria were positive by PCR. In addition, all patients who were rejected by Duke's criteria were PCR negative.

An increasing number of etiologic agents are known to be responsible for culture-negative endocarditis. Table 10-1 lists some of these agents.

Perhaps the most important recent development in the diagnosis of culture-negative endocarditis is the importance of newer serologic methods in the diagnosis of atypical bacteria, including *Coxiella burnetii*, *Bartonella* species and *Chlamydia* species. Lamas and Eykyn, in a recent study of 63 cases of culture-negative endocarditis, found serology to be diagnostic in 15 cases. These included eight *C. burnetii*, six *Bartonella* species, and one *Chlamydia psittaci*. Five of the *Bartonella* cases were confirmed by PCR of the excised valve. In this study, nine cases were diagnosed by culture of the excised valve, even though blood cultures remained negative. Serologic assays appear to be extremely sensitive for both *Coxiella* and *Bartonella* endocarditis.

Another important reason why some cases of endocarditis are culture negative is that some organisms are fastidious and require special culture techniques. A group of slow-growing, gram-negative bacilli, including *Haemophilus aphrophilus*, *Actinobacillus actinomycetemcomitans*, *Cardiobacterium hominis*, *Eikenella corrodens*, and *Kingella* species

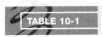

TABLE 10-1	Etiologic Agents in Culture-Negative Endocarditis

Nutritionally-deficient streptococci
HACEK bacteria
Fungi (*Mucor*, *Aspergillus*, and *Histoplasmosis*)
Coxiella burnetii
Chlamydia psittaci
Bartonella quintana
Legionella pneumophila
Tropheryma whippelii

(called as a group the HACEK bacteria), are particularly difficult to grow by standard methods. These organisms require prolonged incubation and subculturing to chocolate agar.

Vitamin B and other nutritionally deficient streptococci cause episodes of endocarditis. These organisms may fail to grow unless the medium is supplemented with pyridoxal hydrochloride or cysteine. These organisms will grow on blood agar streaked with staphylococci as satellite colonies. Nutritionally deficient streptococci show turbid growth in conventional media so that subculturing can then be initiated (such culture methods are now routine in laboratories when endocarditis is suspected). Other unusual bacteria implicated in culture-negative endocarditis include *Brucella* species. The diagnosis is usually suspected by history. Culture requires special media and a carbon dioxide atmosphere. *Legionella*, an unusual cause of culture-negative endocarditis, has occurred almost exclusively in patients with prosthetic heart valves.

Fungal endocarditis frequently presents with negative blood cultures. *Mucor* species, *Aspergillus*, and *Histoplasma* rarely can cause endocarditis. Fungal endocarditis is often right sided and may occur in drug users or patients with prosthetic valves. Vegetations are usually large, and major embolic complications are frequent. Hypertonic media and the use of arterial cultures have been recommended to improve laboratory diagnosis, but these recommendations are unproved.

Shapiro et al. have reported a particularly well-documented case of *C. psittaci* endocarditis. Cultures of blood and pharyngeal specimens were positive, and *Chlamydia* was demonstrated in tissue by immunofluorescent stain. Unusual organisms, such as the murine typhus agent and *Brucella*, have also been diagnosed by serologic methods. The diagnosis of culture-negative enterococcal endocarditis was made in seven patients by using an immunoblotting technique directed against specific enterococcal antigen extracts.

As noted, *Bartonella quintana* has received increasing attention as a potentially important cause of culture-negative endocarditis. Several investigators have used PCR to identify the organism in excised valves. In a multicenter international study, 22 cases of culture-negative endocarditis were reported to be caused by *Bartonella* species. Diagnostic studies included determination of antibody titers to *Bartonella* species by microimmunofluorescence, blood and vegetation culture, and amplification of *Bartonella* DNA from valvular tissue by PCR. Of the 22 patients studied, 13 had preexisting valvular heart disease, 11 were alcoholic, and only 4 owned cats.

Whipple's endocarditis has also been more commonly reported. Fenollar et al. compared 35 cases to other types of endocarditis. Diagnosis must be made by examination of the excised heart valve. Congestive heart failure, previous heart disease, and fever are less likely to be found in Whipple's endocarditis.

In patients with culture-negative endocarditis of native valves, a combination of ampicillin and aminoglycoside has been recommended as empiric therapy. This combination is effective against streptococci, including enterococci, and bacteria of the HACEK group. In patients with prosthetic heart valves and culture-negative endocarditis, both coagulase-positive and coagulase-negative staphylococci may cause the disease. Vancomycin plus aminoglycoside becomes the regimen most often recommended. Rifampin may be added as well. In patients who do not respond to antimicrobial therapy, a reassessment of etiologic agents, including fungi, *Chlamydia, Coxiella,* and other organisms indicated by history and epidemiology, should be pursued. Optimal antibiotic therapy for *Bartonella* endocarditis has not been well established. (SLB)

Bibliography

Abraham AK, et al. Culture-negative infective endocarditis. *Aust N Z J Med* 1984;14:223.
  Among 265 endocarditis cases, 7% were culture negative. All had received prior antimicrobial therapy.
Breathnach AS, et al. Culture-negative endocarditis: contribution of *Bartonella* infections. *Heart* 1997;77:474.
  Describes two cases of Bartonella *endocarditis: one in a homeless man, the other in a patient exposed to fleas. PCR of the excised valves was used to identify the organism.*
Ellner JJ, et al. Infective endocarditis caused by slow-growing fastidious gram-negative bacteria. *Medicine (Baltimore)* 1979;58:145.
  Gives case reports and microbiologic characteristics of fastidious gram-negative organisms, including Cardiobacterium, Actinobacillus, *and* Haemophilus *species.*
Fenollar F, Leipidi H, Raoult D. Whipple's endocarditis: review of the literature and comparisons with Q fever, Bartonella infection, and blood culture positive endocarditis. *Clin Infect Dis* 2001;33:1309.
  Congestive heart failure, fever, and previous valvular heart disease are less frequently found in Whipple's endocarditis.
Goldenberger D, et al. Molecular diagnosis of bacterial endocarditis by broad-range PCR amplification and direct sequencing. *J Clin Microbiol* 1997;35:2733.
  A promising method for diagnosis of culture-negative endocarditis. Allows identification of unusual, nongrowing organisms such as Tropheryma whippelii.
Houpikian P, Raoult D. Diagnostic methods. Current best practices and guidelines for the identification of difficult to culture pathogens in infective endocarditis. *Cardiol Clin* 2003;21:207.
  This paper summarizes the new approach to the workup of a patient with culture-negative endocarditis. It emphasizes the importance of serologic testing, special staining of the excised valve, and PCR for the identification of typical and atypical bacteria.
Kiehn TE, et al. Comparative recovery of bacteria and yeasts from lysis-centrifugation and a conventional blood culture system. *J Clin Microbiol* 1983;18:300.
  The lysis centrifugation system was better than broth for detecting fungi and gram-negative bacilli but was less likely to detect streptococci.
Lamas CC, Eykyn SJ. Blood culture negative endocarditis: analysis of 63 cases presenting over 25 years. *Heart* 2003;89:259.
  Demonstrates the importance of serologic methods in the diagnosis of culture negative endocarditis. A causative organism was identified in 15 of 63 cases using serologic methods for Coxiella, Bartonella, and Chlamydia species. Additionally, nine cases were determined by culture of the excised heart valve.
Lang S, et al. Evaluation of PCR in the molecular diagnosis of endocarditis. *J Infect* 2004;48:269.
  PCR results demonstrated the presence of bacterial DNA in the excised heart valves of some patients with culture negative endocarditis.
McCabe RE, et al. Prosthetic valve endocarditis caused by *Legionella pneumophila. Ann Intern Med* 1984;100:525.
  A case report of endocarditis caused by Legionella pneumophila. *This organism is a potential cause of culture-negative endocarditis in patients with prosthetic valves.*
Millar B, et al. Molecular diagnosis of infective endocarditis- a new Duke's criterion. *Scand J Infect Dis* 2001;33:673.
  PCR amplification of specific gene targets and universal loci for bacteria can be used successfully to determine bacterial and fungal etiology. In this study, all patients with a definite or possible diagnosis by Duke's criteria had a positive PCR for some organism.
Musso D, Raoult D. *Coxiella burnetii* blood cultures from acute and chronic Q-fever patients. *J Clin Microbiol* 1995;33:3129.
  Diagnosis was made by positive blood cultures and serology. Blood cultures must be obtained before the initiation of antibiotic therapy, or results will be negative.

Pesanti EL, Smith IM. Infective endocarditis with negative blood cultures. An analysis of 52 cases. *Am J Med* 1979;66:43.

Compares clinical features of 52 patients having culture-negative endocarditis with those who are culture-positive. Culture-negative patients tend to respond less dramatically to antimicrobial therapy.

Raoult D, et al. Diagnosis of 22 new cases of *Bartonella* endocarditis. *Ann Intern Med* 1996;125:646.

Multicenter, international study suggests that Bartonella *species are an important cause of culture-negative endocarditis. Amplification of* Bartonella *DNA by PCR was performed by using tissue from heart valve. Of the 22 patients, 13 had predisposing valvular heart disease, and 11 were homeless. There was a high level of cross-reacting antibody to* Chlamydia, *making cross-adsorption necessary for proper diagnosis.*

Shapiro DS, et al. Brief report: *Chlamydia psittaci* endocarditis diagnosed by blood culture. *N Engl J Med* 1992;326:1192.

A very well-documented case of C. psittaci *endocarditis. The patient had been exposed to her sister's sick parakeet.*

Rolain JM, Lecam C, Raoult D. Simplified serologic diagnosis of endocarditis due to Coxiella burnetii and Bartonella. *Clin Diagn Lab Immunol* 2003;10:1147.

Serologic assay was 100% sensitive with a positive predictive value of 98% for the diagnosis of endocarditis caused by these organisms.

Tunkel AR, Kaye D. Endocarditis with negative blood cultures. *N Engl J Med* 1992;326:1215.

An editorial accompanying a case report of Chlamydia *endocarditis provides an update on etiologic agents and the diagnostic approach to culture-negative endocarditis.*

Van Scoy RE. Culture-negative endocarditis. *Mayo Clin Proc* 1982;57:149.

Describes an approach to culture-negative endocarditis. Survival is 92% if patient responds to therapy within 1 week.

Walterspiel JN, Kaplan SL. Incidence and clinical characteristics of "culture-negative" infective endocarditis in a pediatric population. *Pediatr Infect Dis* 1986;5:328.

Ten-year pediatric experience with culture-negative endocarditis.

Washington JA II. The role of the microbiology laboratory in the diagnosis and antimicrobial treatment of infective endocarditis. *Mayo Clin Proc* 1982;57:22.

Describes the approach to the diagnostic microbiology of endocarditis, including technique of blood culture, media to use, duration of incubation, and problems with fastidious organisms.

Voldstedlund M, et al. Different polymerase chain reaction-based analyses for culture negative endocarditis caused by Streptococcus pneumoniae. *Scand J Infect Dis* 2003;35:757.

S. pneumoniae was identified by PCR-based analysis in two patients with culture-negative endocarditis.

Wright AJ, et al. The antimicrobial removal device. A microbiological and clinical evaluation. *Am J Clin Pathol* 1982;78:173.

An antimicrobial removal device was of little value in 87 bacteremic patients. Bacteria from 8% of patients grew bacteria in the antimicrobial removal device bottles alone.

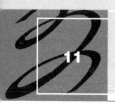

SURGERY IN ACTIVE INFECTIVE ENDOCARDITIS

*I*nfective endocarditis (IE) was uniformly fatal in the preantibiotic era. Since the advent of effective bactericidal antimicrobials, mortality has substantially declined, with survival dependent on factors that include pathogen, host, duration of illness prior to diagnosis, and complications. Although antibiotics form the basis of therapy, it has been recognized for several decades that surgery can contribute to improved outcomes in selected patients. Determination of patients who are candidates for surgery in IE continues to evolve. Appropriate patient selection contributes significantly to patient survivorship in IE.

 ## PREOPERATIVE ASSESSMENT OF THE PATIENT WITH INFECTIVE ENDOCARDITIS

Many patients with IE are infected with organisms amenable to therapy with bactericidal antibiotics, suffer no significant complications, and can be managed successfully medically. However, it is the opinion of the author that patients with IE should be managed at institutions with cardiac surgery capacity, as patients with IE may deteriorate rapidly and unpredictably. In patients requiring surgery, outcomes may be dependent in part on the quality of the facilities and the expertise of surgeons. All persons diagnosed with IE should have standard blood tests performed that include complete blood count (CBC), urinalysis, and tests of hepatic and renal function. They should also have an electrocardiogram (ECG) and (generally) echocardiography performed early in the course of disease to establish a baseline against which to compare future changes and to assess for clinically unrecognized complications. The ECG can document conduction abnormalities that could represent extension of infection into the conducting system. Bundle blocks and first- and third-degree heart block have been reported as complications of IE, most commonly in aortic valve disease. The former is rather common and may indicate only inflammation. However, prolongations of the PR interval also may be associated with high risk of complete heart block and the probability of deep abscess. Thus, patients with prolonged PR intervals should be closely monitored. Complete heart block complicates about 4% of cases of IE. Ischemia or acute myocardial infarction documented by ECG may represent coronary embolization from infected aortic vegetation.

Transesophageal echocardiography (TEE) should be performed on many patients with IE, although absolute indications are not known. In competent hands, a positive study can demonstrate vegetations (and thus define the presence of IE) and identify complications. Investigations indicate, however, that IE and emboli may occur in the setting of (−) echocardiograms, although most data were generated with transthoracic echocardiography (TTE). TEE is a superior test to TTE in visualization of both vegetations and complications, including those of anatomy and hemodynamics. Examples of such complications include valve perforation, abscess, and pericardial effusion. Hemodynamic complications that may be identified include valve incompetence, fistulae, and intracardiac thrombi. It is now considered the most reliable noninvasive test for defining this disease. However, it should not be used as a screening tool for IE. It is the author's opinion that selected patients with IE with prompt response to antibiotics and no evidence of complications may be managed without echocardiography.

TEE is at least 90% sensitive and specific in the diagnosis of IE. As an example, patients with abscess complicating IE were identified on only 13 of 44 TTEs compared with 40 of 44 by TEE. Examples of clinical situations in which TEE may be useful include

(1) follow-up of patients with staphylococcal bacteremia (not initially considered as having IE); (2) assessment of patients with IE who remain febrile or persistently bacteremic; and (3) assessment of patients with IE plus conduction defects, congestive heart failure (CHF), or other potential intracardiac complications. Patients with either bacteremia or clinical findings consistent with IE should undergo TEE if response to antibiotic therapy is suboptimal, generally during the first week.

Cardiac catheterization occasionally may be useful when TEE has not provided adequate diagnostic or anatomic information, or as an adjunct to better assess intracardiac structures or the coronary arteries. The risk of complications is similar to that seen with cardiac catheterization in other groups, and thus is not contraindicated because of the presence of active IE.

SURGERY IN PATIENTS WITH NATIVE VALVE INFECTIVE ENDOCARDITIS

Studies continue to demonstrate improved outcomes of selected patients with IE who have undergone early cardiac surgery. The decision to operate should not be based on duration of prior antibiotics. Appropriate antimicrobial therapy should be initiated before surgery whenever possible, but there is no specified duration of therapy that improves cardiac surgical outcomes. Thus the need for surgery is based on indications and should not be delayed by limited duration of prior antibiotics. Table 11-1 lists reasons for valve replacement in patients with IE.

Congestive Heart Failure

CHF accounts for more than 80% of valve replacements in IE. Most commonly it is a complication of aortic valve endocarditis with resultant cusp perforation, but may also occur in association with mitral valve infection. It may also occur as a result of myocardial abscess, pericardial effusion, fistulae, and other hemodynamic complications of IE. Significant CHF (defined as that requiring more than minimal therapy, generally New York Heart Association Class III/IV) results in death in 50 to 90% of patients treated medically, whereas up to 60% survive with surgery. A recent investigation demonstrated that cardiac surgery in patients with moderate to severe CHF benefited most from cardiac surgery, with a decline in mortality from 51 to 14%. Patients with severe CHF resulting from valve perforation should undergo early valve replacement regardless of duration of antibiotics or continued positive blood cultures. For patients with diseased mitral valves, recent studies suggest that valve repair rather than replacement offers better clinical outcomes. Patients who survive the procedure have good prognoses. Individuals with mild CHF may be treated medically with careful

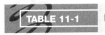

TABLE 11-1   **Indications for Surgery in Infective Endocarditis**

Native valve IE	Prosthetic valve IE
Progressive congestive heart failure	Prosthetic valve dysfunction
Recurrent major vessel embolization	Most cases of early PVE
Major vessel embolization with "at-risk" vegetation	
Fungi	Duration of fever >10 days
Lack of bactericidal agent	Sustained bacteremia
Extravalvular extension of infection	Infection with organisms other than streptococci and HACEK group
Failure of clinical response, generally 7–10 days.	Indications listed under native valve IE
Vegetation >1.5–2.0 cm, especially if within first week of therapy	

observation. Those with moderate CHF may have higher than expected death rates from coronary artery embolization. A common procedure at the time of valve replacement is to obtain Gram's stain and culture of the valve and possibly other removed tissues. The presence of "positive" Gram's stains is common and is related to the duration of antibiotic therapy. However, no relationship with outcome exists. Alternatively, in patients in whom a microbiologic diagnosis has been made preoperatively, intraoperative cultures are of no value in helping to define the microbiology of disease. Successful surgery may truncate duration of antibiotic therapy. In the absence of positive valve cultures, surgery that successfully removes all infected tissue may limit the duration of postoperative antibiotic therapy to 7 to 10 days.

Embolization

Embolization occurs in 10 to 50% of patients with IE and may occur before, during, or after effective medical therapy. It may occur in the absence of echocardiographically defined vegetations, although it is more common when vegetations are identified. Data demonstrate that up to 75% of clinically significant emboli occur before initiation of antibiotics and may therefore not be preventable. The most common site is the cerebral circulation. The risk declines substantially after a week of effective antimicrobial therapy. Complications of embolization are associated with approximately 25% of deaths from IE and are an important cause of long-term morbidity after microbiologic cure. Fungi and fastidious gram-negative organisms (HACEK group) have been associated with large emboli. The enhanced likelihood of embolization also exists with viridans streptococci, *Staphylococcus aureus*, and infected atrial myxomas. Other identified risks include previous embolization, advanced age, and atrial fibrillation. The necessity for valve replacement depends on the timing of embolization plus location and perhaps vegetation size. However, a single embolic event plus echocardiographic evidence of large (>1.0 cm) vegetation may also be an indication for surgery. This is especially true if the vegetation is mobile, on the anterior cusp of the mitral valve, and the patient is within the first week of antibiotic treatment. Operative intervention based only on vegetation size is controversial. Several recent studies imply that patients with vegetations larger than 1.5 to 2 cm carry excess risk for embolization and that surgery should be strongly considered on this basis alone. This may be especially true for disease on left-sided valves, especially if surgery can remove vegetation without valve replacement. It should be emphasized that most vegetations are slow to resolve and may remain present for up to 6 months. A recent report demonstrated that echocardiographic persistence at the end of treatment is not an independent predictor of late sequelae.

Infection with Resistant Organisms

Treatment of IE requires an effective bactericidal agent. Those most commonly used are β-lactams, aminoglycosides, or vancomycin. Others under active investigation include daptomycin and linezolid ("slowly bactericidal"). Unusual cases of IE caused by organisms such as *Chlamydia psittaci, Legionella pneumoniae, Coxiella burnetii,* and *Brucella* species may not be treatable with such compounds. Endocarditis caused by *Pseudomonas aeruginosa* or fungi should generally be managed with early surgical intervention. However, selected patients with right-side endocarditis associated with these organisms may occasionally be managed medically. Although many cases of enteric gram-negative IE will require surgery, each case should be assessed individually. Patients should receive high-dose bactericidal agents and have surgery if persistent bacteremia, CHF, or clinical deterioration occurs.

Extravalvular Extension of Infection

Infection extension beyond the valve generally represents surgical disease and is best defined by TEE. Clinical suspicion is enhanced in the presence of clinical failure to respond, worsening CHF, or heart block. Examples include (1) pericarditis, (2) valve ring abscess, (3) invasion of the conducting system, (4) myocardial abscess, and (5) fistulae. These complications occur most often in aortic valve disease. In unusual circumstances, cardiac catheterization also can be used to obtain quantitative blood cultures from different areas of the heart to try to define the lesion anatomically.

Other Reasons for Operative Intervention

Uncommonly, IE recurs after adequate antimicrobial therapy. This is usually secondary to localized or metastatic abscess or when infection is associated with a more resistant organism. Consideration for heart surgery should be given if no remedial cause can be located in other areas. Transesophageal echocardiography and, possibly, cardiac catheterization should be undertaken to identify occult infectious foci.

 ## SURGERY IN PATIENTS WITH PROSTHETIC VALVE ENDOCARDITIS

Prosthetic valve endocarditis (PVE) complicates valve replacement surgery in 1 to 2% of cases. "Early" PVE occurs within the first 60 days, whereas "late" occurs thereafter. The former is associated with more aggressive pathogens and a less favorable prognosis. Pathologically, PVE usually involves infection around the valve ring with extension into adjacent myocardial tissue. This explains the poor results generally noted with medical therapy alone. Fever for more than 10 days after institution of antimicrobials portends extravalvular extension. The table lists major reasons for cardiac surgery in PVE. Conditions already outlined for native valve IE also necessitate early operative intervention. These include (1) progressive or severe CHF, (2) recurrent major vessel embolization, (3) failure of appropriate medical therapy, and (4) IE caused by fungi and other resistant pathogens. Virtually all cases of early PVE fulfill these criteria, and surgery should generally be considered. Late PVE is a condition that closely mimics subacute native valve IE. For patients who develop PVE more than 12 months after valve replacement and are infected with viridans streptococci or HACEK organisms, attempts at medical therapy alone are reasonable, if reasons for surgery do not exist. A recent 20-year experience with late PVE demonstrated a 52% survivorship at 10 years. However, by the end of the study, only about 25% of patients were alive with the original prosthetic valve.

 ## ENDOCARDITIS ASSOCIATED WITH IMPLANTABLE PACERS/DEFIBRILLATORS

The availability of various devices to assist cardiac function and rhythm has resulted in types of infections not previously noted. All such devices may be complicated by infection involving either the pocket site or the wires leading to the heart. This, in turn, may be complicated by valvular infection, although not necessarily so. Fever in the setting of implantable devices should trigger an assessment for infection. Blood cultures and a careful clinical evaluation of the site should be performed routinely. Any evidence of local infection should result in aspiration of the pocket and, likely, device removal. In the presence of bacteremia but without overt pocket infection, TEE is indicated and, if negative, either gallium or white blood cell scanning to aid with localization of infection. The best therapy is removal of the entire device, including wires, with antibiotic therapy similar to that used for IE. (RBB)

Bibliography

Dinubile MJ. Surgery in active endocarditis. *Ann Intern Med* 1982;96:650–659.
> *This exhaustive review summarizes indications for surgery in native and prosthetic valve endocarditis. It remains extremely important. In addition to classic indications, the author summarizes information on the role of echocardiography and vegetation size in determining surgical need. He provides tables of major and minor criteria for surgical intervention in active endocarditis.*

Eggimann P, Waldvogel F. Pacemaker and defibrillator infections. In: Waldvogel FA, Bisno AL, eds. *Infections Associated with Indwelling Medical Devices.* 3rd ed. Washington, DC; ASM Press; 2000:247–264.
> *This chapter reviews the epidemiology, microbiology, and all clinical issues relevant to the management of infections with these implantable devices. In general, removal of the entire device, including wires, is associated with the highest likelihood of clinical success.*

Morris AJ, et al. Gram stain, culture, and histopathological examination findings for heart valves removed because of infective endocarditis. *Clin Infect Dis* 2003;36:697–704.

The authors retrospectively analyzed more than 400 cases of IE managed with valve removal to assess the value of valve Gram's stain and culture in IE management. They noted that nonviable organisms were regularly encountered and that they may help confirm the diagnosis of IE if preoperative cultures were negative. Positive smears in the absence of positive cultures had no bearing on therapeutic outcome, however. Only positive cultures should be equated with the need for prolonged antibiotics.

Olaison L, Pettersson G. Current best practice guidelines: indications for surgical intervention in infective endocarditis. *Cardiol Clin* 2003;21:235–251.

The authors present contemporary evidence-based information on the value of surgery for IE. Especially good discussions involve issues of embolization and neurologic complications. This manuscript deals primarily with native valve IE, and has an excellent bibliography.

Shively BK, et al. Diagnostic value of transesophageal compared with transthoracic echocardiography in infective endocarditis. *J Am Coll Cardiol* 1991;18:391–397.

These two modes of echocardiography were used in 66 patients with suspected infective endocarditis and compared with a gold standard. TEE was far more sensitive for defining the disease. Neither was associated with false-positive results.

Tornos P, et al. Clinical outcome and long-term prognosis of late prosthetic valve endocarditis: a 20-year experience. *Clin Infect Dis* 1996;24:381–386.

The authors describe their experience with 59 patients with late PVE followed up for 20 years. Only about 25% remained alive and with their original valve. Mortality with nonstreptococcal was significantly higher than that noted with streptococci.

Vikram HR, et al. Impact of valve surgery on 6-month mortality in adults with complicated left-sided native valve endocarditis. *JAMA* 2003;290:3207–3214.

This retrospective investigation demonstrates conclusively that surgery results in lower mortality than medical therapy for patients with complicated left-sided IE. This was especially true for patients with serious CHF. The authors defined "complicated by presence of CHF, new valvular regurgitation, progressive infection, systemic embolization, or vegetation noted by echocardiography. Inclusion of the latter is somewhat controversial, however.

Vuille C, Nidorf M, Picard MH. Natural history of vegetations during successful medical treatment of endocarditis. *Am Heart J* 1994;128:1200–1209.

Echocardiography was used to follow the natural history of vegetations during therapy for IE. At the time of termination of therapy, the majority of patients continued to have vegetations that were generally denser that those seen originally. Presence of vegetations was not an independent predictor of adverse outcome.

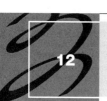

12   ENDOCARDITIS PROPHYLAXIS

*P*atients with certain underlying cardiac lesions should receive prophylactic antimicrobials just before undergoing procedures that might cause a bacteremia resulting in infective endocarditis. The subject of endocarditis prevention, however, continues to stir controversy. Although there is agreement on certain aspects of endocarditis prophylaxis, many issues remain unresolved: Which patients should receive prophylaxis? Which therapeutic and diagnostic procedures require prophylaxis? Which antimicrobial regimens are effective for prophylaxis? Are bactericidal antimicrobials required for prophylaxis? Is antimicrobial prophylaxis for endocarditis cost effective? Data to answer these and other key questions from controlled clinical studies are unavailable and unlikely to be forthcoming. Thus, the current guidelines for the prophylaxis of endocarditis from the American Heart Association and working party of the British Society for Antimicrobial Chemotherapy are empiric. Adherence to these regimens by practicing dentists and physicians is often faulty.

When bacteria invade the bloodstream, persons who have rheumatic heart disease, congenital heart disease, a prosthetic heart valve, mitral valve prolapse, or other cardiovascular disease are at risk for the development of infective endocarditis. The mechanism by which endocarditis occurs is still unclear. Organisms may infect a fibrin clot on a previously diseased valve or adhere to a specific receptor site on a valve leaflet. In either case, a key factor in the pathogenesis of infective endocarditis is the occurrence of a transient bacteremia.

Transient bacteremias develop commonly. They may occur spontaneously, as when a person chews food or defecates. They may result from many procedures that traumatize mucous membranes having an indigenous microbial flora, such as a dental extraction or urethral catheterization. Bacteremias after procedures resulting from mucosal trauma are asymptomatic, usually begin about 1 to 5 minutes after the procedure, and generally last for only 15 to 30 minutes. Quantitative blood cultures usually reveal colony counts of fewer than 10 organisms per milliliter of blood. Transient bacteremias are also associated with local infections, such as those resulting from incision and drainage of an abscess or manipulation of the urinary tract in a patient with asymptomatic bacteriuria. The organisms associated with these bacteremias reflect either the normal flora at the manipulated site or the pathogens causing the local infection.

No data accurately define the incidence of infective endocarditis in patients who undergo invasive procedures without antimicrobial prophylaxis. A history of a predisposing event sometimes can be elicited from patients with endocarditis. Of patients with nonenterococcal streptococcal endocarditis, 15 to 20% had a preceding dental procedure. In another review, only 3.6% of cases of endocarditis were associated with a dental procedure. A preceding genitourinary tract procedure has been reported in up to 42% of patients with enterococcal endocarditis. Thirty-five percent of patients with staphylococcal endocarditis have had a preceding infection of the skin or soft tissue. Endocarditis often occurs without an obvious predisposing event.

The oropharynx is a frequent portal of entry for organisms into the bloodstream. Blood cultures are positive in 18 to 85% of patients after a dental extraction. The frequency of bacteremia correlates with the severity of gingival infection and the extent of tissue trauma. The organisms isolated reflect the normal mouth flora. Viridans streptococci are isolated most frequently, but anaerobic streptococci, coagulase-negative staphylococci, diphtheroids, and *Fusobacterium* also are seen. Strains of viridans streptococci account for 50 to 75% of cases of endocarditis and are usually penicillin sensitive. Streptococci that are relatively resistant to penicillin are found in patients receiving prophylactic penicillin for rheumatic fever and in those given antimicrobial prophylaxis as early as 1 to 2 days before a procedure. Prophylaxis should begin just before a procedure so that serum levels of the antimicrobial are adequate at the time of anticipated bacteremia. Penicillin given just before a dental extraction will decrease the incidence of positive blood cultures after the procedure.

Other dental procedures that may result in a transient bacteremia are periodontal operations, such as gingivectomy, root canal surgery, and dental cleaning. In up to 88% of patients with gum disease, blood cultures are positive, depending on the severity of the disease. The predominant organisms are the same as with dental extraction. Positive blood cultures also are seen after tooth brushing (0 to 26%), the use of oral irrigation devices (7 to 50%) or dental floss (20%), and chewing gum or eating hard candy (0 to 22%). Antimicrobial prophylaxis is impractical for preventing a transient bacteremia secondary to common daily activities. Maintenance of good oral hygiene, however, decreases the amount of gum disease, a key determinant of the frequency of a transient bacteremia after any dental manipulation.

Other procedures involving the oropharynx and respiratory tract may result in bacteremia, including tonsillectomy, nasotracheal intubation, and rigid-tube bronchoscopy. Positive blood cultures, however, rarely are associated with flexible fiberoptic bronchoscopy and lung biopsy.

Diagnostic procedures involving the gastrointestinal tract are another source of transient bacteremias. Positive blood cultures are found in patients undergoing fiberoptic gastrointestinal endoscopy (0 to 10%; 4% overall), rigid sigmoidoscopy (0 to 9.5%; 5% overall), flexible sigmoidoscopy (0%), liver biopsy (3 to 14%), barium enema (11%), and colonoscopy (0 to 27%; 5% overall). Transient bacteremia also occurs in patients having esophageal dilation (mean incidence, 45%), sclerotherapy of esophageal varices (18%), and endoscopic retrograde cholangiopancreatography (6%). The predominant organisms isolated with these procedures are enterococci, a frequent cause of endocarditis, and gram-negative bacilli, organisms rarely involved in native valve endocarditis.

Transient bacteremia and infective endocarditis can occur after urinary tract, obstetric, and gynecologic procedures. The urinary tract is the portal of entry in 20 to 50% of patients with enterococcal endocarditis, whereas 20% of cases caused by this organism are related to obstetric and gynecologic procedures. A transient bacteremia occurs in 8% of patients undergoing urethral catheterization, 24% undergoing urethral dilation, 17% having cystoscopy, and 12 to 31% having transurethral prosthetic resection. The frequency of positive blood cultures increases by several times in patients with infection at the instrumented site, such as a urinary tract infection. Genitourinary tract procedures appear to be the second most common predisposing event.

Transient bacteremia also develops in patients after vaginal delivery, cesarean section, dilation and curettage of the uterus, and insertion or removal of an intrauterine contraceptive device.

Manipulation of an infected focus, such as massage of an infected prostate or incision and drainage of an abscess, is associated with bacteremia and the risk for endocarditis. Transient bacteremia is rare with cardiac catheterization and angiographic procedures. Prevention of endocarditis requires knowledge of both the events likely to produce bacteremia and the patient with predisposing cardiac lesions. Unfortunately, half of patients with endocarditis have no recognized underlying heart disease, making antimicrobial prophylaxis impossible for this group. Rheumatic valvular disease still remains a common form of underlying cardiac disease in patients in whom endocarditis develops. The frequency has declined, however, with the decreasing incidence of rheumatic fever. Patients with a bicuspid aortic valve are predisposed to endocarditis, as are patients with calcific or sclerotic changes in the aortic and mitral valves or annulus (Tables 12-1 to 12-4).

Patients with mitral valve prolapse-click murmur syndrome have been reported to be at increased risk for endocarditis. In a case-control study, the risk for endocarditis in patients with mitral valve prolapse was approximately eight times higher than that for the matched controls. In a study of failures of endocarditis prophylaxis, mitral valve prolapse was the most frequent cardiac abnormality identified, accounting for 33% of cases of endocarditis. Prophylaxis in all patients with mitral valve prolapse would be difficult because of its high incidence (5 to 6% of the American population). One approach is to prescribe prophylaxis to patients with associated mitral insufficiency, thickened mitral leaflets on the echocardiogram, or men older than age 45 with mitral valve prolapse, but not to those who have only a systolic click and are undergoing procedures associated with endocarditis.

Patients with a previous episode of endocarditis also should receive prophylaxis during predisposing events. Patients with prosthetic or bioprosthetic heart valves are also predisposed. Because infection of a prosthesis is often difficult to eradicate and carries a high mortality, antimicrobial prophylaxis is recommended both for the usual predisposing events and for additional procedures associated with a transient bacteremia but a lower risk for infection, such as upper gastrointestinal endoscopy, barium enema, or colonoscopy.

Only estimates are available for the incidence of endocarditis in susceptible persons after exposure to an event associated with transient bacteremia. The incidence is clearly low, because bacteremias often occur after operative procedures, and resultant endocarditis is relatively rare. Similarly, the effectiveness of antimicrobial prophylaxis for infective endocarditis remains unknown. Because a carefully controlled study with a very large number of patients would be required to answer some of the questions on this issue, animals have been used to study the pathogenesis and efficacy of antimicrobial prophylaxis in infective endocarditis. A major criticism of this model is that a high inoculum of bacteria is used to produce infection, in contrast to the low number of organisms associated with a transient bacteremia.

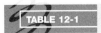 **Endocarditis Prophylaxis Recommended**

For patients with:

- Prosthetic heart valves
- Prior bacterial endocarditis
- Cyanotic congenital heart disease
- Acquired valvular heart disease (e.g., rheumatic heart disease)
- Mitral valve prolapse with mitral regurgitation
- Hypertrophic cardiomyopathy

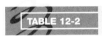 **Endocarditis Prophylaxis Not Recommended**

For patients with:

- Atrial septal defect of the secundum variety
- Coronary artery bypass grafts
- Mitral valve prolapse without regurgitation
- Implanted devices such as cardiac pacemakers, defibrillators

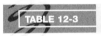 **Procedures in Which Endocarditis Prophylaxis is Recommended**

- Dental extractions
- Periodontal procedures
- Dental procedures associated with bleeding
- Tonsillectomy/adenoidectomy
- Bronchoscopy with rigid but not flexible scope
- Biliary tract surgery
- Surgical operations that involve intestinal mucosa
- Cytoscopy
- Urethral dilation
- Prostate surgery

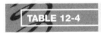 **Procedures in Which Endocarditis Prophylaxis is *Not* Recommended**

- Upper and lower gastrointestinal endoscopy with or without biopsy
- Vaginal delivery
- Vaginal hysterectomy
- Cesarean section
- Cardiac catheterization
- Implantation of cardiac pacemaker, defibrillator or coronary stents

(Modified from Conte C. Endocarditis Prophylaxis yes: endocarditis prophylaxis no. *Clin Cardiol* 2003;26: 255–256.)

Antimicrobial prophylaxis is not indicated for patients at risk for endocarditis who are undergoing cardiac catheterization, pacemaker insertion, or peritoneal dialysis. Effective use of prophylactic antimicrobials requires that adequate drug levels be present at the required site at the time of the event, posing the risk for transient bacteremia. To accomplish this goal, the antimicrobial drug should be given just before the procedure. Initiation of an antimicrobial 1 to 2 days before a procedure can result in the replacement of sensitive strains of bacteria by resistant organisms. Selective pressure is also exerted on the local flora, favoring the emergence of resistant strains. Increasing the duration of treatment beyond one dose after the initial loading dose only raises the cost and increases the possibility of an adverse drug reaction. For dental procedures and other procedures involving the airway, the antimicrobial selected should be directed against viridans streptococci. Genitourinary manipulation and gastrointestinal, gynecologic, and obstetric procedures require that the antimicrobial prophylaxis is directed against enterococci. Antimicrobials should be adequate for penicillinase-producing staphylococci in a predisposed person undergoing incision and drainage of an abscess. A urine culture should be obtained before a genitourinary procedure, so that any infection can be identified and treated before the instrumentation.

Hematogenous seeding of a prosthetic joint implant is a concern in a patient having a procedure associated with a transient bacteremia, as well as for those with an existing infection. No data are available to answer this dilemma, although antimicrobials are frequently administered. Infection of a prosthetic implant has been reported, but the risk appears to be extremely low. Although no medical or legal guidelines exist on this issue, I often recommend antimicrobial prophylaxis, particularly for recently implanted devices (within 2 years, and for immunocompromised patients), but would not fault a physician for not using it. Whether bactericidal antimicrobials are essential for adequate prophylaxis is unclear. Earlier studies in rabbits favored bactericidal drugs, but recent reports show that bacteriostatic antimicrobials may be sufficient to prevent endocarditis under certain circumstances. Similarly, some strains of viridans streptococci are tolerant to penicillin. The relevance of tolerance to successful prophylaxis remains to be determined (Table 12-5).

Antimicrobial regimens for prophylaxis are listed in Table 12-6. The recommendations in the United States are derived from the guidelines proposed by the advisory committee to the American Heart Association. Amoxicillin has replaced penicillin for prophylaxis in patients undergoing dental or upper respiratory tract surgical procedures, and the dose has decreased from 3 g to 2 g orally. No repeated dose after the procedure is recommended. Patients who have recently received penicillin or who are allergic to it should receive oral clindamycin, azithromycin, clarithromycin, or a cephalosporin for dental procedures. For gastrointestinal, genitourinary, and gynecologic procedures, parenteral ampicillin and gentamicin are recommended. Patients with a penicillin allergy should receive parenteral vancomycin plus gentamicin. Because parenteral regimens are often difficult to use in outpatients, amoxicillin may be substituted in low-risk patients. As the recommendations for endocarditis prophylaxis are empiric, clinical judgment must be exercised carefully in selecting which patients should receive antimicrobial prophylaxis for the procedures that might cause a bacteremia. (NMG)

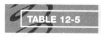

TABLE 12-5	Need for Endocarditis Prophylaxis

1. Base decision on type of underlying heart disease or presence of a prosthetic device.
2. Endocarditis prophylaxis is recommended for patients at high or moderate risk.
3. Endocarditis prophylaxis is not recommended for patients at low risk.
4. Endocarditis prophylaxis is recommended for selected dental, respiratory, gastrointestinal, or gastrourinary tract procedures associated with a transient bacteremia.
5. Endocarditis prophylaxis is *not* recommended for patients having a cardiac catheterization, placement of coronary stents, or for patients with cardiac pacemakers or defibrillators.
6. Endocarditis prophylaxis usually is not recommended for patients with underlying prosthetic orthopedic devices having procedures associated with a transient bacteremia.

TABLE 12-6   **Endocarditis Prophylaxis: Dosage for Adults**

Dental, oral, and upper respiratory tract procedures
Oral

Amoxicillin	2 g 1 hr before procedure
Penicillin allergy	
Clindamycin	600 mg 1 hr before procedure
OR	
Cephalexin* or cefadroxil*	2 g 1 hr before procedure
OR	
Azithromycin or clarithromycin	500 mg 1 hr before procedure

Parenteral**

Ampicillin	2 g IM or IV 30 min before procedure
Penicillin allergy	
Clindamycin	600 mg IV within 30 min before procedure
OR	
Cefazolin*	1 g IM or IV within 30 min before procedure

Gastrointestinal, genitourinary, and gynecologic procedures
Oral

Amoxicillin	2 g 1 hr before procedure

Parenteral

Ampicillin	2 g IM or IV within 30 min before procedure
plus	
Gentamicin	1.5 mg/kg (120 mg maximum) IM or IV 30 min before procedure
Penicillin allergy	
Vancomycin	1 g IV infused *slowly* over 1 hr beginning 1 hr before procedure
plus	
Gentamicin	1.5 mg/kg (120 mg maximum) IM or IV 30 min before procedure

Incision and drainage of skin abscesses caused by coagulase-positive staphylococci, not methicillin-resistant[‡]
Oral

Dicloxacillin	500 mg 1 hr before procedure, then 500 mg q6h

Parenteral

Nafcillin or oxacillin	2 g IV 0.5–1 hr before procedure, then 2 g IV q4h
Cefazolin[§]	1 g IM 1 hr before procedure, then 1 g IV or IM q8h

If methicillin-resistant

Vancomycin[‡,§]	1 g IV over 60 min. Start infusion 1 hr before procedure, then 1 g q12h IV

*Not recommended for patients with history of immediate-type allergy to penicillin.
**Parenteral regimens are recommended for patients with prosthetic or biosynthetic heart valves. Parenteral regimens may be preferred for patients in highest risk groups, although data to support this practice are not available.
[‡]Route and duration of therapy depend on the severity of the infection and on whether the predisposed person is at high risk (e.g., prosthetic heart valve). Results of Gram's stains and cultures should also guide antimicrobial selection.
[§]If patient is allergic to penicillin or receiving continuous oral penicillin, adjust dosage in renal insufficiency for vancomycin and cefazolin.
(Modified from Dejani AS, et al. Prevention of bacterial endocarditis. *JAMA* 1997;277:1794.)

Bibliography

Bayliss R, et al. The bowel, the genitourinary tract, and infective endocarditis. *Br Heart J* 1984;51:339.
Patients with underlying cardiac disease should receive an antimicrobial when they undergo genitourinary or alimentary tract surgery or instrumentation.

Clemens JD, et al. A controlled evaluation of the risk of bacterial endocarditis in persons with mitral valve prolapse. *N Engl J Med* 1982;307:776.
Study supports that mitral valve prolapse is a risk factor for bacterial endocarditis.

Conte C. Endocarditis prophylaxis yes: endocarditis prophylaxis no. *Clin Cardiol* 2003;26:255–256.
Lists patients at risk and procedures in which endocarditis prophylaxis is recommended.

Dajani AS, et al. Prevention of bacterial endocarditis. *JAMA* 1997;277:1794.
Recommendations for antimicrobial prophylaxis from the American Heart Association are outlined. Prophylaxis should be given to patients with moderate-risk to high-risk underlying cardiac lesions who are undergoing procedures associated with a high risk for transient bacteremia.

Devereux RB, et al. Cost effectiveness of infective endocarditis prophylaxis for mitral valve prolapse with or without a mitral regurgitant murmur. *Am J Cardiol* 1994;74:1024.
Administration of amoxicillin to patients undergoing a dental procedure who have mitral valve prolapse and a mitral regurgitant murmur is cost effective.

Durack DT. Prevention of infective endocarditis. *N Engl J Med* 1995;322:38.
Review.

Durack DT, Bisno AL, Kaplan EL. Apparent failures of endocarditis prophylaxis. Analysis of 52 cases submitted to a national registry. *JAMA* 1983;250:2318.
Mitral valve prolapse was the most common underlying cardiac lesion. Symptoms began within 5 weeks of the suspected procedure in about 80% of the cases.

Everett ED, Hirschmann JV. Transient bacteremia and endocarditis prophylaxis. A review. *Medicine (Baltimore)* 1977;56:61.
Classic comprehensive review cites the frequency of transient bacteremias with various procedures.

Fitzgerald RH, et al. Antibiotic prophylaxis for dental patients with total joint replacements. *J Am Dent Assoc* 1997;128:109.
Antibiotic prophylaxis is not indicated for patients undergoing dental procedures who have joint replacements unless there is an increased risk for a hematogenous joint infection. Patients who are at higher risk for infection include those who are immunocompromised, who have undergone implant surgery within the past 2 years or have previously had prosthetic joint infections, and diabetics receiving insulin.

Garrison PK, Freedman LR. Experimental endocarditis I: staphylococcal endocarditis resulting from placement of a polyethylene catheter in the right side of the heart. *Yale J Biol Med* 1970;42:394.
Classic article describing the rabbit model used for experimental endocarditis.

Guntheroth WG. How important are dental procedures as a cause of infective endocarditis? *Am J Cardiol* 1984;54:797.
Dental extractions preceded endocarditis in only 3.6% of cases. Good oral hygiene is the key to preventing endocarditis.

Hall G, et al. Prophylactic administration of penicillins for endocarditis does not reduce the incidence of postextraction bacteremia. *Clin Infect Dis* 1993;17:188.
Amoxicillin did not decrease the frequency of transient bacteremia after extraction when compared with placebo. The effect of antibiotics in preventing endocarditis must be based on other mechanisms.

Hook EW, Kaye D. Prophylaxis of bacterial endocarditis. *J Chronic Dis* 1962;15:635.
A classic review of the portals of entry of organisms and the risk to the susceptible host.

Horsakotte D, et al. Guidelines on prevention, diagnosis and treatment of infective endocarditis. *Eur Heart J* 2004;25:267–276.
Review.

Khandheria BK. Prophylaxis or no prophylaxis before transesophageal echocardiography? *J Am Soc Echocardiogr* 1992;5:285.

Editorial summarizing the frequency of transient bacteremia after common gastrointestinal procedures. Rates are highest with esophageal dilation (45%) and sclerotherapy (18%). Rates are about 5% after transesophageal echocardiography, and it is unclear whether antimicrobial prophylaxis is indicated.

Oliver G, et al. Practice parameters for antibiotic prophylaxis—supporting documentation. *Dis Colon Rectum* 2000;43:1194–2000.
Gastrointestinal procedures rarely cause endocarditis, but prophylaxis is recommended in selected situations.

Oliver R, Roberts GJ, Hooper L. Penicillins for the prophylaxis of bacterial endocarditis in dentistry. *Cochrane Database Syst Rev* 2004;3:1–36.
There is no evidence to support the use of penicillin to prevent endocarditis in at-risk people who are undergoing invasive dental procedures.

Pelletier LL, Durack DT, Petersdorf RG. Chemotherapy of experimental streptococcal endocarditis IV: further observation of prophylaxis. *J Clin Invest* 1975;56:319.
Data from the rabbit model are presented for prophylaxis of streptococcal endocarditis.

Sanders GP, et al. Impact of a specific echocardiographic report comment regarding endocarditis prophylaxis on compliance with American Heart Association recommendations. *Circulation* 2002;106:300–303.
A transthoracic echocardiogram is useful to define the need for prophylaxis.

Seto TB, et al. Specialty and training differences in the reported use of endocarditis prophylaxis at an academic medical center. *Am J Med* 2002;111:657–660.
Most physicians do not recommend prophylaxis. in accordance with the current American Heart Association guidelines.

Seymour RA, Whitworth JM. Antibiotic prophylaxis for endocarditis, prosthetic joints, and surgery. *Dent Clin North Am* 2002;46:635–651.
Review. A controversial subject. Recommend either no prophylaxis or giving antibiotics to immunocompromised patients with prosthetic joints inserted within 2 years.

Shorvan PJ, Eykyn SJ, Cotton PB. Gastrointestinal instrumentation, bacteremia, and endocarditis. *Gut* 1983;24:1078.
A review of gastrointestinal procedures and the risk for endocarditis.

Taran LM. Rheumatic fever in relation to dental disease. *N Y J Dent* 1944;14:107.
In children with rheumatic heart disease, the risk for developing endocarditis after a dental extraction was 1.1%.

van der Meer JTM, et al. Efficacy of antibiotic prophylaxis for prevention of native valve endocarditis. *Lancet* 1992;339:135.
Most cases (87%) of endocarditis were unrelated to any predisposing events.

van der Meer JTM, et al. Awareness of need and actual use of prophylaxis: lack of patient compliance in the prevention of bacterial endocarditis. *J Antimicrob Chemother* 1992;29:187.
By history, antimicrobials were given only 22% of the time to patients at risk for endocarditis and undergoing a procedure associated with a bacteremia.

Gastrointestinal System   IV

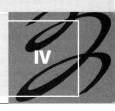

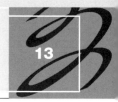

FILLING DEFECTS OF THE LIVER 13

*F*illing defects of the liver will be defined as lesions of sufficient size to be demonstrated by imaging studies that could include standard roentgenograms, computed tomography (CT), magnetic resonance imaging (MRI), or hepatic ultrasound (US). Generally, lesions that are larger than 0.5 to 1.0 cm can be documented by newer imaging techniques. Differential diagnosis includes infection, hematoma, neoplasm, and cysts. Granulomatous processes such as tuberculosis and fungal infection, although capable of involving hepatic parenchyma, are unusual causes of filling defects, as defined above.

 ## CLINICAL PRESENTATION

Clinical presentation is highly variable, depending on cause and patient comorbidities. As an example, uncomplicated hydatid cysts may remain asymptomatic and be documented as an incidental finding when roentgenographic studies are performed for other reasons. Alternatively, pyogenic or amebic abscess may present with high-grade constitutional abnormalities including shock. Many individuals have subtle complaints of right upper quadrant (RUQ) discomfort associated with large lesion size. The severity and acuteness of presentation may provide useful information about etiology.

Radiographic assessment is performed for reasons that include (1) hepatomegaly or RUQ tenderness on physical examination; (2) elevation of hepatic enzymes, most notably alkaline phosphatase; (3) jaundice; (4) fever of undetermined origin; and (5) assessment of metastases in patients with selected known primary malignancies. The choice of imaging procedure will vary with those available within an institution and with clinical suspicions regarding etiology. CT and US have the advantage of allowing aspiration or drainage simultaneously with diagnosis. However, regardless of procedure performed, presence of a lesion usually leads to a procedure for tissue diagnosis, drainage, or both. Exceptions may include "classic" hydatid disease or serologically-confirmed amebic abscess. MRI may be able to distinguish amebic and pyogenic abscess in some circumstances, but microbiologic assessment of aspirated material is always recommended.

 ## PYOGENIC HEPATIC ABSCESS

Hepatic abscess has an incidence of up to 0.2 cases/1,000 hospitalizations and is currently a disease of older individuals. The most common contributory factors are biliary tract infections (33%), direct extension from contiguous infected foci (25%), bacteremia (10%), blunt trauma to the RUQ (15%) (e.g., steering wheel injuries), and retrograde pylephlebitis (6%) (e.g., complication of perforated appendix). The latter was the most common cause in the preantibiotic era. At least 10% are cryptogenic. These etiologies reflect the mechanisms responsible for spread to the liver. Within the past two decades, patients with pyogenic hepatic abscess are more likely to have underlying biliary tract or pancreatic malignancy. About 50% of abscesses are single, and most involve the right lobe of the liver.

Clinical presentation varies with the predisposing factor. Most individuals present subacutely with low-grade constitutional complaints and RUQ discomfort. Fever, chills, and malaise are the most common symptoms, with fever almost universally noted. RUQ discomfort and hepatomegaly are the most common signs, and jaundice occurs in approximately 25% of persons. Up to 20% of individuals have pulmonary complaints that include right-sided pleural effusions, elevation of the right hemidiaphragm, or rales. Pneumonia may be the initial consideration, and sometimes individuals are treated repetitively for this condition before the true diagnosis is considered. Routine laboratory data are generally nonspecific; anemia and leukocytosis are seen in 60% and 70% of individuals, respectively. Elevation of the alkaline phosphatase is noted in 75% of patients and represents the single most common altered liver enzyme. Hyperbilirubinemia is seen in less than 25% of cases and is most commonly associated with biliary tract disease.

Noninvasive imaging techniques are generally used for further assessment. In the absence of contraindications, intravenous contrast-enhanced CT scanning (sensitivity of up to 95%) is more sensitive than ultrasound, but the latter may be preferred for individuals with a high likelihood of biliary tract disease. MRI has also been used, but advantages over CT and US are uncertain and costs are higher. Blood cultures should always be obtained and are positive in approximately 50% of cases. However, sensitivity to identify multiple organisms is less than that seen with direct abscess culture.

Percutaneous drainage of the lesion allows simultaneous diagnosis and therapy. Materials obtained can be sent for Gram's stain, aerobic or anaerobic culture, parasitology, and histopathology. Recent studies document that Gram's stain's sensitivity and specificity are higher for gram-positive than for gram-negative organisms.

Bacteriology of pyogenic hepatic abscesses is often complex and represents the etiology of the underlying condition. Abscess complicating bacteremia from a distant focus may be monomicrobial. Most often associated with biliary tract, trauma and retrograde pylephlebitis are polymicrobial and often include enteric gram-negative bacilli (e.g., *Escherichia coli*, *Klebsiella* sp) and gastrointestinal anaerobes. Trends over the past two decades suggest an increase in hepatic abscesses associated with fungi, streptococci, and *Pseudomonas aeruginosa*. Recent reports also have documented the likelihood of metastatic dissemination of *Klebsiella* sp. infection (often endophthalmitis) from pyogenic abscess. This has been noted especially in diabetics. Sterile abscesses are seen in a small percentage of patients and are likely to reflect either prior antibiotic usage or poor microbiology techniques.

Therapy for pyogenic hepatic abscess includes long-term antibiotics and drainage. Generally, antibiotic therapy should be guided by culture results. The route of administration is controversial. Most clinicians treat intravenously for the first few weeks and then may complete at least a 6-week course with appropriate oral medications. Agents that include metronidazole, fluoroquinolones, and trimethoprim/sulfamethoxazole are bioequivalent by oral and intravenous routes, so there is no benefit to parenteral therapy so long as the gastrointestinal tract is functional. Duration of treatment is guided in part by radiographic resolution. The results of aspiration (occasionally multiple times) of abscess versus ongoing catheter drainage have been conflicting. Some patients have been treated with antibiotics alone, but this should be reserved for those in whom drainage cannot be performed. Open surgical procedures should be done when (1) multiple or septet lesions are identified that cannot be drained percutaneously, (2) surgery is indicated to manage the initiating cause of the abscess (e.g., biliary stones), and (3) the patient has failed to respond to percutaneous drainage. Total surgical extirpation should be considered when hydatid disease is the differential diagnosis.

AMEBIC ABSCESS

Amebiasis afflicts up to 10% of the population, is associated with 50 million cases of invasive disease, and may account for as many as 100,000 deaths. *Entamoeba histolytica* is the only species associated with invasive disease. Amebic abscess is the most common complication of intestinal amebiasis and can occur many years after initial exposure. Best estimates are of more than 20 cases/100,000 population in endemic areas. It should be suspected as a cause of intrahepatic filling defects in patients associated with endemic areas that include Mexico, Central America, and Southeast Asia. Disease is also associated with homosexuality and residence in institutions for the mentally retarded.

	Comparison of Pyogenic and Amebic Liver Abscess[+]

Feature	Amebic	Pyogenic
Male:female	19:1	4:1
Age (median)	28	44
Epidemiology	Endemic area	Any
RUQ pain	59%	27%
Symptoms >14days	14%	37%
RUQ tenderness	67%	42%
(+) Amebic serology	94%	6%
MRI presentation*	Often single lesion. Hyperintense center on T2-weighted images and hypointense center on T1-weighted images. Wall generally thick (>5 mm)	Similar to that seen with amebic abscess. May have proteinaceous debris, hyperintense on T1- and hypointense on T2-weighted images. "Cluster sign" (smaller abscesses surrounding a larger abscess)

*(Adapted from Balci NC, Sirvanci M. MR imaging of infective liver lesions. *MR Clin N Am* 2002;10: 121–135.)
[+](With the exception of MR findings, adapted from Barnes, et al. A comparison of amebic and pyogenic abscess of the liver. *Medicine (Baltimore)* 1987;66:472–483.)

Typically right hepatic lobe involvement is seen, reflecting the most direct route of spread by the portal vein. Table 13-1 provides some ways to help differentiate amebic from pyogenic abscess. Up to 66% of the former present acutely with fever, chills, and new onset RUQ pain. The remainder may have complaints for up to 12 weeks. Some patients present with only an occult febrile syndrome. In all groups, pulmonary complaints such as pleurisy and cough may be noted, and the initial consideration may be pneumonia. About 33% of patients give a history of active diarrhea. Rarely, initial presentation is that of rupture, into either the peritoneum, pleural space, or pericardium. Intra-abdominal rupture is more likely when left-lobe abscesses are present.

For individuals with acute presentations, white blood cell (WBC) count is often elevated; however it may be normal in those with more chronic illness. Both groups may become anemic. Approximately 85% of patients have elevations of alkaline phosphatase; the most reliable chemical test. Hyperbilirubinemia is uncommonly noted.

Indirect hemagglutination testing (serum) is a reliable serologic test for hepatic amebiasis, is positive in at least 85% of patients with extraintestinal disease, and often is greater than 1:256. It should be performed in all patients with space-occupying lesions when a specific diagnosis is uncertain. Elevations are almost always noted less than 2 weeks into disease and may remain high for many years after successful therapy. Antigen detection in either serum (100%), abscess (40%) or stool (40%) may also be valuable and may be especially useful in persons from endemic areas, where antibody is likely to be positive.

Diagnosis can be suspected by hepatic imaging, but there is no pathognomonic picture. A recent review has compared MRI findings of amebic and pyogenic abscesses. Hepatic US or CT scanning provides highly sensitive results and can be repeated to gauge response. Most authors now feel that the former, because of ease of administration and lower expense, is the study of choice for both diagnosis and follow-up. With satisfactory treatment, US should normalize within 20 months. However, lesion size may actually increase during early therapy, and thus some authorities do not recommend immediate follow-up if the patient is clinically responding. Up to 50% of cases demonstrate multiple space-occupying lesions. Most common sites remain within the right lobe. Results of hepatic US are variable and include round or oval hypoechoic lesions, often containing debris, cystic lesions, or solid or heterogeneous masses. The average size of abscesses is 7 to 10 cm, but 33% are larger than 10 cm. In acute case (fewer than 5 days of symptoms), initial US may be negative.

The role of percutaneous lesion aspiration for either diagnosis or treatment remains controversial. A recent prospective investigation of metronidazole alone versus metronidazole plus abscess aspiration for lesions of 7 to 10 cm. demonstrated a limited advantage of aspiration and recommended that most persons can be treated with medication alone. However, aspiration is indicated if (1) alternative diagnoses are considered (excluding hydatid disease); (2) lesions are larger than 10 cm; (3) patients fail to respond to standard therapy within 72 hours; or (4) left-sided lesions are at risk of rupture. Surgical intervention is rarely indicated but may be lifesaving if rupture has occurred. Material obtained at aspiration or surgery should be evaluated for the presence of organisms. Typical fluid is not foul-smelling and is brownish ("anchovy paste"), often devoid of organisms, and typically without polymorphonuclear leukocytes. Standard cultures (aerobic and anaerobic) and histopathology should be carried out in all cases.

Medical therapy for amebic abscess consists of oral or intravenous metronidazole, 750 mg three times daily for 5 to 10 days. A regimen of 2.4 g daily by mouth for several days has also been successfully used. Up to 90% of patients respond clinically within 72 hours. More toxic regimens that are uncommonly indicated consist of dehydroemetine 1 to 1.5 mg/kg per day for 5 days plus either diloxanide furoate or paromomycin.

 ## ECHINOCOCCAL CYST (HYDATID DISEASE)

Hydatid disease is endemic in areas of southern Europe, the Middle East, and Australia, and represents the larval stage of the canine tapeworm *Echinococcus granulosus*. Cases reported in the United States are primarily imported. Human disease is generally asymptomatic and identified during hepatic imaging for other reasons. Sixty percent to 75% of all cysts occur in the liver; 20 to 40% of individuals have multiple cysts.

Clinical presentation is most often chronic and generally represents that of an enlarging, space-occupying lesion in the absence of significant constitutional symptomatology. Symptoms are vague abdominal pain and pressure. At least 33% of patients remain asymptomatic. Complaints are generally not noted until cysts reach more than 7 cm; average cyst size at surgery is approximately 11 cm. Hepatic enlargement may be noted, often in association with a palpable mass. Leakage and rupture are potentially lethal complications and can occur spontaneously, after trauma, or at surgical removal. Material is "allergenic," and leakage may be associated with anaphylaxis.

Diagnosis should be suspected in patients with RUQ symptoms and a history of travel to an endemic area. Routine laboratory data are not useful. About 60% of patients will have an elevation of alkaline phosphatase, and 33% demonstrate eosinophilia. An indirect hemagglutination titer of more than 1:64 is seen in about 50% of cases. CT scan, US, or routine abdominal films often demonstrate single or multiple cystic areas, generally with partial calcification. Intracystic septation with partial calcification of the cyst is pathognomonic.

Therapy is surgical extirpation under controlled conditions to avoid spillage of cyst contents. Percutaneous aspiration is contraindicated for this reason. In patients for whom surgical extirpation cannot be performed, either albendazole (10–15 mg/kg per day for 1 month) or mebendazole (50–150 mg/kg per day for 3 months) can be used, but with poorly documented and uncertain outcomes.

NEOPLASM AND OTHER CAUSES OF HEPATIC FILLING DEFECTS

Neoplasms often involve the liver. Most common primary neoplasms are hepatocellular carcinoma and cholangiocarcinoma. Hepatic metastases from lung, breast, large intestine, stomach, pancreas, and melanoma are commonly observed. One investigation demonstrated that 39% of adults dying with solid tumors had hepatic metastases. Clinical presentation varies and overlaps with that seen in infections. The presence of ascites is distinctly unusual for infections. Alternatively, patients with pyogenic abscess are more likely to have at least three of the following: leukocytosis, fever, risk factors for pyogenic abscess, shorter clinical course, and normal hepatic size.

CT scanning is considered the best screening test for hepatic metastases larger than 0.5 cm. Sensitivity is better than 90%, but specificity is low. Hepatic US is generally considered the next most important test and (like CT) can distinguish solid from cystic lesions. Lesions, including cavernous hemangioma, focal fatty deposits, and nodular hyperplasia can often be diagnosed by characteristic CT scan plus radionucleotide imaging. Both US and CT scanning often can discriminate between simple cysts and other lesions. Although one or another study can provide clues to etiology, ultimate diagnosis usually requires tissue or fluid sampling.

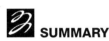 **SUMMARY**

Hepatic filling defects have many etiologies. Clinical presentation is variable, and diagnosis is usually made by noninvasive radiographic assessment plus sampling of the lesion. In the absence of hydatid disease concerns, percutaneous biopsy/aspiration of the lesion provides a direct and relative safe initial approach. (RBB)

Bibliography

Balci NC, Sirvanci M. MR imaging of infective liver lesions. *Magn Reson Imaging Clin N Am* 2002;10:121–135.
The authors present a review of MR findings in a variety of liver infections. They claim that pyogenic and amebic abscess may be able to be differentiated, but still note the need for further studies to confirm diagnosis.
Barakate MS, et al. Pyogenic liver abscess: a review of 10 years' experience in management. *Aust N Z J Surg* 1999;69:205–209.
The authors present a recent retrospective review of a relatively large (98 patients) patient population with pyogenic liver abscess. Presentations and initial laboratory data were as historically described. Most persons were treated with antibiotics plus percutaneous drainage; several with small abscesses were given antibiotics alone. Reasons for failure of the regimens, requiring surgical intervention, included unresolved jaundice, severe renal dysfunction, rupture, multiloculation, and biliary communication.
Barnes PF, et al. A comparison of amebic and pyogenic abscess of the liver. *Medicine (Baltimore)* 1987;66:472–483.
The authors compare the clinical characteristics of 96 patients with amebic abscess to those of 48 patients with pyogenic abscess. Features that included Latin American birthplace, younger age, abdominal pain with RUQ tenderness, symptoms for fewer than 14 days, and selected hepatic enzyme determinations helped predict amebic abscess. Ultrasonographic features of round or oval shape and "hypoechoic appearance with fine, homogeneous low-level echoes at high gain" were also statistically more common with amebic abscess.
Blessmann J, et al. Treatment of amoebic liver abscess with metronidazole alone or in combination with ultrasound-guided needle aspiration: a comparative, prospective and randomized study. *Trop Med Internat Health* 2003;8:1030–1034.
The authors studied 39 matched patients with hepatic amoebic abscess, diagnosis corroborated by serum antibody studies. Abscess size was 6 to 10 cm, and patients were untreated before the study. More complete resolution of liver tenderness by day 3 in the group with drainage was the only difference between the two groups, and does not justify this procedure. The authors conclude that metronidazole alone is adequate therapy for most persons with amebic abscess less than 10 cm.
Cady B. Natural history of primary and secondary tumors of the liver. *Semin Oncol* 1983;10:127–134.
This review provides an excellent overview of the likely causes of hepatic neoplasia and their clinical presentation.

Chemaly RF, et al. Microbiology of liver abscesses and the predictive value of abscess Gram's stain and associated blood cultures. *Diagn Microbiol Infect Dis* 2003;46:245–248.

The authors reviewed 40 episodes of hepatic abscess with culture confirmation to assess value of Gram's stain from aspirated contents and blood cultures drawn within the week prior to drainage. Fifty percent of patients had (+) blood cultures, and almost 80% had a (+) Gram's stain. The latter was more sensitive/specific for Gram (+) organisms, whereas blood cultures missed some organisms in polymicrobial infections subsequently confirmed by abscess culture. Despite these limitations, the authors conclude that both modalities are valuable in the microbiologic assessment of pyogenic hepatic abscess.

Haque R, et al. Amebiasis. *N Engl J Med* 2003;348:1565–1573.

An excellent contemporary overview of amebiasis, not specifically liver abscess. Dosing recommendations for all agents useful in amebic abscess are provided, including pediatric dosing.

Klotz SA, Penn RL. Clinical differentiation of abscess from neoplasm in newly diagnosed space-occupying lesions of the liver. *South Med J* 1987;80:1537–1541.

The authors recognized the difficulty in differentiating malignant from pyogenic intrahepatic lesions by imaging techniques alone and looked critically at clinical presentations. Those with pyogenic abscesses had shorter prodromes, risk factors for abscess, fever, leukocytosis, and normal hepatic size. Presence of at least three of these correctly predicted all abscesses.

Rajak CL, et al. Percutaneous treatment of liver abscesses: needle aspiration versus catheter drainage. *Am J Roentgenol* 1998;170:1035–1039.

The authors conducted a prospective randomized trial of percutaneous versus catheter drainage in 50 patients with liver abscess. Twenty patients had amebic abscess and 19 were of "indeterminate" origin (secondary to prior treatment). Thirty had signs of impending rupture. If limited to two aspirations, measured outcomes of duration of hospitalization and clinical improvement were better with catheter drainage (mean duration of drainage was 7 days). However, the authors did not discriminate between those with hepatic versus amebic abscess.

Ravdin JI. Amebiasis. *Clin Infect Dis* 1995;20:1453–1466.

The author provides an excellent overview of recent developments in amebiasis. Biology, epidemiology, diagnosis, management, and prevention are explored. Much practical information, obviously provided by a "hands on" clinician is given in this article.

Schaefer JW, Khan Y. Echinococcosis (hydatid disease): lessons from experience with 59 patients. *Rev Infect Dis* 1991;13:243–247.

This paper reports the experience from Saudi Arabia with almost 60 patients with hydatid disease. Currently, diagnosis can be made by US or CT presentation. Serologic diagnosis is specific but insensitive. Surgery is the management strategy of choice and should be reserved for symptomatic cases. Outcomes were uniformly satisfactory when performed electively, but morbidity and mortality were encountered when rupture had occurred.

Seeto RK, Rockey DC. Pyogenic liver abscess. Changes in etiology, management, and outcome. *Medicine* 1996;75:99–113.

The authors provide an excellent review of the subject, summarizing information about epidemiology, bacteriology, and management. The central role of CT and US in both the diagnosis and management of pyogenic hepatic abscess is stressed. The authors feel that drainage rather than aspiration of abscess is the therapy of choice. This therapeutic regimen has cure rates of up to 75%—and up to 90% within the past 5 years.

Tanyuksel M, Petri WA Jr. Laboratory diagnosis of amebiasis. *Clin Microbiol Rev* 2003;16:713–729.

The authors present an excellent overview of amebiasis and the roles for various microbiologic and serologic testing modalities. They point out limitations of antibody testing in persons from endemic regions and discuss the value of the antigen-detection methodologies currently available.

Yu SCH, et al. Treatment of pyogenic liver abscess: prospective randomized comparison of catheter drainage and needle aspiration. *Hepatology* 2004;39:932–938.

The authors prospectively compared outcomes for two groups of matched patients with pyogenic hepatic abscess. One group received percutaneous drainage while the second had catheter drainage. Abscess size was generally smaller than 7 cm. All received the same antibiotics. For those who received percutaneous drainage, almost 60% required more than one procedure, and almost 20 received more than three aspirations. Catheters were left in place for a median of 13 days. Although no statistically significant differences were noted, those treated with repeated aspiration had slightly shorter durations of hospitalization (11 days vs. 15 days), and lower mortality rates (1 patient vs. 4 patients). The authors conclude that percutaneous drainage is a preferred alternative to catheter drainage in patients with pyogenic hepatic abscess.

COMMUNITY-ACQUIRED PERITONITIS   14

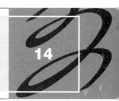

eritonitis represents an inflammatory condition of the abdominal cavity. Three major types are spontaneous (primary) bacterial peritonitis (PBP), peritonitis complicating visceral perforation, ("secondary" bacterial peritonitis), and that complicating continuous ambulatory peritoneal dialysis (CAPD). An additional type, "tertiary peritonitis," is a complication of surgery for visceral perforation. However, as the latter is generally hospital acquired, it will not be further discussed. Organisms encountered and management strategies differ. Rarely, peritonitis may be associated with recurrence of granulomatous disease, such as tuberculosis or fungal infections. Additionally, clinical peritonitis unassociated with infection may occur as a result of peritoneal studding from malignancy, chemical irritants, and others.

ANATOMY AND PHYSIOLOGY OF THE PERITONEAL SPACE

The peritoneum is a closed space with many invaginations and outpockets. In the female, the fallopian tubes breech this closure. Upper and lower peritoneal areas are connected by left and right gutters; these are potential conduits for infected material. The most dependent of these areas is the pelvis. Other candidates for accumulation of drainage are the left and right subdiaphragmatic spaces. The lesser sac, one of the largest of the potential spaces, is bounded by the pancreas and stomach and has an opening called the *foramen of Winslow*. Because of its unique location, it may be spared from general peritoneal infection. Alternatively it may become infected as an isolated area.

The peritoneal cavity is lined by a single-layered serous membrane that allows rapid bidirectional transfer of materials. Physical forces, including oncotic and hydrostatic pressure, determine flow rate and direction. Most commonly employed antibiotics penetrate the inflamed peritoneum and can rapidly achieve therapeutic concentrations. Lymphatics remove proteins and particulate matter. Those of the peritoneum freely associate with those above the diaphragm and allow the rapid dispersal of particulate matter into the pleura. The diaphragmatic surface is covered with specialized lymphatics bearing stoma of 8 to 12 μm. Bacteria and proteins can be removed through pores of this size.

Removal of potential pathogens occurs primarily by lymphatics. Organisms are taken up through peritoneal lining cells, absorbed by lymphatics, and ultimately enter the bloodstream through the thoracic duct. Containment of infection is aided by production of fibrin secondary to inflammation. Normal anatomic barriers such as omentum, abdominal organs, and the diaphragm may allow actively infected areas to remain sequestered from the remainder of the peritoneal cavity. Finally, host defenses that include peritoneal macrophages, polymorphonuclear leukocytes (PMNs), complement, and immunoglobulins can be activated to opsonize, phagocytize, and kill microorganisms.

 ## PRIMARY BACTERIAL PERITONTIS

PBP is not associated with an identifiable intra-abdominal source. At-risk adults generally have underlying cirrhosis with ascites. PBP is one of the major considerations in patients with liver disease who clinically deteriorate. In-hospital mortality reaches 50%; 1-year death rate is up to 60%. Relapse rates up to 43% at 6 months and 69% at 1 year have been described. Symptoms include worsening hepatic failure, abdominal discomfort, and fever. Risks for PBP include severity of underlying liver disease (e.g., Pugh class C), presence of gastrointestinal bleeding, history of prior PBP, and iatrogenic manipulations such as Foley catheterization or intravenous lines.

Primary bacterial peritonitis is generally caused by a single pathogen; identification of multiple organisms should prompt a search for perforated viscus. *Escherichia coli* or *Klebsiella* sp. (40–60%) and streptococci/enterococci (30%) are most often detected. Anaerobes are rarely identified and, if noted, should prompt a search for perforation. Within the past 5 years, emerging resistance of *Streptococcus pneumoniae* to β-lactam antibiotics has been noted, but has not been associated with increased mortality in patients with PBP. A variant of spontaneous peritonitis, culture-negative neutrocytic ascites, exists when there is ascitic fluid leukocytosis (>250/mm^3), no prior antibiotics, and negative cultures. Presentation and natural history are the same as with PBP. Proposed reason for culture negativity is immune response of ascitic fluid.

Patients suspected of PBP should have blood cultures and diagnostic paracentesis. This can be performed in the presence of coagulopathy, as risks are minimal. Blood cultures are positive in about one-third of patients. Within ascitic fluid, cell count and differential demonstrate primarily PMNs and more than 250 to 500 cells/mm^3. Other parameters that help define PBP include ascitic fluid/serum lactic dehydrogenase ratio greater than 0.4 and ascitic fluid/serum glucose ratio less than 1.0, Gram's stain typically demonstrates a single morphology, but is irregularly positive. Fluid obtained by paracentesis should be injected into blood culture bottles in an amount according to manufacturer's specifications.

Therapy consists of appropriate antimicrobials and support. The choice of agent can be based on Gram's stain if positive, plus knowledge of local resistance patterns. Gram-positive cocci in chains represent streptococci. Ceftriaxone or cefotaxime as monotherapy for initial treatment is generally appropriate. Gram-negative bacilli demonstrated on Gram's stain can be managed similarly with monotherapy. The choice depends primarily on knowledge of local susceptibility patterns, cost, ease of administration, and host factors. Recommendations for empiric therapy, if treatment cannot be guided by Gram's stain, are generally a third-generation cephalosporin or a β-lactam/β-lactamase combination, or ertapenem. Aztreonam has been well studied for PBP, and although it works well for illness caused by gram-negative bacilli, gram-positive superinfection has been noted, and resistance of Enterobacteriaceae is emerging regionally. For susceptible enteric gram-negative bacilli in patients considered for oral therapy, oral fluoroquinolones or trimethoprim-sulfamethoxazole (TMP-SMX) could be considered. Oral ofloxacin has been well studied, with results that compare favorably with parenterally administered third-generation cephalosporins in patients without septic shock and capable of being managed on oral medications.

For persons with a good initial response to therapy and a single "typical" pathogen isolated, follow-up paracentesis is not necessary. However it should be performed after 48 hours of treatment if there are any considerations of secondary peritonitis, or if response is not satisfactory. Duration of therapy is generally 5 days.

Peritonitis caused by *Mycobacterium tuberculosis* or fungi needs to be considered in patients with negative bacterial cultures, and failure to respond to standard therapies. Most have evidence of exudative ascites. Tuberculous peritonitis comprises more than 50% of cases of abdominal tuberculosis, is most common in women (71%), and can mimic an acute abdomen, spontaneous bacterial peritonitis (SBP), or tumor. Many cases have no evidence of disease elsewhere (46%), and skin tests may be negative (17%). Most cases are associated with exudative ascites and more than 500 lymphocytes/mm^3. Diagnosis is best made by peritoneal biopsy for smear, culture, and histopathology. Failure to initially identify patients with this condition leads to enhanced mortality. Diagnosis and treatment must be made before final culture reports. Fungal peritonitis is most commonly associated with either *Candida* species or *Cryptococcus neoformans*. The former should be considered in patients with previous intra-abdominal surgery and recent broad-spectrum antimicrobials. The latter usually represents a component of disseminated cryptococcosis and generally is diagnosed by aspiration of ascitic fluid.

Antibiotic prophylaxis should be given to all patients who survive an initial bout or who are at high risk for SBP (e.g., variceal bleeding, low ascitic protein concentrations, or prolonged prothrombin times). Oral fluoroquinolones and TMP/SMX have been used, but either may predispose to emergence of resistance, and long-term mortality benefits are uncertain. Diuresis to decrease ascitic fluid volume (and therefore raise ascitic fluid protein) is also indicated.

 # SECONDARY BACTERIAL PERITONITIS

Secondary bacterial peritonitis generally results from spillage of the contents of a hollow viscus. Common causes are penetrating trauma, malignancy, diverticular and appendiceal infections, cholecystitis, and pyloric ulcer disease. Consequences depend in part on the bacteriologic composition of the spilled material. Clinical presentation often involves well-defined symptom complexes. Older patients and those on high doses of corticosteroids may have subtle symptoms. As a result, symptoms may last longer before diagnosis, and patients may therefore be sicker upon presentation.

Normal Gastrointestinal Flora

Organisms colonizing the gastrointestinal tract vary qualitatively and quantitatively among different sites (Table 14-1). Such differences have important clinical implications. Polymicrobial contamination with three to five species often follows large-bowel spillage. Anaerobes including *Bacteroides fragilis* predominate. Summarized results from animal and human trials indicate that (1) early mortality from peritonitis approaches 40% and is caused primarily by gram-negative sepsis from *E. coli*; (2) most survivors develop intra-abdominal abscesses with a complex flora that include *B. fragilis, E. coli,* enterococci, and other anaerobes; (3) the capsule of *B. fragilis* is independently abscessogenic; and (4) a pecking order of antimicrobial agents exists that vary considerably in their ability to improve survival and decrease abscess formation. Conclusions from these studies demonstrate the need for antimicrobials that target both enteric gram-negative and anaerobic (including *B. fragilis*) organisms. However, there is no advantage to multiple agents, compared with monotherapy.

 TABLE 14-1   **Comparative Bacteriology of the Intact Gastrointestinal Tract**

Anatomic area	Enteric gram (−) bacilli	*Bacteroides* sp.	Streptococci	Other anaerobes
Empty stomach	0.0*	0.0	0.0	0.0
Full stomach	1.5	1.5	0.0	0.0
Gallbladder	0.0	0.0	0.0	0.0
Jejunum	1.0	1.0	2.4–4.2	1.0
Distal ileum	3.3–5.6	5.2–5.7	2.5–4.9	2.5–5.7
Colon	6.0–7.6	8.5–10.0	4.0–7.0	5.0–10.5

*log$_{10}$ bacteria/mL gastrointestinal contents.

In community-acquired peritonitis, the roles of enterococci and *Candida* sp. are controversial. The former is identified in up to 20% of infections, and some recent data identify documentation of enterococcal species as a risk factor for adverse outcome when not targeted in therapy. However, there are no data demonstrating enhanced outcomes when it is treated, especially in persons who are otherwise relatively healthy. In general, neither organism needs to be empirically covered unless believed to be a predominant pathogen on Gram's stain, associated with positive blood cultures, or noted in pure culture. Vancomycin-resistant enterococci (VRE) are unlikely to be identified in community-acquired disease. However, both become important considerations following antimicrobial therapy or reoperation for complications.

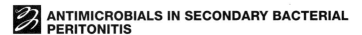

ANTIMICROBIALS IN SECONDARY BACTERIAL PERITONITIS

Antibiotics used in secondary bacterial peritonitis should take into account likely pathogens; this is based in part on initial site of infection. As an example, perforation of the previously healthy stomach is likely to result in either sterile peritonitis or infection associated with low numbers of oropharyngeal flora. Alternatively, peritoneal contamination from the colon will be associated with a complex flora involving enteric bacilli and anaerobes. Numerous antibiotics (when coupled with drainage) administered as monotherapy or combinations are effective and appropriate for the management of secondary bacterial peritonitis. The author prefers monotherapy when possible, as it is generally easier to manage and may be less expensive. Table 14-2 summarizes some initial treatment regimens. Choice among them requires knowledge of local resistance problems, host factors (allergy, end organ function), cost, and availability on hospital formularies.

Optimal length of therapy for secondary bacterial peritonitis is unknown. Traumatic injuries repaired within 12 hours require antibiotics for fewer than 24 hours. For persons with established peritonitis, 5 to 7 days of IV therapy is recommended. Patients who remain febrile or who otherwise fail to respond during this time frame should be studied for complications. Use of oral agents for part of the course is indicated for patients with good initial response and functional gastrointestinal tracts.

Removal of necrotic tissue, drainage of abscesses, and closure of perforations are major goals of surgery. Percutaneous catheter drainage of abscesses should be used when feasible,

TABLE 14-2 Selected Antimicrobials Useful in Secondary Community-Acquired Bacterial Peritonitis

Antibiotic(s): single agents	Dosage (IV)[†]
Cefotetan	2 g q 12 hr
Imipenem/cilastatin	500 mg q 6 hr
Piperacillin/tazobactam	3.375 g q 6 hr
Ertapenem	1 g q 24 hr
Antibiotics: combinations	
Ceftriaxone + metronidazole	1–2 g q 24 hr + 500 mg q 8 hr
Gentamicin + metronidazole	5 mg/kg q 24 hr + 500 mg q 8 hr
Gentamicin + clindamycin	5 mg/kg q 24 hr + 900 mg IV q 8 hr
Ciprofloxacin (or levofloxacin)	400 mg q 12 hr (or 750 mg q 24 hr)
plus metronidazole	plus 500 mg q 8 hr

(Adapted from Solomkin JS, et al. Guidelines for the selection of anti-infective agents for complicated intra-abdominal infections. *Clin Infect Dis* 2003;37:997–1005.)
[†] Duration of therapy variable, generally 5 to 7 days; use of oral or stepdown to oral dependent on functional gastrointestinal system.

but this technique has little value in acute secondary peritonitis where a source control site must be accomplished. For isolated abscesses, percutaneous drainage is associated with success rates higher than 85%. It can also be used for poor surgical candidates.

PERITONEAL DIALYSIS

Peritoneal dialysis (PD) remains an important management strategy for end-stage renal disease, and catheter-related infections continue to be a complication. Peritoneal dialysis may be performed either by CAPD or automated (APD) modalities; the latter has seen increasing favor. Peritonitis incidence appears to be decreasing and is now recognized in approximately 1 in 24 patient treatment months. Relationship between peritonitis and mortality is most noted in Caucasian, nondiabetic, older patients. Peritonitis contributes to mortality in about 15% of patients and is most notable with gram-negative bacilli and fungi. Selected patients on long-term CAPD do not develop peritonitis, presuming a role for host defenses or meticulous care. Most common pathogenetic mechanisms are bacterial migration along the dialysis catheter or breaks in sterile technique during dialysis exchanges. Dialysis fluid inside the peritoneal cavity can support the growth of many pathogens including most enteric bacilli, *Staphylococcus aureus,* and *Pseudomonas aeruginosa.* Patients identified as nasal carriers of *S. aureus* are at higher risk than noncarriers for the development of *S. aureus* peritonitis.

In the context of PD, peritonitis is defined as the presence of turbid dialysate for which etiologies other than infection cannot be identified. It most often is associated with more than 100 white blood cells (WBC)/mm^3, primarily polymorphonucleocytes. Risk factors include advanced age, use of CAPD, and initiation of CAPD earlier in its history. Reasons why up to 50% of patients never develop peritonitis whereas others have recurrent episodes are uncertain; however, chronic nasal carriage of *S. aureus* has been identified as a risk factor in some patients with recurrent infections associated with this organism.

The most common clinical presentation is cloudy peritoneal dialysate. Fever is noted in only 33% of patients, whereas abdominal pain and tenderness are seen in the majority. Up to one-third of patients will be sick enough to require hospitalization, but in general, therapy is rendered in an outpatient setting. It is uncommon for infections to disseminate beyond the peritoneal cavity.

The bacteriology of peritonitis complicating PD is monomicrobial; the presence of polymicrobial infection should prompt an assessment for perforated viscus. *S. aureus* and *Staphylococcus epidermidis* are responsible for approximately 50% of infections. *P. aeruginosa* is associated with 5 to 10% of cases but causes significant mortality and morbidity. Miscellaneous organisms including fungi (mostly *Candida* species) and mycobacteria (not *M. tuberculosis*) and sterile specimens are noted in 10 to 20% of cases. Fungal peritonitis causes 3 to 4% of all cases of peritonitis, is mostly caused by *Candida* sp., and is associated with prior use of antibiotics. Etiology can usually be suspected from Gram-stained specimens of fluid. This information should be used for antibiotic decision making. Culture for aerobic and anaerobic organisms should always be obtained, and special cultures for acid-fast bacilli and fungi should be sought if standard Gram's stain fails to demonstrate bacteria.

The linchpin of management is the administration of appropriate antimicrobials. Most cases are unlikely to be complicated by bacteremia and can be managed by intraperitoneal antimicrobials and preservation of the dialysis catheter. Therapy should be immediately initiated as rapidly as feasible, but always within 3 hours. The "best" agent(s) is based on likely organisms and their resistance patterns. Pending culture confirmation, intraperitoneal cefazolin plus ceftazidime has been recommended. However, methicillin-resistant *S. aureus* (MRSA) and vancomycin-resistant enterococci (VRE) have complicated PD and will not respond to β-lactam antibiotics. They are most likely to be noted in the setting of heavy antibiotic administration and prior infections. *P. aeruginosa* infections are generally managed with two effective agents. Table 14-3 summarizes treatment recommendations for selected antibiotics and is based in part on residual renal function. Vancomycin, linezolid, quinupristin/dalfopristin, or daptomycin may be used for resistant gram (+) organisms; however, limited data in PD exist for many of these. Best data suggest that linezolid can

TABLE 14-3   Antibiotics for Use in Peritonitis Complicating CAPD

Antibiotic	Route	Dose
Cefazolin	Intraperitoneal*	15 mg/kg
Ceftazidime	Intraperitoneal	1 g
Cefotaxime	Intraperitoneal	2 g
Aztreonam	Intraperitoneal	1 g
Ciprofloxacin	Oral or iv	500 mg bid
Gentamicin/tobramycin	Intraperitoneal	0.6 mg/kg
Imipenem/cilastatin	Intravenous	1 g q 12 hr
Vancomycin	Intraperitoneal	15–30 mg/kg q 5–7 days
Metronidazole	Oral or IV	500 mg tid
Fluconazole	Oral or IV	200 mg q 24 hr

*Intraperitoneal: add dose to one of the daily bags. Dosage may need to be modified based on residual urine output and whether CAPD is intermittent or continuous.

continue to be dosed at 600 mg q 12 hours, but it is suggested that a dose be given after dialysis, when possible.

Catheter removal is not generally needed. It should be performed, however, if tunnel infection or failure to respond within 48 to 72 hours is noted, or if there is evidence of perforated viscus. Parenteral antimicrobials are initially indicated if bacteremia or sepsis is suspected. The duration of treatment may be as short as 7 to 10 days (gram-positive infection) to 2 to 3 weeks (gram-negative or fungal infection). Azoles such as fluconazole are replacing amphotericin in the management of fungal infections caused by susceptible organisms.

Prevention of peritonitis in CAPD is difficult and best associated with patient education and strict adherence to technique and infection control procedures. Antibiotic prophylaxis does not work well and is generally not recommended. However, use of nasal mupiricin appears to decrease the risk of *S. aureus* infection in patients undergoing peritoneal dialysis. A recent meta-analysis demonstrated an overall reduction of *S. aureus* of infections of 63% when this product was used, with reductions seen in both peritonitis and catheter exit site infections. *S. aureus* peritonitis may also be preventable with use of daily mupiricin at the catheter exit site or by use of rifampin, 600 mg 5 days of every 3 months. Antibiotic prophylaxis, generally with cefazolin, has been shown to decrease the risk of infection after catheter replacement. (RBB)

Bibliography

Capdevila O, et al. Pneumococcal peritonitis in adult patients. *Arch Intern Med* 2001; 161:1742–1748.
> *The authors present retrospective data on 45 cases of pneumococcal peritonitis demonstrated over approximately 20 years. Compared with other pathogens, patients with* S. pneumoniae *peritonitis had more bacteremia and higher mortality. Hematogenous dissemination from the lower respiratory tract was a primary source of peritonitis. Despite increasing β-lactam resistance, there was no appreciated impact on mortality.*

Inadomi J, Sonnenberg A. Cost-analysis of prophylactic antibiotics in spontaneous bacterial peritonitis. *Gastroenterology* 1997;113:1289–1294.
> *The authors conclude that prophylactic antibiotics are a cost-effective strategy for patients with cirrhosis and ascites. Issues addressed include development of PBP, subsequent mortality, and the cost of the drugs. Agents primarily assessed with norfloxacin and TMP/SMX. Prophylaxis is cost effective when compared with placebo.*

Keane WF, et al. Adult peritoneal dialysis-related peritonitis treatment recommendations: 2000 update. *Perit Dial Int* 2000;20:396–411.
> *The authors provide an update on issues regarding peritoneal dialysis-related peritonitis, including antibiotic recommendations for therapy and prevention, and dosing regimens.*

Numerous tables are provided, and concerns about resistant organisms are addressed. Of particular interest is a change in philosophy about catheter removal. Catheters may be left in place regardless of organism so long as the patient is responding rapidly to therapy. The authors also address reasons for surgery and the evolving role of azoles for the treatment of fungal peritonitis.

Solomkin JS, et al. Guidelines for the selection of anti-infective agents for complicated intra-abdominal infections. *Clin Infect Dis* 2003;37:997–1005.

These guidelines result from collaboration among the Infectious Disease Society of America, American Society of Microbiology, the Surgical Infection Society, and others. Issues related to timing of antibiotics, choice, and duration of therapy are addressed in depth. Recommendations regarding culture techniques and need for Gram staining are given. The latter is not recommended for community-acquired secondary peritonitis. The authors do not recommend routine therapy for Candida or enterococci (even if identified) unless specific immunosuppression or recurrent infection is documented. I disagree with this, although cases need to be individualized.

Such J, Runyon BA. Spontaneous bacterial peritonitis. *Clin Infect Dis* 1998;27:669–676.

The authors present a robust review of etiology, pathophysiology, diagnosis/treatment, and prevention. An excellent single review of the topic.

Tacconelli E, et al. Mupirocin prophylaxis to prevent Staphylococcus aureus infection in patients undergoing dialysis: a meta-analysis. *Clin Infect Dis* 2003;37:1629–1638.

The authors performed a meta-analysis to determine the role of mupiricin in decreasing likelihood of S. aureus *infections complicating dialysis. Both hemodialysis and peritoneal dialysis were investigated. Risk reduction was seen in both groups, but the authors comment that optimal regimens least likely to result in emergence of mupiricin resistance need to be established.*

INFECTIONS OF THE HEPATOBILIARY TRACT

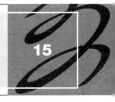

15

*I*nfections of the hepatobiliary tract are common and mostly related to gallstone disease. At autopsy, approximately 20% of women and 8% of men age 40 and older have gallstones. Both prevalence of gallstones and morbidity and mortality associated with biliary infections increase with age. Despite improvements in biliary tract imaging and interventions with endoscopic and radiographically guided therapy, adverse outcomes from hepatobiliary infections continue. One reason for this is that biliary disease and infection frequently present without "classic" signs or symptoms related to the biliary fossa. In the elderly, critically ill, diabetic, or immunocompromised patient, fever may be the sole presentation. Overwhelming sepsis and death lie at the other end of the spectrum. HIV-infected patients can be difficult to diagnose as well, because of their blunted inflammatory response and because causative pathogens may be atypical. A high index of suspicion must be maintained in all febrile patients, especially in those without an obvious alternative cause.

 ## BACTERIOLOGY OF THE BILIARY TRACT

The normal biliary tract is sterile. Several factors believed to maintain sterility include (1) the sphincter of Oddi and antegrade bile flow, which prevent bacteria from moving from the duodenum into the biliary tree; (2) biliary IgA; and (3) bile salts, which are believed to be

| TABLE 15-1 | Bacteriology of Pyogenic Hepatobiliary Infections |

Category	Organism
Gram-negative aerobes	Most common: *E. coli, Klebsiella* spp.
	Other: *P. aeruginosa, Proteus* spp.,
	Enterobacter spp., *Citrobacter* spp.,
	Morganella spp., *Serratia marcescens*
Gram-positive aerobes	Most common: *Enterococcus* spp.
	Other: *S. aureus*, viridans streptococci
Anaerobes	Most common: *Bacteroides* spp.
	Other: *Fusobacterium* spp., anaerobic
	streptococci, *Clostridium* spp.
Microaerophilic	*Streptococcus milleri*

(Adapted from Johannsen E, Sifri C, Madoff L. Pyogenic liver abscesses. *Infect Dis Clin North Am* 2000;14:547–563.)

necessary in preventing colonization of the upper small bowel with pathogenic bacteria. The other major source of bacteria that seed the biliary tract is the portal venous system. In animal models, bile can become infected when bacteria are introduced into the portal venous system after the common duct has been ligated. Whatever the route, bile stasis promotes bacterial growth, and increased biliary pressure facilitates release of bacteria, endotoxin, and inflammatory cytokines into the circulation.

Because the gut is the most likely source of bacteria, it follows that the most common pathogens are aerobic gram-negative enteric bacilli, with *Escherichia coli*, and *Klebsiella* sp. most frequently isolated. Table 15-1 depicts bacteriology of pyogenic hepatobiliary infections. Of the gram-positive cocci, *Enterococcus* sp. is most frequently isolated. Anaerobes may be found in up to 50% of biliary infections, usually as a component of mixed infection. *Bacteroides* spp. are the most common isolates, followed by *Clostridium* sp. Approximately 1% of patients undergoing cholecystectomy demonstrate *Candida*. These cases generally involve patients who are immunocompromised or in intensive care units. Prolonged antibiotic use and total parenteral nutrition are additional risk factors. Choledocholithiasis is much more likely to result in infected bile than cystic duct obstruction, with rates approaching 100% in patients with ascending cholangitis. Most cultures of bile in cholangitis reveal polymicrobial infection. Blood cultures are frequently positive in the presence of hepatobiliary infection and bacterial isolates are consistent with bile cultures.

 GENERAL CONSIDERATIONS

Disorders of the hepatobiliary tract generally present in similar fashion. Distention and inflammation of the gallbladder or common bile duct (CBD) result in right upper quadrant (RUQ) pain that may radiate to the back or ipsilateral clavicle or scapula. Nausea and vomiting are frequent, and eating may exacerbate pain, as biliary pressure increases in response to cholecystokinin from the duodenum. When cystic duct or CBD obstruction is absent, the term *biliary colic* is used. In this case, symptoms last for several hours at most, and fever is rare. When either duct is obstructed, fever is the rule and symptoms last more than 4 hours. RUQ tenderness is present in most patients. In those with cystic duct obstruction, Murphy's sign (inspiratory arrest when manual pressure is applied to the RUQ) or a palpable RUQ mass indicating a distended gallbladder may be present. When biliary disease or infection is present in elderly, diabetic, or immunocompromised patients, fever may be absent and RUQ tenderness subtle. Acute cholecystitis in the older patient is usually associated with higher morbidity and mortality. Up to 40% of the elderly have gangrene, perforation, or empyema at the time of surgical intervention. Differential diagnosis includes acute cholecystitis, acute cholangitis, and acute pancreatitis.

Other diagnoses include pyelonephritis, retrocecal appendicitis, perforated duodenal ulcer, right lower lobe pneumonia, pulmonary infarction, acute hepatitis or an acute coronary syndrome.

 ## ACUTE CALCULUS CHOLECYSTITIS

In the United States, most cases of acute cholecystitis are caused by cystic duct obstruction by gallstones with subsequent proliferation of colonizing bacteria. Gallbladder ischemia and inflammation ensue. If obstruction continues and ischemia lasts sufficiently long, tissue necrosis may develop, sometimes resulting in gangrene and perforation. Diagnosis of acute cholecystitis is usually made clinically and should be confirmed radiographically. Plain films of the abdomen reveal a gallstone in approximately 15% of patients.

RUQ ultrasound is the procedure of choice. It is highly sensitive and specific and may be able to predict perforation. If it cannot be obtained, computed tomography (CT) provides similar information. Biliary scintigraphy is also highly accurate in diagnosing acute calculus cholecystitis with sensitivity and specificity greater than 94% in most studies.

Leukocytosis is present in most patients, averaging 12,000/mm^3. Levels higher than 15,000 suggest empyema or perforation. Hepatic enzymes may be normal or only mildly elevated, and bilirubin is increased in 45% of patients. If transaminase levels are greater than three times the upper limit of normal, or the bilirubin is greater than 3 mg/dL, choledocholithiasis and cholangitis must be suspected. Mild elevations in amylase and alkaline phosphatase are not uncommon.

Management of acute cholecystitis consists of supportive care, appropriate antimicrobials, and surgery. Antimicrobial therapy is guided by likely causative organisms. "Penetration" of antimicrobials into the biliary tract has received attention in the literature; however, little clinical data confirm its importance. Additionally, most agents fail to penetrate bile in the presence of total biliary tract obstruction. In all cases of acute cholecystitis, high-dose, broad-spectrum, parenteral antimicrobials are initially indicated, as bacteremia is common and may be polymicrobial. The regimen should cover most enteric gram-negative bacilli. Although the need to treat for enterococci and anaerobes is controversial, the authors recommend that initial therapy should include them. Table 15-2 provides authors' recommendations for antibiotic management. Combination agents such as piperacillin-tazobactam, ertapenem, or imipenem-cilastatin are adequate in most cases. Monotherapy with fluoroquinolones has been found to be effective in some trials, but these agents may not be effective against anaerobes and enterococci, so we do not recommend them as initial therapy. Antibiotics should be adjusted once culture results are known. When *Candida* is present, limited to the gallbladder, and believed to be pathogenic, cholecystectomy without antifungal therapy is curative in nonneutropenic patients.

The timing of surgical intervention remains controversial, but most authorities recommend prompt cholecystectomy (within days of admission) after initial medical stabilization. Delaying surgery in those patients whose symptoms remit results in increased morbidity (but not mortality), as 25% will go on to develop recurrent episodes of acute cholecystitis within 1 year of the initial event. Laparoscopic or open cholecystectomy is the definitive therapy for acute cholecystitis. For patients who are too ill to tolerate major surgery, percutaneous cholecystostomy may prove lifesaving, and results in clinical improvement in up to 90% of cases. Patients who fail to stabilize within 24 hours or who demonstrate clinical deterioration should be operated on promptly.

 ## ACUTE ACALCULOUS CHOLECYSTITIS

In 2 to 15% of cases, cholecystitis is acalculous. Severe burns, residence within intensive care units, the postoperative state, hypotension, total parenteral nutrition, and cardiac arrest have been implicated. There is a predilection for men. Gallbladder ischemia and reperfusion injury is likely the final common pathway that leads to inflammation and disease. Mortality is 30 to 50%, many times higher than that seen in calculus disease, because gangrene

TABLE 15-2   **Selected Therapies for Hepatobiliary Infections**

	Antibiotic	Maximum dose and/or *comments*
Monotherapy	Imipenem/cilastatin	500 mg q 6 hr.
	Piperacillin/tazobactam	4.475 g q 6 hr. *This dose should be used if P. aeruginosa considered*
Multidrug therapies	FQ plus metronidazole	FQ dose depends on agent selected. Metronidazole 500 mg q 6–8 hrs. *Indicated for patients with severe β-lactam allergy. Metronidazole also advantageous in liver abscess if amoebiasis suspected.*
	Ampicillin plus clindamycin plus Ag	Ampicillin 2–3 g q 4–6 hr, clindamycin 900 mg q 8 hr, Ag (generally gentamicin or tobramycin) 5 mg/kg q 24 hr.
Miscellaneous	Linezolid	600 mg q 12 hr. *Should be considered for VRE*

FQ, Fluoroquinolone; Ag, Aminoglycoside; VRE, Vancomycin-resistant enterococci.

(>50%) and perforation (>10%) are more common. Diagnosis of acalculous cholecystitis is difficult, in part because of the severity of the patient's illness. Many individuals cannot be adequately assessed and may be receiving medications that dull response. Fever, leukocytosis, and vague abdominal discomfort may be the sole presentation, and even these may not be present simultaneously. Diagnosis is generally made by RUQ ultrasound, which shows a thickened gallbladder wall (>3.5 mm) and pericholecystic fluid. Abdominal CT scanning provides similar information and may suggest alternative diagnoses but is less available to critically ill patients. Laparoscopy can be lifesaving in selected cases and may obviate the need for formal laparotomy. Alternatively, follow-up ultrasound 24 hours after a nondiagnostic initial test may be used when suspicion remains; progressive thickening of the gallbladder wall is consistent with acalculous cholecystitis. Therapy consists of percutaneous cholecystostomy, which leads to improvement in more than 85% of cases. Cholecystectomy is generally not required in these cases. Cholecystectomy should be performed if this treatment is unsuccessful. Antibiotics are given parenterally and should cover the likely enteric flora of an intensive care unit. The agents listed for acute calculus cholecystitis are also generally effective in acalculous disease.

COMPLICATIONS OF ACUTE CHOLECYSTITIS

Gallbladder perforation occurs in 10 to 15% of cases and should be suspected in patients after delays in diagnosis and in men older than age 70. Three forms of perforation are (1) free perforation into the peritoneal cavity, (2) rupture with local containment, and (3) rupture into an adjacent viscus. The first carries the worst prognosis. Perforation with local containment often occurs several days after clinical cholecystitis is evident and usually presents as antimicrobial treatment failure. A palpable mass may become obvious. Rupture into an adjacent viscus, often the stomach, may be at first associated with dramatic clinical improvement. Management of perforation is surgical.

Emphysematous cholecystitis is an uncommon condition associated with air in either the gallbladder wall or lumen. Clinical presentation mimics "typical" acute cholecystitis, but has a higher occurrence in elderly diabetic males and a higher mortality rate (15% versus 3–8%). *C. perfringens* is frequently implicated (45% versus 10–15%). Early surgical intervention and broad-spectrum antibiotics that cover anaerobes are necessary. Empyema of the gallbladder is documented at the time of operation and usually presents in the severely ill patient with RUQ discomfort. At the time of surgery, a pus-filled organ is demonstrated.

ASCENDING CHOLANGITIS

Ascending cholangitis results from infection within the CBD and is most often caused by an obstructing stone. Other causes of CBD obstruction include CBD stricture from trauma during surgery or endoscopy, sclerosing cholangitis, and pancreatic or choledochal neoplasms. Rarely, *Ascaris lumbricoides, Clonorchis sinensis,* and *Echinococcus* spp. have rarely been identified in the CBD as the cause of obstruction in patients with appropriate travel histories.

Fever (>90%), RUQ pain (>70%), and jaundice (>60%) are generally observed. All three (Charcot's triad) are present in more than 50% of patients. The addition of delirium (10–20%) and hypotension (30%; Reynolds's pentad) occurs in approximately 10% of patients. Charcot's intermittent fever represents recurrent cholangitis, usually caused by a partially obstructing stone or a series of stones passing through the common duct. This occurs in less than 20% of patients with cholangitis.

Ascending cholangitis is the most common cause of polymicrobial bacteremia, and the isolation of multiple enteric pathogens from blood cultures should prompt consideration of the biliary tract as a primary source. Overall, approximately 30% of patients with cholangitis will demonstrate positive blood cultures, and of these 25% will be polymicrobial. The bacteriology of cholangitis is the same as that for cholecystitis.

Diagnosis is confirmed by radiographic studies that include ultrasound, CT, endoscopic retrograde cholangiopancreatography (ERCP), magnetic resonance cholangiopancreatography (MRCP), and percutaneous transhepatic cholangiography (PTC). Ultrasound is generally the first modality used because it is widely available, cheap, and effective in evaluating for cholecystitis, the most common alternative clinical diagnosis. CBD dilatation or a CBD stone in the appropriate clinical setting suggests the diagnosis of cholangitis and provides the rationale for proceeding directly to ERCP for biliary decompression. CT scanning provides information similar to the ultrasound and may be more accurate at determining the level of the obstruction and in suggesting alternative diagnoses. It is limited, however, when the CBD is not dilated because many gallstones are radiolucent. MRCP and CT cholangiography rival ERCP with respect to their ability to delineate biliary abnormalities and, in some institutions, have replaced ERCP as the imaging modality of choice when ultrasound is equivocal. MRCP is frequently used when the results of ERCP are equivocal. PTC is highly accurate in determining the cause and site of biliary obstruction, but concerns about its safety have limited its use.

Treatment of acute cholangitis consists of supportive care, antimicrobial therapy, and biliary decompression to prevent septic shock, hepatic abscesses, secondary biliary cirrhosis, and relapsing cholangitis. Standard definitive therapy consists of endoscopic sphincterotomy, stone retrieval, and biliary stent placement. The success rate with this modality is higher than 90%. When patients are too unstable to undergo endoscopy, or when endoscopy is unsuccessful, percutaneous transhepatic biliary drainage or open surgical techniques can be used. Antibiotic therapy for 3 days after definitive decompression has been found recently to be as effective as longer durations of therapy. The presence of yeast on Gram's stain or heavy growth of *Candida* spp. on culture merits antifungal therapy. Although amphotericin B deoxycholate has historically been used, the authors prefer fluconazole. This agent has been demonstrated to be a suitable alternative to amphotericin B deoxycholate for candidemia and is generally safe and well tolerated.

Biliary Tract Infections in Patients with HIV/AIDS

Recognition of hepatobiliary complications in patients with AIDS dates back to the early 1980s when patients with biliary tract cryptosporidiosis and obstruction were identified. Although individuals with HIV/AIDS may develop typical bacterial diseases as described above, two syndromes specific to this population are AIDS-related cholangiopathy syndrome and acalculous cholecystitis.

Acalculous cholecystitis generally presents with subacute or chronic RUQ pain and fever in the setting of advanced AIDS. Noninvasive imaging depicts gallbladder wall thickening and pericholecystic fluid. Although gall stones may be found in up to 25% of patients, these are not thought to be causative. Laboratory data frequently demonstrate significant elevations of alkaline phosphatase and an absence of leukocytosis unless secondary bacterial infection has occurred. Transaminases and bilirubin are often normal. The organisms implicated most commonly are *Cryptosporidium* or cytomegalovirus (CMV). Other identified opportunists include *Microsporidia* and *Isospora*. Cholecystectomy, either laparoscopic or open, is indicated. This procedure is very effective in reducing pain, unless there is concomitant involvement of the common bile duct. Cholecystectomy is safe in this population.

AIDS-related cholangiopathy is seen in patients with advanced AIDS (typical CD4 count $<100/mm^3$), who may present with symptoms that are identical to those of acalculous cholecystitis, but cholangiopathy is more likely to present with severe pain, nausea, and high fevers. In spite of this, fevers, nausea and vomiting are seen in only about 50% of cases. Jaundice is distinctly unusual, with only 15% of patients having a bilirubin higher than 2 mg/dL. Alkaline phosphatase can be significantly elevated, whereas transaminases remain normal or marginally increased. Diagnosis should be suspected in patients with advanced AIDS and RUQ pain. The microbiology of AIDS-related cholangiopathy is the same as that for acalculous cholecystitis in this population, with *Cryptosporidium* and CMV found in up to 62% and 42% of cases, respectively. It is believed that these organisms cause an intense inflammatory response in the wall of the common bile duct, resulting in narrowing of the lumen, which precipitates the clinical syndrome.

Ultrasound is the initial imaging modality of choice and effectively visualizes CBD dilatation and strictures. If seen, ERCP may be performed because it provides the best visualization of the common duct bile for microscopy and culture, biopsy of the ducts and of any masses that are seen, and for sphincterotomy as needed. A confident diagnosis of this disorder can be made when typical cholangiographic findings are found in a patient with RUQ pain and advanced AIDS and whose bile or stool contains typical pathogens. Treatment with sphincterotomy, with or without stenting of the common bile duct, provides symptomatic relief in most patients. Pathogen-directed antimicrobial therapy is unrewarding. Unless there is bacterial superinfection, patients rarely die because of AIDS-related cholangiopathy. Median survival of patients at diagnosis is 7 to 9 months, owing to their advanced HIV infection. Highly active antiretroviral therapy is associated with reduced mortality in these patients.

PYOGENIC HEPATIC ABSCESS

Pyogenic hepatic abscess is uncommon, with 8 to 22 cases reported per 100,000 hospital admissions. In the pre-antibiotic era, the most common cause was seeding of the liver through the portal vein from complicated appendicitis or diverticulitis. Most cases now occur from common bile duct obstruction and cholangitis. The liver can also be seeded through (1) the hepatic artery during septicemia, (2) blunt trauma, and (3) contiguous spread from adjacent infected foci. However, some cases remain cryptogenic. As opposed to amebic liver abscesses, which occur most frequently in younger patients (often male) from underdeveloped countries, those that are pyogenic generally appear in the fifth and sixth decades without a predilection for either sex. The right lobe of the liver is most often affected and there is a single lesion in about 50% of cases.

Clinical presentation is variable. When associated with generalized sepsis, hectic chills and fever may occur in conjunction with RUQ tenderness and jaundice. This very helpful constellation of signs only occurs in 10% of patients and points to common bile duct obstruction as a cause. Localizing findings are as likely to be present as not, and constitutional symptoms such as malaise, fatigue, anorexia, and weight loss frequently predominate. More commonly, hepatic abscess presents as vague RUQ discomfort in the absence of major constitutional complaints. Patients may present within a few days of symptom onset, but equally common is symptomatology lasting longer than 1 month.

Routine hematologic and microbiologic studies are not generally useful, except if blood cultures are positive. The most common clue is elevation of serum alkaline phosphatase out of proportion to other liver function tests, which in the proper clinical context suggests infiltrative disease of the liver. Abnormalities of other liver function tests are common, but elevations are not notable unless there is concomitant acute or serious biliary disease.

The cornerstone of the diagnostic workup is radiographic imaging with ultrasound or CT. These procedures are positive in more than 90% of cases but may miss lesions smaller than 1 cm in diameter. CT scanning is more sensitive than ultrasound and is generally preferred for guiding drainage procedures when the use of intravenous contrast is not an issue and the biliary tract is not being evaluated. Differential diagnosis of a space-occupying lesion in the liver includes tumors, amebic abscess, and cysts in immunocompetent patients. In patients with AIDS, space-occupying lesions may be associated with Kaposi's sarcoma, lymphoma, CMV, and opportunistic fungi or mycobacteria. Up to 80% of patients will have an abnormal chest radiograph showing atelectasis, elevation of the right hemidiaphragm, or an effusion. When pleuropulmonary manifestations predominate, strong consideration must be given to amebic liver abscess. In this case, an enzyme immunoassay for IgG is the most sensitive and specific test for invasive disease, and results are obtained within several days. Regarding pyogenic diseases, blood cultures are positive in about 50% of cases and abscess cultures in 80 to 90%. Recent reports suggest that approximately 40% of abscess aspirates are monomicrobial, 40% are polymicrobial, and 20% are sterile. Anaerobes are involved in 20 to 30% of cases. Bacteriology most commonly includes aerobic enteric gram-negative bacilli, especially *E. coli* and *Klebsiella* spp., enterococci, viridans streptococci, *Staphylococcus aureus*, and anaerobes, most notably *Bacteroides* spp. Septic metastatic complications, often involving the eye or lung, are frequently associated with *K. pneumoniae* and underlying diabetes. Liver abscesses complicating bacteremia are often due to *Streptococcus pyogenes* or *S. aureus*. In recent years, as the use of myeloablative chemotherapy and bone marrow transplantation has increased in frequency, *Candida* spp. have become more common and may account for up to 20% of cases in institutions where this procedure is performed.

Therapy consists of appropriate antimicrobials and drainage. Empiric antibiotic choice should include coverage for common enteric bacilli and anaerobes, including *B. fragilis*. If the source of the bacteria that seeded the liver is known, antimicrobial choice should be modified to cover the bacterial flora of that site. A potential advantage of clindamycin in a regimen is its ability to achieve therapeutic levels within hepatic tissue, but no controlled studies have been done that compared various antimicrobial agents or regimens. Metronidazole is an attractive option for anaerobic coverage when amebic disease is suspected. Currently the standard of care is to also treat patients with CT-guided percutaneous drainage of all accessible abscesses, with the drainage catheters left in place until output is minimal. Drainage plus antimicrobials results in a 70 to 90% success rate. Intravenous antimicrobial therapy should be continued for at least 4 weeks with adequate drainage and at least 8 weeks if drainage is not performed or is incomplete. Oral therapy has not been well studied, but many consider starting oral antibiotics after 3 to 4 weeks of intravenous treatment. Alternatively, a totally oral regimen may be indicated if antibiotics with 100% oral bioavailability can be used and the patient has a functional GI tract. A follow-up CT scan of the liver at 2 to 4 weeks helps to determine the effectiveness of treatment and the need for extending the course of antimicrobial therapy. Percutaneous aspiration without catheter drainage and conservative management with antimicrobials alone have been less well studied and currently are not considered the standard of care. (RBB)

Bibliography

Calvo MM, et al. Role of magnetic resonance cholangiopancreatography in patients with suspected choledocholithiasis. *Mayo Clin Proc* 2002;77:422–428.
A recent study that supports the use of MRCP as a diagnostic tool in patients at low to moderate risk for choledocholithiasis. The performance of MRCP as a diagnostic tool was similar to that of ERCP. The investigators used a risk stratification model (Cotton criteria), based on clinical, laboratory, and other imaging findings prior to MRCP or ERCP. They suggest MRCP is an effective way of avoiding the risk of diagnostic ERCP in patients at low to moderate risk for choledocholithiasis.
Chandler CF, et al. Prospective evaluation of early versus delayed laparoscopic cholecystectomy for treatment of acute cholecystitis. *Am Surg* 2000;66:896–900.
Only the latest in a series of studies that have confirmed that early in this case, as soon as the operating schedule allowed laparoscopic cholecystectomy (LC is superior to interval LC because early LC reduces the length of hospital stay and hospital charges,

without increasing operative time, conversion to an open procedure, or complication rate.)

Cullen JJ, et al. Effect of endotoxin on opossum gallbladder motility: a model of acalculus cholecystitis. *Ann Surg* 2000;232:202–207.

A fascinating study in which opossum gallbladders were examined histologically after endotoxin was infused into adult animals. Endotoxin resulted in mucosal hemorrhage, coagulation necrosis, fibrin deposition, and mucosal loss, consistent with an ischemic insult and similar to that seen in acute acalculus cholecystitis (AAC). This provides a mechanism for the development of AAC, at least in those who have suffered septic shock.

Johannsen EC, Sifri CD, Madoff LC. Pyogenic liver abscesses. *Infect Dis Clin North Am* 2000;14:547–563.

An excellent systematic review of the topic that includes some interesting information on the use of percutaneous aspiration without catheter drainage and antimicrobial therapy alone in the management of this disease.

Ko WF, et al. Prognostic factors for the survival of patients with AIDS cholangiopathy. *Am J Gastroenterol* 2003;98:2176–2181

In this retrospective study of 94 patients with AIDS cholangiopathy, the median survival from diagnosis of cholangiopathy was 9 months. A history of a prior opportunistic infection and a high serum alkaline phosphatase level were associated with decreased survival. The CD4 count, type of cholangiopathy, and the performance of sphincterotomy were not associated with survival. Highly active antiretroviral therapy (HAART) was associated with prolonged survival.

Menezes N, et al. Prospective analysis of a scoring system to predict choledocholithiasis. *Br J Surg* 2000;87:1176–1181.

Determining which patients with symptoms of acute cholecystitis should be evaluated for CBD stones with MRCP or ERCP is important. This study presents a point-based risk stratification model, based on clinical, biochemical, and radiographic findings, that was 86% sensitive and 82% specific for the finding of CBD stones, as determined by ERCP.

Nash JA, Cohen SA. Gallbladder and biliary tract disease in AIDS. *Gastroenterol Clin North Am* 1997;26:323–335.

The authors review the principles of diagnosis and treatment of biliary tract syndromes unique to AIDS. They stress acalculus cholecystitis and cholangiopathy syndromes and point out that most cases occur in patients with advanced AIDS who have limited lifespans. Drainage procedures are often indicated, but therapy targeted at offending opportunists is generally unrewarding.

Ryu JK, Ryu KH, Kim KH. Clinical features of acute acalculous cholecystitis. *J Clin Gastroenterol* 2003;36:166–169.

An interesting study that challenges the notion that AAC is a disease of the critically ill. Of 156 patients with acute cholecystitis, 22 ultimately were diagnosed with AAC, and 20 of these presented from the outpatient setting. Most patients were male, the average age was 63, and 35% had atherosclerotic vascular disease confirming these common associations.

Van Lent AU, et al. Duration of antibiotic therapy for cholangitis after successful endoscopic drainage of the biliary tract. *Gastrointest Endosc* 2002;55:518–522.

The optimal duration of antibiotic therapy after biliary decompression for acute cholangitis is unknown. This study retrospectively identified 80 patients who had been successfully treated for acute cholangitis with ERCP, and then followed up with them for 6 months. Forty-one patients received antibiotic therapy for 3 days or less, 19 for 4 or 5 days, and 20 patients received therapy for more than 5 days (range: 0–42 days). Recurrent cholangitis occurred with equal frequency in the three well-matched groups. The authors suggest that 3 days of therapy is sufficient.

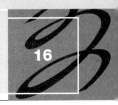

MANAGEMENT OF INFECTIOUS DIARRHEA

16

*C*linically, *diarrhea* means that the patient has passed three or more watery stools, or one or more bloody stools in 24 hours. Viruses account for 50 to 70% of causes of acute infectious diarrhea, bacteria 15 to 20%, parasites 10 to 15%, and it appears that 5 to 10% of cases are of unknown etiology. Definitions of the types of diarrhea are shown in Table 16-1. Specific indications for medical evaluation include profuse watery diarrhea with dehydration; dysentery; passage of many small-volume stools containing blood and mucus; fever (temperature of 38.5°C [101.3°F] or higher); passage of six or more unformed stools every 24 hours or a duration of illness longer than 48 hours; diarrhea with severe abdominal pain in a patient older than age 50; diarrhea in the elderly (age 70 or older) or the immunocompromised patient (AIDS, after transplantation, or receipt of cancer chemotherapy).

 DIAGNOSIS

From a study at the University Hospital of Geneva, the culture positivity rate of 6.1% decreased to 2.7% when patients received antimicrobial agents (P <.001). The positivity rate for patients hospitalized for 3 days or fewer was 12.6%, whereas it dropped to 1.4% for patients hospitalized for longer than 3 days (P <.001). Stool studies will be more useful in those patients who have a history of bloody diarrhea; have traveled to an endemic area; or have recently had antibiotics, immunosuppression, or exposure to infants in day care centers. The bacterial enteropathogens identified by normal stool culture are *Shigella*, *Salmonella*, *Campylobacter*, *Aeromonas*, and usually *Yersinia*. As an alternative, a rectal swab can be placed in transport media and then cultured. Please note that some pathogens will not be detected by routine stool culture. One should alert the laboratory to look for these microbes: *Escherichia coli* 0157:H7 and other Shigatoxin-producing *E. coli*, *Vibrios cholerae*, other noncholera *Vibrios*, and possibly *Yersinia*.

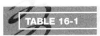 **TABLE 16-1**   **Definitions of Types of Diarrhea**

Entity	Days	Comments
Diarrhea		Defined as stool weight greater than 200 *g* in 24 hours. The average stool output is 100 g of stool per day.
Acute	<14	
Persistent	>14	
Chronic	>30	
Severe		The patient will have one or more of the following: volume depletion, fever, six or more stools in 24 hours, an illness lasting longer than 48 hours, or be immunocompromised.

Positive fecal leukocyte, lactoferrin, and occult blood tests lend support toward using empiric antimicrobial therapy. Conversely, when negative, they will eliminate the need for stool cultures. The most commonly identified pathogens in patients with these positive test results include *Shigella, Salmonella, Campylobacter, Aeromonas, Yersinia*, noncholera *Vibrios*, and *Clostridium difficile*.

Several studies have shown that the *routine* ordering for ova and parasites is not cost effective in severe acute diarrhea. Eliminating routine stool cultures and ova and parasite examinations on hospitalized patients would significantly reduce hospital and patient costs without altering patient care. Nationwide, such a policy might achieve a cost savings of up to 30 million per year according to one study. A travel history is important to help define who might benefit from such testing. Infection by *Cryptosporidium, Giardia*, or both, should be suspected whenever one returns from Russia; *Cyclospora* should be considered in travelers to Nepal; and *Giardia* should be suspected in persons who have recently traveled to the mountainous areas of North America. In day care centers, *Giardia* and *Cryptosporidium* are common causes of diarrhea. Also note that homosexual males will often have positive results for *Giardia* and *Entamoeba histolytica*. See Tables 16-2 and 16-3 for information about persistent and/or parasitic causes of diarrhea.

 ## TREATMENT OF COMMON PATHOGENS

In all patients with diarrhea requiring medical evaluation, fluid and electrolyte therapy and alteration of the diet should be part of the management. When nonspecific therapy is desired, loperamide is the drug of choice for most cases of diarrhea. Loperamide is the recommended agent for most cases of diarrhea because of its safety and efficacy of approximately 80%. Diphenoxylate possesses central opiate effects, which can be problematic. The antimotility drugs should not be given to patients with moderate to severe *C. difficile* related diarrhea. Bismuth subsalicylate is the preferred agent when vomiting is the important clinical manifestation of enteric infection. Bismuth subsalicylate, however, should not be given to immunocompromised patients with diarrhea to prevent the taking of excessive doses. In some cases of severe, refractory cases, octreotide may be effective. Consultation with a gastrointestinal (GI) specialist is advised. Table 16-4 includes information on treatment of common bacterial pathogens.

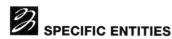 ## SPECIFIC ENTITIES

Clostridium difficile

C. difficile diarrhea is becoming increasingly more common in hospitalized patients. See Table 16-5 for information regarding the diagnosis of this condition. Response to oral therapy with vancomycin or metronidazole is better than 95%. Vancomycin should be reserved for patients who fail to respond to metronidazole. Intravenous metronidazole might be effective. It should be considered if the oral route is unavailable. Vancomycin, on the other hand, is not effective intravenously. First recurrences will usually respond to retreatment with the same drug for another 10-day course. The organism is a spore former and recurrence does not necessarily imply resistance. The antibiotics are not effective against the spores, only the vegetative organisms. Relapse occurs in about 25% of cases. Assays for *C. difficile* toxin are usually unnecessary immediately after the completion of treatment. Note that about one third of patients for whom therapy is successful have positive assays. *Saccharomyces boulardii*; bacitracin and *Lactobacillus* GG, and rifampin have been used with vancomycin or metronidazole to treat recurrences. The anion-exchange resin, cholestyramine, also has been used to bind the toxin. A tapering course of vancomycin over 3 to 6 weeks has been used to treat patients with multiple recurrences. Administration of vancomycin by nasogastric tube or rectal enema has been used in refractory cases. Intravenous immunoglobulin therapy has been used with success in a

TABLE 16-2   Acid-Fast Negative Protozoans

Organism	Geography	Transmission	Clinical features	Diagnosis	Treatment
Giardia lamblia	Anywhere but notably acquired in St. Petersburg, and the mountainous regions in North America	Waterborne and person to person Boil drinking water, or if not possible, use halogenated water purification tablets Patients with common variable immunodeficiency or X-linked agammaglobulinemia are at increased risk of infection	1–2 wk incubation period. The clinical spectrum of giardiasis is broad, including asymptomatic cyst passage; acute, often self-limited diarrhea; and chronic severe diarrhea with malabsorption and weight loss. In addition to diarrhea, a majority of symptomatic patients report bloating, cramping, and foul-smelling, greasy stools	Identification of cysts or motile trophozoites in stool or duodenal aspirate. Sensitivity is around to 85 to 90% after three stools. Newer antigen detection assays range in sensitivity from 85 to 98%	Metronidazole 250–500 t.i.d. for 1–2 wks Tinidazole 2 g P.O. × one dose Furazolidone is widely used in children in the United States, 100 mg q.i.d. × 10 days Paromomycin 25–30 mg/kg per day in three doses for 5–10 days Avoid milk products if there is a transient lactase deficiency
Microsporidia E. bieneusi and Encephalito-zoon (formerly Septata) intestinalis	Diverse locations	Any immunocompromised patient presenting with persistent unexplained diarrhea. HIV	Persistent diarrhea	Calcofluor White and Uvitex stains lack specificity Polymerase chain reaction techniques hold promise for improved detection of microsporidia in stool.	Albendazole 400–800 mg P.O. b.i.d. for 3 or more weeks Other therapies besides albendazole under study include metronidazole, atovaquone, thalidomide, and nitazoxanide Albendazole is not effective for *E. bieneusi*
E. histolytica	Diverse locations	Fecal-oral	Persistent diarrhea	Stool studies or serological tests. Serologic tests such as enzyme-linked immunosorbent assay and agar gel diffusion are more than 90% sensitive, but these tests often become negative within a year of initial infection	Metronidazole, 750 mg t.i.d. × 5–10 days, plus either diiodohydroxyquin, 650 mg t.i.d. × 20 days, or paromomycin, 500 mg t.i.d. × 7 days

Parasite	Treatment	Comments
Cryptosporidium	If severe, consider paromomycin, 500 mg t.i.d. × 7 days	5 μm. Yellow under auramine. Fluorescence with monoclonal antibody to Cryptosporidium
Isospora spp	Bactrim DS, b.i.d. × 7–10 days	20–30 μm long containing two visible sporocysts that are acid-fast. Eosinophilia is possible.
Cyclospora	Bactrim DS b.i.d. × 7 days	10 μm in diameter. Bright blue under ultraviolet light

small number of patients as well. See Tables 16-6 and 16-7 for more information regarding therapy.

 TRAVELER'S DIARRHEA

General Concerns

The most common travel disease is traveler's diarrhea (TD), affecting between 20 and 75% of those who vacation abroad. The onset of TD usually occurs within the first week of travel but may occur at any time while traveling, and even after returning home. The risk of TD varies according to the itinerary of the tourist. Risk also varies according to the underlying health status and age of the host, with the highest incidence occurring in small children and young adults aged 20 to 30. Certain conditions may predispose patients to a higher risk of acquiring TD, including those with HIV and other immunocompromising conditions.

Choice of cuisine also affects a traveler's risk. Particularly risky would be food bought from a street vendor. Higher risk foods include uncooked vegetables, salads, unpeeled fresh fruit; raw or undercooked meat or shellfish. Safe drinks include bottled carbonated beverages; beer or wine; and boiled or treated water. Tap water and unpasteurized milk carry an increased risk of infection. A common mistake is to put ice into a glass to cool a soft drink, thereby contaminating the beverage with infected water. Water should be brought to a boil or chemically purified using tincture of iodine (5 drops per quart), tetraglycine hydroperiodide tablets, or iodinizing filters. To kill viruses at altitudes above 2,000 m (6,562 ft), water should be boiled for 3 minutes or chemical disinfection should be used after the water has boiled for 1 minute. Chemical disinfection with iodine is an alternative method of water treatment when it is not feasible to boil water. However, this method cannot be relied on to kill Cryptosporidium unless the water is allowed to sit for 15 hours before it is drunk. Two well-tested methods for disinfection with iodine are the use of tincture of iodine and tetraglycine hydroperiodide tablets (e.g., Globaline, Potable-Aqua, or Coghlan's).

A guide to buying water filters for preventing cryptosporidiosis and giardiasis can be found at www.cdc.gov/ncidod/dpd/parasites/cryptosporidiosis/factsht_crypto_prevent_water.htm. These two organisms are either highly (Cryptosporidium) or moderately (Giardia) resistant to chlorine; so conventional halogen disinfection may be ineffective. Boiling water or filtration can be used as an alternative to disinfection.

Many filters that remove parasites may not be able to kill or remove smaller organisms. More details are available at http://www.cdc.gov/travel/food-drink-risks.htm.

Organisms That Cause Traveler's Diarrhea

Bacterial enteropathogens cause approximately 80% of TD cases. (See Table 16-8.) Five major groups of E. coli cause enteric infections: enterotoxigenic E. coli (ETEC), enteropathogenic E. coli (EPEC), enterohemorrhagic E. coli (EHEC), enteroaggregative E. coli (EaggEC), and enteroinvasive E. coli (EIEC). Of the offending bacteria, ETEC accounts for the majority of infections, although Shigella species, Campylobacter species, Salmonella

| | TABLE 16-4 | Treatment of Common Bacterial Pathogens | | |

Etiology	Treatment	Dose	Comments
Shigellosis (febrile dysentery)	FQ (possibly Bactrim or azithromycin)	500 mg P.O. b.i.d. × 3 days. Bactrim DS P.O. b.i.d. × 3 days	Up to 10 days if immunocompromised
Moderate to severe TD	FQ	Cipro 500 mg P.O. b.i.d. × 3–5 days or Bactrim DS P.O. b.i.d. × 3 days	Treat for longer if ill enough. One dose may be helpful in mild cases.
Enteropathogenic E. coli diarrhea (EPEC)	Treat as febrile dysentery		
Enterotoxigenic E. coli diarrhea (ETEC)	Treat as for mod-severe TD		
Enteroinvasive E. coli diarrhea (EIEC)	Treat as for Shigella		
Enterohemorrhagic E. coli diarrhea (EHEC)	Avoid if possible. May increase HUS risk		Avoid antimotility agents
Salmonella	Cipro (Azithro and ceftriaxone also effective)	500 mg P.O. b.i.d. × 5–7 days.	Treat if immunocompromised or ill.
Campylobacteriosis	Azithromycin or Cipro (FQ)	500 mg q day × 3 days, or 500 mg b.i.d. × 3 days	FQ resistance occurs. Emycin may be used as well
Aeromonas	FQ, Bactrim or third generation cephalosporin	Treat as febrile dysentery	
Yersinia	For most cases, treat as febrile dysentery, for severe cases give ceftriaxone	1 g IV q 24 hours for 5 days	
Listeria	Ampicillin (plus gentamicin if severe)	200 mg/kg per day IV, divided q 6 hours.	Bactrim is an alternative

FQ, Fluoroquinolone; HUS, Hemolytic uremic syndrome.

species, *Aeromonas* species, *Plesiomonas shigelloides*, and noncholera *Vibrios* all have been isolated from travelers.

ETEC produces a watery diarrhea, especially during warmer, wetter months. Diarrheal symptoms are associated with cramps and low-grade or no fever. ETEC is the most common cause of diarrhea in travelers to Latin America, whereas *Campylobacter jejuni* is relatively more common in Southeast Asia, particularly Thailand. *V. parahaemolyticus* has been isolated with increased frequency in travelers to Southeast Asia. EPEC was the first recognized *E. coli* capable of causing outbreaks of diarrhea in infants. Effective treatment is important because of mortality rates of 25 to 50% and the potential for prolonged diarrhea. Unfortunately resistance to trimethoprim-sulfamethoxazole (TMP-SMX) is increasing. EaggEC has been associated with prolonged diarrhea in children in developing countries and in HIV-infected adults. EaggEC has been shown to have significant resistance to TMP-SMX (57%) and ampicillin (65%). EIEC is closely related to *Shigella* and appears to respond to treatment directed against that organism. Resistance to TMP-SMX and ampicillin is common,

TABLE 16-5 Comparison of *C. difficile* Tests

Test	% Sensitivity	% Specificity	Comments
EIA	63–99*	75–100	A few hours. A/B toxins. There is a false-negative rate of 10–20%
Toxin, culture assay	90	98	Better than culture alone but takes 3–4 days
Cytotoxin	80–100	99–100	Toxin B. Takes 48 hours
Latex	58–92	80–96	Detects glutamate dehydrogenase. Not sensitive enough.
PCR	92–97	100	*C. difficile* toxin A or B, or both. Not commercial

PCR, Polymerase chain reaction.
Note that endoscopy is ~50 % sensitive.
*Performing enzyme immunoassays on two to three specimens increases the diagnostic yield by 5–10%.

unlike resistance to quinolones, which continues to be low at present. *EHEC*, especially *E. coli* O157:H7, are responsible for an estimated 20,000 infections each year in the United States, but unfortunately, studies do not support a role for antibiotic therapy, either in the treatment of the diarrheal syndrome or in the prevention of hemolytic-uremic syndrome.

Clinically, features of *C. jejuni* infection range from an absence of symptoms to rare fulminant sepsis and death.*Campylobacter* species are found in fowl and many wild and domestic animals, and most human infections probably result from contamination of milk and other animal food sources, especially poultry. The most common clinical manifestation is diarrhea, but most patients also have fever, abdominal pain, nausea, and malaise. Diarrhea lasts for about 1 week in most travelers without antimicrobial therapy, but symptoms may persist for 1 to 3 weeks in 20% of ill persons. Reactive arthritis has been reported in association with this infection, and Guillain-Barré syndrome occurs about 1 to 3 weeks after the intestinal infection. However, no relation between the severity of the gastrointestinal symptoms and the chance of developing Guillain-Barré syndrome has been demonstrated,

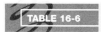

TABLE 16-6 Treatment of *C. difficile*

Drug	Dose
Oral metronidazole	250 mg q.i.d. or 500 mg t.i.d. times 10 days
Intravenous metronidazole	500 mg IV every 8 hours. Treatment failures have occurred. The oral route is preferred if possible.
Oral vancomycin	125 mg four times per day for 10 days is the preferred dose. May consider increasing the dose to 500 mg four times per day if the patient is critically ill or has a mild ileus, colonic dilation, or perforation.
Colonic vancomycin	If the patient has a paralytic ileus, one can give the drug via a tube directly into the cecum or ileostomy. May give 500 mg vancomycin in 500 mL up to four times per day. Some rectal tubes allow giving the vancomycin through the tube directly as well
Bacitracin	500 mg P.O. q 6 hours for 10 days
Cholestyramine	2–4 g P.O. b.i.d. to q.i.d. Must be spaced from other drugs. Difficult to use if the patient is on other medications.

TABLE 16-7	Treatment of Relapsed *C. difficile*

Drug	Dose
Saccharomyces boulardii	500 mg orally twice daily for 1 month, if the patient is not immuno-compromised, beginning 4 days before a 10-day course of specific antibiotic therapy has been completed.
Vancomycin or metronidazole	After a second 10-day course is given, if a second relapse occurs consider giving these drugs orally for 1–2 months in a tapering fashion such as every other day. May combine with Questran, Lactobacillus, Saccaromyces as well
Oral yogurt, Lactobacillus GG.	Lactobacillus GG, one capsule b.i.d.
Human immune globulin	Intravenous infusion, for patients with documented deficiencies.
Oral vancomycin plus rifampin	Watch for drug interactions with other drugs. Rifampin 300 mg b.i.d.

and even asymptomatic infections can trigger Guillain-Barré syndrome. Erythromycin is the drug of choice for most cases of *Campylobacter* enteritis, but clindamycin also can be used. Erythromycin has not altered the duration of gastrointestinal symptoms in multiple clinical trials, although it does reduce the duration of fecal carriage of *Campylobacter*. In contrast, ciprofloxacin has been shown to reduce the duration of clinical symptoms and to eradicate *Campylobacter* from the stool, but resistance is a concern. Studies have shown azithromycin to be superior to ciprofloxacin in decreasing the excretion of *Campylobacter* spp. and as effective as ciprofloxacin in shortening the duration of illness. Azithromycin therapy may be an effective alternative to ciprofloxacin therapy in areas where ciprofloxacin-resistant *Campylobacter* spp. are prevalent.

Norwalk virus, rotavirus, and enteric adenoviruses have been isolated from between 2 and 27% of returning travelers with diarrhea. Among parasites, *Giardia lamblia* is an important cause of diarrhea in travelers to St. Petersburg, Russia, and the mountainous regions of North America. Of note, *E. histolytica*, *Cryptosporidium parvum*, and *Cyclospora cayetanensis* are less common causes of diarrhea in travelers. Cyclosporiasis especially should be considered in travelers returning from Peru and Nepal, whereas cryptosporidiosis occurs with increased frequency in travelers to Russia. An important clue to a possible parasitic etiology is that a prolonged visit (longer than 2 months) is often required to acquire a parasite as opposed to a bacterial etiology.

Treatment of Traveler's Diarrhea

Bismuth subsalicylate (BSS) (Pepto-Bismol) taken in the form of two 262-mg tablets four times a day with meals and qhs, lowers the attack rates of traveler's diarrhea from 40 to 14% compared with a placebo. The dosage of two tablets of BSS four times daily (2.1 g/day) appears to be a safe and effective means of reducing the occurrence of TD among persons at risk for periods up to 3 weeks. Caution is advised for patients taking salicylate-containing medications or anticoagulants, as well as those with chronic renal insufficiency and gout. BSS may produce tinnitus and blackened stools, and may also interfere with the absorption of doxycycline. Comparisons of BSS with loperamide have shown similar efficacy, but less stools are passed in those taking loperamide. Loperamide might also be beneficial when added to TMP-SMX or ciprofloxacin, particularly during the first 24 hours of therapy. *Lactobacillus* preparations have been used to prevent TD, but their efficacy remains uncertain. Diphenoxylate plus atropine (Lomotil) is not as effective as loperamide and may actually prolong symptoms of infection secondary to *Shigella*, and may cause urinary retention and central nervous system toxicity.

TABLE 16-8 Traveler's Diarrhea

Pathogen	Clinical symptoms	Stool findings	Treatment	Other
ETEC Heat-stable toxins (Sta; STb)	Abdominal cramps, headache, myalgias Vomiting Low-grade fever	Watery diarrhea (No WBCs)	FQ if needed	Boil it, cook it, peel it–or forget it
EHEC	Blood, pain and fever	Specialized testing	Probably avoid antibiotics and antimotility agents	Associated with hamburger consumption
Salmonella	Abdominal cramps, headache, myalgias Fever	Watery or inflammatory* Culture serology	FQ, cephalosporin	Beef, poultry, pork, eggs, dairy products, vegetables, fruit
Shigella	Abdominal cramps and bloody diarrhea Fever	Inflammatory or watery Culture	Loperamide decreases the number of unformed stools and shortens the duration of diarrhea in adults treated with ciprofloxacin	Potential reactive arthropathy or Reiter syndrome sequelae
Campylobacter	Abdominal cramps, bloody diarrhea, myalgias Fever	Watery or inflammatory	In patients who have moderate-to-severe dysentery, who are elderly, who are presumed to be bacteremic with chills and systemic symptoms, or who are at increased risk of complications, such as immunocompromised or pregnant patients, treatment may be of significant benefit FQ or azithromycin	Poultry is the primary source of Campylobacter
V. parahaemolyticus	Abdominal cramps, headache Bloody diarrhea on occasion	Inflammatory or watery	Doxycycline, TMP-SMX and quinolones	Raw or poorly cooked seafood Caribbean cruise ships and in people traveling in Asia

FQ, Fluoroquinolone; WBC, White blood cells;
*Inflammatory may have fecal WBCs.

Antibiotic Prophylaxis

Patients for whom antibiotic prophylaxis might be considered include those who are at increased risk of developing severe or complicated disease, such as the immunocompromised; those with inflammatory bowel disease; insulin-dependent diabetics; and patients taking either diuretics or proton pump inhibitors.

When used as prophylaxis, antibiotics should be taken daily as a single dose while in an area of risk and continued from 1 to 2 days after leaving. Quinolones have emerged as the drugs of choice, but resistance may limit their long-term usefulness. Ciprofloxacin given at a dose of 500 mg daily has been shown to be up to 95% effective in preventing diarrhea, but perhaps azithromycin should be considered if *Campylobacter* is endemic in the proposed destination.

Therapy of Traveler's Diarrhea

For travelers with significant diarrhea (more than 3 stools during an 8-hour period, particularly if associated with nausea, vomiting, abdominal cramping, fever, or bloody stools), antibiotic therapy is recommended either with or without loperamide. Until recently, TMP/SMX was the drug of choice for the treatment of TD but resistance has limited its effectiveness, except in areas where *Cyclospora* is a significant cause of diarrhea.

Fluoroquinolones, either alone or in combination with loperamide, reduce the duration of diarrhea by more than 50% compared with a placebo. In instances where the use of a fluoroquinolone is appropriate, a 3-day course is effective in most cases. Single-dose therapy may be adequate in most cases; however, for bacteria such as *Campylobacter* and *Shigella dysenteriae*, concerns have been raised that single-dose therapy may be inadequate, especially if the potential for invasive disease exists. In areas where fluoroquinolone-resistant *Campylobacter jejuni* has been found, azithromycin might be considered the drug of choice. (JWM)

Bibliography

American Gastroenterological Association medical position statement: guidelines for the evaluation and management of chronic diarrhea. *Gastroenterology* 1999;116:1461–1463.
This document presents the official recommendations of the American Gastroenterological Association (AGA) on the evaluation and management of chronic diarrhea.

Risk of enteric illness associated with travel: a case review of gastroenteritis among Canadian travellers: January to April, 2000. *Can Commun Dis Rep* 2001;27:45–49.

Adachi JA, et al. Empirical antimicrobial therapy for traveler's diarrhea. *Clin Infect Dis* 2000;31:1079–1083.
Preliminary clinical results for patients with diarrhea predominantly caused by Campylobacter spp. have shown that azithromycin may be an effective alternative to fluoroquinolones for the treatment of traveler's diarrhea.

Ansdell VE, Ericsson CD. Prevention and empiric treatment of traveler's diarrhea. *Med Clin North Am* 1999;83:945–73.
This article discusses the cause of diarrheal illness in travelers, as well as epidemiology, prevention, treatment, and a general approach to self-treatment.

Diemert DJ. Prevention and self-treatment of travelers' diarrhea. *Prim Care* 2002;29:84–855.
Excellent discussion of organisms.

DuPont HL. Guidelines on acute infectious diarrhea in adults. The Practice Parameters Committee of the American College of Gastroenterology. *Am J Gastroenterol* 1997;92:1962–1975.
These guidelines were developed under the auspices of the American College of Gastroenterology and its Practice Parameters Committee.

DuPont HL, Ericsson CD. Prevention and treatment of traveler's diarrhea. *N Engl J Med* 1993;328:1821–1827.

DuPont HL, et al. Prevention of travelers' diarrhea by the tablet formulation of bismuth subsalicylate. *JAMA* 1987;257:1347–1350.
The dosage of two tablets of bismuth subsalicylate four times daily (2.1 g/day) appears to be a safe and effective means of reducing the occurrence of travelers' diarrhea among persons at risk for periods up to 3 weeks.

DuPont HL, et al. Rifaximin: a nonabsorbed antimicrobial in the therapy of travelers' diarrhea. *Digestion* 1998;59:708–714.
Discussion of a new antibiotic for traveler's diarrhea. Rifaximin shortened the duration of travelers' diarrhea compared with TMP/SMX and two earlier studied placebo-treated groups. A poorly absorbed drug, if effective in treating bacterial diarrhea, has pharmacologic and safety advantages over the existing drugs.

DuPont HL, et al. Comparative efficacy of loperamide hydrochloride and bismuth subsalicylate in the management of acute diarrhea. *Am J Med* 1990;88:15S–19S.
Both treatments were well tolerated, and none of the minor adverse effects reported resulted in discontinuation of therapy. It was concluded that loperamide is effective at a daily dosage limit of 8 mg (40 mL) for the treatment of acute nonspecific diarrhea and provides faster, more effective relief than bismuth subsalicylate.

Ericsson CD. Travelers' diarrhea. Epidemiology, prevention, and self-treatment. *Infect Dis Clin North Am* 1998;12:285–303.
Current therapeutic options, in order of increasing effectiveness, include attapulgite, BSS-containing compounds, loperamide, antimicrobial agents such as the fluoroquinolones, and the combination of loperamide and an antimicrobial agent. Under study are a nonabsorbed antimicrobial agent, rifaximin, and a novel calmodulin inhibitor, zaldaride. Development and evaluation of vaccines against enterotoxigenic E. coli and Shigella are proceeding apace but are not yet available for routine use.

Ericsson CD, et al. Single dose ofloxacin plus loperamide compared with single dose or three days of ofloxacin in the treatment of traveler's diarrhea. *J Travel Med* 1997;4:3–7.
The combined use of a single dose of ofloxacin with loperamide is safe and more efficacious in the treatment of TD than use of ofloxacin alone.

Ericsson CD, et al. Treatment of traveler's diarrhea with sulfamethoxazole and trimethoprim and loperamide. *JAMA* 1990;263:257–261.
The combination of sulfamethoxazole-trimethoprim plus loperamide is highly recommended for the treatment of most patients with TD.

Ericsson CD. Safety and efficacy of loperamide. *Am J Med* 1990;88:10S–14S.
Loperamide is safe and effective for the treatment of acute diarrhea. Efficacy data suggest that loperamide is more effective than the prescription drug diphenoxylate and an over-the-counter bismuth subsalicylate preparation.

Fekety R. Guidelines for the diagnosis and management of Clostridium difficile-associated diarrhea and colitis. American College of Gastroenterology, Practice Parameters Committee. *Am J Gastroenterol* 1997;92:739–750.

Goldsweig CD, Pacheco PA. Infectious colitis excluding E. coli O157:H7 and C. difficile. *Gastroenterol Clin North Am* 2001;30:709–733.
Excellent review article.

Goodgame R. Emerging causes of traveler's diarrhea: Cryptosporidium, Cyclospora, Isospora, and Microsporidia. *Curr Infect Dis Rep* 2003;5:66–73.
Effective treatment is available for Cyclospora, Microsporidia, and Isospora.

Guerrant RL, et al. Practice guidelines for the management of infectious diarrhea. *Clin Infect Dis* 2001;32:331–351.
Excellent review article.

Johnson PC, et al. Comparison of loperamide with bismuth subsalicylate for the treatment of acute travelers' diarrhea. *JAMA* 1986;255:757–760.
We conclude that loperamide is a safe and effective alternative to bismuth subsalicylate for the treatment of nondysenteric TD.

Juckett G. Prevention and treatment of traveler's diarrhea. *Am Fam Physician* 1999;60:119–124, 135–136.
Excellent review article.

Kuschner RA, et al. Use of azithromycin for the treatment of Campylobacter enteritis in travelers to Thailand, an area where ciprofloxacin resistance is prevalent. *Clin Infect Dis* 1995;21:536–541.

Azithromycin is superior to ciprofloxacin in decreasing the excretion of Campylobacter spp. and as effective as ciprofloxacin in shortening the duration of illness. Azithromycin therapy may be an effective alternative to ciprofloxacin therapy in areas where ciprofloxacin-resistant Campylobacter spp. are prevalent.

Okhuysen PC. Traveler's diarrhea due to intestinal protozoa. *Clin Infect Dis* 2001;33:110–114.

The microbiology, epidemiology, clinical presentation, and treatment of the most common intestinal parasites found in travelers are presented in this minireview.

Oldfield EC 3rd, Wallace MR. The role of antibiotics in the treatment of infectious diarrhea. *Gastroenterol Clin North Am* 2001;30:817–836.

Excellent review article.

Ramzan NN. Traveler's diarrhea. *Gastroenterol Clin North Am* 2001;30:665–678.

This article presents a review of causes, presentation, and diagnosis of TD. Treatment and prevention of this common problem are described in some detail. Finally, a practical and cost-effective approach to evaluating and treating a returning traveler is presented.

Rendi-Wagner P, Kollaritsch H. Drug prophylaxis for travelers' diarrhea. *Clin Infect Dis* 2002;34:628–633.

In conclusion, there is no satisfactory prophylactic option, and worldwide monitoring of antimicrobial susceptibility patterns and the search for novel antimicrobial agents, such as nonabsorbed antibiotics, and nonantibiotic medications should continue.

Siegel DL, et al. Inappropriate testing for diarrheal diseases in the hospital. *JAMA* 1990;263:979–982.

Eliminating routine stool cultures and ova and parasite examinations in hospitalized patients would significantly reduce hospital and patient costs without altering patient care. Nationwide, such a policy might achieve a cost savings of $20 to $30 million per year.

Taylor DN, et al. Treatment of travelers' diarrhea: ciprofloxacin plus loperamide compared with ciprofloxacin alone. A placebo-controlled, randomized trial. *Ann Intern Med* 1991;114:731–734.

In a region where enterotoxigenic E. coli was the predominant cause of travelers' diarrhea, loperamide combined with ciprofloxacin was not better than treatment with ciprofloxacin alone. Loperamide appeared to have some benefit in the first 24 hours of treatment in patients infected with enterotoxigenic E. coli. Both regimens were safe.

HEPATITIS C—DIAGNOSIS AND MANAGEMENT

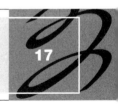

17

*H*epatitis C remains an important infectious disease in the United States with a prevalence of about 1.8%. About 75% of those infected with the virus develop chronic liver disease. The disease causes 10,000 to 12,000 deaths per year. The chronic liver disease that is caused by hepatitis C may range from mild, asymptomatic infection to fulminant liver failure. Hepatitis C is among the most common causes of liver transplantation in the United States and one of the most common causes of hepatic carcinoma.

EPIDEMIOLOGY

Currently, most patients with hepatitis C infection—about 65%—have a history of intravenous drug abuse. About 15% of patients became infected by blood transfusions, but these transfusions occurred before 1989 when tests and screenings became available. Patients with frequent exposure to blood products, such as those with hemophilia or those on dialysis with chronic renal failure, are also at risk for hepatitis C. Healthcare workers may become hepatitis C positive from needlestick injuries, although such transmission is less likely to occur than with hepatitis B.

Maternal fetal transmission is uncommon, as is sexual transmission between monogamous partners. However, people with multiple sex partners and those who have sexually transmitted disease are at increased risk. Unsanitary health conditions, such as poorly sterilized equipment, contaminated needles, syringes, and infusions can contribute to the spread of hepatitis C infection.

 THE HEPATITIS C VIRUS

The hepatitis C virus (HCV) is an RNA, single-stranded virus with an envelope and belongs in the family of Flaviviridae. The virus has six major genotypes. Because it mutates rapidly, there are numerous subpopulations with slight genomic differences. These mutations change the envelope proteins and may let the virus evade the immune system.

In recent years, genomic differences have been found to result in differences in response to interferon-α. Treatment recommendations now depend on genotypic typing. Genotype 1 makes up about 75% of virus infections, genotypes 2 and 3, about 10% each. Genotypes do not predict prognosis or mode of transmission, but they do effect ease of treatment.

HCV antibody is detected by a third-generation enzyme immunoassay (EIA-3) that is highly sensitive and specific. The recombinant immunoblot assay can be used to confirm anti-HCV reactivity but is not frequently used at this time because of the improved predictive value of the EIA. Direct assays for HCV RNA are available. Qualitative tests using polymerase chain reaction (PCR) or branched chain DNA assays detect serum HCV at low concentrations, confirming active disease. This test is particularly useful when liver enzymes are normal or when several potential causes of liver disease need to be differentiated. A PCR assay approved by the Food and Drug Administration (FDA) will detect HCV RNA in serum at low levels—50 to 100 copies per milliliter. Quantitative tests are used to determine viral load. Viral load is now used in making treatment decisions about continuing versus stopping treatment. Genotypic testing is now necessary in planning treatment schedules. Patients with genotypes 2 or 3 are more likely to respond to interferon than patients with genotype 1. Dosages and duration of treatment will depend on genotype.

 CLINICAL SIGNS AND SYMPTOMS OF HEPATITIS C

Most acute cases are asymptomatic. Chronic infection is also often asymptomatic or patients may have vague, nonspecific symptoms. Table 17-1 lists signs and symptoms of chronic hepatitis C infection. Extrahepatic manifestations of the disease are rare, occurring in 1 to 2% of patients with hepatitis C. Table 17-2 lists theses complications.

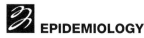 **MEDICAL MANAGEMENT OF HEPATITIS C**

Treatment has evolved to become more effective and more complicated since the initial protocols with interferon-α. Treatment must take into consideration individual patient motivation, severity of disease, contraindications, and likelihood of successful response. As noted, HCV genotype must be determined before therapy, as protocols now vary with

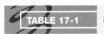

TABLE 17-1	Signs and Symptoms of Hepatitis C Infection

Fatigue
Right upper quadrant discomfort
Nausea, decreased appetite
Arthralgia
Hepatosplenomegaly
Ascites
Peripheral edema
Excoriations

genotype. HCV RNA level must also be determined to assess outcome. Figure 17-1 describes a detailed treatment algorithm based on the fact that the regimen of pegylated interferon-α and ribavirin will be 48 weeks for genotype 1 and 24 weeks for genotype 2 or 3. Responses are evaluated at weeks 12 and 24. Nonresponse, based on viral load, will result in cessation of therapy. It is known that if HCV RNA titers do not decline by more than 2 logs by week 12, then no future response is likely. Pegylated interferon is an alpha interferon with an inert polyethylene glycol that changes the uptake, distribution, and excretion of interferon-α.

Pegylated interferon can be given once weekly subcutaneously. There are two forms of pegylated interferon: alfa-2a and alpha-2b, which are equivalent in safety and effectiveness but have different dosing protocols. Ribavirin is an oral agent that has synergy with alpha interferon against hepatitis C, improving response twofold to threefold. Patients with genotype 1 have sustained response rates with the two-drug regimen of 42 to 46% with the optimal 48-week course of therapy. Patients with genotype 2 or 3 have a response rate of 78 to 82% and need only a 24-week course for optimal response.

 WHO SHOULD BE TREATED?

The best candidates for treatment will have HCV antibody, HCV RNA, elevated serum aminotransferase, and evidence of chronic hepatitis on liver biopsy. The National Institutes of Health Consensus Development Conference Panel has recommended that treatment be limited to those who have pathologic evidence of progressive disease, including fibrosis or severe degrees of inflammation and necrosis. Patients with evidence of cirrhosis should be evaluated on an individual basis. Those with jaundice, ascites, encephalopathy and gastrointestinal bleeding would not be good candidates for treatment with interferon/ribavirin.

Older patients are generally not good candidates for therapy but must be evaluated on an individual basis. Benefits are not well documented in the elderly and side effects are more common. In children, interferon therapy has been used as monotherapy. Ribavirin has not been evaluated with respect to toxicity or dosing guidelines. Because HCV is particularly severe in patients with HIV disease, treatment should be considered in those with dual infection unless there are contraindications.

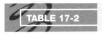

TABLE 17-2	Extrahepatic Manifestations of Hepatitis C

Skin rashes (purpura, vasculitis, urticaria, lichen planus, porphyria cutanea tarda)
Mixed cryoglobulinemia
Neuropathy
Membranoproliferative glomerulonephritis
B cell lymphoma
Sjögren's syndrome

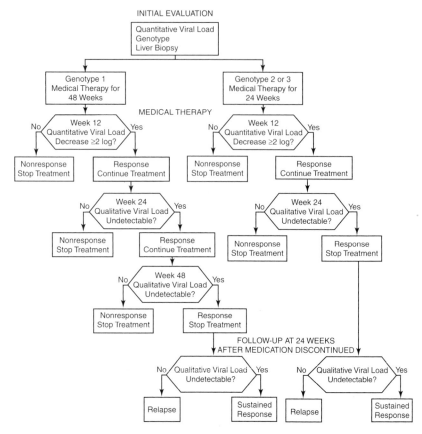

Figure 17-1. Treatment Algorithm for Chronic Hepatitis C Virus Infection.

Therapy is not advisable for those with decompensated cirrhosis, normal liver function tests, or transplant patients. Treatment is difficult for those with poorly controlled diabetes, coronary heart disease, seizures, and severe psychiatric disease particularly depression. Table 17-3 lists the most common adverse effects of pegylated interferon and ribavirin.

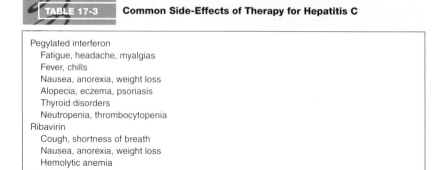

TABLE 17-3	Common Side-Effects of Therapy for Hepatitis C

Pegylated interferon
    Fatigue, headache, myalgias
    Fever, chills
    Nausea, anorexia, weight loss
    Alopecia, eczema, psoriasis
    Thyroid disorders
    Neutropenia, thrombocytopenia
Ribavirin
    Cough, shortness of breath
    Nausea, anorexia, weight loss
    Hemolytic anemia

Future treatment developments may include vaccine development and molecular interventions, such as RNA polymerase, and helicase or protease inhibitors. (SLB)

Bibliography

Colin C, et al. Sensitivity and specificity of third-generation hepatitis C virus antibody detection assays: an analysis of the literature. *J Viral Hepat* 2001;8:87.
There has been great improvement in the sensitivity and specificity of the enzyme immunoassays, making the immunoblot assays unnecessary in most cases.
DiBisceglie AM, et al. Recombinant interferon alpha therapy for chronic hepatitis C: a randomized, double-blind, placebo-controlled trial. *N Engl J Med* 1989;321:1506.
Recombinant interferon-α reduced disease activity in chronic hepatitis C, as assessed by serial testing of serum aminotransferase activities and histology of liver biopsy specimens.
Everhart JE, et al. Risk for non-A, non-B (type C) hepatitis through sexual or household contact with chronic carriers. *Ann Intern Med* 1990;112:544.
Conclusive evidence of HCV transmission to family members or sexual contacts of adult patients with well-documented disease was not demonstrated in this study.
Flamm SL. Chronic hepatitis C virus infection. *JAMA* 2003;289:2413.
Update on the diagnosis and treatment of hepatitis. Includes an algorithm for treatment based on genotype.
Fried MW, et. al. Peg interferon alpha-2a plus ribavirin for chronic hepatitis C virus infection. *N Engl J Med* 2002;347:975.
Describes current preferred regimen. HCV viral load is followed and treatment is discontinued if no response is demonstrated.
Hoofnagle JH. Course and outcome of hepatitis C. *Hepatology* 2002;36:S21.
Describes clinical signs and symptoms including extrahepatic manifestations of hepatitis C.
Lumreras C, et al. Clinical, virological, and histologic evolution of hepatitis C virus infection in liver transplant recipients. *Clin Infect Dis* 1998;26:48.
Prospective study to define the clinical course of hepatitis C in liver transplant patients. Hepatitis C was often associated with early graft hepatitis.
Marcellin P, et al. Long-term histologic improvement and loss of detectable intrahepatic HCV RNA in patients with chronic hepatitis C and sustained response to interferon-α therapy. *Ann Intern Med* 1997;127:825.
Patients with hepatitis C who have been treated with interferon-α and have persistently normal ALT levels with no HCV RNA after 6 months usually have a sustained response, histologic improvement, and no intrahepatic HCV RNA.
McHutchison JG, Patel K. Future therapy for hepatitis C. *Hepatology* 2002;36:S245.
Describes newer developments in therapy, including vaccines, helicase inhibitors, protease inhibitors.
National Institute of Health Consensus Development Conference Statement: management of hepatitis C 2002-June 10–12,2002. *Hepatology* 2002;36:S3.
Gives recommendations on who should be treated with combination therapy, including histology based on liver biopsy.
Osmond DH, et al. Risk factors for hepatitis C virus seropositivity in heterosexual couples. *JAMA* 1993;269:361.
Provides little evidence for sexual transmission of HCV.
Pereira BJG, et al. Prevalence of hepatitis C virus RNA in organ donors positive for hepatitis C antibody and in the recipients of their organs. *N Engl J Med* 1992;327:910.
Recipients of organs from HCV antibody-positive patients became infected with HCV.
Terada S, Katayama K. Minimal hepatitis C infectivity in semen. *Ann Intern Med* 1992;117:171.
HCV RNA was not detected in the semen of seropositive patients.
Yeung LT, King SM, Roberts EA. Mother to infant transmission of hepatitis C virus. *Hepatology* 2001;34:223.
Transmission of the virus occurs in only 3 to 7% of infants born to mothers with active infection.

Urinary Tract

V

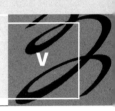

URINARY TRACT INFECTIONS— BASIC PRINCIPLES OF THERAPY

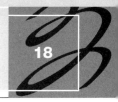

The management of urinary tract infections will depend on several basic questions, as outlined in Table 18-1.

Most bacteria in the urine are gram-negative bacilli. Many different antibiotics have a broad range of activity to these organisms. The commonly used antibiotics all attain adequate levels in the urine even with oral therapy. Choice of therapy will include issues such as drug allergy and relative contraindications, antibiotic cost, and potential for resistance. Under some circumstances, organisms such as enterococci and staphylococci also will need to be covered.

TREATMENT OF PYELONEPHRITIS

Most patients, both men and women, with pyelonephritis will present with fever and may have costovertebral tenderness. Other systemic complaints, such a nausea and vomiting, are common. In some cases, however, the symptoms will be subtle and difficult to distinguish from cystitis.

The Infectious Disease Society of America has provided guidelines for the treatment of uncomplicated pyelonephritis (Table 18-2).

For mild to moderate symptoms, 7 to 14 days of oral therapy is recommended using a fluoroquinolone or trimethoprim-sulfamethoxazole (TMP-SMX). Sulfonamides, ampicillin, and amoxicillin are no longer adequate for initial therapy because of their decreasing spectrum of activity against gram-negative bacilli. When enterococci is suspected by Gram's stain or grown from culture, amoxicillin is recommended. When symptoms are more severe or the patient appears septic, broader spectrum regimens are recommended, including fluoroquinolones, aminoglycoside and ampicillin, or cephalosporin and aminoglycoside.

Hospitalized patients with pyelonephritis are usually treated with parenteral antibiotics for several days, then switched to oral agents based on susceptibility data.

In patients with hospital-acquired pyelonephritis, a history of recurrent infection, or prior infection with a resistant organism, initial antimicrobial therapy must have an antipseudomonal spectrum. Depending on the institution's antimicrobial resistance profile, agents such as ceftazidime, tobramycin, or amikacin, imipenem, ticarcillin-clavulanic acid, or ciprofloxacin may be initiated. When results of antimicrobial susceptibility tests become available, therapy can be revised. If aminoglycoside therapy was begun in an older patient or one with renal insufficiency, a safer antimicrobial should be chosen once susceptibility results define all options.

TABLE 18-1 Major Factors in the Classification and Treatment of Urinary Tract Infection

1. Patient's age and gender
2. Site of infection: upper versus lower
3. Symptomatic or asymptomatic
4. Likely causative agent
5. Recurrent infection

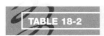 **International Diseases Society of America (IDSA) Guidelines: Acute Uncomplicated Pyelonephritis**

1. Mild or moderate symptoms, compliant patient: outpatient treatment (total of 7–14 days)
   —May require >12–24 hours' initial observation in emergency department (parenteral or oral Rx)
   —Oral treatment
   • Fluoroquinolone
   • TMP-SMX, if uropathogen known to be susceptible
   • If gram-positive pathogen: amoxicillin or amoxicillin-clavulanate
2. Severe symptoms or noncompliant patient: inpatient treatment
   —Parenteral therapy until afebrile
   • Aminoglycoside + ampicillin
   • Fluoroquinolone
   • Extended-spectrum cephalosporin + aminoglycoside
   —Change to oral agent to finish course once patient is stable and signs and symptoms are improving, usually 48–72 hours. Usually, the oral regimen can be selected on the basis of pretherapy urine culture and susceptibility.

Rx, Therapy.
Recommendations based on clinical presentation of patient.

Bacteria should be cleared from the urine within 24 to 48 hours of therapy. If bacteriuria persists, antimicrobial therapy should be changed based on susceptibility results.

Patients with persistent fever or toxicity despite appropriate antimicrobial therapy should be investigated for perinephric or renal cortical abscess.

 TREATMENT OF LOWER URINARY TRACT INFECTION

The Infectious Disease Society of America has provided guidelines for the treatment of acute, uncomplicated lower urinary tract infection (Table 18-3). These guidelines apply to nonpregnant women with cystitis. They are based on the knowledge of susceptibility patterns of pathogens in the community, particularly the susceptibility pattern to TMP-SMX. They do not apply to patients who have had frequent urinary tract infections who have been on prior antibiotic therapy. These guidelines do not apply to men with presumed prostatitis, treatment for which is described in another chapter.

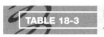 **Infectious Diseases Society of America (IDSA) Guidelines: Acute Uncomplicated Urinary Tract Infections**

Resistance	Recommended drug dosage
TMP-SMX resistance <20%	TMP-SMX × 3 days 160–800 mg b.i.d.
	TMP × 3 days 200 mg b.i.d.
TMP-SMX resistance >10–20%	Fluoroquinolone × 3 days
	Norfloxacin 400 mg b.i.d.
	Ciprofloxacin 250 mg b.i.d.
	Ofloxacin 200 mg b.i.d.
	Nitrofurantoin 50–100 mg q.i.d. × 7 days
	Macrocrystals 100 mg q.i.d. × 7 days
	Monohydrate/macrocrystals 100 mg b.i.d. × 7 days
	Fosfomycin tromethamine 3 g SDT

SDT, Single-dose treatment.

Many studies have found that short-course therapy for lower urinary tract infection (3 days or even 1 dose) is as effective as a 7- to 14-day course. These studies have generally been performed in young women with symptoms of cystitis. Many different oral regimens have been used, including TMP-SMX, norfloxacin, ciprofloxacin, cephalexin, and amoxicillin-clavulanate (Augmentin). Recent reviews have warned that single-drug therapy for cystitis is somewhat less effective than 3-day regimens. Men with cystitis generally receive at least 7 days of antibiotic therapy because of concern for complicating factors, particularly prostatitis.

Cystitis in older women has not been well studied. Long-term eradication of bacteriuria is less likely to be seen in older women, particularly if their functional status is poor. Older women with typical symptoms of cystitis should be treated for 3 days with a quinolone or TMP-SMX. Relapse after 3 days should be considered evidence for upper tract disease, and treatment guidelines, as previously described, should be followed.

Urinary tract infection in pregnant women is a common problem and can result in premature delivery and low-birth-weight infants. Pregnant women should be screened for asymptomatic bacteriuria and treated if positive. Cephalosporin and amoxicillin-clavulanic acid (Augmentin) are good choices for asymptomatic bacteriuria or cystitis. TMP-SMX is avoided in the first trimester. Pregnant women with pyelonephritis are admitted to the hospital and treated with ampicillin and gentamicin or another broad-spectrum regimen, such as ureidopenicillin, aztreonam, or broad-spectrum cephalosporin. There is some concern about aminoglycoside's effect on the fetus, so aminoglycosides are avoided when possible.

When urinary tract infection is complicated by an abnormal urinary tract, underlying host factors, or recurrence, treatment requires more individualization. Resistant and unusual organisms are more likely to be encountered, for example in diabetic patients, patients with spinal cord injuries, and patients with a history of renal stones. Review of urine Gram's stain and evaluation of urine culture and sensitivity become important in the management of urinary tract infection in these patients and empirical therapy will require a broader regimen, based on an evaluation of the likely pathogens and their susceptibility.

Prospective studies have confirmed the value of in vitro antimicrobial susceptibility testing. The initial disappearance of bacteriuria is closely correlated with the susceptibility of the microorganism to the concentration of the antimicrobial agent achieved in the urine. (SLB)

Bibliography

Dembry LM, Andriole VT. Renal and perirenal abscesses. *Infect Dis Clin North Am* 1997; 11:663.
  Renal carbuncles and corticomedullary abscesses usually resolve after 1 week of antibiotic therapy. The patient should then be evaluated by an appropriate imaging technique.
Fihn SD, et al. Trimethoprim-sulfamethoxazole for acute dysuria in women: a single-dose or 10-day course. A double-blind, randomized trial treatment. *Ann Intern Med* 1985;108:350.
  A history of urinary tract infection, use of spermicide, and the presence of more than 10^5 bacteria correlate with failure of the single-treatment regimen.
Hooton TM, Stamm WE. Diagnosis and treatment of uncomplicated urinary tract infection. *Infect Dis Clin North Am* 1997;11:551.
  Detailed literature review of treatment for cystitis and uncomplicated pyelonephritis in both men and women.
Manges AR, Dietrich PS, Riley LW. Multidrug-resistant Escherichia coli clonal groups causing community-acquired pyelonephritis. *Clin Infect Dis* 2004;38:329.
  Describes a clonal group of Escherichia coli *that is increasingly responsible for resistant community-acquired infection. This* E. coli *is resistant to TMP-SMX.*
Mombelli G, et al. Oral versus intravenous ciprofloxacin in the initial empiric management of severe pyelonephritis or complicated urinary tract infection. *Arch Intern Med* 1999;159:53.
  Outcome was equivalent regardless of the route of therapy.
Nicolle LE. Urinary tract infection: traditional pharmacologic therapies. *Am J Med* 2002; 133S:35S.

Basic recommendations for uncomplicated urinary tract infection including discussion of the use of TMP-SMX as first-line therapy.

Norby SR. Short-term treatment of uncomplicated lower urinary tract infections in women. *Rev Infect Dis* 1990;12:458.
Reviews of large numbers of patients indicate that short-course therapy for cystitis is not as effective as traditional regimens.

Raz R, et al. Comparison of single-dose administration and 3-day course of amoxicillin with clavulanic acid for treatment of uncomplicated urinary tract infection in women. *Antimicrob Agents Chemother* 1991;35:1688.
A 3-day regimen is better than single-dose therapy only in the population with recurrent urinary tract infection.

Ronald AR, et al. Complicated urinary tract infection. *Infect Dis Clin North Am* 1997;11:583.
Urinary tract infections may be complicated by structural abnormalities, metabolic abnormalities, immunologic deficiencies, or unusual organisms. Complicated infections usually require longer periods of therapy, although better data are needed to make definitive recommendations.

Stamey TA. Recurrent urinary tract infections in female patients: an overview of management and treatment. *Rev Infect Dis* 1987;9(suppl 2):S195.
Single-dose therapy is not effective in all patients with lower urinary tract infection; a 3-day course gives better overall results.

Stamm WE, McKevitt M, Counts GW. Acute renal infection in women: treatment with trimethoprim-sulfamethoxazole or ampicillin for 2 or 6 weeks. A randomized trial. *Ann Intern Med* 1987;106:341.

Talan DA, et al. Comparison of ciprofloxacin and trimethoprim sulfamethoxazole for acute, uncomplicated pyelonephritis in women: a randomized trial. *JAMA* 2000;283:1583.
Ciprofloxacin was superior in this trial, probably because of organisms resistant to TMP-SMX.

Trienekens TA, et al. Different lengths of treatment with co-trimoxazole for acute uncomplicated urinary tract infections in women. *BMJ* 1989;299:1319.
Three days of therapy for cystitis was as effective as 7 days.

Warren JW, et al. Guidelines for antimicrobial treatment of uncomplicated acute bacterial cystitis and acute pyelonephritis in women. *Clin Infect Dis* 1999;29:745.
The Infectious Disease Society of America guidelines are presented for both cystitis and pyelonephritis. In the treatment of cystitis, TMP-SMX is recommended if resistance is less than 20% in the community. Otherwise, quinolones, nitrofurantoin, or fosfomycin are considered. For pyelonephritis, recommendations are made based on severity of symptoms.

Yoshikawa TT, Nicolle LE, Norman DC. Management of complicated urinary infection in older patients. *J Am Geriatr Soc* 1996;44:1235.
Describes treatment for recurrent urinary tract infection and catheter-related bacteriuria, including the special considerations in the elderly.

ASYMPTOMATIC BACTERIURIA 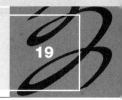 19

*H*ow does one approach a patient who has significant bacteriuria but is asymptomatic? Significant bacteriuria is defined as greater than 10^5 bacteria per milliliter of urine obtained by sterile technique on consecutive samples. Patients with significant bacteriuria who have urinary tract symptoms require antimicrobial therapy.

 ASYMPTOMATIC BACTERIURIA

Asymptomatic bacteriuria occurs when a patient with more than 10^5 bacteria per milliliter of urine on two consecutive occasions does not have symptoms of urinary tract infection.

In some patients with asymptomatic bacteriuria, including pregnant women and patients with obstructive uropathy, treatment is recommended. Treatment is felt to help prevent symptomatic upper urinary tract infection. The benefits of treatment in children and diabetics with asymptomatic bacteriuria is not as clear. Asymptomatic bacteriuria in the elderly is generally benign and does not require therapy.

Older men and women have a higher incidence of bacteriuria than younger adults, for the following reasons: (1) prostatic hypertrophy in men, (2) loss of bactericidal prostatic secretions in men, (3) perineal soiling in women, (4) bladder dysfunction and genitourinary instrumentation, and (5) loss of hormone-dependent protection against introital colonization in postmenopausal women. The incidence of bacteriuria increases with the degree of debility and institutionalization, from 2% in some ambulatory elderly to 59% in some hospitalized patients.

Because of this high incidence, the role of antimicrobial therapy in this setting has become an area of interest and controversy. In at least two studies, older nursing home patients with asymptomatic bacteriuria died earlier than those with sterile urine. Other studies have found no correlation of bacteriuria with longevity. The concern that chronic bacteriuria will cause chronic pyelonephritis is not supported by longitudinal studies. Patients with chronic pyelonephritis have underlying uropathy, hypertension, or diabetes mellitus, but not bacteriuria alone. Patients with asymptomatic bacteriuria do not develop progressive abnormalities on intravenous pyelogram. Randomized controlled trials of antimicrobial therapy for asymptomatic bacteriuria in older men and women could demonstrate no effect on mortality. Recent studies, however, have shown that in patients with asymptomatic bacteriuria studied by a bladder washout technique, localization of bacteria to the kidney is commonly found. Patients with asymptomatic bacteriuria treated with antimicrobials do not maintain urine sterility. Such therapy is associated with side effects, cost, and the development of resistant organisms. Hence, antimicrobials are generally not recommended for asymptomatic bacteriuria in the elderly. Asymptomatic bacteriuria is not in itself an indication for anatomic assessment of the urinary tract. Patients with asymptomatic bacteriuria and obstructive uropathy should receive antimicrobial therapy, as well as those with asymptomatic bacteriuria prior to genitourinary instrumentation.

In the older patient with bacteriuria whose general condition has acutely deteriorated, the term *asymptomatic bacteriuria* loses its usefulness. Urinary tract infection can present in a more subtle manner in the elderly, and patients with urosepsis may remain afebrile

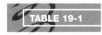

TABLE 19-1	Treating Asymptomatic Bacteriuria

A. Treatment Recommended:
   Pregnant women
   Patients with urinary tract obstruction
B. Treatment not recommended:
   The elderly
   Young women
C. Treatment controversial:
   Children—usually treated
   Diabetic patients—no evidence for efficacy

or demonstrate only mental status changes. A patient with a history of bacteriuria who becomes septic will often need to be treated for urosepsis if no definite focus of infection can be found.

Patients who require external condom catheters have a bacteriuria rate of as high as 87%. In patients with long-term Foley catheters, bacteriuria is inevitable.

Asymptomatic bacteriuria is common in young sexually active women, but it rarely persists and more than 90% of cases resolve without developing infection. Asymptomatic bacteriuria lasting more than 2 months is rare. Treatment would clearly not be indicated in this group unless symptoms occur.

The pregnant woman with asymptomatic bacteriuria represents a special situation in which the benefits of treatment outweigh risks. Reflux and resulting pyelonephritis occurs in this group. Preterm delivery and low birth weight appear to be bona-fide associations with asymptomatic bacteriuria.

The consequences of asymptomatic bacteriuria in patients with diabetes mellitus are not as well defined. The rates of asymptomatic bacteriuria in diabetic women may be similar to nondiabetics unless control of blood sugar is poor. Rates for diabetic versus nondiabetic men are similar. The overall benefits of treatment remain unproved (see Table 19-1).

Screening children for asymptomatic bacteriuria is widely recommended in the hope of preventing pyelonephritis. However, such detection has not been proved to prevent pyelonephritis or renal scarring and is now controversial. (SLB)

Bibliography

Baldassarre JS, Kaye D. Special problems of urinary tract infection in the elderly. *Med Clin North Am* 1991;75:375.
   Describes the rationale for conservative management of asymptomatic bacteriuria.
Bendall MJ. A review of urinary tract infection in the elderly. *J Antimicrob Chemother* 1984;13(suppl B):69.
   Excellent review of the international literature, particularly with respect to patterns of bacteriuria over time.
Bondadio M, et al. Asymptomatic bacteriuria in women with diabetes: influence of metabolic control. *Clin Infect Dis* 2004;38:41.
   A similar incidence of bacteriuria was found in women with and without diabetes. However, severe impairment of metabolic control did increase the incidence of bacteriuria.
Boscia JA, et al. Epidemiology of bacteriuria in an elderly ambulatory population. *Am J Med* 1986;80:208.
   Different patterns of bacteriuria occur in the elderly. Bacteriuria may be persistent or episodic.
Dontas AS, et al. Bacteriuria and survival in old age. *N Engl J Med* 1981;304:939.
   In a Greek nursing home, survival is shortened by presence of asymptomatic bacteriuria.
Geerlings SE, et al. Asymptomatic bacteriuria may be considered a complication in women with diabetes. Diabetes Mellitus Women Asymptomatic Bacteriuria Utrecht Study Group. *Diabetes Care* 2000;23:744.

Incidence of asymptomatic bacteriuria was 26% in nonpregnant women. Did not correlate with hemoglobin AC levels.

Hooten TM, et al. A prospective study of asymptomatic bacteriuria in sexually active young women. *N Engl J Med* 2000;343:992.
More than 90% of cases of asymptomatic bacteriuria in these women resolved without causing symptoms.

Kemper KJ, Avner ED. The case against screening urinalyses for asymptomatic bacteriuria in children. *Am J Dis Child* 1992;146:343.
Screening children for asymptomatic bacteriuria is considered costly and ineffective in this review.

Mims AD, et al. Clinically inapparent (asymptomatic) bacteriuria in ambulatory elderly men: Epidemiological, clinical and microbiological findings. *J Am Geriatr Soc* 1990;38: 1209.
Twenty-nine of 238 ambulatory older men had asymptomatic bacteriuria. Patients were followed up from 1 to 4.5 years. Gram-positive organisms were commonly isolated.

Mittendorf R, Williams MA, Kass EH. Prevention of preterm delivery and low birth weight associated with asymptomatic bacteriuria. *Clin Infect Dis* 1992;14:927.
Meta-analysis is used to confirm association of bacteriuria in pregnant women with preterm delivery and low-birth-weight infants.

Nicolle LE, Mayhew WJ, Bryan L. Prospective randomized comparison of therapy and no therapy for asymptomatic bacteriuria in institutionalized elderly women. *Am J Med* 1987;83:27.
A randomized trial of antimicrobial therapy in older women with asymptomatic bacteriuria. Despite a lowered prevalence of bacteriuria, no difference in genitourinary morbidity or mortality was found. Antimicrobial therapy was associated with recurrent infection, adverse drug effects, and increasingly resistant organisms.

Nicolle LE, et al. The association of bacteriuria with resident characteristics and survival in elderly institutionalized men. *Ann Intern Med* 1987;106:682.
No difference was found in the survival of older men who were bacteriuric versus nonbacteriuric.

Nicolle LE, et al. Localization of urinary tract infection in elderly, institutionalized women with asymptomatic bacteriuria. *J Infect Dis* 1988;157:65.
Using bladder washout technique, it was found that 67% of women with asymptomatic bacteriuria had upper tract infection.

Ooi ST, Frazee LA, Gardner WG. Management of asymptomatic bacteriuria in patients with diabetes mellitus. *Ann Pharmacother* 2004;38:490.
Review article that concludes that antimicrobial treatment for asymptomatic bacteriuria in the diabetic patient is not indicated.

Ouslander JG, Greengold B, Chen S. External catheter use and urinary tract infections among incontinent male nursing home patients. *J Am Geriatr Soc* 1987;35:1063.
Reports a high incidence of bacteriuria in patients with external condom catheters.

Pels RJ, et al. Dipstick urinalysis screening of asymptomatic adults for urinary tract disorders. II. Bacteriuria. *JAMA* 1989;262:1221.
Recommends that urine culture alone be used to screen pregnant women for bacteriuria. Dipstick screening may be adequate with diabetic patients.

Raz R. Asymptomatic bacteriuria. Clinical significance and management. *Int J Antimicrob Agents* 2003;22(suppl 2):45.
Review article concludes that asymptomatic bacteriuria should not be treated in the elderly, healthy school girls, diabetic women, or patients with indwelling Foley catheters.

Ronald AR, Pattullo ALS. The natural history of urinary infection in adults. *Med Clin North Am* 1991;75:299.
Reviews definitions and data on asymptomatic bacteriuria and renal function.

U.S. Preventive Services Task Force. Screening for asymptomatic bacteriuria, hematuria, and proteinuria. *Am Fam Physician* 1990;42:389.
Recommends leukocyte esterase and nitrate tests for bacteriuria screening in pregnant women, diabetic patients, and, perhaps, schoolchildren.

Zhanel GG, Harding GK, Guay DR. Asymptomatic bacteriuria. Which patients should be treated? *Arch Intern Med* 1990;150:1389.
   The authors recommend that neonates, preschool children, pregnant women, and nonelderly men be treated for asymptomatic bacteriuria.
Zhanel GG, Harding GK, Nicolle LE. Asymptomatic bacteriuria in patients with diabetes mellitus. *Rev Infect Dis* 1992;13:150.
   Excellent review of the implications of bacteriuria in diabetic patients. A 2-week course of antimicrobials is effective in initial eradication.

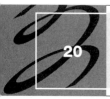

20   THE SIGNIFICANCE OF PYURIA

yuria is an important laboratory parameter in at least two different settings:

   It is extremely important in the assessment of bacterial infection of the urinary tract. It is present in almost all such infections; therefore, its absence must suggest another diagnosis.

   It is present as a nonspecific reaction to inflammation of the urinary tract. The differential diagnosis for sterile pyuria is, therefore, a broad one.

Pyuria is often arbitrarily defined as greater than 10 leukocytes per high-power microscopic field from a centrifuged specimen. This method clearly represents only a crude quantitative assessment for several reasons:

1. Initial urine volumes are variable.
2. Centrifugation is not standardized with respect to time or speed.
3. The amount of urine placed on the slide is variable.
4. With no grid for reference, there is observer bias in the area to be counted.

   Several methods for quantifying pyuria are more accurate and useful in clinical studies, though impractical for office evaluation. Measurement of pyuria as the leukocyte excretion rate has been used as a more accurate quantitative method. Rates of excretion greater than 400,000 leukocytes/hour correlate with symptomatic urinary tract infection. Measurements of pyuria by hemocytometer have correlated greater than 10 leukocytes/mm^3 with greater than 10^5 bacteria per colony forming unit (CFU).

   More recently, rapid methods to determine pyuria have received widespread use. Measurement of leukocyte esterase, an enzyme in neutrophil granules, can be determined within 1 to 2 minutes using an enzyme-impregnated dipstick. It correlates well with significant pyuria as defined by greater than 10 white blood cells (WBC)/mm^3 urine. Correlation with dipstick and microscopy is variable, depending on patient population. In one large study, the combination of negative leukocyte esterase and negative nitrate test ruled out urinary tract infection. The leukocyte esterase test need be only 80 to 90% sensitive for infection by itself.

   Stamm (1983) concluded that accurate estimation of pyuria is important for the following reasons: (1) 10 leukocytes/mm^3 or greater occurs in less than 1% of asymptomatic, nonbacteriuric patients but in more than 96% of symptomatic patients with significant bacteriuria; (2) most symptomatic women with pyuria but without significant bacteriuria do

TABLE 20-1	Causes of Sterile Pyuria

Perinephric abscess
Urethral syndrome
Chronic prostatitis
Renal tuberculosis
Fungal infection
Renal papillary necrosis
Heavy metal toxicity
Sarcoidosis
Systemic lupus erythematosus
Genitourinary malignancy
Interstitial nephritis
Transplant rejection
Transurethral prostatectomy

have urinary tract infection, either with uropathogens less than 10^5/mL or with *Chlamydia trachomatis;* (3) patients with catheter-associated bacteriuria and pyuria are more likely to have true infection. Several studies in spinal–cord-injured patients with indwelling catheters have confirmed that pyuria is a risk factor for increased morbidity secondary to untreated urinary tract infection.

Any inflammatory reaction in the urinary system can result in sterile pyuria greater than 10 WBCs/mm^3 of urine or greater than 10 WBCs per high-power microscopic field.

Pyuria may be the result of inflammation anywhere along the urinary tract, from renal parenchyma to urethra. Urinary tract infections produce a mucosal inflammatory reaction and cytokine-induced neutrophil influx. Interleukin 8 is produced by urinary tract epithelial cells.

The patient's history is important in the evaluation of pyuria, particularly with respect to prior urinary tract infections or predisposing factors for urinary tract infection. Elements that predispose to pyuria include:

> Recurrent urinary tract infection
> Recent sexual intercourse in young women
> Use of spermicide in young women
> Urinary catheterization or other instrumentation
> Diabetic women—more likely to have pyuria in some studies
> Male patients with AIDS

Sterile pyuria has become a commonly used misnomer; it used to describe pyuria in which urine cultures for bacteria are negative (Table 20-1).

Sterile pyuria can occur in chronic prostatitis, in that bladder urine will usually have less than 10^5 bacteria/mL of urine. Prostatic secretions will have high numbers of the etiologic agent. Renal papillary necrosis should be suspected in patients with sterile pyuria who have diabetes, sickle cell disease, or chronic alcoholism. Urethral inflammation may also cause pyuria. Genital herpes can cause dysuria and pyuria. Infection with *C. trachomatis* causes an acute urethral syndrome with dysuria and frequency. Patients with peripheric or renal cortical abscesses may present with signs and symptoms of upper urinary tract infection and pyuria, but negative urine cultures.

Other noninfectious causes of pyuria are uric acid and hypercalcemic nephropathy, lithium and heavy metal toxicity, genitourinary malignancy, sarcoidosis, transplant rejection, interstitial cystitis, and polycystic kidney disease. Pyuria may persist for several months after transurethral prostatectomy. (SLB)

Bibliography

Agace WW, et. al. Interleukin-8 and the neutrophil response to mucosal gram-negative infection. *J Clin Invest* 1993;92:780.

Describes how urinary tract infection induces cytokine stimulation and neutrophil influx.

Christensen WI. Genitourinary tuberculosis. Review of 102 cases. *Medicine (Baltimore)* 1974;53:377.
Ninety percent of patients with renal tuberculosis have hematuria or pyuria.

Deville WL, et al. The urine dipstick test useful to rule out infections. A meta-analysis of accuracy. *BMC Urol* 2004;4:4.
Dipstick can be used to exclude presence of infection, but the combination of leukocyte esterase and nitrate are needed. The predictive value varies with the patient population.

Dieter RS. Sterile pyuria: a differential diagnosis. *Comp Ther* 2000;26:150.
Gives categories of disease that may be responsible for pyuria.

Johnson CC. Definitions, classification, and clinical presentation of urinary tract infection. *Med Clin North Am* 1991;75:241.
Good brief descriptions of acute urethral syndrome and perinephric abscess.

Komaroff AL. Urinalysis and urine culture in women with dysuria. *Ann Intern Med* 1986;104:2.
Describes the value of the urinalysis (including urine culture and WBC in urine in various disease states).

Menon EB, Tan ES. Pyuria: index of infection in patients with spinal cord injuries. *Br J Urol* 1992;69:144.
Spinal cord patients with indwelling catheters who have more than 100 WBC per high-power field are more likely to have morbidity from urinary tract infection.

Murray T, Goldberg M. Analgesic abuse and renal disease. *Annu Rev Med* 1975;26:537.
Analgesic nephropathy as a cause of sterile pyuria is discussed.

Pappas PG. Laboratory in the diagnosis and management of urinary tract infections. *Med Clin North Am* 1991;75:313.
Describes laboratory methods for defining pyuria.

Patterson JE, Andriole VT. Renal and perirenal abscesses. *Infect Dis Clin North Am* 1987;1:907.
Renal abscesses can cause pyuria without positive cultures. Corticomedullary abscesses usually are a complication of reflux or obstruction.

Pels RJ, et al. Dipstick urinalysis screening of asymptomatic adults for urinary tract disorders. II. Bacteriuria. *JAMA* 1989;262:1221.
Describes the leukocyte esterase screening test and its correlation with WBCs in urine.

Petersen EA, et al. Coccidioiduria: clinical significance. *Ann Intern Med* 1976;85:34.
Discusses infection with Coccidioides immitis as a cause of sterile pyuria.

Pfaller MA, Koontz FP. Laboratory evaluation of leukocyte esterase and nitrite tests for the detection of bacteriuria. *J Clin Microbiol* 1985;21:840.
Reports 92% negative predictive value for urinary tract infection using leukocyte esterase screening test.

Randall RE, et al. Cryptococcal pyelonephritis. *N Engl J Med* 1968;279:60.
Discussion of infection with Cryptococcus neoformans as a cause of sterile pyuria.

Rothberg MB, Wong JB. All dysuria is local. A cost-effectiveness model for designing site-specific management algorithms. *J Gen Intern Med* 2004;19:433.
Describes all combinations of urinalysis, urine culture, pelvic exam, Chlamydia cultures, and empiric therapy in the evaluation of dysuria in office practice.

Stamm WE. Measurement of pyuria and its relation to bacteriuria. *Am J Med* 1983;75(suppl):53.
Compares methods of measuring urine leukocytes. An excellent summary of the significance of pyuria and its sensitivity and specificity in several clinical contexts.

Stamm WE, et al. Causes of the acute urethral syndrome in women. *N Engl J Med* 1980;303:409.
Describes the syndrome of dysuria and pyuria in young women. About a third of the women studied had C. trachomatis infection.

Teklu B, Ostrow JH. Urinary tuberculosis: a review of 44 cases treated since 1963. *J Urol* 1976;115:507.
Documents sterile pyuria as a frequent finding in renal tuberculosis.

Thorley JD, Jones SR, Sanford JP. Perinephric abscess. *Medicine (Baltimore)* 1974;53:441.
A review of the clinical and radiographic features of perinephric abscess.
Van Norstrand JD, Junkins AD, Bartholdi RK. Poor predictive ability of urinalysis and
microscopic examination to detect urinary tract infection. *Am J Clin Path* 2000;113:
709.
*In this study there was a lack of sensitivity for the detection of urinary tract infection
using the leukocyte esterase dipstick test even using nitrate test concomitantly.*

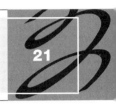

PROSTATITIS 21

rostatitis is a common but poorly understood inflammatory process in male adults. A
recent national survey estimates that almost 2 million visits are made annually in the United
States for prostatitis. Eight percent of all urology visits and 1% of all primary care visits
are for prostatitis. It is the most common urologic diagnosis in men older than age 50. The
standard classification of prostatitis as acute bacterial and chronic bacterial is now clearly
inadequate, as the majority of patients with prostatitis have a chronic condition for which
no evidence of infection can be found. The NIH Consensus Conference on Prostatitis divides the disease into six categories. Categories I and II represent the traditional syndromes
of acute and chronic bacterial prostatitis. Category III describes a chronic pelvic pain syndrome and is divided into subcategories A and B. Category III A is an inflammatory pelvic
pain syndrome evidenced by white blood cells (WBCs) in semen, expressed prostatic secretions, or postmassage urine. This category also may be described as a nonbacterial chronic
prostatitis. Category III B is a noninflammatory pelvic pain syndrome most consistent with
the term *prostatodynia*. Category IV is asymptomatic prostatitis in which inflammation is
noted as part of a workup for prostatic cancer or infertility. Table 21-1 summarizes these
categories.

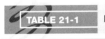 **ACUTE BACTERIAL PROSTATITIS**

The clinical diagnosis of acute bacterial prostatitis is usually straightforward. An acute
illness develops with chills, fever, and local symptoms of back or perineal pain. Symptoms

TABLE 21-1	**NIH Consensus Definition of Prostatitis**

I. Acute Bacterial Prostatitis
II. Chronic Bacterial Prostatitis
III. Chronic Prostatitis/Chronic Pelvic Pain
A. Inflammatory
B. Noninflammatory
IV. Asymptomatic Inflammatory Prostatitis

of frequency and dysuria are also present. Malaise, generalized myalgias, and prostration have been described. On rectal examination, the prostate is tender, swollen, and indurated. Urinary retention resulting from bladder outlet obstruction may be recognized by bladder percussion. Laboratory data will show an elevated peripheral WBC count. A midstream urine sample will usually have WBCs and more than 10^5 bacteria per milliliter on culture. Macrophages laden with fat droplets also may be seen. In the setting of acute bacterial prostatitis, prostatic massage may lead to bacteremia and is contraindicated.

As in other acute bacterial infections, identification of the etiologic agent is crucial to therapy. Most cases of acute bacterial prostatitis are caused by gram-negative enteric bacilli. *Escherichia coli* causes most community-acquired infections; more resistant gram-negative bacilli, such as *Klebsiella* and *Pseudomonas*, may cause hospital-acquired infection. *Enterococcus faecalis* is the only gram-positive coccus that frequently causes prostatitis. Staphylococci have been reported in some studies. In the antimicrobial era, *Neisseria gonorrhoeae* is only rarely isolated.

These organisms causing acute bacterial prostatitis are also implicated in urinary tract infection. Hypotheses on routes of infection explain this commonality. The several routes of infection in prostatitis are as follows: (1) reflux of infected urine into ejaculatory and prostatic ducts, (2) ascending urethral infection, (3) spread of colonic bacteria through the lymphatic system, and (4) hematogenous spread. Bacterial infections of the prostate are more common in patients with indwelling Foley catheters and condom catheters. Acute prostatitis has occurred in men after transurethral prostatic resection.

Recently, several investigators have described both a systemic and a local immune response in prostatitis. High levels of antigen-specific IgA become detectable immediately on diagnosis. A serum IgG response to specific antigen also occurs and declines slowly over months. Measurement of antigen-specific antibody also may be useful in determining response to therapy.

Patients with acute bacterial prostatitis should have blood cultures and urine Gram's stain and culture before antimicrobial therapy. Gram-positive cocci seen in chains suggest enterococcal infection. Ampicillin plus an aminoglycoside is a regimen of choice. Most patients will have gram-negative bacilli on smear.

Trimethoprim-sulfamethoxazole is commonly used for community-acquired infection, as it provides broad coverage for most gram-negative bacilli. Although only lipid-soluble and basic antimicrobials penetrate the normal prostate gland, diffusion into an acutely inflamed prostate is less of a problem. The severe inflammation of acute prostatitis allows agents that normally diffuse poorly into prostatic secretions to attain therapeutic levels. Quinolones, particularly ciprofloxacin, the monobactam aztreonam, aminoglycosides, and third-generation cephalosporins have all been used successfully. Antimicrobial doses should attain therapeutic levels in the serum. Response is usually dramatic. Analgesia, hydration, bed rest, and stool softener are also recommended.

Complications of acute bacterial prostatitis include septicemia, prostatic abscess, and epididymitis. Chronic prostatitis may occur after infection in some patients. Prostatic abscess results from a mixed gram-negative and anaerobic infection. Treatment of prostatic abscess may require transurethral prostatectomy.

 CHRONIC BACTERIAL PROSTATITIS

There is increasing evidence that relatively few cases of chronic prostatitis are caused by bacterial infection. National Institutes of Health (NIH) category II prostatitis represents only about 7% of cases. Chronic bacterial prostatitis is, however, a major cause of recurrent urinary tract infection in men.

Patients may have dysuria or other voiding symptoms. Chronic pain in the perineum, low back, penis, or scrotum is also described. Chills and fever are not common. Patients may give a prior history of acute bacterial prostatitis. On physical examination, the prostate may be tender, boggy, and indurated, or it may be normal.

The etiologic agents responsible for chronic prostatitis are generally those that cause urinary tract infection. *E. coli* is the most important community-acquired pathogen; more resistant gram-negative bacilli such as *Pseudomonas aeruginosa* are more likely to be hospital acquired. *E. faecalis* also is responsible for chronic prostatitis, but usually as part of a mixed infection with gram-negative bacilli. Series of patients with *Staphylococcus epidermidis* have been reported. *Mycoplasma hominis* and *Ureaplasma urealyticum* were cultured in 82 of 597 patients in one series. Higher concentrations of these organisms were found in expressed prostatic secretions than in first-voided specimens. *Chlamydia* species have not been as well established as etiologic agents. Granulomatous prostatitis is usually caused by tuberculosis or fungal infection, but may occur without a clear-cut etiology.

There is a consensus that the diagnosis of chronic prostatitis is best made by quantitative cultures of concomitantly obtained specimens from urethra, midstream bladder urine, and prostatic secretions. Quantitative cultures of four carefully collected specimens are compared, including first-voided 10 mL (VB1), midstream urine (VB2), prostatic secretions obtained after prostatic massage (expressed prostatic secretions), and first-voided 10 mL after prostatic massage (VB3). In bacterial prostatitis, bacteria in the prostatic specimens (expressed prostatic secretions and VB3) are tenfold higher than in the first two specimens. The test may be simplified by comparing bacterial growth before and after prostatic massage.

The pharmacokinetics of antimicrobials in the prostate is complex. Many antimicrobials with activity against gram-negative bacilli diffuse poorly into prostatic tissue. Trimethoprim-sulfamethoxazole appears to achieve the best prostatic fluid levels. The quinolones also achieve good levels. In general, antimicrobial bases achieve better levels than acids. To diffuse through the prostate, the antimicrobial must be lipid soluble and not bound to plasma proteins.

Trimethoprim-sulfamethoxazole has been the best studied antimicrobial for chronic prostatitis. With full-dose therapy for 4 weeks or more, a relapse rate of at least 40% is reported. Some clinicians recommend a more extensive period of therapy—as long as 6 months. Direct injection of antimicrobials into the prostate has been reported to be successful in Belgium and Sweden but it is controversial and rarely used in the United States. Quinolones are now most commonly used, but precise success versus failure rates vary from study to study.

 ## CHRONIC ABACTERIAL PROSTATITIS

It is now commonly accepted that nonbacterial prostatitis is much more common than chronic bacterial prostatitis and more difficult to categorize.

The NIH classification describes type III prostatitis as a chronic abacterial prostatitis with chronic pelvic pain syndrome. Type IIIA is an inflammatory chronic pelvic pain syndrome and type IIIB is noninflammatory. Type IIIA will show white blood cells in semen or prostatic secretions, whereas type IIIB will not.

Collins et al. examined evidence for various causation theories. These include occult infection, autoimmune disease, psychological factors, zinc levels, and various anatomical abnormalities. There is certainly no gold standard diagnostic test for this category of prostatitis, nor is it clear that this NIH classification system will be useful in treatment recommendations. Therapies for chronic abacterial prostatitis are unproven but include certain categories (Table 21-2).

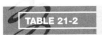 **Potential Treatments for Abacterial Prostatitis**

Medications used to treat benign prostatic hypertrophy
• Anti-inflammatory agents
• Antibiotics
• Thermotherapy
• Allopurinol
• Quercetin

Adequately powered, randomized controlled trials will be needed before treatment recommendations can be made. Evidence is currently not adequate to recommend routine antibiotics or alpha blocker treatment.

The NIH classification also includes a category for patients who are asymptomatic but have evidence of inflammation either by prostatic biopsy for elevated prostate-specific antigen (PSA) or semen analysis for infertility study. The implications of such asymptomatic inflammation is not known. (SLB)

Bibliography

Barbalias GA, et al. Alpha-blockers for the treatment of chronic prostatitis in combination with antibiotics. *J Urol* 1998;159:883.
   Alpha blockers were found to be beneficial in bacterial prostatitis, nonbacterial prostatitis, and prostatodynia. Patients with nonbacterial prostatitis did better with alpha blockers than with a combination of antibiotics and alpha blockers.

Becopoulos T, et al. Acute prostatitis: which antibiotic to use first. *J Chemother* 1990;2: 244.
   Describes serum and prostatic tissue concentrations of six antimicrobials administered to 48 patients just before prostatectomy.

Collins MM, MacDonald, R, Wilt TJ. Diagnosis and treatment of chronic abacterial prostatitis. A systematic review. *Ann Intern Med* 2000;133:367–381.
   Extensive review article that includes theories of causation and analysis of treatment trials. The paucity of good data is emphasized.

Hua VN, Schaeffer AJ. Acute and chronic prostatitis. *Med Clin North Am* 2004;88:483–494.
   Detailed comparison of old versus new NIH classification of prostatitis syndromes.

Krieger JN, Egan KJ. Comprehensive evaluation and treatment of 75 men referred to chronic prostatitis clinic. *Urology* 1991;38:11.
   The authors describe their clinical experience with a chronic prostatitis clinic. A comprehensive approach to diagnosis led to specific treatment in 49% of patients.

Krieger JN. Prostatitis revisited. New definitions, new approaches. *Infect Dis Clin North Am* 2003:17:395–407.
   Emphasizes the role of research to determine whether differences in classification measures will make practical difference in diagnosis and treatment. Includes new definitions.

Krieger JN, Ross SO, Riley DE. Chronic prostatitis. Epidemiology and role of infection. *Urology* 2002;60:8–13.
   Documents high incidence of prostatitis worldwide.

Lipsky BA. Urinary tract infections in men. Epidemiology, pathophysiology, diagnosis, and treatment. *Ann Intern Med* 1989;110:138.
   Gram-negative bacilli are responsible for 75% of cases of acute bacterial prostatitis.

Litwin MS, et al. The National Institutes of Health chronic prostatitis symptom index. Development and validation of a new outcome measure. *J Urol* 1999;162:369–375.
   Thirteen items used to quantify symptoms and quality of life in prostatitis.

Meares EM Jr. Prostatitis. *Med Clin North Am* 1991;75:405.
   Detailed review of types of prostatitis and their diagnosis and treatment. Includes discussion of immune response in bacterial prostatitis. Recommends 30 days of therapy for acute prostatitis.

Naber KG. Use of quinolones in urinary tract infections and prostatitis. *Rev Infect Dis* 1989;11(suppl 1321):37.
   Quinolones are shown to achieve good concentrations in prostatic tissue and seminal fluid.

Naber KG. The role of quinolones in the treatment of chronic bacterial prostatitis. *Infection* 1991;19(suppl 3):S170.
   A review of 23 studies of the efficacy of quinolones in bacterial prostatitis. Most were not randomized, and many did not include adequate follow-up.

Nickel JC, et al. Prevalence of prostatitis-like symptoms in a population based study using the NIH chronic prostatitis symptom index. *J Urol* 2001;165:842–845.

Overall, 9.7% of men were classified as having some type of NIH prostatitis syndrome in this survey study.

Roberts RO, et al. Prevalence of a physician-assigned diagnosis of prostatitis: the Olmsted County study of urinary symptoms and health status among men. *Urology* 1998;51:578.
Community-based prevalence of physician-assigned diagnosis of prostatitis is high, similar to that of ischemic heart disease. Men who have a single episode of a prostatitis syndrome had a 20 to 50% chance of a second episode.

Wolfson JS, Hooper DC. Fluoroquinolone antimicrobial agents. *Clin Microbiol Rev* 1989; 2:378.
Reviews the efficacy of quinolones in prostatitis.

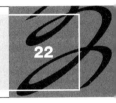

COMPLICATED URINARY TRACT INFECTIONS

22

A complicated urinary tract infection (UTI) is defined as either pyelonephritis or a urinary tract infection with a structural or functional abnormality. Traditionally, infections in men and children have been defined as complicated UTIs, but others also may be at risk, as shown in Table 22-1.

Imaging studies (ultrasound, computed tomography [CT]) should be ordered to evaluate for obstruction. Obstruction may cause a change in intrarenal blood flow and affect antibiotic delivery. Of course, one should obtain a urine analysis with microscopic examination, along with urine culture and sensitivity testing. The white blood cell (WBC) count will often remain elevated for several days in complicated cases, and the serum creatinine might deteriorate despite appropriate therapy.

 ## URINARY TRACT OBSTRUCTION

As mentioned previously, diagnostic imaging is extremely important in diagnosing most of these conditions. Along with broad-spectrum antibiotics, urgent consultation with a urologist should be undertaken to help diagnose and relieve obstruction. If ureteral

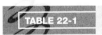 **TABLE 22-1** **Patients at Risk for a Complicated UTI**

Structural or functional abnormalities	Other
Spinal cord lesion	Diabetes
Neurogenic bladder	Those with persistent fever
Indwelling Foley	Urea Splitting Organisms/Tuberculosis
Stones	Those with bacterial persistence
Papillary necrosis	Men
Pregnancy	Children
	Transplants
	Nosocomial acquisition

TABLE 22-2	Cause of Obstruction		
Congenital	**Intrinsic**	**Extrinsic**	**Microbiologic**
Posterior urethral valves	Urethral strictures, bladder outlet obstruction, cystocele, stone, fungus ball, papillary necrosis	Retroperitoneal mass/cancer	Urea splitting organisms producing struvite stones

obstruction is present and the patient is otherwise stable, cystoscopy should be performed with placement of an indwelling ureteral stent. If stent placement cannot be achieved or the patient has an underlying lesion not easily amenable to stent placement, percutaneous nephrostomy tube (PNT) placement should be considered. Generally PNT is a safe procedure. One study noted that there were 22 major complications (4%) in 569 procedures, including cardiac arrest, bleeding requiring transfusion or embolization, septicemia, hydrothorax, or pneumothorax. Thirty-eight percent of complications were minor, including UTI, catheter dislodgement, catheter obstruction by debris, urinary leakage, and inflammation of the skin at the site of insertion of the percutaneous catheter. Shockwave lithotripsy is contraindicated during pregnancy because of theoretical risks to the fetus and ovaries. Causes of urinary tract obstruction are shown in Table 22-2.

URINARY TRACT INFECTIONS IN PREGNANCY

Elevated progesterone levels of pregnancy lead to a decreased ureteral peristalsis and increased bladder capacity. The urinary bladder is physically displaced superiorly and anteriorly by the gravid uterus, leading to urinary stasis. The more commonly reported risk factors for UTI during pregnancy are a medically indigent status, sickle cell hemoglobin, diabetes, a history of UTI, and a neurogenic bladder. Asymptomatic bacteriuria is the most common UTI encountered during pregnancy, occurring in 2 to 7% of all pregnant women. Less than 1% of women actually acquire bacteriuria during pregnancy if their initial screening culture is negative, unless they have one of the risk factors listed previously. Organisms causing UTIs during pregnancy are usually gram-negative Enterobacteriaceae and group B streptococcus (GBS).

All pregnant women should undergo a urine analysis with microscopy and culture early in pregnancy to evaluate for asymptomatic bacteriuria. Asymptomatic bacteriuria in pregnancy is associated with prematurity and low birth weight, maternal anemia, and maternal hypertension. Other screening techniques that have been used for the detection of bacteriuria during pregnancy include leukocyte esterase activity, the nitrite test, and microscopic examination of a drop of unspun urine for bacteria. It is now generally accepted that routine urinalysis is inaccurate and should not be used alone as a screening tool for bacteriuria during pregnancy. Generally the nonculture tests lack sufficient sensitivity compared to culture. If the initial urine culture reveals no organisms, a repeat urine culture should be performed at 16 weeks' gestation. Acute pyelonephritis will develop in approximately one fourth of all pregnant women with untreated bacteriuria in comparison with 3 to 4% of women who are treated. Treatment options for these patients can be seen in Table 22-3. A follow-up urine culture should be performed to check for eradication of the organism. Approximately one third of women will have a recurrent UTI, so they should be recultured frequently. Pregnant females with a diagnosis of pyelonephritis are at an increased risk of premature labor. The initiation of antibiotics for the treatment of acute pyelonephritis actually may initiate uterine activity and also increase the risk of adult respiratory distress syndrome. Third-generation cephalosporins or broad-spectrum penicillin antibiotics are generally used for initial therapy. Follow-up cultures are important to ensure eradication.

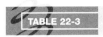

TABLE 22-3   Treatment of Asymptomatic Bacteriuria of Pregnancy

3-Day regimens (preferred)	Relapse of infection or lack of eradication	Suppression	Antibiotics to be avoided if possible*
Ampicillin 250 mg q.i.d. Amoxicillin 500 mg t.i.d. Cephalexin 250 mg q.i.d. Bactrim DS b.i.d. Nitrofurantoin 100 mg b.i.d.	For relapse, an extended course based on culture and sensitivity results is suggested, such as a 10- to 21-day course of nitrofurantoin 100 mg twice a day. Base on sensitivities.	Nitrofurantoin, 100 mg orally every night for the remainder of pregnancy is one option. Base on sensitivities.	Quinolones Tetracycline Aminoglycosides Third trimester use of Bactrim and nitrofurantoin

*Sulfa-containing antibiotics will compete for fetal bilirubin-binding sites on albumin, predisposing the fetus to kernicterus, especially in premature infants. Nitrofurantoin can cause hemolytic anemia in those with glucose-6-phosphate dehydrogenase deficiency, so caution is advised.

URINARY TRACT INFECTIONS IN PATIENTS WITH SPINAL CORD INJURY AND NEUROPATHIC BLADDER

Because of altered sensation, these patients often present with complaints of cloudy urine, vague abdominal discomfort, malaise, lethargy, or just fever. Studies have shown that intermittent catheterization is preferred over indwelling catheterization. Neither the technique of intermittent catheterization (sterile or nonsterile) nor the type of catheter appears to change the incidence of UTI. Silver oxide catheters may decrease the risk of infection, but this is controversial. If indwelling catheters are used, there is a chance of forming a biofilm on the catheter. As this biofilm worsens with time, it has been recommended that long-term catheters be changed at least monthly (2 weeks to 3 months).

UTIs in this population frequently are asymptomatic, polymicrobial, caused by antibiotic-resistant bacteria, and very likely to recur or relapse. Asymptomatic bacteriuria in spinal cord-injured patients is generally not treated because of the fear of resistance. Typically fluoroquinolones are chosen as initial therapy because of their broad spectrum of activity. The optimal duration of therapy has not been established, but I recommend a 7- to 14-day course. Follow-up cultures should be obtained to ensure eradication, but long-term surveillance cultures are not necessary in most patients, as they are frequently colonized with bacteria. Prophylactic antibiotics are of limited usefulness because of the fear of emerging resistance. The regular use of antimicrobial prophylaxis for most patients who have neurogenic bladder caused by spinal cord dysfunction is not supported.

For those patients who require persistent treatment, obstruction should be ruled out. PNL in patients with neurogenic voiding dysfunction is safe and effective, with outcomes comparable to that of patients without such lesions. The complication rate is small but statistically significant. It is important to obtain adequate urine cultures, because renal pelvis and bladder culture data may differ and affect the outcome. Risk factors for recurrent stone disease include a high spinal cord lesion, indwelling urinary catheter, and ureterosigmoidostomy. In patients who are found to have high intravesical pressures (>40 cm H_2O), interventions to decrease storage pressures (i.e., anticholinergics, bladder augmentation) should be considered. Urinary diversion surgery may be indicated in selected patients as well.

URINARY TRACT INFECTIONS IN PATIENTS WITH URINARY DIVERSION

When UTI is suspected, patients should have the conduit urine obtained by catheterization through a sterile catheter for culture, as these patients are frequently colonized by bacteria. Infectious disease and urologic consultations are advised.

 URINARY TRACT INFECTIONS IN DIABETIC PATIENTS

Complicated UTIs are more common in diabetic patients. These patients are at an increased risk for pyelonephritis, papillary necrosis, renal carbuncle, renal and perinephric abscesses, and, as noted below, emphysematous pyelonephritis. The clinician should have a low threshold to order appropriate imaging studies. Asymptomatic bacteriuria occurs in diabetic women more commonly than in nondiabetics and is associated with an increased risk of symptomatic UTI among patients with type 2 diabetes. Symptomatic UTIs tend to follow a more complicated course in diabetics. Despite these independent observations, antimicrobial therapy has not been shown to reduce symptomatic UTIs, pyelonephritis, or hospitalization for UTI. Broad-spectrum antibiotics are indicated. Trimethoprim-sulfamethoxazole can lead to hypoglycemic episodes. Patients should have follow-up urine cultures to ensure eradication.

 EMPHYSEMATOUS PYELONEPHRITIS

Emphysematous pyelonephritis is a life-threatening acute necrotizing parenchymal and perirenal infection caused by gas-forming bacteria (facultative anaerobes, such as *Escherichia coli*, *Proteus*, and *Klebsiella*). It occurs primarily in diabetics and patients with papillary necrosis and renal obstruction. CT scan is the diagnostic imaging of choice.

Treatment includes broad-spectrum antimicrobial therapy and relief of obstruction if present. Urgent urologic consultation is advised. Traditionally, a nephrectomy is recommended for all patients. Percutaneous drainage has been used as well in selected patients.

 PERINEPHRIC ABSCESS

Historically perinephric abscesses were hematogenously spread and, therefore, caused by *Staphylococcus aureus*. More recently, ascending gram-negative organisms are the major cause, with gram-positive organisms seen less often. Yeast may also cause these infections in immunocompromised patients. A high index of suspicion is advised, especially in patients with a history of stone disease, genitourinary surgery, severe diabetes, polycystic renal disease of dialysis, urinary tract obstruction, cancer, or immunosuppression. Patients who do not respond after a few days of appropriate antibiotics need an imaging study, and CT is the procedure of choice. Abscesses may be intrarenal, cortical, perinephric or paranephric (outside Gerota's fascia).

Small abscesses may resolve spontaneously with antimicrobial therapy alone, but most patients need a urologic or interventional radiologist to see the patient. PNT placement or percutaneous drainage of the abscess may be required. Severe cases may require a nephrectomy. (JWM)

Bibliography

Delzell JE Jr, Lefevre ML. Urinary tract infections during pregnancy. *Am Fam Physician* 2000;61:713–721.
  Recurrent infections are common during pregnancy and require prophylactic treatment. Pregnant women with urinary GBS infection should be treated and should receive intrapartum prophylactic therapy.
Dunn SR, et al. Emphysematous pyelonephritis: report of 3 cases treated by nephrectomy. *J Urol* 1975;114:348–350.

Incision and drainage are reserved for poor surgical risk patients. All patients should remain on antibacterial therapy and have frequent follow-up examinations.

Garcia Leoni ME, Esclarin De Ruz A. Management of urinary tract infection in patients with spinal cord injuries. *Clin Microbiol Infect* 2003;9:780–785.

The classic symptoms of UTI are unreliable indicators in spinal cord injury patients with neurogenic bladder. Lack of pyuria reasonably predicts the absence of UTI in patients with spinal cord injury. Asymptomatic bacteriuria need not be treated with antibiotics. Symptomatic UTI warrants therapy in all patients.

Gilstrap LC 3rd, Ramin SM. Urinary tract infections during pregnancy. *Obstet Gynecol Clin North Am* 2001;28:581–591.

Excellent review article. Pregnant women with UTIs should be followed up closely after treatment, because as many as one third will experience a recurrence.

Harding GK, et al. Antimicrobial treatment in diabetic women with asymptomatic bacteriuria. *N Engl J Med* 2002;347:1576–1583.

Treatment of asymptomatic bacteriuria in women with diabetes does not appear to reduce complications. Diabetes itself should not be an indication for screening for, or treatment of, asymptomatic bacteriuria.

Hoepelman A I, et al. Pathogenesis and management of bacterial urinary tract infections in adult patients with diabetes mellitus. *Int J Antimicrob Agents* 2003;22(suppl 2): 35–43.

The recommended treatment of acute pyelonephritis does not differ from that in nondiabetic patients. Clinical trials specifically dealing with the treatment of UTIs in diabetic patients, comparing the optimal duration and choice of antimicrobial agent, are needed.

Maynard FM, Diokno AC. Clean intermittent catheterization for spinal cord injury patients. *J Urol* 1982;128:477–480.

Clean intermittent catheterization appears to be a safe and satisfactory alternative for long-term management of the neurogenic bladder of selected patients with spinal cord injury, as the incidence of serious renal complications is low.

Morton SC, et al. Antimicrobial prophylaxis for urinary tract infection in persons with spinal cord dysfunction. *Arch Phys Med Rehabil* 2002;83:129–138.

The regular use of antimicrobial prophylaxis for most patients who have neurogenic bladder caused by spinal cord dysfunction is not supported. A clinically important effect, however, has not been excluded. Future research should focus on randomized trials in those patients who have recurrent UTIs that limit their daily functioning and well-being.

Naber KG, et al. EAU guidelines for the management of urinary and male genital tract infections. Urinary Tract Infection (UTI) Working Group of the Health Care Office (HCO) of the European Association of Urology (EAU). *Eur Urol* 2001;40:576–588.

The topics include classification, diagnosis, treatment, and follow-up of uncomplicated UTI, UTI in children, UTI in diabetes mellitus, renal insufficiency, renal transplant recipients and immunosuppression, complicated UTI caused by urologic disorders, sepsis syndrome, urosepsis, urethritis, prostatitis, epididymitis, orchitis, and principles of perioperative prophylaxis in urology.

Nicolle LE. Asymptomatic bacteriuria: when to screen and when to treat. *Infect Dis Clin North Am* 2003;17:367–394.

Different populations have unique risk factors, and the benefits and risks of different management approaches for asymptomatic bacteriuria must continue to be addressed systematically in appropriate clinical trials.

Ooi ST, et al. Management of asymptomatic bacteriuria in patients with diabetes mellitus. *Ann Pharmacother* 2004;38:490–493.

A review of the literature regarding the management of asymptomatic bacteriuria (ASB) in patients with diabetes mellitus. Available evidence does not support antimicrobial treatment of ASB among patients with diabetes mellitus.

Patterson JE, Andriole VT. Bacterial urinary tract infections in diabetes. *Infect Dis Clin North Am* 1997;11:735–750.

Diabetes mellitus has a number of long-term effects on the genitourinary system. Ultrasonography or further radiographic studies, such as CT scanning, may also be warranted, depending on the clinical picture, to identify upper urinary tract complications early for appropriate intervention.

Radecka E, Magnusson A. Complications associated with percutaneous nephrostomies. A retrospective study. *Acta Radiol* 2004;45:184–188.

Percutaneous nephrostomy is a gentle procedure associated with high technical success and low morbidity. However, the risk of the procedure has to be weighed against the expected benefit.

Rubenstein JN, Schaeffer AJ. Managing complicated urinary tract infections: the urologic view. *Infect Dis Clin North Am* 2003;17:333–351.

Comprehensive, excellent review. Appropriate urinary tract imaging, antimicrobials, medical and surgical therapies, and follow-up are required to avoid potentially devastating outcomes.

Siroky MB. Pathogenesis of bacteriuria and infection in the spinal cord injured patient. *Am J Med* 2002;113(suppl 1A):67S–79S.

Spinal cord injury produces profound alterations in lower urinary tract function. Incontinence, elevated intravesical pressure, reflux, stones, and neurologic obstruction, commonly found in the spinal cord-injured population, increase the risk of urinary infection. The overall rate of urinary infection in spinal cord injured patients is about 2.5 episodes per patient per year. Guidelines for selecting antimicrobial agents in spinal cord injured patients are similar to guidelines for the treatment of complicated urinary infections in the general population. Characteristics of the quinolones make them well suited to treating UTI in the spinal cord injured patient.

Stapleton A. Urinary tract infections in patients with diabetes. *Am J Med* 2002;113(suppl 1A):80S–84S.

Treatment of asymptomatic bacteriuria in patients with diabetes is often recommended to prevent the risk of symptomatic UTI. However, the management of asymptomatic bacteriuria in patients with diabetes is complex, with no single preferred approach. Compare to the article by Harding, above.

Watson RA, et al. Percutaneous nephrostomy as adjunct management in advanced upper urinary tract infection. *Urology* 1999;54:234–239.

In particular, this review focuses attention on the clinically important insight that urine cultures from percutaneous nephrostomy drainage often identify pathogens that differ from those detected in concurrent bladder cultures.

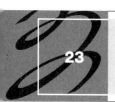

23 CANDIDURIA

*M*ost positive *Candida* urine cultures are isolated or transient findings of little significance and represent colonization rather than true infection. *Candida* urinary tract infections (UTIs) are important nosocomial infections.

Candiduria is usually defined as the presence of greater than 10^5 fungal colony-forming units (cfu)/mL urine. The prevalence of candiduria can occur in up to 20% of hospitalized patients, and it is often uncertain as to whether one is dealing with colonization alone or an infection. The absence of pyuria and low colony counts tend to rule out *Candida* infection, but the low specificity of pyuria and colony counts of more than 10^3 cfu/mL of urine require that results be interpreted in the proper clinical context. Probably only 3 to 4% of cases of candiduria lead to candidemia, but 10% of all cases of candidemia are associated with a prior episode of candiduria. Microscopy for the presence of white blood cells and casts may be useful in differentiating colonization from UTI. If the patient has not been catheterized nor had urologic instrumentation recently, it is prudent to screen for diabetes mellitus and renal insufficiency by biochemical testing and for anatomic anomalies using ultrasound. Ultrasound of the renal tract also can demonstrate the presence of fungal balls in patients who have persistent candiduria. Reasonable tests to screen for the possibility of disseminated candidiasis would include a chest radiograph, abdominal ultrasound, C-reactive protein, cultures of other potentially infected sites (e.g., tracheal aspirate or bronchial lavage, bile, surgical drains, intravascular line tips) and blood cultures.

Candiduria can arise in several ways; colonization of the urinary tract may occur in the catheterized patient. Common factors predisposing to such infections include ongoing broad-spectrum antibiotic therapy, diabetes mellitus, renal insufficiency and anatomic anomalies of the urinary tract. Patients may seed their urinary tract from bloodstream spread as well. Many infections are associated with the use of Foley catheters, internal stents, and percutaneous nephrostomy tubes. Diabetic patients, especially when their diabetes is poorly controlled, are particularly at risk, primarily because of increased instrumentation, urinary stasis, and obstruction secondary to autonomic neuropathy. Antimicrobials similarly play a critical role, in that candiduria almost always emerges during or immediately after antibiotic therapy. Antibiotics, especially broad-spectrum agents, act by suppressing protective indigenous bacterial flora in the gastrointestinal (GI) tract and lower genital tract, facilitating *Candida* colonization of these sites with ready access to the urinary tract.

It is clear that colonization usually can be treated by simply replacing the urinary catheter or removing it permanently if possible. True infection of the urinary tract should be treated with a short, definitive course of an antifungal agent, usually fluconazole, in addition to catheter removal. Prognosis depends on the anatomic site of *Candida* infection and the presence of urinary drainage tubes, obstruction, and concomitant renal failure. Candiduria is often a marker of severe disease. A high mortality rate of 20% is found in candiduria patients, which is a reflection of the multiple serious illnesses found in these patients. *Candida albicans* is usually the most common species isolated from the urine, whereas non-*albicans Candida* species account for almost half the *Candida* urine isolates. *C. glabrata* is responsible for 25 to 35% of infections. Risk factors for *C. glabrata* UTI are similar to those that predispose patients to *C. albicans* infections.

 ## ASYMPTOMATIC CANDIDURIA

Usually, no antifungal therapy is required for asymptomatic candiduria. An exception is the presence of asymptomatic candiduria after renal transplantation. In catheterized patients, *removal of the catheter* often results in cessation of candiduria (40%). *Change of catheter* results in elimination of candiduria in only 20% of patients. However, persistent candiduria in noncatheterized patients should be investigated because the likelihood of obstruction is high. Also, those patients who are about to undergo urologic instrumentation or surgery should have candiduria eliminated before the procedure. Successful elimination can be achieved by amphotericin B irrigation using a concentration of 50 μg/dL of sterile water for 5 days or with systemic therapy using amphotericin B, flucytosine, or fluconazole. Fluconazole, 200 mg/day, as oral therapy should continue for at least 7 days.

 ## *CANDIDA* CYSTITIS

Symptomatic cystitis requires treatment with either amphotericin B bladder irrigation (50 μg/dL) or systemic therapy. The quantity and duration of bladder irrigations with amphotericin B remain a matter of controversy. Some clinical studies advocate daily irrigation of a 50 mg/L solution of amphotericin B administered for 7 days, whereas other investigators advocate daily instillation of 200 to 300 mL of amphotericin B given for 60 to 90 minutes.

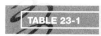

TABLE 23-1	Treatment Options for Candiduria	
Asymptomatic candiduria	**Candida cystitis**	**Candida pyelonephritis or sepsis**
Do not treat	Fluconazole 200 mg daily for	Fluconazole
Consider changing the	14 days	Systemic amphotericin B
catheter or	Less often amphotericin	Caspofungin
discontinuation, if possible	irrigation of 50 mg/L	Treat until blood cultures are
If treatment is indicated (very	solution of amphotericin B	negative for at least
rare), consider fluconazole	administered for 2–7 days.	2 weeks
first or perhaps	Usually given for 5 days.	
amphotericin irrigation	Rarely systemic	
Treatment might be indicated	amphotericin as a single	
in renal transplants or	dose of 0.3 mg/kg IV	
other	? flucytosine	
immunocompromised	*Non-albicans species will	
individuals, or those	still often respond to	
undergoing invasive	Diflucan but might require	
procedures	other therapy	
Candida krusei is usually resistant to fluconazole.		

Studies comparing bladder irrigations and oral fluconazole in older patients noted that amphotericin B irrigation had an initial success rate of 96% versus 73% for fluconazole. A repeat course of therapy was necessary in 24% of the amphotericin B group and 18% of the fluconazole group. One month after treatment, the eradication rate was similar for both groups (84% for the amphotericin B group and 80% for the fluconazole group). Of the oral azole agents, both ketoconazole and itraconazole are poorly excreted in the urine and there is limited and suboptimal clinical experience only. The usual dose of fluconazole of 200 mg/day is prescribed for 7 to 14 days. Single-dose IV amphotericin B, 0.3 mg/kg, also has been shown to be useful in the treatment of lower urinary tract candidiasis. Some physicians use flucytosine, 25 mg/kg per day given orally for 7 to 14 days. Resistance and toxicity limit the use of flucytosine. *C. glabrata* is somewhat resistant to fluconazole. Fluconazole, in contrast to other azoles, achieves a high concentration in the urine, which is usually tenfold higher than its concentration in the serum. Therefore, a 400-mg dose of fluconazole results in urine concentrations in excess of 100 μg/mL in patients with normal renal function. The MIC_{50} of *C. glabrata* for fluconazole is usually approximately 8 μg/mL; therefore, patients might respond to this agent if isolated in the urine but caution is advised (see Table 23-1).

ASCENDING PYELONEPHRITIS AND *CANDIDA* UROSEPSIS

An upper UTI requires systemic antifungal therapy, as well as an investigation to rule out obstruction, papillary necrosis, or a fungus ball. The fungus ball may complicate ascending or descending infections and tends to be found in dilated areas of the urinary tract, especially in the presence of obstruction and stasis. An ultrasound or computed tomogram (CT) often shows these fungus balls. Irrigation of nephrostomy tubes with either amphotericin B or fluconazole may serve to achieve high concentrations of antifungal agents at the site of infection. Urologic consultation is advised. Management of renal candidiasis secondary to hematogenous spread is the same as systemic candidiasis, including IV amphotericin B, 0.6 to 1.0 mg/kg per day, or IV fluconazole, 5 to 10 mg/kg per day for several weeks. (JWM)

Bibliography

Agustin J, et al. Failure of a lipid amphotericin B preparation to eradicate candiduria: preliminary findings based on three cases. *Clin Infect Dis* 1999;29:686–687.

Ayen O, et al. Clinicians' reaction to positive urine culture for Candida organisms. *Mycoses* 1999;42:285–289.

These findings show that clinicians nowadays do not follow current guidelines for the management of candiduria. Efforts to increase clinicians' awareness of these guidelines, which are intended to confirm the diagnosis and stratify treatment according to patient risk factors, appear to be necessary.

Castiglia M, et al. Fluconazole therapy for candiduria. *J Fam Pract* 1995;416:536.

Chakrabarti A, et al. Does candiduria predict candidaemia? *Indian J Med Res* 1997;106: 513–516.

The authors evaluated the reliability of candiduria as an indicator of systemic candidosis. The sensitivity and specificity of urine culture for predicting candidemia were 65.8% and 60.4%, respectively, positive predictive value was 54.3%, and negative predictive value 71.1%. Therefore, candiduria is not a reliable indicator of candidemia. However, the isolation of non-albicans Candida *species from urine was a better indicator for candidemia compared with isolation of* C. albicans *as 59.5% of patients with non-albicans* Candida *species in urine had candidemia compared with 33.3% with* C. albicans.

Chiew YF. Candidal renal papillary necrosis: report of a case and review. *Singapore Med J* 1996;37:119–121.

Renal papillary necrosis (RPN) due to Candida *is a rare disease with only 19 cases reported over the past 37 years. Indeed, patients with underlying diseases who develop persistent candiduria should have radiographic investigation of the urinary tract to detect candidal RPN so that early remedial measures can be carried out.*

de Oliveira RD, et al. [Nosocomial urinary tract infections by Candida species]. *Rev Assoc Med Bras* 2001;47:231–235.

Isolation of a yeast in urine does not necessarily indicate infection, but Candida *urinary tract infection is an increasing nosocomial problem. The overall mortality in the 60 days after the candiduria episode was 40%. Conclusions: The non-albicans species of* Candida *were the major agents of candiduria and are emergent pathogens of the urinary tract in critically ill patients. The underlying illnesses, risk factors, and high mortality commonly associated with* Candida *UTI also were observed in a Brazilian university hospital.*

Fisher JF. Candiduria: when and how to treat it. *Curr Infect Dis Rep* 2000;2:523–530.

The clinical finding of candiduria is often an enigmatic problem for the evaluating physician. The significance of yeast in the urine can range from procurement contamination to a sign of a life-threatening, opportunistic fungal infection. Proper evaluation requires validation of funguria, consideration of the setting in which it occurs, and the status of the patient. Provided that the patient is clinically stable, asymptomatic candiduria usually need not be treated with an antifungal agent. Rather, management should be directed at the elimination of predisposing factors, if feasible. When treatment is required, appropriate agents include amphotericin B (AmB), various lipid preparations of AmB (L-AmB), azoles, and flucytosine. Parenteral AmB is most useful against life-threatening infections in which the urinary tract is but one component of a widespread infection, or when resistant Candida *are causative. Shorter courses of therapy may be preferable in certain cases. L-AmB treatment has been less successful. Intravesical AmB is a time-honored approach, but is best used diagnostically rather than therapeutically. Fluconazole is currently the agent of first choice for susceptible fungi, but dosage and duration of therapy have not been established. Flucytosine is a useful alternative, especially for resistant* Candida, *but its toxicity must be closely monitored.*

Fong IW. The value of a single amphotericin B bladder washout in candiduria. *J Antimicrob Chemother* 1995;36:1067–1071.

The sensitivity of a positive urine culture for Candida *species after a single amphotericin B bladder washout in predicting kidney infection or invasive candidiasis was 100% (confidence interval [CI] = 63–100%); but the specificity was only 81% (CI = 47–100%) and the positive predictive value only 44%.*

Gross M, et al. Unexpected candidemia complicating ureteroscopy and urinary stenting. *Eur J Clin Microbiol Infect Dis* 1998;17:583–586.

Candiduria may present a risk for dissemination during invasive, relatively simple urologic procedures.

Gubbins PO, et al. Current management of funguria. *Am J Health Syst Pharm* 1999;56:1929–1935; quiz 1936.

Recent findings on the epidemiology and treatment of funguria are reviewed. Studies indicate that intravesical amphotericin B and oral fluconazole therapy are each effective in clearing funguria. Intravesical amphotericin B appears to act more rapidly; however, the effect of systemic fluconazole therapy often persists longer than that of amphotericin B irrigation, and oral therapy is more convenient and less expensive. Oral fluconazole appears to have a more delayed but more lasting effect on funguria than amphotericin B bladder irrigation. Studies are needed to determine whether intravesical amphotericin B still has a role in the treatment of funguria and to refine strategies involving fluconazole.

Harris AD, et al. Risk factors for nosocomial candiduria due to Candida glabrata and Candida albicans. *Clin Infect Dis* 1999;29:926–928.

In conclusion, patients receiving fluconazole treatment are at risk of developing C. glabrata candiduria.

Hsu CC, Ukleja B. Clearance of Candida colonizing the urinary bladder by a two-day amphotericin B irrigation. *Infection* 1990;18:280–282.

The minimum duration of continuous amphotericin B irrigation (50 mg/L per day) required to clear the Candida colonizing the urinary bladder was investigated. Because of the relatively short irrigation time, the protocol may be useful in clinical evaluation of the site of urinary candidiasis.

Huang CT, Leu HS. Candiduria as an early marker of disseminated infection in critically ill surgical patients. *J Trauma* 1995;39:616.

Johnson JR. Should all catheterized patients with candiduria be treated? *Clin Infect Dis* 1993;17:814.

Lundstrom T, Sobel J. Nosocomial candiduria: a review. *Clin Infect Dis* 2001;32:1602–1607.

Comprehensive review article. This review summarizes the state of the art of diagnosis and management of candiduria.

Pappas PG, et al. Guidelines for treatment of candidiasis. *Clin Infect Dis* 2004;38:161–189.

Sobel JD. Management of asymptomatic candiduria. *Int J Antimicrob Agents* 1999;11:285–288.

Reference is made to a recent placebo-controlled prospective study in which fluconazole was significantly more effective than placebo in short-term eradication of asymptomatic candiduria. Nevertheless, follow-up of these asymptomatic patients revealed identical candiduria rates within 1 month of cessation of therapy. In most studies, evidence of clinical benefit in asymptomatic patients by the eradication of candiduria has not been evident. In conclusion, the majority of hospitalized patients, particularly those with continued catheterization, do not require local or systemic antifungal therapy for asymptomatic candiduria.

Sobel JD, et al. Candiduria: a randomized, double-blind study of treatment with fluconazole and placebo. The National Institute of Allergy and Infectious Diseases (NIAID) Mycoses Study Group. *Clin Infect Dis* 2000;30:19–24.

Management of candiduria is limited by the lack of information about its natural history and lack of data from controlled studies on the efficacy of treating it with antimycotic agents. We compared fungal eradication rates among 316 consecutive candiduric (asymptomatic or minimally symptomatic) hospitalized patients treated with fluconazole (200 mg) or placebo daily for 14 days. In an intent-to-treat analysis, candiduria cleared by day 14 in 79 (50%) of 159 patients receiving fluconazole and 46 (29%) of 157 patients receiving placebo (P < .001), with higher eradication rates among patients completing 14 days of therapy (P < .0001), including 33 (52%) of 64 catheterized and 42 (78%) of 54 noncatheterized patients. Pretreatment serum creatinine levels were inversely related to candiduria eradication. Fluconazole initially produced high eradication rates, but cultures at 2 weeks revealed similar candiduria rates among treated and untreated patients. Oral fluconazole was safe and effective for short-term eradication of candiduria, *especially after catheter removal. Long-term eradication rates were disappointing and not associated with clinical benefit.*

Sobel JD, Lundstrom T. Management of candiduria. *Curr Urol Rep* 2001;2:321–325.

This review attempts to summarize the diagnosis and management of candiduria.

Talluri G, et al. Polymerase chain reaction used to detect candidemia in patients with candiduria. *Urology* 1998;51:501–505.

Candiduria has been shown to be an early marker of disseminated fungal infection in critically ill patients who have undergone surgery. The management of candidemia and disseminated candidiasis depends on rapid and definitive identification of Candida. Candiduria manifests as an early sign of candidemia, and systemic antifungal therapy timed appropriately based on the clinical condition and onset of candiduria will improve outcome. Detection of fungal DNA in blood by polymerase chain reaction is of value in establishing the diagnosis. Additional studies with a larger sample size are required to evaluate the specificity and sensitivity of polymerase chain reaction as a routine diagnostic test for candidemia.

Talluri G, et al. Immune response in patients with persistent candiduria and occult candidemia. *J Urol* 1999;162:1361–1364.

Levels of Th1 (proinflammatory interleukin [IL]-1, IL-2 and tumor necrosis factor-α) and Th2 (anti-inflammatory IL-4 and IL-10) cytokines were measured in the sera of patients with persistent candiduria. Th1 cytokines were within normal limits or slightly decreased in all patients with persistent candiduria with or without candidemia. These observations indicate that an abnormal immune response develops in patients with persistent candiduria with or without candidemia.

Tokunaga S, et al. Clinical significance of measurement of serum D-arabinitol levels in candiduria patients. *Urol Int* 1992;482:195–199.

D-Arabinitol, a major candidal metabolite, is reported to be a useful parameter to diagnose disseminated candidiasis. These results suggest that knowledge of the serum D-arabinitol concentration may help to diagnose promptly invasive candidiasis, particularly Candida pyelonephritis. In addition, enzymatic fluorometric assay kits are considered to be advantageous, in that they require little time and are simple to use, as compared with gas-liquid chromatography.

Tokunaga S, et al. D-arabinitol versus mannan antigen and candidal protein antigen as a serum marker for Candida pyelonephritis. *Eur J Clin Microbiol Infect Dis* 1995; 142:118–121.

To evaluate serum markers for the diagnosis of Candida pyelonephritis, levels of D-arabinitol, candidal mannan antigen and candidal protein antigen were measured using an enzymatic fluorometric assay, an enzyme immunoassay, and a latex agglutination assay, respectively. These results suggest that the D-arabinitol/creatinine ratio is the most useful marker of Candida pyelonephritis.

Genital Tract VI

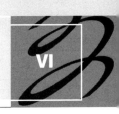

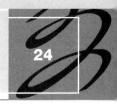
rethral discharge is the most frequent sexually transmitted disorder occurring in men. In the majority of patients, the discharge has an infectious pathogenesis. If the urethral discharge is not caused by *Neisseria gonorrhoeae*, the patient has nongonococcal urethritis (NGU). These two forms of urethritis, however, are not mutually exclusive, as coinfection with *N. gonorrhoeae* and *Chlamydia* or *Ureaplasma* occurs in 15 to 25% of heterosexual men with urethritis.

NGU is the most common sexually transmitted disease in men and results in about 4 to 6 million visits yearly in the United States. The Centers for Disease Control estimates that there are 2 1/2 times as many cases of NGU as cases of gonorrhea in men. Whereas the incidence of gonorrhea has declined recently, significant increases in gonorrhea have been reported in men who have sex with men. Which type of infection is present depends on the population studied. The highest proportion of NGU cases occurs in college students seen at student health clinics, with rates of 80 to 90% reported. In sexually transmitted disease clinics, cases of gonorrhea appear to be slightly more numerous.

Several organisms are implicated as causes of acute NGU. *Chlamydia trachomatis* is isolated in 30 to 40% of patients with NGU. *Chlamydia* is also recovered from the endocervix of about 70% of women whose partners have chlamydial NGU. *Ureaplasma urealyticum* is thought to be responsible for 20 to 25% of cases of NGU. There is a higher incidence of *U. urealyticum* in men having their first episode of NGU. Other, infrequent infectious causes of NGU, which account for 1 to 5% of cases, are *Trichomonas vaginalis*, herpes simplex virus, *Mycoplasma genitalium*, and *Candida*. *M. genitalium* has been found to cause some cases of urethritis, but the rates are not well defined, because specific testing is not widely available. The cause of the remaining 20 to 30% of NGU cases is unknown. Thirty to 40% of patients who do not have intercourse with a new or untreated partner have recurrent urethral discharge within 6 weeks of appropriate therapy for NGU. Most men with recurrent NGU are culture negative for *Chlamydia* and *Ureaplasma*, and the cause remains unknown. Resistant *Ureaplasma* is implicated as a cause of urethritis that fails to improve after a course of tetracycline. *Chlamydia* appears to be an infrequent cause of persistent or recurrent urethritis. *T. vaginalis* accounts for only a minority of cases of persistent NGU.

Clinically, gonococcal urethritis has an abrupt onset, with an incubation period of 1 to 7 days. The discharge tends to be purulent, and dysuria is a frequently associated syndrome. The clinical picture of NGU is different, with a gradual onset, an incubation period of 10 to 14 days, and mucoid discharge. The symptoms are milder, and patients often wait several days before seeking care. NGU has a tendency to recur, and a prior history of urethritis is common. There is overlap between the symptoms of the two conditions, and a Gram's stain, culture, DNA probe test, or nucleic acid amplification tests of the discharge are essential for diagnosis. Both *N. gonorrhoeae* and *Chlamydia* can cause asymptomatic urethral infections. About 10% of NGU cases are asymptomatic.

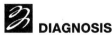

DIAGNOSIS

When a male patient presents with a discharge or dysuria, or both, the physician should obtain material for Gram's stain and culture by stripping the distal urethra. If no discharge is present, or if asymptomatic gonorrhea is suspected, a calcium alginate nasopharyngeal swab should be inserted 2 cm into the urethra to obtain a specimen for Gram's stain and culture. Voiding within 2 hours of the examination may interfere with obtaining material for smear. The Gram's-stained specimen shows neutrophils that contain several intracellular gram-negative diplococci in 95% of patients with gonorrhea. The Gram's-stained smear may require a careful search, as the distribution of organisms is uneven. Most neutrophils contain no organisms, and a few cells are loaded with gram-negative diplococci. The hallmark of urethritis is the presence of polymorphonuclear leukocytes (PMNs) on a Gram's-stained smear of urethral discharge. The presence of at least four PMNs per oil immersion field (1,000×) indicates urethral inflammation.

Patients who are symptomatic but have no evidence of a urethral discharge should have their first 10 mL of urine examined for the presence of PMNs. The urine sample should be centrifuged and the sediment examined for PMNs. Pyuria is defined as the presence of 15 or more PMNs per high-dry field (400×). In some patients with *Chlamydia* isolated, however, urethral Gram's-stained smears and first-voided urine lack enough PMNs to fulfill these criteria for urethral inflammation. In two studies, nearly one third of the patients who had *Chlamydia* isolated did not show evidence of urethral inflammation.

The Gram's stain is also highly sensitive (95%) in the diagnosis of NGU. The smear shows neutrophils without intracellular diplococci; this is confirmed by a culture that is negative for the gonococcus. For many clinicians, the diagnosis of NGU depends on the exclusion of gonococcal infection. The swab should be inoculated into an appropriate selective medium (e.g., Thayer-Martin, Martin-Lewis) at room temperature, or inoculated onto a transport system (e.g., Jembec) that yields a carbon dioxide-containing environment. A serologic test for syphilis should always be obtained. In patients with persistent or recurrent NGU, a wet preparation of the urethral discharge may reveal *Trichomonas*.

In addition to the traditional methods of diagnosing gonorrhea by using Gram's stain and culture, rapid diagnostic tests have become commercially available. For asymptomatic urethral gonorrhea, the Gram's stain has a sensitivity of only 40% in comparison with the culture. The sensitivity of a single endocervical culture for gonorrhea is about 85%.

One rapid test uses a nonisotopic DNA probe to detect *C. trachomatis* and *N. gonorrhoeae* from the same specimen. The nucleic acid probes are highly specific and can screen large numbers of specimens. With first-voided urine samples, the leukocyte esterase test can be used to screen for both gonorrhea and NGU. The sensitivity of this nonspecific test is about 80%, and it can be used to identify patients who need further testing.

A number of rapid tests have been developed for diagnosing chlamydial infections. One, a direct immunofluorescent test (Micro Trak), uses a monoclonal antibody conjugated with fluorescein isothiocyanate. The test, which takes about 30 minutes, requires expertise with immunofluorescent microscopy. In one report, the test had a 93% sensitivity and 96% specificity. Tests using the polymerase chain reaction (PCR) and ligase chain reaction (LCR) and transcription-mediated amplification (TMA) are also available to detect *C. trachomatis* and *N. gonorrhoea* using a first voided urine or urethral or endocervical swab. The highly sensitive PCR- and LCR-based assays appear to be useful to screen the urine of asymptomatic men. Patients prefer noninvasive tests on urine to the use of urethral swab specimens.

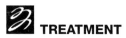 TREATMENT

Because 15 to 20% of heterosexual men with gonococcal urethritis have simultaneous chlamydial urethritis, therapy must be directed against both pathogens. Penicillin-resistant and tetracycline-resistant strains of *N. gonorrhoeae* occur frequently, so that penicillin, ampicillin, and tetracycline are no longer recommended. Ceftriaxone administered in a dose of 125 mg intramuscularly is the drug of choice. Ceftriaxone is also likely to be effective against incubating syphilis. A single 400-mg dose of cefixime, administered orally, appears to be as effective as ceftriaxone. Alternatives for penicillin- and cephalosporin-allergic patients with genital or rectal gonorrhea include 2 g spectinomycin IM or an oral quinolone, such as ciprofloxacin (500 mg once) or ofloxacin (400 mg once). Spectinomycin is not recommended for the treatment of pharyngeal gonorrhea, but ceftriaxone and ciprofloxacin appear effective. Men treated with ceftriaxone, cefixime, a single dose of a quinolone, or spectinomycin, which are adequate drugs for gonorrhea, have a persistent mucoid discharge (so-called postgonococcal urethritis) if *Chlamydia* or *Ureaplasma* infection is also present.

After treatment of gonorrhea with one of the single-dose regimens, patients should be given a single dose of azithromycin or a 7-day course of doxycycline or tetracycline for coexisting chlamydial infection. Azithromycin is preferred because a single dose improves compliance. Erythromycin (1 g/day) may be substituted for tetracycline. Ofloxacin, but not ciprofloxacin, administered for a 7-day course is another alternative drug for *Chlamydia* infection. *M. genitalium* responds to doxycycline, azithromycin, or erythromycin. A repeated culture is not necessary after treatment unless the patient remains symptomatic or has a recurrence.

Unfortunately, about 33% of patients have persistent or recurrent NGU within 6 weeks of initiation of therapy. The rate of recurrence is the same after 3 weeks of initial therapy as with 1 week. The results of therapy are best if *Chlamydia* is isolated initially, not as good if *Ureaplasma* is present, and poor if neither organism is present initially. Tetracycline-resistant *Chlamydia* is not a problem with recurrent NGU, but resistant *Ureaplasma* has been reported. Erythromycin (2 g/day orally) administered for 7 days is effective against *Chlamydia* and tetracycline-resistant *Ureaplasma*. Trimethoprim-sulfamethoxazole is effective against *Chlamydia* but lacks activity against *Ureaplasma*. Every effort should be made to treat both male and female sex partners of infected patients to prevent reinfection.

Management of recurrent NGU is a difficult problem. The cause is usually unknown. The following must be considered as possible causes of failure to respond or of recurrence: (a) reinfection, (b) patient noncompliance, (c) mixed infection, (d) *T. vaginalis* urethritis, (e) resistant *Ureaplasma*, (f) herpes simplex virus infection, (g) foreign bodies, and (h) trauma (mainly "milking" the urethra). Optimal management is unclear. A urologic evaluation may be beneficial for a minority of patients with unresponsive urethritis. If the patient was compliant with the initial regimen and renewed exposure can be excluded, then metronidazole (2 g orally in a single dose) plus erythromycin (2 g/day) for 1 week is recommended. (NMG)

Bibliography

Bowie WR. Approach to men with urethritis and urologic complications of sexually transmitted diseases. *Med Clin North Am* 1990;74:1543.
Review.

Calvet HM. Sexually transmitted diseases other than human immunodeficiency virus infection in older adults. *Clin Infect Dis* 2003;36:609–614.
Consider a sexually transmitted disease in the sexually active elderly.

Centers for Disease Control and Prevention. Sexually transmitted diseases treatment guidelines 2002. *MMWR Morb Mortal Wkly Rep* 2002;51:1–80.
Treatment guidelines.

Davies PO, Ridgway GL. The role of polymerase chain reaction and ligase chain reaction for the detection of *Chlamydia trachomatis. Int J STD AIDS* 1997;8:731–738.
About 60% of men and 75% of women with Chlamydia *are asymptomatic. These new tests (PCR and LCR) are more sensitive than enzyme-linked immunosorbent assays, but at two to three times the cost.*

Deguchi T, et al. Comparison among performances of a ligase chain reaction-based assay and two enzyme immunoassays in detecting *Chlamydia trachomatis* in urine specimens from men with nongonococcal urethritis. *J Clin Microbiol* 1996;34:1708–1710.
Use of an LCR assay had a sensitivity of 94%, which was better than the Chlamydia *culture yield (85%).*

Holmes KK, et al. Etiology of nongonococcal urethritis. *N Engl J Med* 1975;292:1199.
Evidence is given that Chlamydia *is a frequent cause of NGU.* Chlamydia *organisms were isolated from 42% of patients with NGU and from 7% of controls.*

Hook EW, Holmes KK. Gonococcal infections. *Ann Intern Med* 1985;102:229.
Classic review.

Hooton TM, et al. Erythromycin for persistent or recurrent nongonococcal urethritis. *Ann Intern Med* 1990;113:21.
A 3-week course of erythromycin (2 g/d) was more effective than placebo for male patients with persistent or recurrent NGU.

Horner P, Thomas B, Gilroy CB, et al. Role of mycoplasma genitalium and ureaplasma urealyticum in acute and chronic nongonococcal urethritis. *Clin Infect Dis.* 2001;32:995–1003.
Review.

Horner PJ, et al. Association of *Mycoplasma genitalium* with acute non-gonococcal urethritis. *Lancet* 1993;342:582–585.
Another cause of NGU.

Iwen PC, Blair TMH, Woods GL. Comparison of the Gen-Probe PACE 2 system, direct fluorescent antibody and cell culture for detecting *Chlamydia trachomatis* in cervical specimens. *Am J Clin Pathol* 1991;95:578.
Uses a nonisotopic DNA probe for the direct detection of organisms based on a chemiluminescent detection system.

Jacobs NF Jr, Arum ES, Kraus SJ. Nongonococcal urethritis: the role of *Chlamydia trachomatis*. *Ann Intern Med* 1977;86:313.
Classic. Mycoplasma hominisdoes not appear to be a major cause of NGU.

Jacobs NF Jr, Kraus SJ. Gonococcal and nongonococcal urethritis in men: clinical and laboratory differentiation. *Ann Intern Med* 1975;82:7.
Gram's stain is highly sensitive in the diagnosis of gonococcal urethritis and NGU.

Judson FN, Ehret JM, Handsfield HH. Comparative study of ceftriaxone and spectinomycin for treatment of pharyngeal and anorectal gonorrhea. *JAMA* 1985;253:1417.
Ceftriaxone is highly effective for urethral, pharyngeal, and rectal gonococci, including β-lactamase–positive strains.

Martin DH, et al. A controlled trial of a single dose of azithromycin for the treatment of chlamydial urethritis and cervicitis. *N Engl J Med* 1992;327:921.
A single 1-g dose of azithromycin was highly effective for the treatment of genital chlamydial infections.

Palmer HM, et al. Detection of *Chlamydia trachomatis* by the polymerase chain reaction in swabs and urine from men with nongonococcal urethritis. *J Clin Pathol* 1991;44:321.
A PCR for C. trachomatis from urethral swabs compared favorably with a direct immunofluorescence test using monoclonal antibodies (Micro Trak).

Peipert JF. Genital chlamydial infections. *N Engl J Med* 2003;349:2424–2430.
Review.

Plourde PJ, et al. Single-dose cefixime versus single-dose ceftriaxone in the treatment of antimicrobial-resistant *Neisseria gonorrhoeae* infection. *J Infect Dis* 1992;166:919.
Cefixime in a dose of 400 mg orally was highly effective (98%) for the treatment of uncomplicated gonococcal urethritis in men and cervicitis.

Podgore JK, Holmes KK, Alexander ER. Asymptomatic urethral infections due to *Chlamydia trachomatis* in male U.S. military personnel. *J Infect Dis* 1982;146:828.
Asymptomatic Chlamydia infection was noted in 11% of male personnel.

Schachter J, et al. Noninvasive tests for diagnosis of *Chlamydia trachomatis* infection: application of ligase chain reaction to first-catch urine specimens of women. *J Infect Dis* 1995;172:1411–1414.
An LCR assay was better than the chlamydial culture in diagnosing infection in women by means of first-voided urine specimens.

Stamm WE, et al. Azithromycin for empirical treatment of the nongonococcal urethritis syndrome in men. A randomized double-blind study. *JAMA* 1995;274:545–549.
Use of a single dose of azithromycin was as effective as 1 week of doxycycline for NGU.

Stimson JB, et al. Tetracycline-resistant *Ureaplasma urealyticum*: a cause of persistent nongonococcal urethritis. *Ann Intern Med* 1981;94:192.
A cause of persistent but not recurrent NGU.

Swartz SL, et al. Diagnosis and etiology of nongonococcal urethritis. *J Infect Dis* 1978;138:445.
Criteria for the diagnosis of NGU included at least four neutrophils per high-power field in Gram's-stained smears of urethral discharge and a negative culture for N. gonorrhoeae. Gardnerella, group B streptococci, and yeasts were not found as causative organisms of NGU.

Taylor-Robinson D. Mycoplasma genitalium—an update. *Int J STD AIDS* 2002;13:145–151.
A cause of persistent and recurrent urethritis.
Wong ES, et al. Clinical and microbiological features of persistent or recurrent nongonococcal urethritis in men. *J Infect Dis* 1988;158:1098.
Ninety percent of patients with urethritis caused by C. trachomatis *and 70% of cases caused by* U. urealyticum *responded to antimicrobials. When neither organism is involved, more than 50% of cases persist or relapse. The physician should culture or treat for* T. vaginalis *when a second course of antimicrobials fails.*
Yoshida T, et al. Rapid detection of Mycoplasma genitalium, Mycoplasma hominis, Ureaplasma parvum, and Ureaplasma urealyticum organisms in genitourinary samples by PCR-microtiter plate hybridization assay. *J Clin Microbiol* 2003;41:1850–1855.
Review.

SEROLOGIC TESTS FOR SYPHILIS

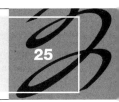 25

*M*ost cases of syphilis are diagnosed with a serologic test rather than by darkfield microscopic examination of a skin lesion. The causative agent, *Treponema pallidum*, has yet to be grown on artificial culture medium. The darkfield microscopic examination in some cases may not be readily available or is not applicable. It is useful only with moist lesions of primary and secondary syphilis, and the lesions of syphilis may be atypical. Serologic tests for syphilis are invaluable not only for diagnosis but as a measure of response to therapy. Unless the serologic test results are interpreted carefully, however, they can be highly misleading.

Serologic tests for syphilis are of two types: nontreponemal and treponemal. The nontreponemal tests detect an antibody to a cardiolipin-lecithin-cholesterol antigen. The antibodies detected in the nontreponemal tests, called reagins, are immunoglobulins (IgG and IgM). These should not be confused with IgE antibodies, which occur in allergic disorders and are also called reagins. These tests are easy to perform, highly sensitive, and moderately specific. The results are reported as reactive, weakly reactive, and nonreactive, and they are reported quantitatively as the highest dilution of the patient's serum that reacts positively. The test results tend to become negative or at least to demonstrate a drop in titer after treatment. Examples of currently used nontreponemal tests include the Venereal Disease Research Laboratory (VDRL) slide test and various rapid reagin tests, such as the rapid plasma reagin circle card test (RPR-CT). They are used to aid in the diagnosis of symptomatic infections, screen asymptomatic persons, and follow titers in treated cases to determine the effectiveness of therapy. The VDRL slide test and the RPR-CT are the two most frequently used nontreponemal tests. Treponemal tests measure specific antitreponemal antibody against treponemal components. These tests are highly sensitive and specific and are the standard laboratory tests that establish the diagnosis of syphilis or confirm the possibility of a false-positive nontreponemal test. The most widely used treponemal tests include the fluorescent treponemal antibody absorption (FTA-ABS) test and the microhemagglutination assay for *T. pallidum* antibodies (MHA-Tp). The hemagglutination test uses antigens of *T. pallidum* adsorbed to erythrocytes. The erythrocytes used in the various tests differ, but the data fail to show that any one hemagglutination test is superior to another. The most specific test available to diagnose congenital syphilis is the FTA-ABS performed on the purified 19S-IgM fraction of neonatal serum. The diagnosis of congenital neurosyphilis

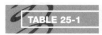 **TABLE 25-1** Interpretation of the EIA Treponemal Test

Setting	IgM	IgG
Primary syphilis	+	−
Secondary syphilis	+	−
Latent syphilis	−	+
Past treated syphilis (<10 yrs)	−	+
Past treated syphilis (>10 yrs)	−	−
Tertiary syphilis	−	±

is difficult because standard tests are lacking. A potential test uses Western blot analysis to detect IgM antibodies to *T. pallidum* in the cerebrospinal fluid (CSF). New tests need to be compared with the recovery of *T. pallidum* by rabbit inoculation or detection of the organism by the polymerase chain reaction (PCR) technique. Most physicians have been taught that an FTA-ABS test with a positive result usually remains reactive for life, even with adequate therapy, and should not be used to monitor the effectiveness of treatment. Results of a study, however, have demonstrated seroreversal of the treponemal tests after therapy for syphilis in some patients infected with HIV. Another report noted a reversion to seronegativity in the FTA-ABS test of normal hosts in some patients treated for primary syphilis.

For years, treponemal tests, such as the FTA-ABS, have been used to confirm the diagnosis of syphilis. These tests are labor intensive and require subjective interpretation of laboratory personnel. Another treponemal test is available that detects *T. pallidum* IgG and IgM antibodies. The test, called an enzyme immunoassay (EIA), can be used for screening and to confirm the diagnosis of syphilis. The test may be negative in severely immunosuppressed patients, such as those with HIV disease, and cannot be used to monitor response to therapy, such as the RPR. False-positive IgM antibody results can occur in patients with acute Epstein-Barr virus infection or systemic lupus erythematosus. Table 25-1 lists information on how to interpret the results of the syphilis EIA treponemal test.

The results of the FTA-ABS test depend on the degree of fluorescence and are reported as negative, minimally reactive (1+), and positive (2+ to 4+). This is a qualitative test, and the degree of positivity does not indicate the stage of illness. All patients with an equivocal (formerly designated borderline) FTA-ABS test result should be retested. If the result of the repeated test is again equivocal or negative, syphilis is unlikely. A positive test result indicates past or present infection. A patient with an FTA-ABS test result of 1+ is called a minimal reactor, and this result is considered negative unless the patient has clinical features to suggest syphilis. For patients with an FTA-ABS test result of 1+, the test should be repeated on another specimen. Caution is essential in interpreting the results of any fluorescent test, as laboratory errors may occur. The FTA-ABS test should be performed on serum, and its use on CSF remains controversial. The first treponemal test developed was the *T. pallidum* immobilization test (TPI), which is no longer in clinical use. The rabbit intratesticular infectivity test is the oldest and most sensitive test to identify *T. pallidum*. The newest technique is the PCR. The PCR test is used in research settings but could be valuable in the diagnosis of congenital syphilis, neurosyphilis, and early primary syphilis.

In general, treponemal tests are more sensitive than nontreponemal tests. With primary syphilis, nontreponemal tests are positive in 76% of patients, compared with 86% for the FTA-ABS or MHA-Tp test. In secondary syphilis, reactivity is 99 to 100% for both nontreponemal and treponemal tests. In latent and late syphilis, the reactivity of nontreponemal tests is 73%, compared with 96% for treponemal tests. Thus, because the treponemal tests (e.g., the FTA-ABS) are highly sensitive and specific, they are useful in suspected primary or, especially, tertiary syphilis, as the nontreponemal test results are occasionally negative in these patients.

Treponemal tests help identify false-positive reactors (positive nontreponemal test and negative treponemal test). The causes of false-positive nontreponemal test results include technical errors, presence of other treponemal diseases, such as yaws (not really false positives), and true, biologically false-positive reactions. Titers in false-positive reactions are usually low (<1:8), and the reactivity is classified as acute (<6 months of reactivity) or chronic (>6 months). The causes of transiently false-positive nontreponemal test results include a variety of acute viral illnesses, pregnancy (rarely), malaria, and some immunizations. Chronic false-positive reactions may be noted with collagen vascular diseases, drug addiction, advanced age, Hansen's disease, malignancy, thyroiditis, and certain drugs for hypertension. Infrequently (<1% of cases), a test result is false positive in cases of systemic lupus erythematosus, drug addiction, and pregnancy. A beaded fluorescence pattern (i.e., fluorescence limited to a few portions of the fixed treponeme) is described in patients with systemic lupus erythematosus and a false-positive treponemal test result (the usual pattern being homogeneous fluorescence). A false-positive MHA-Tp test is rarely reported in pregnancy, infectious mononucleosis, and Hansen's disease.

The diagnosis of syphilis in the HIV-infected patient can be a problem. For many patients infected with HIV-1, the serologic tests for syphilis are useful to establish the diagnosis. In selected patients, however, the serologic test results will be negative, and if clinical findings suggest the disease, then darkfield microscopy or a direct fluorescent antibody test for *T. pallidum* (DFA-Tp) should be performed on exudate from a lesion, or a tissue biopsy specimen should be examined with DFA-Tp or a silver stain.

Examination of the CSF is essential for the diagnosis of symptomatic neurosyphilis. The necessity of a lumbar puncture to examine CSF is controversial in regard to immunocompetent patients who are asymptomatic but may have neurosyphilis. Examination of the CSF is essential in an HIV-infected patient with a positive syphilis serology. The gold standard for the laboratory diagnosis of neurosyphilis is the VDRL slide test performed on CSF. The value of tests such as the FTA-ABS or RPR-CT on CSF remains unclear, and therefore they should not be performed on CSF. Unfortunately, results of the CSF VDRL slide test may be negative in 40 to 73% of patients with neurosyphilis. The VDRL cannot be used on CSF to follow response to therapy as it can on serum. The clinician is usually faced with two situations. First, the physician must determine which serologic test is indicated and what the likely result will be for each patient with suspected syphilis. Second, if the laboratory reports a positive test for syphilis, the physician must decide how to interpret this result and how to manage the patient.

Primary syphilis is a consideration in patients presenting with ulcerative genital or extragenital lesions. Darkfield examination of moist lesions or the DFA-Tp test may be useful in establishing the diagnosis. The DFA-Tp test, which uses a specific fluorescein-labeled antibody against *T. pallidum,* is performed particularly on smears from oral lesions. Nontreponemal test results are positive in 76% of patients, and the FTA-ABS test is positive in 86%. If the initial serologic test result is negative for a patient with a suspected lesion, therapy should be started and the test repeated weekly for 1 month. The clinical manifestations of secondary syphilis are varied, but it is usually suspected on the basis of skin or mucous membrane lesions. Results of the VDRL slide test are positive in all patients at this stage of the illness, usually with high titers (>1:32). A negative test excludes the diagnosis. A prozone reaction may result in a false-negative VDRL test result. In late-stage syphilis, the VDRL slide test is positive in about 70% of patients, and the FTA-ABS test is positive in 96%. Congenital syphilis occasionally can be confirmed by positive findings on darkfield examination. Because the VDRL slide test result may be positive as a result of passive transfer of IgG treponemal antibodies from mother to healthy newborn, presumptive evidence for the diagnosis requires either a significant rise in titer (fourfold) or a stable titer at 3 months of age. Performance of the FTA-ABS test on the purified 19S-IgM fraction of neonatal serum is helpful in the diagnosis of congenital syphilis.

A frequent clinical problem is the management of an asymptomatic patient with an unexpectedly positive nontreponemal test result. The first step is to repeat the test to exclude the possibility of laboratory error. If the repeated test result is positive, a treponemal test is indicated to exclude a false-positive reaction. Then, if the treponemal test result is positive, the clinician should consider the following possibilities: (a) congenital syphilis, (b) treated or untreated acquired syphilis, which can be clarified by the history, and (c) nonvenereal treponemal infection, such as yaws.

Four serologic patterns are observed:

1. Nontreponemal and FTA-ABS tests can be positive with untreated or treated syphilis at any stage, with congenital diseases, or with other spirochetal infections, such as yaws. Clues from the history and physical examination should be helpful.
2. A negative nontreponemal test and a positive FTA-ABS test can indicate adequately treated syphilis, untreated early primary or late infection, Lyme disease, or rarely (<1%) a false-positive FTA-ABS test. Patients with Lyme disease will have a negative VDRL slide test result but may have a positive FTA-ABS test caused by antibody to *Borrelia burgdorferi*, which cross-reacts with *T. pallidum* antigens.
3. A positive nontreponemal test with a negative FTA-ABS test is a false-positive reaction.
4. A negative nontreponemal test and negative FTA-ABS test are seen in incubating syphilis, in the absence of syphilis, and at times in the HIV-infected patient with syphilis. In the future, nucleic acid amplification tests may have a role in the diagnosis of syphilis. (NMG)

Bibliography

Catteral RD. Systemic disease and the biological false-positive reaction. *Br J Vener Dis* 1972;48:1.
Lists the causes of false-positive reactions.

Dattner B, Thomas EW, DeMello L. Criteria for the management of neurosyphilis. *Am J Med* 1951;10:463.
Classic. After appropriate therapy for neurosyphilis, the VDRL slide test may remain reactive for years. CSF cell count and protein should be followed to monitor response.

Donovan B. Sexually transmissible infections other than HIV. *Lancet* 2004;363:545–556.
Review.

Erbelding EJ, et al. Syphilis serology in human immunodeficiency virus infection: evidence for false-negative fluorescent treponemal testing. *J Infect Dis* 1997;176:1397–1400.
Some HIV patients with a positive RPR-CT result and a negative FTA-ABS test result, classified as biologic false-positive reactors, may have syphilis based on history and immunoblot testing.

Fiumara NJ. Biologic false-positive reactions for syphilis: Massachusetts, 1954–1961. *N Engl J Med* 1963;268:402.
Classic. Found in 20% of patients and usually with a titer of 1:1 to 1:4.

Fiumara NJ. Treatment of primary and secondary syphilis: serological response. *JAMA* 1980;243:2500.
All patients with primary syphilis had a negative RPR-CT result within 12 months, and all patients with secondary syphilis were negative by 24 months. (See also Guinan ME. Treatment of primary and secondary syphilis: defining failure at 3- and 6-month follow-up. JAMA 1987;257:359. At the 3-month follow-up visit, cured patients had a fourfold drop in VDRL slide test titer.)

Flood JM, et al. Neurosyphilis during the AIDS epidemic, San Francisco, 1985–1992. *J Infect Dis* 1998;177:931–940.
The median age of patients with neurosyphilis was 39, and early symptomatic disease (e.g., acute syphilitic meningitis, uveitis, or meningovascular syphilis) was common.

Hook EW, Marra CM. Acquired syphilis in adults. *N Engl J Med* 1992;326:1060.
Review. Lyme disease may be associated with a positive FTA-ABS test but a negative RPR or VDRL test.

Hoshmand H, Escobar MR, Kopf SW. Neurosyphilis: a study of 241 patients. *JAMA* 1972; 219:726.
Nontreponemal tests were reactive in only 48.5% of patients with neurosyphilis when serum was used but in 56.7% when performed on CSF.

Lukehart SA, et al. Invasion of the central nervous system by *Treponema pallidum*: implications for diagnosis and treatment. *Ann Intern Med* 1988;109:855.
T. pallidum was isolated from the CSF in 30% of patients with untreated primary or secondary syphilis. The CSF should be examined in all patients with syphilis who are positive for HIV.

Nandwani R, Evans DT. Are you sure it's syphilis? A review of false-positive serology [Review]. *Int J STD AIDS* 1995;6:241–248.

Biologic false-positive reactions are classified as acute if they persist for less than 6 months or chronic if they last longer.

Rawstron SA, et al. Congenital syphilis: detection of *Treponema pallidum* in stillborns. *Clin Infect Dis* 1997;24:24–27.

The use of a fluorescent antibody stain against T. pallidum *was superior to silver staining to identify treponemes in tissue.*

Rolfs RT, et al. A randomized trial of enhanced therapy for early syphilis in patients with and without human immunodeficiency virus infection. *N Engl J Med* 1997;337:307–314.

Current therapy for neurosyphilis with benzathine penicillin is adequate for HIV-positive patients.

Sanchez PJ, Wendel GD, Norgard MV. IgM antibody to *Treponema pallidum* in cerebrospinal fluid of infants with congenital syphilis. *Am J Dis Child* 1992;146:1171.

By means of Western blot analysis, the diagnosis of congenital neurosyphilis was supported by detection of IgM antibody to T. pallidum *in the CSF.*

Scheck DN, Hook EW III. Neurosyphilis [Review]. *Infect Dis Clin North Am* 1994;8:769.

Only 30 to 70% of patients with central nervous system syphilis have a positive CSF VDRL test result.

Schmidt BL, Edjlalipour M, Lugar A. Comparative evaluation of nine different enzyme linked immunosorbent assays for determination of antibodies against *Treponema pallidum* in patients with primary syphilis. *J Clin Microbiol* 2000;38:1279–1282.

Newer EIA tests are useful to confirm the diagnosis of syphilis.

Schroeter AL, et al. Treatment for early syphilis and reactivity of serological tests. *JAMA* 1972;221:471.

A positive treponemal test usually remains so for life, even with adequate therapy.

Sparling PF. Diagnosis and treatment of syphilis. *N Engl J Med* 1971;284:642.

Classic. Compares the reactivity of various serologic tests in the different stages of syphilis. The VDRL slide test usually will become negative 6 to 12 months after treatment of primary syphilis, or 12 to 24 months after treatment of secondary syphilis.

Timmermans M, Carr J. Neurosyphilis in the modern era. *J Neurol Neurosurg Psychiatry* 2004;12:1727–1730.

Half of the patients presented with delirium and dementia.

PELVIC INFLAMMATORY DISEASE

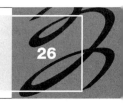

26

*P*elvic inflammatory disease (PID) refers to a range of inflammatory disorders of the structures of the upper genital tract, causing any combination of endometritis, salpingitis, tubo-ovarian abscess, or pelvic peritonitis. Pathogens causing these infections are usually sexually transmitted and community acquired, particularly *Neisseria gonorrhoeae* and *Chlamydia trachomatis*. However, organisms also may be part of the normal flora of the vagina, including anaerobes, gram-negative bacilli, group B streptococci, and *Gardnerella vaginalis*.

Pelvic inflammatory disease is a very common problem, in both the outpatient setting and as a disease requiring hospitalization. It is responsible for more than 2.5 million outpatient visits, 200,000 hospitalizations and more emergency room visits than any other

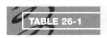 **TABLE 26-1** Risk Factors for Pelvic Inflammatory Disease

Age younger than 35	Multiple sexual partners
Nonbarrier contraception	Previous episode of PID
New sexual partner	Attending STD clinic

gynecologic cause. It includes a spectrum of severity and has an array of signs and symptoms that make definitive diagnosis sometimes difficult.

 ## CLINICAL PRESENTATION

PID usually appears with lower abdominal pain than may be unilateral or bilateral. The pain may worsen with coitus or after menses. Most women will complain of 1 to 2 weeks of pain. Pain may radiate to the back and even down the legs. The symptoms in patients who are HIV positive are often more severe. Abnormal uterine bleeding occurs in one third of patients. Bowel and bladder symptoms suggest an alternate diagnosis. Right upper quadrant pain may occur as part of a picture of concomitant perihepatitis. The Centers for Disease Control and Prevention guidelines emphasize that cases go unrecognized for failure to appreciate mild or nonspecific symptoms, such as dyspareunia, vaginal discharge, and abnormal bleeding. Healthcare providers should maintain a low threshold of suspicion for this disease. An appreciation of risk factors will help maintain an aggressive approach to diagnosis. Table 26-1 describes risk factors for PID.

 ## PHYSICAL EXAMINATION FINDINGS

Lower abdominal tenderness, with adnexal and cervical motion tenderness will be present in most patients with PID. A finding of mucopurulent discharge also is very suggestive of the diagnosis. Rectovaginal examination will reveal evidence of adnexal and uterine tenderness. Diffuse tenderness will be greatest in the lower quadrants and may be symmetrical. Rebound tenderness and decreased bowel sounds are also common. Right upper quadrant tenderness suggests perihepatitis. Fever is present in some patients.

CDC guidelines describe minimal criteria for empiric treatment of PID in sexually active young women. These include only:

> Uterine/adnexal tenderness
> Cervical motion tenderness

Table 26-2 includes additional criteria that may be useful in supporting the diagnosis of PID.

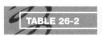 **TABLE 26-2** Additional Criteria for the Diagnosis of PID

Oral temperature greater than 101°F
Abnormal vaginal discharge
Presence of white cells on saline microscopy of vaginal secretions
Elevated erythrocyte sedimentation rate
Documentation of cervical infection by *N. gonorrhoeae* or *C. trachomatis*

DIAGNOSIS BY LABORATORY AND IMAGING

The diagnosis of PID can be made most specifically by additional evaluation. These include:

Endometrial biopsy, which shows evidence of endometritis
Laparoscopic abnormalities consistent with PID
Transvaginal sonography showing thickened, fluid-filled tubes

Laparoscopy would be appropriate for a patient in whom other inflammatory etiologies have not been ruled out, or for a patient who has failed treatment for PID or is not improving on maximum therapy. Ultrasound is useful to exclude adnexal masses and identify pelvic or tubo-ovarian abscesses. Endometrial biopsy appears to correlate well with PID, as plasma cell endometritis is present in most women with PID. Sensitivity and specificity appear to vary significantly from study to study.

 TREATMENT OF PELVIC INFLAMMATORY DISEASE

Most treatment regimens for PID will be empiric. They will have to cover both gonococci and *Chlamydia* but should also have spectrum of activity for anaerobes, gram-negative bacilli, and streptococci. Treatment should be initiated as soon as the diagnosis is made. Local antibiotic susceptibility data, antibiotic safety based on the patient's individual profile, past history of infection and ability to tolerate oral therapy are some important issues in antibiotic selection.

Parenteral therapy is begun if the patient is ill enough to require hospitalization. Hospitalization will be preferred when the patient is pregnant, when a high fever, nausea, or vomiting is present, when a concomitant illness or surgical emergency cannot be ruled out, and when the patient has failed oral therapy. Table 26-3 lists the parenteral antibiotic regimens recommended by the 2002 CDC guidelines.

The quinolones, with or without metronidazole for anaerobic coverage, also have been used successfully and should cover the most important pathogens. Ampicillin-sulbactam with doxycycline is another good, empiric regimen.

For oral therapy, ofloxacin or levofloxacin have been shown to be adequate in many clinical trials. Metronidazole can be added to improve anaerobic coverage. The CDC also recommends an empiric outpatient regimen using parenteral antibiotics. This regimen is as follows:

Ceftriaxone 250 mg IM in a single dose
or
Cefoxitin 2 g IM with 1 g of probenecid
or
Third-generation parenteral cephalosporin
plus

 CDC-Recommeded Parenteral Antibiotic Regimens

Regimen A	Regimen B
Cefotetan 2 g IV every 12 hours	Clindamycin 900 mg IV every 8 hours
or	plus
Cefoxitin 2 g IV every 6 hours	Gentamicin
plus doxycycline 100 mg orally or IV every 12 hours	

Doxycycline 100 mg orally twice per day for 14 days
with or without
Metronidazole 500 mg orally twice per day for 14 days.

Male sex partners should be evaluated and treated if they have had sex with the PID patient within 60 days. The regimen must be effective against both *Chlamydia* and gonococci. (SLB)

Bibliography

Aral SO, Mosher WD, Cates W Jr. Self-reported pelvic inflammatory disease in the United States, 1988. *JAMA* 1991;266:2570.
   A discussion of risk factors associated with PID: age, race, vaginal douching, age at first intercourse, sexually transmitted disease history, and number of lifetime sexual partners.
Barbosa C, et al. Pelvic inflammatory disease and human immunodeficiency virus infection. *Obstet Gynecol* 1997;89:65–70.
   HIV-positive patients who had PID had longer hospital stays and persistent fever compared with HIV-negative patients who had PID.
Boardman LA, et al. Endovaginal sonography for the diagnosis of upper genital tract infection. *Obstet Gynecol* 1997;90:54–57.
   A negative vaginal ultrasound examination does not exclude a diagnosis of PID.
Bowie WR, Jones H. Acute pelvic inflammatory disease in outpatients: association with *Chlamydia trachomatis* and *Neisseria gonorrhoeae. Ann Intern Med* 1981;95:685.
   Chlamydia *was isolated from 22% of patients and* N. gonorrhoeae *from 10%.*
Centers for Disease Control. Guidelines for sexually transmitted diseases. Pelvic inflammatory disease *MMWR Morb Mortal Wkly Rep* 2002;51:48–51.
   Comprehensive review of diagnosis and management. Emphasizes importance of a low threshold of suspicion for the disease, minimum criteria for initiating treatment, and new treatment regimens.
Curtis KM, et al. Visits to emergency departments for gynecologic disorders in the United States 1992–1994. *Obstet Gynecol* 1998;91:1007.
   PID was the most common cause among gynecologic disorders for visits to the emergency room.
Eschenbach DA, et al. Polymicrobial etiology of acute pelvic inflammatory disease. *N Engl J Med* 1975;293:166.
   Discusses the two forms of PID: gonococcal and nongonococcal. Anaerobes and aerobic species are important in the latter.
Hemsell DL, et al. Comparison of three regimens recommended by the Centers for Disease Control and Prevention for the treatment of women hospitalized with acute pelvic inflammatory disease. *Clin Infect Dis* 1994;19:720–727.
   Three regimens (cefotetan-doxycycline, cefoxitin-doxycycline, clindamycin-gentamicin) were equally effective for hospitalized women with PID.
Kahn JG, et al. Diagnosing pelvic inflammatory disease: a comprehensive analysis and considerations for developing a new model. *JAMA* 1991;266:2594.
   Comprehensive review of diagnostic studies. There is no ideal test for diagnosis of PID.
McCormack WM. Pelvic inflammatory disease. *N Engl J Med* 1994;330:115–119.
   Review. Clinical presentation is often silent or with atypical features. Infertility occurs in about 25% of patients.
Muller-Schoop JW, et al. *Chlamydia trachomatis* as a possible cause of peritonitis and perihepatitis in young women. *Br Med J* 1978;1:1022.
   Chlamydia *infection may mimic the Fitz-Hugh–Curtis syndrome.*
Peipert JF, et al. Performance of clinical and laparoscopic criteria for the diagnosis of upper genital infection. *Infect Dis Obstet Gynecol* 1997;5:291.
   Low sensitivity, high specificity in diagnosis of PID by laparoscopy.
Peipert JF, et al. Evaluation of ofloxacin in the treatment of laparoscopically documented acute pelvic inflammatory disease. *Infect Dis Obstet Gynecol* 1999;138:44.
   Oral regimen of ofloxacin was effective therapy in these patients with well-documented PID.

Rolfs RT, Galaid EI, Zaidi AA. Pelvic inflammatory disease: trends in hospitalizations and office visits, 1979 through 1988. *Am J Obstet Gynecol* 1992;166:983.
Hospitalization rates decreased by 36% and were highest for women ages 15 to 29.

Safrin S, et al. Long-term sequelae of acute pelvic inflammatory disease. *Am J Obstet Gynecol* 1992;166:1300.
In a retrospective study of PID, 24% of patients had pelvic pain for at least 6 months, 43% had a subsequent episode of PID, and 40% were infertile.

Sweet RL, Schachter J, Robbie MO. Failure of β-lactam antibiotics to eradicate *Chlamydia trachomatis* in the endometrium despite apparent clinical cure of acute salpingitis. *JAMA* 1983;250:2641.
Treatment of acute salpingitis should include an antimicrobial that eradicates Chlamydia, *such as doxycycline.*

Walker Ck, et al. Pelvic inflammatory disease: meta analysis of antimicrobial regimen efficacy. *J Infect Dis* 1993;168:969.
Oral and parenteral regimens appeared to be equally effective in the treatment of PID.

Walters MD, Gibbs RS. A randomized comparison of gentamicin-clindamycin and cefoxitin-doxycycline in the treatment of acute pelvic inflammatory disease. *Obstet Gynecol* 1990;75:867.
The comparison shows similar clinical and microbiologic cure rates in acute PID with both agents.

Washington AE, et al. Assessing risk for pelvic inflammatory disease and its sequelae. *JAMA* 1991;266:2581.
A discussion of risk markers, such as socioeconomic status, and risk factors, such as contraceptive practices.

Wendel GD Jr, et al. A randomized trial of ofloxacin versus cefoxitin and doxycycline in the outpatient treatment of acute salpingitis. *Am J Obstet Gynecol* 1991;164:1390.
Oral ofloxacin given for 10 days was equal in efficacy to cefoxitin plus doxycycline.

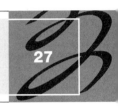

THERAPY OF GENITAL HERPES   27

*F*ew diseases other than AIDS have attracted such an enormous amount of media attention as genital herpes. The major consequence of genital herpes infection, excluding the emotional toll, is transmission of the virus from mother to infant during birth. Neonatal herpes simplex virus (HSV) infection is a life-threatening illness that occurs in babies up to 4 to 6 weeks of age. If the mother is known to be infected at the time of delivery, transmission of HSV to the newborn can be prevented by delivering the baby by cesarean section. However, neonatal herpes infection develops in most cases because the disease is unsuspected at the time of delivery, as the mother often has no history of genital herpes virus infection. Serial viral cultures are not indicated for most women during late gestation.

It is estimated that 5 to 20 million people in the United States suffer from recurrent genital HSV infections. Because this is not a reportable disease, nationwide statistics are unavailable. In one study of residents of Rochester, Minnesota, the overall incidence was 50 cases per 100,000 population, with a peak incidence of 128 cases per 100,000. Approximately 25% of the adult population is positive for HSV-2 antibody. The incubation period for genital HSV-1 or HSV-2 is about 4 days (range 2 to 12).

After the first episode of genital herpes infection, the major morbidity of the disease consists of frequent recurrences. One report shows that most patients with symptomatic recurrent genital herpes have five to eight recurrences yearly. The rate of recurrence of genital herpes varies with the HSV type. Only 14% of patients with genital HSV-1 note a recurrence after their first episode, compared with 60% of patients with HSV-2. The recurrence rate is 77% for patients who have a prior history of genital herpes. Recurrences occur slightly more frequently in men than in women. The median time to the next recurrence is approximately 40 days in patients with recurrent episodes of genital herpes and about 4 months in patients with first episodes.

Few data are available to define the triggering factors responsible for recurrences. One report noted that the recurrence rate diminished with time for some patients, but another shows no difference in recurrence rate between persons who have had the disease for more than 5 years and those who have had the disease for fewer than 5 years. Most patients cite emotional stress as a triggering factor, and one study noted that recurrence is more frequent 5 to 12 days before menses. Others find no relationship between recurrences and menses or sexual activity. The majority of recurrences result from the endogenous reactivation of latent virus rather than from reinfection.

First episodes of genital herpes can be divided into primary (absence of neutralizing antibody to HSV-1 or HSV-2) and nonprimary initial episodes (serologic evidence of past HSV infection). About 60% of patients who present with a first episode of genital herpes have primary infection with either HSV-1 or HSV-2. Approximately 30 to 70% of patients with a first episode of genital herpes (nonprimary infection) have preexisting antibody to HSV-2, indicating an earlier, asymptomatic infection. Among homosexual men with HSV-2 antibody, 70% denied any history of genital or rectal herpes infection. Eighty-five percent of first-episode genital herpes lesions are produced by HSV-2 and the remainder by HSV-1. The frequency of oral-genital sex may alter these rates.

Primary genital herpes is characterized by both systemic and local symptoms. Constitutional complaints consisting of low-grade fever, headache, malaise, and myalgias usually subside after 1 week. Local symptoms include pain, itching, dysuria, tender adenopathy, and genital lesions, which are initially single or multiple small vesicles on an erythematous base; these become intensely painful, ulcerative sores. The lesions persist for 2 to 3 weeks and become crusted before healing. The primary infection may also be asymptomatic. The mean duration of viral shedding is about 12 days.

Nonprimary first-episode genital herpes refers to illness in patients with antibody to HSV. The disease is milder and of shorter duration than primary genital herpes. Systemic symptoms are generally absent. Recurrent genital herpes is a local disease without systemic complaints. Both the severity and duration of the symptoms are significantly less than in primary or nonprimary first-episode disease. Pain in patients with recurrent herpes usually lasts 3 to 4 days, and the lesions resolve in about 1 week.

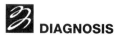 **DIAGNOSIS**

In the United States, HSV is the most frequent infectious cause of genital ulcers. Laboratory confirmation of the diagnosis is usually based on identifying the virus using polymerase chain reaction (PCR) or growing the virus in tissue culture. Isolation of the virus generally requires only 1 to 3 days. Multinucleated giant cells are characteristic of herpesvirus, and these cells can be seen by opening a vesicle with a scalpel and taking a scraping from the base of the lesion. The material is smeared on a slide (Tzanck preparation), fixed in alcohol, and stained with either Wright's or Giemsa stain. Vesicles are more likely to be positive on viral culture or Tzanck smear than are crusted ulcer lesions. Results of viral culture for herpes are positive in about 80% of cases, and the positivity rate for the Tzanck smear is 50%. PCR and viral culture are still the best laboratory tests.

The clinician should be aware that the laboratory tests for HSV IgG 1 and 2 are reliable. The PCR is a highly sensitive and specific test for identifying HSV in clinical specimens.

TABLE 27-1	Treatment of Genital Herpes
Drug	**Dose and schedule**
Primary Genital Herpes	
Acyclovir	400 mg orally three times/day 7–10 days
Valacyclovir	1000 mg orally two times/day 7–10 days
Famciclovir	250 mg orally three times/day 7–10 days
Recurrent Disease*	
Acyclovir	800 mg orally two times/day 5 days
Valacyclovir	1000 mg orally once daily 5 days
Famciclovir	125 mg orally two times/day 5 days
Suppressive Therapy†	
Acyclovir	400 mg twice daily
Valacyclovir	500 mg once daily
Valacyclovir	1000 mg once daily (for ≥10 recurrences 1 year)
Famciclovir	250 mg two times/day

*The recommendations for episodic treatment in HIV-infected persons are as follows: acyclovir, 200 mg five times per day for 5 to 10 days or 400 mg three times per day for 5 to 10 days; valacyclovir, 1000 mg twice daily for 5 to 10 days; or famciclovir, 500 mg twice daily for 5 to 10 days.
†The recommendations for suppressive therapy in HIV-infected persons are as follows: acyclovir, 400 to 800 mg two or three times per day; valacyclovir, 500 mg twice daily; or famciclovir, 500 mg twice daily.
(Modified from Kimberlin DW, Rouse DJ. Genital herpes. *N Engl J Med* 2004;350:1970–1977.)

TREATMENT

Acyclovir has been the drug of choice for genital herpes since 1982 and has a record of efficacy and safety. The drug is now available in generic formulations. Two other drugs available for the treatment of genital herpes include famciclovir and valacyclovir; they offer the advantage of less-frequent dosing compared with acyclovir (Table 27-1). Topical therapy is of limited value for genital herpes and is not indicated if systemic therapy is administered. Rarely, patients may have an acyclovir-resistant HSV infection, and foscarnet is the drug of choice in this situation. Acyclovir inhibits replication of both HSV-1 and HSV-2. It is converted to acyclovir triphosphate, an inhibitor of DNA polymerase, by viral thymidine kinase. The presence of viral thymidine kinase is not necessary for foscarnet activity because this drug does not undergo phosphorylation. Three formulations of acyclovir are available: topical, oral, and IV preparations.

Topical acyclovir is available as a 5% ointment in polyethylene glycol. Topical use usually does not result in serum levels of the drug. Intravaginal use should be avoided. Except for some decrease in viral shedding, topical acyclovir has little therapeutic value in recurrent herpes.

IV acyclovir is effective in the treatment of primary genital herpes. The drug is administered for 5 days as 5 mg/kg of body weight given at 8-hour intervals intravenously over 1 hour. Both systemic and local symptoms resolve more rapidly with IV acyclovir in comparison with placebo. Adverse effects are minimal. Bone marrow depression has not been a problem in normal hosts. Rapid bolus injections should be avoided and adequate hydration maintained. No effect on the recurrence rate is noted. The dosage of the drug should be reduced in patients with renal failure. The IV drug is not indicated for recurrent herpes infections.

Orally administered acyclovir has been found to be effective in treating both primary and recurrent genital herpes. For first-episode genital herpes, the drug is given as 200-mg capsules five times daily or 400 mg three times daily for 10 days; for recurrent disease, it is administered as 200-mg capsules five times daily or 400 mg three times daily for 5 days. The drug is effective in decreasing viral shedding and shortening the healing time. Results are more impressive than expected with primary in comparison with nonprimary first-episode or recurrent disease. Self-initiated therapy is more effective than physician-initiated treatment. There are no significant differences in duration of pain or time to subsequent recurrence between treatment with oral acyclovir and placebo in patients with recurrent genital herpes. Oral acyclovir is well tolerated, and adverse effects are uncommon.

Famciclovir is a prodrug of penciclovir and lacks antiviral activity. The drug is well absorbed (70%) after oral administration and rapidly converted to penciclovir. The intracellular half-life of penciclovir triphosphate ranges from 7 to 20 hours, which permits less-frequent dosing in comparison with acyclovir. In patients whose renal function is moderately or severely reduced, dose reduction is recommended. An IV preparation is not available.

Valacyclovir, the L-valine ester of acyclovir, is a prodrug of acyclovir. The drug is rapidly converted to acyclovir after oral absorption. The bioavailability of valacyclovir is about 55%, which is far better than that of acyclovir, which is only 15 to 21%. An IV formulation of valacyclovir is not available. However, the area under the curve (AUC) of oral valacyclovir is similar to that of IV acyclovir.

Table 27-1 lists the doses of acyclovir, famciclovir, and valacyclovir for primary disease, recurrent or episodic disease, and suppression. Except for the cost, long-term suppression of recurrent herpes has been well tolerated. The emergence of resistant strains of HSV has not been a problem. Patients should be given a 1- to 2-month drug holiday each year to assess the recurrence rate.

Condoms appear to decrease the transmission of herpesvirus infection, and their use should be promoted. Intercourse should be avoided during symptomatic episodes of HSV infection. There is also a risk of transmitting herpes when patients are asymptomatic. A vaccine for HSV is under study. A vaccine would be useful for both prevention and treatment. A cure for HSV is still eagerly awaited by millions of genital herpes sufferers. (NMG)

Bibliography

Boggess KA, et al. Herpes simplex virus type 2 detection by culture and polymerase chain reaction and relationship to genital symptoms and cervical antibody status during the third trimester of pregnancy. *Am J Obstet Gynecol* 1997;176:443–451.
PCR was more sensitive than culture for detecting asymptomatic genital HSV.

Brock BV, et al. Frequency of asymptomatic shedding of herpes simplex virus in women with genital herpes. *JAMA* 1990;263:418.
Asymptomatic viral shedding occurs commonly and is not related to the menstrual cycle.

Corey L, et al. Once-daily valacyclovir to reduce the risk of transmission of genital herpes. *N Engl J Med* 2004;350:11–20.
Once-daily valacyclovir reduces viral shedding and transmission of HSV-2 infection to a susceptible partner.

Corey L, et al. Genital herpes simplex virus infections: clinical manifestations, course, and complications. *Ann Intern Med* 1983;98:958.
Review. Twenty-five percent of recurrent episodes were asymptomatic.

Cowan FM, et al. Relationship between antibodies to herpes simplex virus (HSV) and symptoms of HSV infection. *J Infect Dis* 1996;174:470–475.
The majority of HSV infections are asymptomatic and unrecognized.

DeJesus E, et al. Valacyclovir for the suppression of recurrent genital herpes in human immunodeficiency virus-infected subjects. *J Infect Dis* 2003;188:1009–1016.
Valacyclovir was safe in HIV infected patients.

Gottlieb SL, et al. Incidence of herpes simplex virus type 2 infection in 5 sexually transmitted disease (STD) clinics and the effect of HIV/STD risk-reduction counseling. *J Infect Dis* 2004;190:1059–1067.
Only 10% of new HSV-2 infections were diagnosed clinically.

Gold D, Corey L. Acyclovir prophylaxis for herpes simplex virus infection. *Antimicrob Agents Chemother* 1987;31:361.
Review of prophylaxis. The physician should stop acyclovir after 9 months to see if the recurrence rate warrants continued prophylaxis.

Guerry SL, et al. Recommendations for the selective use of herpes simplex virus type 2 serological testing. *Clin Infect Dis* 2005;40:38–45.
Type-specific HSV-2 testing is useful for high–risk, asymptomatic patients, such as those with HIV positivity.

Guinan ME, Wolinsky SM, Reichman RC. Epidemiology of genital herpes simplex virus infection. *Epidemiol Rev* 1985;7:127.
Disease may affect 20 million persons in the United States, with less than 25% of those infected being symptomatic.

Johnson RE, et al. A seroepidemiologic survey of the prevalence of herpes simplex virus type 2 infection in the United States. *N Engl J Med* 1989;321:7.
The prevalence of HSV-2 antibodies was from less than 1% in the group younger than age 15 to 20% for those ages 30 to 44 years.

Kimberlin DW, Rouse DJ. Genital herpes. *N Engl J Med* 2004;350:1970–1977.
Management guidelines.

Koutsky LA, et al. Underdiagnosis of genital herpes by current clinical and viral-isolation procedures. *N Engl J Med* 1992;326:1533.
The history or clinical examination identified only 39% of women with past or current genital HSV infections. That most cases of genital herpes are unrecognized is a factor in the continued spread of this infection.

Major CA, et al. Expectant management of preterm premature rupture of membranes complicated by active recurrent genital herpes. *Am J Obstet Gynecol* 2003;188:1551–1555.
The risk of developing neonatal herpes with premature rupture of the membranes was 10%. Expectant management of patients in this setting with recurrent genital herpes at 31 weeks or less is recommended.

Mertz GJ, et al. Transmission of genital herpes in couples with one symptomatic and one asymptomatic partner: a prospective study. *J Infect Dis* 1988;157:1169.
Asymptomatic and unrecognized acquisition of HSV-2 infection was common.

Mertz GJ, et al. Risk factors for the sexual transmission of genital herpes. *Ann Intern Med* 1992;116:197.
In 69% of patients, transmission occurred from sexual contact during periods of asymptomatic viral shedding. Risk of acquisition of HSV was higher in women than men.

Mertz GJ, et al. Oral famciclovir for suppression of recurrent genital herpes simplex virus infection in women. A multicenter, double-blind, placebo-controlled trial. *Arch Intern Med* 1997;157:343–349.
The most effective dose of famciclovir for suppression of recurrent genital HSV was 250 mg twice a day. Emergence of resistant strains to penciclovir was not a problem.

Randolph AG, Hartshorn RM, Washington AE. Acyclovir prophylaxis in late pregnancy to prevent neonatal herpes: a cost-effectiveness analysis. *Obstet Gynecol* 1996;88:603–610.
Based on decision analysis, oral acyclovir prophylaxis in late pregnancy is more cost effective than cesarean section for women with recurrent genital herpes.

Reeves WC, et al. Risk of recurrence after first episodes of genital herpes. *N Engl J Med* 1981;305:315.
The recurrence rate is 77% for those with a past history of herpes.

Rouse DJ, Stringer JS. An appraisal of screening for maternal type-specific herpes simplex virus antibodies to prevent neonatal herpes. *Am J Obstet Gynecol* 2000;183:400–406.
More data are needed before type-specific herpes screening in pregnancy can be recommended.

Sacks SL, et al. Patient-initiated, twice-daily oral famciclovir for early recurrent genital herpes. A randomized, double-blind multicenter trial. *JAMA* 1996;276:44–49.
Oral famciclovir (125 mg twice daily for 5 days) was effective for recurrent or episodic genital herpes. The intracellular half-life of penciclovir is 10 to 20 hours, compared with 0.7 hours for acyclovir, permitting dosing twice a day.

Scott LL. Perinatal herpes: current status and obstetric management strategies. *Pediatr Infect Dis* 1995;14:827.
Review. Weekly genital HSV cultures are not indicated. Route of delivery should be based on the presence of identifiable lesions and symptoms.

Scott LL, et al. Acyclovir suppression to prevent recurrent genital herpes at delivery. *Infect Dis Obstet Gynecol* 2002;10:71–77.
Acyclovir given after 36 weeks of gestation to term decreased HSV viral shedding and symptomatic disease.

Scott LL, et al. Acyclovir suppression to prevent cesarean delivery after first-episode genital herpes. *Obstet Gynecol* 1996;87:69–73.
Use of acyclovir from 36 weeks of gestation until delivery may have a role in reducing the cesarean section rate.

Solomon AR, et al. The Tzanck smear in the diagnosis of cutaneous herpes simplex. *JAMA* 1984;251:633.
This test has a sensitivity of about 50%.

Wald A, et al. Virologic characteristics of subclinical and symptomatic genital herpes infection. *N Engl J Med* 1995;333:770–775.
Most new HSV infections are acquired from partners with unrecognized or subclinical disease. Subclinical viral shedding of HSV-2 is common.

Wald A, et al. Suppression of subclinical shedding of herpes simplex virus type 2 with acyclovir. *Ann Intern Med* 1996;124:8–15.
Acyclovir suppresses shedding of genital HSV.

Wald A, et al. Frequent genital herpes simplex virus 2 shedding in immunocompetent women. Effect of acyclovir treatment. *J Clin Invest* 1997;99:1092.
PCR was more sensitive than viral culture in detecting genital HSV-2 shedding, which was noted in 28% of days. Oral acyclovir reduced shedding by 80%.

Watts DH, et al. A double-blind, randomized, placebo-controlled trial of acyclovir in late pregnancy for the reduction of herpes simplex virus shedding and cesarean delivery. *Am J Obstet Gynecol* 2003;188:836–843.
Viral shedding still occurs with acyclovir, and neonatal infection is an issue.

Whitley RJ, et al. The natural history of herpes simplex virus infection of mother and newborn. *Pediatrics* 1980;66:489.
Only 20% of mothers of infants infected with HSV gave a history of recurrent genital herpes infection.

Whitley RJ, et al. Herpes simplex viruses. *Clin Infect Dis* 1998;26:541–555.
Review.

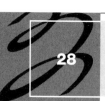

28 VAGINITIS

*V*aginal discharge is a common gynecologic complaint and accounts for half of patient visits to private gynecologists. Vaginitis, or inflammation of the vagina, is usually associated with an increase in vaginal secretions or discharge. Vaginal discharge may be normal or pathologic. Normal or physiologic vaginal discharge, called *leukorrhea,* is not associated with vulvar discomfort, is usually nonpruritic, has no offensive odor, contains few white cells, and has normal vaginal flora. The predominant organisms comprising normal vaginal flora are lactobacilli, which are gram-positive rods. Normal vaginal secretions have an acidic pH of about 4.0. Common causes of an increase in physiologic discharge are ovulation, pregnancy, and oral contraceptive use. Discharge may also increase before normal menstruation. An abnormal vaginal discharge usually has an offensive odor, often contains many polymorphonuclear leukocytes, has an abnormal vaginal microflora, and is frequently accompanied by dysuria, dyspareunia, and vulvar itching and soreness.

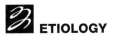 ETIOLOGY

There are many causes, both infectious and noninfectious, for an abnormal vaginal discharge. Extravaginal disease may mimic vaginal discharge. Dermatologic and psychosomatic disorders may result in vaginal complaints. Rectovaginal or vesicovaginal fistulae may result in the passage of either feces or urine through the vagina. Patients with proctitis may have a discharge that simulates a vaginal discharge. Noninfectious causes of vaginal discharge include chemical irritation or allergy from contraceptive foams or feminine hygiene products, a foreign body, such as a forgotten vaginal tampon or device used for masturbation, and atrophic vaginitis. The vaginal mucosa in postmenopausal women may be deficient in estrogen, resulting in a thin, scanty discharge that is sometimes accompanied by vulvar soreness and pruritus. The atrophic vaginal mucosa also may become secondarily infected. Vaginal discharge is sometimes seen with gynecologic neoplasms. The discharge may be scanty and tinged with blood.

The majority of cases of vaginal discharge have an infectious cause, and numerous organisms have been implicated. The three most frequent forms of infectious vaginitis are candidal vaginitis, trichomoniasis, and bacterial vaginosis caused by *Gardnerella vaginalis* and a variety of anaerobes. *Neisseria gonorrhoeae* rarely infects the adult vagina, and the discharge caused by the gonococcus originates in the endocervix. The discharge passes through the introitus and is perceived by the patient as vaginal discharge. Similarly, chlamydial or herpetic cervicitis may be associated with an excessive cervical discharge, which the patient observes as an abnormal vaginal discharge.

The symptoms of vaginitis are vaginal discharge, dysuria, dyspareunia, and foul vaginal odor. Dysuria can indicate infection at a number of different sites: the urethra (acute urethral syndrome), bladder (cystitis), kidneys (pyelonephritis), vulva and vagina (vulvovaginitis), and cervix (cervicitis). A patient may be able to localize the dysuria as either internal (felt inside the body), indicating urinary tract infection, or external (felt over the vaginal labia as urine is passed), suggesting vaginitis. In a large study of women presenting to a primary care clinic with a complaint of dysuria, vaginitis was found far more often than a urinary tract infection (70% vs. 12%). Therefore, women with dysuria should be asked about symptoms of vaginal discharge and vulvar irritation, as well as the presence of internal or external dysuria.

 CANDIDIASIS

The most frequent causes of vaginal infection, depending on the population studied, are vulvovaginal candidiasis and bacterial vaginosis. Most of the fungi isolated from patients with vaginitis are *Candida albicans*. Approximately 10 to 15% of cases are caused by other *Candida* species, such as *Candida glabrata*. Although vaginal candidiasis can be transmitted sexually, sexual acquisition is of limited importance; therefore, there is no need to treat asymptomatic male sexual partners of women with vaginal candidiasis. Moreover, patients can continue intercourse during therapy. Predisposing risk factors for vaginal candidiasis are antimicrobials, pregnancy, oral contraceptives, corticosteroids, exogenous hormones, diabetes mellitus, local allergy to perfumes, HIV, and nylon underwear. The data supporting the importance of some of the risk factors, such as oral contraceptives, remain controversial, and further evidence is needed. Host factors must be involved to explain why some women have infrequent episodes of vaginal candidiasis and others suffer from recurrent infections. Rectal colonization with yeasts is often blamed for recurrent vaginal candidiasis, but in one study the rate of relapse was not related to rectal carriage of *Candida*. The cause of most episodes of recurrent vaginal candidiasis is unknown because the usual predisposing factors are often absent.

As reported for vaginitis of other causes, the clinical features of candidiasis are not distinct enough to permit an accurate etiologic diagnosis. Self-diagnosis is often inaccurate. A curdlike discharge suggests the diagnosis, but a thin discharge occurs as well. The diagnosis can usually be confirmed with a 10% potassium hydroxide preparation or Gram's-stained vaginal smear. Vaginal pH is normal in patients with candidiasis. The diagnosis, however, is not ruled out by a negative result on wet preparation or Gram's-stained smear for yeasts. A culture for *Candida* may be helpful in symptomatic patients when microscopic examination for yeasts is negative. Some 25 to 50% of normal women have yeast as part of their vaginal flora; therefore, for most patients a vaginal culture for *Candida* is not indicated. The diagnosis is made by microscopic examination, and empiric antifungal therapy should be administered.

Various antifungal agents (clotrimazole, miconazole, terconazole, butoconazole, tioconazole, nystatin, ketoconazole, itraconazole, and fluconazole) are used successfully to treat vulvovaginal candidiasis. Cure rates with the different preparations are similar, but duration of therapy varies. Nystatin is administered intravaginally for 14 days, miconazole for 3–7 days, and clotrimazole for 1–14 days, depending on the dose. Single-dose intravaginal therapy with clotrimazole (500 mg) also yields comparable results. A single oral dose of 150 mg of fluconazole is effective, convenient, and preferred. Women with complicated infections are less likely to respond to short-course therapy and require fluconazole for 10 to 14 days. Fluconazole can also be given as 150 mg every 72 hours for 3 doses to eradicate *Candida*. One study shows that even powdered boric acid (600 mg) in gelatin capsules inserted intravaginally produces cure rates better than 90%. Unfortunately, boric acid capsules are not commercially available and must be prepared by a pharmacist or by the patient. Oral ingestion of yogurt containing *Lactobacillus acidophilus* or other *Lactobacillus* preparations may decrease the rate of vaginal candidiasis in comparison with placebo.

Although the various intravaginal preparations can achieve excellent results for an isolated episode of vulvovaginal candidiasis, management of recurrent disease, defined as four or more episodes per year, is a frustrating problem for both patient and clinician. Current therapy has limited value. Use of preparations to decrease *Candida* in the stool and treatment of the male partner do not affect the recurrence rate. In one controlled trial, after inducing clinical remission with fluconazole, patients were given either fluconazole (100 mg weekly) for 6 months or placebo. At 12 months about half the patients were asymptomatic as compared with 27% who received placebo. Fluconazole was well tolerated, and developing resistant *Candida* was not an issue. Management of patients who stop suppressive fluconazole therapy and have a recurrence of *Candida* is unknown and requires further study. Other drugs for recurrent disease after an initial induction regimen has resulted in negative cultures include ketoconazole (100 mg daily) and clotrimazole (500-mg vaginal suppositories once weekly). Liver function tests should be obtained monthly for patients receiving long-term ketoconazole. Further studies are needed to help solve the difficult problems of recurrent vaginal candidiasis.

 ## TRICHOMONIASIS

Trichomonas vaginalis, a flagellate protozoan, is a well-recognized and frequent cause of vaginitis. The organism is usually, but not invariably, transmitted by sexual intercourse. Trichomoniasis facilitates the transmission of HIV. The textbook description of trichomoniasis as vaginitis with frothy discharge and "strawberry appearance" of the cervix is rarely seen. Trichomoniasis, like vaginitis of other causes, cannot be reliably diagnosed by the clinical presentation. Vaginal pH is increased to about 5.0 to 5.5, as in patients with nonspecific vaginitis. In symptomatic patients, a wet mount of vaginal secretions obtained from the posterior vaginal fornix establishes a diagnosis for about 70% of patients. The wet mount is less sensitive in patients with asymptomatic infections. The culture in which modified Diamond's medium is used diagnoses 95% of cases, but this technique requires 2 to 7 days. Another useful diagnostic test, called the InPouch system, consists of two chambers—one for wet preparation and the other for culture. Papanicolaou's smear detects about 70% of infections, depending on the expertise of the cytologist. A test using nucleic acid amplification (polymerase chain reaction) can detect *Trichomonas* from vaginal fluid and urine. The test has a sensitivity of 64 to 91%, but it is not yet commercially available. Secretions for diagnosis should be obtained not from the endocervical canal but from the posterior vaginal fornix.

Both symptomatic and asymptomatic women with trichomoniasis should receive treatment. If trichomoniasis is untreated in pregnancy, there is an increase in premature rupture of the membranes and premature birth. In addition, the regular sexual partners of patients need to be treated to prevent reinfection. A single 2-g dose of metronidazole is highly effective. Male partners also can be treated with a 2-g dose of metronidazole. Alcohol should be avoided for 24 hours after metronidazole is taken. In the first trimester of pregnancy, metronidazole is not recommended, and clotrimazole can be prescribed for intravaginal use, although this drug is less effective than metronidazole. Metronidazole can be used in the last two trimesters of pregnancy without adverse effects. A few patients have intractable trichomoniasis, which usually responds to 2 g of metronidazole taken orally for 7 days. Rarely, IV metronidazole is required to treat this infection when a patient cannot tolerate the oral drug. Paromomycin can be used for the rare patients who fail to respond to metronidazole. Tinidazole also may be used to treat resistant strains of *Trichomonas*.

 BACTERIAL VAGINOSIS

Bacterial vaginosis, formerly "nonspecific vaginitis," accounts for at least 40% of cases of vaginitis. The origin of the syndrome is polymicrobic; causative organisms include G. *vaginalis* (a small gram-variable coccobacillus) and a variety of anaerobes, such as *Bacteroides* species and *Peptococcus* species. A curved, gram-variable to gram-negative anaerobic organism (*Mobiluncus* species) has also been isolated as part of the polymicrobial flora. Confusion has arisen about the taxonomic position of G. *vaginalis*. The former designations were *Haemophilus vaginalis* and *Corynebacterium vaginalis*. Bacterial vaginosis also is associated with a decrease in the lactobacilli that produce hydrogen peroxide.

Features of this diagnosis include a thin, homogeneous vaginal discharge; vaginal pH greater than 4.5; a fishy amine odor after 10% potassium hydroxide is added to a drop of vaginal discharge; vaginal odor resulting from the abnormal amines released; and the presence of clue cells, which are vaginal epithelial cells covered with gram-variable coccobacilli. These cells are noted in 90% of patients with this disease, whereas only 10% of uninfected women have them. A culture for G. *vaginalis* is invariably positive, but 50% of uninfected persons also have this organism as part of the normal vaginal flora. There is little need, therefore, to obtain a culture to confirm the diagnosis. In addition, aerobic lactobacilli and white cells are generally absent from the vaginal smear. A DNA probe for G. *vaginalis* is available for diagnosis, but it is expensive.

The mode of disease transmission is not clear, and sexual transmission is unproven. Treatment of the male sexual partner usually is not indicated. Studies of sexual transmission found no beneficial effects on cure rates when partners of women with bacterial vaginosis were treated. However, this issue is still controversial, and partners of women with intractable or recurrent disease should be treated. Studies have reported an increased risk for prematurity linked to chorioamnionitis in women with bacterial vaginosis.

Metronidazole is the drug of choice for this disease. Various treatment schedules may be used, including administering 500 mg orally twice daily for 7 days, or a 2-g single dose. There is no difference in cure rates obtained with a single dose of metronidazole or with a more prolonged course, but the recurrence rate is higher with single-dose therapy. Clindamycin administered in a dosage of 300 mg twice daily for 7 days also is efficacious. Topical intravaginal treatment with 5 g of 2% clindamycin vaginal cream once daily for 7 days, clindamycin vaginal ovules (100 mg) for 3 days, or 5 g of metronidazole vaginal gel once a day for 5 days is also effective. Metronidazole (250 mg three times daily) or clindamycin (300 mg twice daily) given for 7 days is recommended in pregnancy. Asymptomatic women from whom clue cells are obtained on a wet mount do not require therapy, except in pregnancy and before elective gynecologic surgery. Future studies are needed to define the natural history of asymptomatic disease, identify complications, develop strategies to manage patients with intractable disease, and discover the best screening approaches and treatment in pregnancy. (NMG)

Bibliography

Anderson MR, Klink K, Cohrssen A. Evaluation of vaginal complaints. *JAMA* 2004; 291:1368–1379.
Symptoms alone are not adequate to distinguish the different causes of vaginitis.

Amsel R, et al. Nonspecific vaginitis: diagnostic criteria and microbial and epidemiologic associations. *Am J Med* 1983;74:1368–1379.
Diagnostic criteria for bacterial vaginosis include a vaginal pH greater than 4.5; a fishy odor from the vaginal discharge with the addition of 10% potassium hydroxide; clue cells; and a thin, homogeneous vaginal discharge.

Brunham RC, et al. Mucopurulent cervicitis—the ignored counterpart in women of urethritis in men. *N Engl J Med* 1984;311:1.
Illustration of mucopurulent cervicitis caused by Chlamydia.

Centers for Disease Control and Prevention. Sexually transmitted disease treatment guidelines 2002. *MMWR* 2002;51:1–78.
Treatment recommendations.

Cerikcioglu N, Beksac MS. Cytolytic vaginosis: misdiagnosed as candidal vaginitis. *Infect Dis Obstet Gynecol* 2004;12:13–16.
An entity due to overgrowth of lactobacilli that may be confused with candidiasis.

Ferris DG, et al. Over-the-counter antifungal drug misuse associated with patient-diagnosed vulvovaginal candidiasis. *Obstet Gynecol* 2002;99:419–425.
In women who purchased over-the-counter antifungal medication, the diagnosis was correct only one third of the time.

Fouts AC, Kraus SJ. *Trichomonas vaginalis:* reevaluation of its clinical presentation and laboratory diagnosis. *J Infect Dis* 1980;141:137.
A frothy discharge is not pathognomonic for trichomoniasis.

Hager WD. Treatment of metronidazole-resistant *Trichomonas vaginalis* with tinidazole: case reports of three patients. *Sex Transm Dis* 2004;31:343–345.
Tinidazole can be used to treat metronidazole-resistant trichomoniasis.

Hauth JC, et al. Reduced incidence of preterm delivery with metronidazole and erythromycin in women with bacterial vaginosis. *N Engl J Med* 1995;333:1732–1736.
In pregnant women with bacterial vaginosis, use of erythromycin plus metronidazole decreased the rates of prematurity.

Heine RP, et al. Polymerase chain reaction analysis of distal vaginal specimens: a less invasive strategy for detection of *Trichomonas vaginalis. Clin Infect Dis* 1997;24:985–987.
Polymerase chain reaction testing had a yield of 92% for trichomoniasis when a swab was inserted about 1 inch into the vagina.

Hilton E, et al. Ingestion of yogurt containing *Lactobacillus acidophilus* as prophylaxis for candidal vaginitis. *Ann Intern Med* 1992;116:353.
Daily ingestion for 6 months of 8 oz of yogurt with Lactobacillus acidophilus *decreased the rate of vaginal candidal colonization and infection. (See also Drutz DJ.* Lactobacillus *prophylaxis for* Candida *vaginitis.* Ann Intern Med *1992;116:419.*

Holley RL, et al. A randomized, double-blind clinical trial of vaginal acidification versus placebo for the treatment of symptomatic bacterial vaginosis. *Sex Transm Dis* 2004;31;236–238.
Vaginal acidification was not effective to treat bacterial vaginosis.

Joesoef MR, Schmid G. Bacterial vaginosis. *Clin Evid* 2004:11:2054–2063.
Concise review.

Komaroff AL, et al. Management strategies for symptoms of urinary and vaginal infections. *Arch Intern Med* 1978;138:1069.
Internal dysuria suggests that the patient has a urinary tract infection, and external dysuria favors a diagnosis of vaginitis.

Lugo-Miro VI, Green M, Mazur L. Comparison of different metronidazole therapeutic regimens for bacterial vaginosis: a meta-analysis. *JAMA* 1992;268:92.
There is no difference between the cure rates of patients with bacterial vaginosis treated with metronidazole as a 2-g single dose, a 2-g single dose given for 2 days, 400 mg three times daily for 5 days, or 500 mg twice daily for 7 days.

Milne JD, Warnock DW. Effect of simultaneous oral and vaginal treatment on the rate of cure and relapse in vaginal candidiasis. *Br J Vener Dis* 1979;55:362.
Relapse of vaginal candidiasis was unrelated to rectal carriage of yeast.

Nyirjesy P, et al. Over-the-counter and alternative medicines in the treatment of chronic vaginal symptoms. *Obstet Gynecol* 1997;90:50–53.

The most frequent alternative medicines used were Acidophilus *products or yogurt. Most of the yogurt products lack hydrogen peroxide-producing* Lactobacillus *strains that might be of benefit.*

Paterson BA, et al. The tampon test for trichomoniasis: a comparison between conventional methods and a polymerase chain reaction for *Trichomonas vaginalis* in women. *Sex Transm Infect* 1998;74:136–139.

Polymerase chain reaction testing on a tampon specimen was useful for diagnosis of trichomoniasis.

Schaaf VM, Perez-Stable EJ, Borchardt K. The limited value of symptoms and signs in the diagnosis of vaginal infections. *Arch Intern Med* 1990;150:1929.

An etiology of vaginitis was identified in only half the patients. Symptoms did not differ for the three diagnoses.

Schmitt C, Sobel JD, Meriwether C. Bacterial vaginosis: treatment with clindamycin cream versus oral metronidazole. *Obstet Gynecol* 1992;79:1020.

Cure rate with clindamycin vaginal cream was 72%. No data exist regarding the use of clindamycin cream in pregnancy.

Sobel J, Peipert JF, Mcgregor JA, et al. Efficacy of clindamycin vaginal ovule (3-day treatment) vs. clindamycin vaginal cream (7-day treatment) in bacterial vaginosis. *Infect Dis Obstet Gynecol* 2001;9:9–15.

Similar cure rates were seen using clindamycin vaginal ovule (100 mg) for 3 days compared with the clindamycin vaginal cream for 7 days.

Sobel JD, Chaim W. Treatment of *Torulopsis glabrata* vaginitis: retrospective review of boric acid therapy. *Clin Infect Dis* 1997;24:649–652.

In patients with Torulopsis (Candida) glabrata *vaginitis who fail azole therapy, vaginal boric acid may be effective.*

Sobel JD, et al. Maintenance fluconazole therapy for recurrent vulvovaginal candidiasis. *N Engl J Med* 2004;351:876–883.

Weekly treatment with fluconazole (150 mg) for 6 months was more effective than placebo in preventing recurrent vaginal candidiasis.

Sobel JD, et al. Single oral dose fluconazole compared with conventional clotrimazole topical therapy of *Candida* vaginitis. *Am J Obstet Gynecol* 1995;172:1263–1268.

A single oral dose of fluconazole (150 mg) was effective for vaginal candidiasis.

Sobel JD, et al. Vulvovaginal candidiasis: epidemiologic, diagnostic, and therapeutic considerations. *Am J Obstet Gynecol* 1998;178:203–211.

Review.

Spence MR, et al. The minimum single oral metronidazole dose for treating trichomoniasis: a randomized, blinded study. *Obstet Gynecol* 1997;89:699–703.

The minimum effective dose of metronidazole was 1.5 g.

Swygard H, et al. Trichomoniasis: clinical manifestations, diagnosis and management. *Sex Transm Infect* 2004;80:91–95.

Review.

Van Slyke KK, Michel VP, Rein MF. Treatment of vulvovaginal candidiasis with boric acid power. *Am J Obstet Gynecol* 1981;141:145.

Boric acid powder (600 mg) in a gelatin capsule inserted intravaginally at bedtime had a 91% cure rate.

Wendel KA, et al. *Trichomonas vaginalis* polymerase chain reaction compared to standard diagnostic and therapeutic tools for detection and treatment of vaginal trichomoniasis. *Clin Infect Dis* 2002;35:576–580.

The polymerase chain reaction and culture have a sensitivity of about 80% in diagnosing vaginal trichomoniasis.

Wolner-Hanssen P, et al. Clinical manifestations of vaginal trichomoniasis. *JAMA* 1989;261:571.

Excellent review of the clinical manifestations. Colpitis macularis (strawberry cervix) had a sensitivity of 44% with an odds ratio of 241; a frothy discharge had a sensitivity of 8% with an odds ratio of 21. Overall, the sensitivity of the symptoms and signs of trichomoniasis is low.

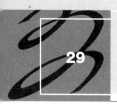

29 HUMAN PAPILLOMAVIRUS

$\mathcal{H}$uman papillomavirus (HPV) is perhaps the most common sexually transmitted infection in the United States. Infected persons are usually asymptomatic, and many infections clear spontaneously. Mild disease includes genital warts, verruga, or cytologically evident dysplasia of the cervix or anus. Persistent anogenital infection is strongly associated with advanced cervical neoplastic disease and invasive carcinoma of the cervix. High-risk genotypes of HPV are likely to be responsible for a high proportion of squamous-origin carcinomas of the cervix, vagina, vulva, anus, and penis worldwide. Cofactors, such as tobacco use, ultraviolet radiation, pregnancy, folate deficiency, and immune suppression have been implicated in this process as well.

There are 5.5 million new cases of HPV every year, and approximately 20 million Americans are infected. There are more than 100 types of HPV, and approximately 20 to 30 types infect the female genital tract. Certain HPV types are closely associated with certain clinical conditions. HPV 6 and 11 commonly cause genital warts, whereas HPV 16 and 18 cause cervical dysplasia and invasive cancer. Women with a history of a cervical high-grade squamous intraepithelial lesion (HGSIL) or invasive squamous cell carcinoma (SCC) of the cervix are at increased risk for subsequent development of invasive cancer in other tissues of the anogenital/mucosal category, particularly vaginal and anal carcinoma. In these patients, the relative risk (RR) of vaginal carcinoma is 5.6, and the risk of anal carcinoma is 4. Anal cancer (RR of 33) has been strongly associated with male homosexuality and specific male practices, such as engaging in receptive anal intercourse.

HPV cannot be cultured by traditional microbiologic techniques in a clinical laboratory. HPV lesions are thought to arise from the proliferation of infected basal keratinocytes. Infection typically occurs when basal cells are exposed to infectious virus through a disturbed epithelial barrier, as would occur during sexual intercourse or after minor skin abrasions. HPV infections have not been shown to be cytolytic; rather, viral particles are released as a result of degeneration of desquamating cells.

The genome of HPV is small, with approximately 8000 base pairs and a limited number of genes. Most HPV genotypes have a similar organization consisting of a transcription and replication control region; an *early region* encoding proteins for replication, regulation, and modification of the host cytoplasm and nucleus; and a *late region* encoding capsid proteins. These genes have been divided into "early" and "late" genes based on when and where they are expressed in the diseased epithelium. Two late genes, L1 and L2, encode for capsid proteins. These proteins have been the basis of prophylactic HPV vaccines. Three early genes are involved in oncogenesis. E6 and E7 proteins bind to and degrade p53 and retinoblastoma family proteins, respectively. The net effect of HPV inactivating these host proteins is that the host cell is primed for proliferation and unchecked growth.

 ## EPIDEMIOLOGY OF HPV INFECTIONS

An estimated 500,000 new cervical cancer cases and 300,000 deaths occur worldwide each year, and 75% of the deaths are in developing countries. It appears that HPV 16 was identified in approximately half of all cases of cervical cancers. HPV 18 is detected in about 15% of tumors. Studies have demonstrated that most women are infected with HPV within the first few years of becoming sexually active, and that most sexually active adults are infected with HPV during their lifetimes. Possible associated risk factors for HPV infection include more than one sex partner, tobacco use, and use of oral contraceptives. Most initial infections occurred without symptoms or clinical signs of HPV infection. People infected with HIV, cancer chemotherapy recipients, renal transplant patients, and other immunosuppressed persons have impaired ability to clear virus, permitting longer duration of infection and increased likelihood of oncogenic integration. It also should be noted that transmission between partners of the same-sex is possible, and that screening for cervical dysplasia is indicated for lesbian women.

 ## DIAGNOSIS OF HPV INFECTIONS

These lesions have been described as "cauliflower like." Biopsy of suspected genital warts can be useful in cases in which there is an unusual presentation, such as hyperpigmentation, ulceration, or if there is a suspicion of cancer. The traditional method for detection of high-risk HPV is the Papanicolaou-stained (Pap) smear. *The Bethesda System 2001* classifies squamous cell abnormalities into four categories: (1) ASC (atypical squamous cells); (2) LSIL (low-grade squamous intraepithelial lesions); (3) HGSIL; and (4) SCC. False-negative rates as high as 30% have been reported.

New methods of collection and processing of specimens for Pap smears have been developed recently to help reduce the number of false-negative results. In these methods, the specimen is collected in a preservative solution rather than being spread directly on the microscope slide by hand. The uniform monolayer created by these methods is easier for a technician to read. The FDA also has approved some computerized systems that display potentially abnormal cells on a screen for review and analysis. Either conventionally prepared or monolayer Pap smear slides can be screened by using these computer-assisted systems. The *AutoPap 300QC* has been FDA approved for both primary screening and rescreening of Pap smears. The *PapNet system* is approved for rescreening only.

The *Digene Hybrid Capture* test detects HPV DNA by hybridizing it with known matching RNA sequences. The *Digene Hybrid Capture II (HC2) System* uses a specific HPV RNA probe cocktail to detect target DNA in patient specimens. The resulting RNA:DNA hybrids are captured onto the surface of a microplate well coated with antibodies specific for RNA:DNA hybrids. Immobilized hybrids are then reacted with alkaline phosphatase-conjugated antibodies specific for the RNA:DNA hybrids. Hybridization is detected with a chemiluminescent substrate. As the substrate is cleaved by the bound alkaline phosphatase, light is emitted. The light is measured as relative light units (RLUs) by a luminometer. The intensity of light that is emitted denotes the presence or absence of target DNA in the specimen.

In March 2000, the Food and Drug Administration (FDA) approved the use of Digene HC2 HPV DNA testing as a follow-up test for women with abnormal Pap tests. In September 2002, the ASCCP Consensus Guidelines for the Management of Women with Cervical Cytological Abnormalities listed Digene HC2 HPV DNA testing as the preferred management protocol for women with a cytologic diagnosis of ASC-US as a triage prior to

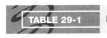 **Digene Test Internet Resources**

Type of Web resource	Location
Clinician oriented	http://www.paml.com/Files/TestUpdates/HPV%20Testing.pdf
Clinician oriented	http://www.thedoctorsdoctor.com/labtests/The_pap.htm
Company site	http://www.digene.com/clinician_1.html

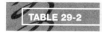 **Interpretation of Hybrid Capture Results in Patients With ASCUS Pap Smear***

Digene hybrid HPV result	capture	Refer to colposcopy[†]	Result interpretation
Probe A Negative	Probe B Negative	No	There is a high probability that a higher disease stage will not be found at colposcopy
Positive Negative Positive	Negative Positive Positive	Yes	Progression to high-grade disease is probable

*Data from the Digene Corporation HPV Test Hybrid Capture II product insert.
[†]Results are not meant to deter women from colposcopy.

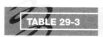 **Cytotoxic Agents for HPV**

Agent	Apply	Comments	Efficacy
Trichloroacetic acid	80–90% solution applied weekly to genital warts in the clinic The treatment can be applied weekly for 4 weeks	Not absorbed Can be used in pregnancy Burning and pain Allow sufficient drying time	Effective in 63–70% Rate of recurrence is unclear
Podophyllin	Applied weekly in the clinic to warts as a 10–25% suspension in benzoin Applications should be <0.5 mL Not to be used in areas >10 mm²	Wash off in 4 hr. Not to be used in pregnancy. Bone marrow suppression Absorbed systemically.	Efficacy similar to podofilox 23–65% recurrences
Podofilox Gels, cream, solutions	Apply 0.5% to warts twice a day for 3 days, followed by 4 days without treatment The treatment is repeated for 2–4 cycles	Not to be used in pregnancy Self application Burning and itching	48–77% clearance within 4–6 weeks Recurrences of 4–38%
5 Fluorouracil	Apply as a 5% cream A thin layer of cream is spread over the lesions one to three times per week	For treatment of multifocal or extensive vulvar or vaginal intraepithelial neoplasia For self application Local irritation Not to be used in pregnancy	Some experts do not recommend the use of this drug in the primary care setting

(Adapted from Wiley DJ, et al. External genital warts: diagnosis, treatment, and prevention. *Clin Infect Dis* 2002;35(suppl 2):S210–224 and Zanotti KM, et al. Update on the diagnosis and treatment of human papillomavirus infection. Human papillomavirus: a review. *Clev Clin J Med* 2002;69:948, 951–955, 956 passim.)

colposcopy. In April 2003, the FDA cleared the use of Digene HC2 as a screening test to be used in conjunction with a liquid-based Pap test for women older than age 30.

When Is the Test Used?

The HPV-DNA test is used only in conjunction with Pap testing. The test is used:

1. When a woman's Pap test results are mildly abnormal. The HPV-DNA Test is then used to tell whether HPV is present at high enough levels to indicate that an HPV infection exists. If she has an HPV infection, she may be tested further to be sure that she does not have serious cervical abnormalities.
2. When women older than age 30 have HPV infections that do not disappear over time. These women may be at greater risk for developing cervical disease. Women older than age 30 with a positive Pap test and a positive HPV-DNA test have a higher than average risk of cervical cancer and may need to be tested more frequently. Only a small percentage of HPV infections, however, lead to cancer.

The test has a negative predictive value of 99% and has a greater than 95% sensitivity. See Tables 29-1 and 29-2 for more information regarding the assay.

TREATMENT OF HPV INFECTIONS OF THE LOWER GENITAL TRACT

No treatment is 100% effective and, unfortunately, relapse is common. The main indication for therapy is the removal of symptomatic lesions. Many small warts resolve without therapy, and usually HPV-induced cervical cell changes are transient. Around 90% regress spontaneously within 12 to 36 months as the immune system eliminates the virus. Please see Table 29-3 for a discussion of the individual agents. When using ablative therapies, consider

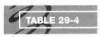

TABLE 29-4   **Physical Ablation for HPV**

Modality	Use	Methods	Other information	Efficacy estimates
Laser ablation	For destruction of extensive genital warts or treatment of extensive or multifocal vulvar lesions or VIN	CO^2 laser vaporizes tissue No pathologic assessment	Destructive method requiring general anesthesia Postoperative discomfort	More costly? 23–52% effective 60–77% recurrence
Surgery	For large exophytic *Condylomata* or confluent vulva or vaginal lesions	Excision Pathologic assessment possible	Anesthesia required Multifocal disease is problematic	35–72% clearance 19–29% recurrence at 1 year
LEEP	Excise CIN or genital warts	Loop electrode excision	Depth of excision might be difficult to control	61–94% clearance 14–22% recurrence
Cryotherapy	Freeze genital warts	Liquid nitrogen		40% clearance at 3 months; 27% at 6 months

LEEP, Loop electrocautery excision procedure.
Treatment options for intra-anal pathology include trichloroacetic acid, cryotherapy, electrosurgery, and laser treatment.
(Adapted from Wiley DJ, et al. External genital warts: diagnosis, treatment, and prevention. *Clin Infect Dis* 2002;35(suppl 2):S210–224 and Zanotti KM, et al. Update on the diagnosis and treatment of human papillomavirus infection. Human papillomavirus: a review. *Clev Clin J Med* 2002;69:948, 951–955, 956 passim.)

TABLE 29-5 Immunomodulation for HPV

Agent	Mechanism	Apply	Other	Efficacy
Imiquimod (Aldara)	Modifies the immune response Potent inducer of interferon-α and enhances cell-mediated cytotoxic activity	Self application 5% cream is applied overnight three times per week for up to 16 weeks Wash with soap and water on awakening	Not recommended for mucosal surfaces, such as the vagina Mild to moderate inflammation	30–60% clearance Women >men?
Interferons	Immunomodulation and direct antiviral?	Intralesional injections at the base of the wart three times a week for 3 weeks	Flulike symptoms and leukopenia	30–50% clearance Not widely used or even recommended by most experts

(Adapted from Wiley DJ, et al. External genital warts: diagnosis, treatment, and prevention. *Clin Infect Dis* 2002;35(suppl 2):S210–224 and Zanotti KM, et al. Update on the diagnosis and treatment of human papillomavirus infection. Human papillomavirus: a review. *Clev Clin J Med* 2002;69:948, 951–955, 956 passim.)
Aldara website http://www.3m.com/us/healthcare/pharma/aldara/hcp_resources.jhtml

using acetic acid first to help define the area of interest. Recurrence rates are high because these methods often fail to eradicate the latent reservoir of HPV remaining behind.

Imiquimod, podophyllin, and podofilox should not be used during pregnancy; furthermore, treatment for subclinical genital HPV infection and lower grade cervical intraepithelial neoplasia (CIN) during pregnancy is not recommended, as spontaneous improvement postpartum is not uncommon. Cesarean delivery is indicated only if the genital warts block the vaginal opening. The effect of cesarean delivery on perinatal transmission is unknown and should not be performed solely for this indication. Perinatal transmission of HPV is a rare event (Table 29-4).

Condom use may reduce the risk of spread, but exposure is still possible given the ability of the virus to affect nearby epithelium. Routine examination of asymptomatic partners is not recommended. Simultaneous treatment of the asymptomatic partner does not lead to a reduced likelihood of recurrence in the patient.

VACCINATION

Key HPV gene products have been used as subunit vaccines, similar to the approach used for the hepatitis B vaccine. One large efficacy trial was recently reported in the *New England Journal of Medicine*. There were no cases of HPV 16-persistent infection or HPV 16-related cervical dysplasia in women who received the experimental vaccine. Calculated vaccine efficacy was 90 to 100% (Table 29-5). (JWM)

Bibliography

Agnantis NJ, et al. The current status of HPV DNA testing. *Eur J Gynaecol Oncol* 2003;24:351–356.
Although there is a lack of randomized controlled trials in this field, data from observational studies indicate that HPV DNA testing after conservative surgical treatment for CIN may be very sensitive and may detect early residual and recurrent disease.
Apgar BS, et al. The 2001 Bethesda System terminology. *Am Fam Physician* 2003;68:1992–1998.

The 2001 Bethesda System for reporting cervical or vaginal cytologic diagnoses is an incremental change in the uniform terminology introduced in 1988 and revised in 1991.

Ault KA, et al. Human papillomavirus infections: diagnosis, treatment, and hope for a vaccine. *Obstet Gynecol Clin North Am* 2003;3:809–817.

HPV infections are common, with millions of Americans infected. Common gynecologic manifestations of HPV infection include genital warts and cervical neoplasia. Excellent overall review article.

Bolick DR, et al. Laboratory implementation of human papillomavirus testing. *Arch Pathol Lab Med* 2003;127:984–990.

Which methodology is the best fit for the laboratory? Is it better to develop an in-house testing service or to send it out? How do I get started? What are the financial and economic issues, and how should they be managed?

Burd EM. Human papillomavirus and cervical cancer. *Clin Microbiol Rev* 2003;16:1–17.

Superb review article. Good overall summary. A valuable resource.

Castellsague X, Munoz N. Chapter 3: cofactors in human papillomavirus carcinogenesis—role of parity, oral contraceptives, and tobacco smoking. *J Natl Cancer Inst Monogr*: 2003;(31):20–28.

If confirmed, our conclusions may imply that multiparous women, women who are smokers, and women on long-term oral contraceptives use may need closer surveillance for cytologic abnormalities and HPV infections than women in the general population.

Cohn SE, et al. Sexually transmitted diseases, HIV, and AIDS in women. Update on the diagnosis and treatment of human papillomavirus infection. *Med Clin North Am* 2003;87:971–995.

Current therapies do not reliably eradicate HPV infection, and benign genital warts and genital tract intraepithelial neoplasia often recur after treatment. We discuss the pathogenesis, clinical manifestations, detection, and treatment of HPV infections of the anogenital tract.

Devaraj K, et al. Development of HPV vaccines for HPV-associated head and neck squamous cell carcinoma. *Crit Rev Oral Biol Med* 2003;14:345–362.

Should they fulfill their promise, these vaccines may prevent HPV infection or control its potentially life-threatening consequences in humans.

Galloway DA. Papillomavirus vaccines in clinical trials. *Lancet Infect Dis* 2003;3:469–475.

A firm grasp of the molecular pathogenesis of HPVs and the natural history of genital HPV infections, combined with greater understanding of how to trigger effective immune responses, offers hope for the elimination of HPV-associated diseases.

Garland SM. Imiquimod. *Curr Opin Infect Dis* 2003;16:85–89.

In the future, imiquimod and newer generations of imidazoquinolines (resiquimod) require further investigation for potential clinical utility in treating other cutaneous and mucosal viral infections, dysplasias and neoplasia, as well as potential vaccine adjuvants.

Herzog TJ. New approaches for the management of cervical cancer. *Gynecol Oncol* 2003;90:S22–S27.

Vaccines against HPV are being developed and clinically tested and hopefully, in the future, it may be possible to eradicate cervical cancer.

Hubbard RA. Human papillomavirus testing methods. *Arch Pathol Lab Med* 2003; 127:940–945.

Review article.

Jin XW, et al. New advances transform the management of women with abnormal pap tests. *Cleve Clin J Med* 2003;70:641–648.

New advances in Papanicolaou test technology, human papillomavirus DNA testing, and revisions in the Bethesda terminology for cervical cytology have transformed the management of abnormal Pap tests. This approach has been validated by a recent randomized clinical trial and, in some instances, can reduce the number of colposcopies by 50%.

Kahn JA, Bernstein DI. Human papillomavirus vaccines. *Pediatr Infect Dis J* 22:443–445.

Review article.

Kim JJ, et al. Cost-effectiveness of alternative triage strategies for atypical squamous cells of undetermined significance. *JAMA* 2002;287:2382–2390.

Reflex HPV DNA testing uses either residual liquid-based cytologic specimens or samples co-collected at the time of the initial screening for conventional cytology. Reflex HPV DNA testing provides the same or greater life expectancy benefits and is more cost effective than other management strategies for women diagnosed as having ASC-US.

Klencke BJ, Palefsky JM. Anal cancer: an HIV-associated cancer. *Hematol Oncol ClinNorth Am* 2003;17:859–872.

Although not yet included in the Centers for Disease Control and Prevention definition of AIDS, anal cancer clearly occurs more commonly in HIV-infected patients. An effective screening program for those groups who are at highest risk might be expected to impact rates of anal cancer just as significantly as did cervical Pap screening programs for the incidence of cervical cancer. Large, prospective studies will be required before solid conclusions about the impact of various factors on anal cancer prognosis and outcome can be drawn.

Koutsky LA, et al. A controlled trial of a human papillomavirus type 16 vaccine. *N Engl J Med* 2002;347:1645–1651.

Administration of this HPV-16 vaccine reduced the incidence of both HPV-16 infection and HPV-16–related cervical intraepithelial neoplasia. Immunizing HPV-16–negative women may eventually reduce the incidence of cervical cancer.

Lowy DR, Frazer IH. Chapter 16: prophylactic human papillomavirus vaccines. *J Natl Cancer Inst Monogr* 2003;(31):111–116.

Review article.

Lozano R. Successfully integrating human papillomavirus testing into your practice. *Arch Pathol Lab Med* 2003;127:991–994.

Integrating HPV testing into the practice of cervical cancer screening is a continuous process that begins and ends with education. Additional logistical issues, often laboratory specific or state specific, are addressed here.

Manhart LE, Koutsky LA. Do condoms prevent genital HPV infection, external genital warts, or cervical neoplasia? A meta-analysis. *Sex Transm Dis* 2002;29:725–735.

Mathews WC. Screening for anal dysplasia associated with human papillomavirus. *Top HIV Med* 2003;11:45–49.

Anal dysplasia is detectable by Pap screening and colposcopic biopsy; because Pap testing results have relatively low reproducibility, two baseline tests may be prudent. Screening should also ascertain risk factors for dysplasia, degree of immunosuppression, and history of prior anal disease. Treatment options for anal dysplasia are limited by morbidity and high recurrence rates; however early detection may permit better tolerance of therapy, and current estimates indicate that routine screening for the condition would be cost-effective.

Palefsky JM, Holly EA. Chapter 6: immunosuppression and co-infection with HIV. *J Natl Cancer Inst Monogr* 2003;(31): 41–46.

Understanding HPV infection in those who are immunocompromised offers the potential to better understand its pathobiology in the putatively immunocompetent host.

Schiffman M, Kjaer SK. Chapter 2: natural history of anogenital human papillomavirus infection and neoplasia. *J Natl Cancer Inst Monogr* 2003;(31):14–19.

This chapter suggests promising areas of future epidemiologic research on HPV and anogenital cancer, organized around our understanding of cervical carcinogenesis.

Schiffman M, Solomon D. Findings to date from the ASCUS-LSIL Triage Study (ALTS). *Arch Pathol Lab Med* 2003;127:946–949.

Controversy exists in the United States regarding the proper evaluation and management of LSIL and equivocal (atypical squamous cells of undetermined significance [ASCUS, now ASC-US]) cervical cytologic interpretations. To address this issue, the National Cancer Institute initiated the ASCUS-LSIL Triage Study (ALTS). ALTS is a multicenter, randomized clinical trial designed to evaluate three alternative methods of management, namely, immediate colposcopy, cytologic follow-up, and triage by HPV DNA testing. This article summarizes the major findings of ALTS that have been published to date.

Sedlacek TV, et al. Advances in the diagnosis and treatment of human papillomavirus infections. *Clin Obstet Gynecol* 1999;42:206–220.

Review article.

Among 27 estimates from 20 studies, there was no consistent evidence that condom use reduces the risk of becoming HPV DN positive. However, risk for genital warts, CIN of grade II or III (CIN II or III), and invasive cervical carcinoma (ICC) was somewhat reduced. Available data are too inconsistent to provide precise estimates. However, they suggest that while condoms may not prevent HPV infection, they may protect against genital warts, CIN II or III, and ICC.

Smith KJ, et al. The imidazoquinolines and their place in the therapy of cutaneous disease. *Expert Opin Pharmacother* 2003;4:1105–1119.

Imiquimod, the first FDA-approved imidazoquinoline, has been marketed as a 5% cream, which is approved for the therapy of genital warts. The advantage of imiquimod therapy over other therapies for genital warts is the decrease in recurrence rate with the establishment of an adaptive immunologic response or immunologic memory/surveillance response.

Stanley M. Chapter 17: genital human papillomavirus infections—current and prospective therapies. *J Natl Cancer Inst Monogr* 2003;(31):117–124.

Review chapter.

Verdon ME. Issues in the management of human papillomavirus genital disease. *Am Fam Physician* 1997;55: 1813-6, 1819, 1822.

Wiley DJ, et al. External genital warts: diagnosis, treatment, and prevention. *Clin Infect Dis* 2002;35(suppl 2):S210–224.

Biopsy is indicated when external genital warts (EGWs) are fixed to underlying structures or discolored, or when standard therapies are not effective. Recurrences are common, and no single treatment is superior to others. Among women with atypical squamous cells, molecular HPV testing may be useful in determining who should be referred for colposcopy. Condoms may provide some protection against HPV-related diseases and thus are recommended in new sexual relationships and when partnerships are not mutually monogamous. Because the efficacy of cesarean section in preventing vertical transmission of HPV infection from women with EGWs to their progeny has not been proved, it is not recommended.

Winer RL, et al. Genital human papillomavirus infection: incidence and risk factors in a cohort of female university students. *Am J Epidemiol* 2003;157:218–226.

Incidence data on HPV infection are limited, and risk factors for transmission are largely unknown. The authors followed 603 female university students in Washington State at 4-month intervals between 1990 and 2000. The data show that the incidence of HPV associated with acquisition of a new sex partner is high and that nonpenetrative sexual contact is a plausible route of transmission in virgins.

Wright TC Jr, et al. 2001 Consensus guidelines for the management of women with cervical intraepithelial neoplasia. *Am J Obstet Gynecol* 2003;189:295–304.

The study was undertaken to provide consensus guidelines for the management of women with histologically confirmed CIN that can act as a precursor to invasive cervical cancer and represents one of the most significant gynecologic diseases of women of reproductive age. Conclusion: evidence-based guidelines have been developed for the management of women with biopsy-confirmed CIN.

Zanotti KM, et al. Update on the diagnosis and treatment of human papillomavirus infection. Human papillomavirus: a review. *Cleve Clin J Med* 2002;69:948,951–955, 956 passim.

Comprehensive review article with excellent tables.

Nervous System 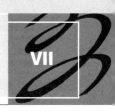 VII

*W*e typically produce about 500 cc of cerebrospinal fluid (CSF) a day, with approximately 150 cc in the central nervous system. Normal CSF pressure is between 70 and 180 mm H_2O.

If a spinal tap is performed, the analysis will usually show less than five white cells/mm^3 (only one of which can be a polymorphonuclear [PMN] cell). As many as 30% of patients may exhibit CSF pleocytosis after a generalized or focal seizure. Eosinophils are always abnormal and most commonly represent a parasitic infestation of the central nervous system (CNS). They also may be seen after myelography, pneumoencephalography, and other infectious and allergic conditions.

Glucose enters the CSF by way of the choroid plexus, as well as by transcapillary movement into the extracellular space of the brain and the cord by carrier-mediated transport. Typically about 2 hours are required before the CSF glucose reaches a steady state with blood glucose changes. This can cause confusion if iatrogenic hyperglycemia from administered glucose is present for several hours before performing a lumbar puncture (LP). CSF glucose is normally between 50 and 80 mg/dL, which is only 60% of the glucose concentration in the blood. Note that the ventricular fluid glucose levels are 7 mg/dL higher than those values found in lumbar fluid.

The normal range of the lumbar CSF protein level is 15 to 45 mg/dL. The concentration is lower in the ventricles (5 to 15 mg/dL) and the basilar cisterns (10 to 25 mg/dL), reflecting a gradient in the permeability of capillary endothelial cells to proteins in the blood. Levels higher than 500 mg/dL are uncommon and are seen mainly in meningitis, subarachnoid bleeding, and with spinal tumors. The high levels seen with cord tumors result from an increase in local capillary permeability. With high levels (generally 1,000 mg/dL), CSF may clot. Hemorrhage into the CSF or the introduction of blood by a traumatic tap will most likely raise CSF protein levels. The CSF protein should typically rise by 1 mg for every 1,000 red cells, but this is variable.

Xanthochromia is defined as a yellow-orange discoloration produced by red cell lysis and is caused by one or more of the following pigments: oxyhemoglobin, bilirubin, and methemoglobin. Oxyhemoglobin is seen within 2 hours of subarachnoid bleeding and red cell lysis. It reaches a peak in approximately 48 hours after hemorrhage and it disappears in 3 to 30 days. The appearance of bilirubin in the CSF results from the conversion of oxyhemoglobin by the enzyme heme oxygenase. Enzyme activity appears approximately 12 hours after the hemorrhage occurs. Bilirubin may persist for 2 to 4 weeks. Note that bilirubin in CSF caused by hepatic or hemolytic disease will not appear until a serum level of 10 to 15 mg total bilirubin per 100 mL is reached. Also note that xanthochromia may be seen with CSF protein values above 150 mg/dL. Xanthochromia can be detected as well after a traumatic tap if the red blood cell (RBC) counts exceed 150,000 cells/cc.

In traumatic punctures the fluid generally clears between the first and third tubes as the needle is washed by CSF. Decreasing cell counts on the first and third tubes help confirm this. Often the RBCs are greater than 1,000 cells. The presence of a clot in one of the tubes strongly favors a traumatic tap. In subarachnoid hemorrhage, clotting does not occur because blood is defibrinated at the site of the hemorrhage. The white blood cell (WBC):RBC ratios in the CSF to serum can be compared. If greater than 1, the pleocytosis usually cannot be accounted for by a traumatic tap.

MENINGITIS

Meningitis is defined as an inflammation of two of the membranes that surround the brain and spinal cord. These membranes (the pia and arachnoid mater) are called the meninges and form the subarachnoid space, which is filled with spinal fluid. When bacterial meningitis occurs, WBCs flow into the spinal fluid and are usually detectable on examination of the fluid. When bacterial meningitis appears with typical symptoms of fever, headache, and meningismus, there often is little doubt regarding the nature of the problem. However, the presentation and clinical features of other types of meningitis is variable, and analysis of the CSF can be helpful in forming a differential diagnosis. Details regarding specific infections can be found in Tables 30-1 through 30-5.

Because of the low prevalence of lesions that contraindicate LP, a screening cranial computed tomogram (CT) solely to establish the safety of performing an LP typically provides limited additional information. Physicians can use their overall clinical impression and three clinical predictors to identify patients with the greatest risk of having intracranial lesions that may contraindicate LP. These three predictors are papilledema, focal neurologic findings, and altered mentation. One should not delay antibiotics while awaiting a cranial CT.

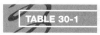 **CSF Analysis by Type of Pathogen**

Type of meningitis	Staining	Cell count	Protein	Glucose	Opening pressure (mm H₂O)	Culture positive
Bacterial	60–90% Gram's stain positive	100–20K Usually PMNs	100–500	<40	Can be >180	75–80%
Viral		<300 Mostly lymphs	Often normal	>40	Normal	Variable <50%*
Lyme		Usually <100, mostly lymphs	May be elevated	Usually >40	Normal	
Syphilis		Usually increased lymphs	May be elevated	May be elevated	Normal	
Rickettsia		Increased in one-third of patients PMNs or Lymphs	Increased in one-third of patients	Low in 8%	Normal	
Fungal	50% India ink positive with *Cryptococcus*	20–500 Usually lymphs	Usually elevated	Usually <40	*Cryptococcus* may have elevated pressures	Variable 25–50% depending on the species
TB	20–80%	50–4000 Usually lymphs	150–200	<40	Can be >180	50–80%

*Compared with CSF viral culture, the Enterovirus (EV) RT-PCR has a sensitivity and specificity of 97% and 100% for the diagnosis of aseptic meningitis.

TABLE 30-2	Differential Diagnosis by Cell Type		

PMN	Lymphocyte	Eosinophils
Actinomycosis	Borrelia	*Angiostrongylus*
Aspergillosis		*Baylisascaris*
Brucella	Brucella	
Candida	CMV	*Coccidioides*
Drugs		Drugs
Entamoeba		
Leptospirosis	LCV	Hodgkin's
Lupus	Malignancy	
Nocardia		
Parameningeal focus	Parameningeal focus	Schistosomiasis
	Sarcoid	Syphilis
TB (early)	TB (later)	TB
	Taenia	Taenia
	Toxoplasmosis	

BACTERIAL MENINGITIS

The yield from CSF cultures in bacterial meningitis is from 70 to 85%. Initially positive CSF cultures will typically become sterile in 90% of patients within 24 to 36 hours of antibiotic therapy. Findings in the CSF that are characteristic for bacterial meningitis include a glucose concentration of 45 mg/dL or below, a protein concentration above 500 mg/dL, and a WBC count above 1000/mm³. If the lumbar puncture is delayed for even a few hours after antibiotic therapy is started, the Gram's stain and cultures might be negative. In contrast, abnormalities in the cell count, protein, and glucose will persist for at least several days. Starting empiric therapy for suspected bacterial meningitis is the first priority of the clinician and should not be delayed for diagnostic tests. Gram's stain of the CSF is useful because it may quickly reveal the nature of the organism in 80% of culture-positive cases and in up to 10% in culture-negative specimens. Gram's stain has a sensitivity of 60 to 90% and a specificity approaching 100%. A repeat analysis 24 to 36 hours later may be useful in patients who are not responding to treatment or have resistant organisms.

STREPTOCOCCUS PNEUMONIAE

Noncultural methods have been investigated in the diagnosis of *S. pneumoniae*. Polymerase chain reaction (PCR) amplification may be relatively sensitive and very specific in CSF and less sensitive in blood. The NOW *S. pneumoniae* antigen test in CSF yields a rapid and very reliable diagnosis of pneumococcal meningitis, enabling prompt and adequate treatment.

TABLE 30-3	PCR testing of Viral Infections		

Pathogen	Sensitivity%	Specificity%
HSV	95	99
JC (PML)	75–90	85–90
Enterovirus	95	99
West Nile virus	55 CSF/10 serum	
CMV	80–100	75–95

TABLE 30-4	Causes of Chronic and Recurrent Meningitis

Chronic	Recurrent
Cryptococcus, Histoplasmosis,	Mollaret's
Coccidioides	HSV
Sporothrix schenckii	
M. tuberculosis	Behçet's
Syphilis	Posttraumatic (CSF leak)
Hypogammaglobulinemic/enteroviral infections	Tumor
Brucella	Drugs
Benign chronic lymphocytic meningitis	Systemic lupus erythematosus
Behçet's	
Granulomatous angiitis	
Tumor	
Sarcoid	
Uveomeningoencephalitis (Vogt-Koyanagi-Harada syndrome)	
Systemic lupus erythematosus, Sjögren's syndrome, polyarteritis nodosa	
Wegener's granulomatosis	

Its low sensitivity in urine indicates that this mode of testing is not particularly useful for the diagnosis of pneumococcal meningitis.

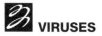 **VIRUSES**

Enterovirus

Usually these patients will present with an abrupt onset of headache, fever, nausea, vomiting, malaise, photophobia, meningismus, and occasionally a rash. The CSF will typically have a lymphocytic prominence of less than 250 cells/mm^3, a normal glucose, and a mildly elevated protein of usually less than 150 mg/dL. It should be noted, however, that some patients will have an early (8–48 hr) predominance of polymorphonuclear white cells. A repeat lumbar puncture will show a shift toward the typical pattern of lymphocytes within 24 to 48 hours later.

The polymerase chain reaction (PCR) test for enteroviruses can help confirm the diagnosis, decrease the cost of unnecessary antibiotics, and shorten hospital stays, according to recent studies. Enteroviral PCR has a sensitivity of 92 to 100% and a specificity of 97 to 100% in CSF. To be truly cost effective, it needs to be performed within the first 24 hours in most cases. When compared to CSF PCR, CSF viral culture is able to detect 14 to 24%

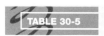

TABLE 30-5	Internet Resources

Website	Address
ARUP	http://www.arup-lab.com/index.jsp
Specialty Labs	http://www.specialtylabs.com/main.html
Mayo Clinic	http://www.mayoclinic.org/labmed-pathology-rst/index.html
CDC/ West Nile	http://www.cdc.gov/ncidod/dvbid/westnile/index.htm
IDSA meningitis guidelines	http://www.journals.uchicago.edu/IDSA/guidelines/

of cases of viral meningitis. Although culture of virus from the CSF is diagnostic of viral meningitis, culture of virus from the throat or rectum is not diagnostic, but only supportive in value.

Herpes Simplex

Because this disease affects the frontal and medial temporal lobes, it is associated with taste and smell hallucinations, speech disorders, and strange behavior. Culture of the CSF is not very helpful, so PCR is considered the test of choice for diagnosis of herpes simplex infections. In a previous study, HSV DNA was detected by PCR in CSF of 53 (98%) of 54 patients with biopsy-proven herpes simplex encephalitis (HSE) and was detected in all 18 CSF specimens obtained before brain biopsy from patients with proven HSE. Four of 19 CSF specimens were positive after 2 weeks of antiviral therapy. Positive results were found in three (6%) of 47 patients whose brain tissue was culture negative. Untreated HSV-1 encephalitis has a mortality rate of 70%, but patients generally will respond to a dose of acyclovir of 10 mg/kg IV every 8 hours for 10 to 14 days

Cytomegalovirus

In HIV-infected patients with low CD4 counts, cytomegalovirus (CMV) may cause polyradiculitis, myelitis, encephalitis, or multifocal neuritis. On imaging studies, periventricular enhancement often is seen. Of note, the CSF often will reveal a polymorphonuclear pleocytosis or hypoglycorrhachia. CSF CMV PCR has a sensitivity of 80 to 100% and a specificity of 75 to 100% for detecting CMV infection of the CNS in patients also infected with HIV.

Varicella Zoster Virus

CSF DNA can be detected in patients with postvaricella cerebellitis, and other neurologic symptoms. Varicella zoster virus (VZV) DNA might be detected alone or as part of a multiplex PCR.

Epstein-Barr Virus

In persons infected with HIV, Epstein-Barr virus (EBV) is associated with nearly 100% of primary CNS lymphomas. In a recent study, PCR for EBV DNA in CSF was 100% sensitive and 98.5% specific for AIDS-associated primary CNS lymphoma.

JC Papovavirus

Progressive multifocal leukoencephalopathy (PML) is a demyelinating disease of the CNS caused by JC papovavirus (JCV). JCV DNA detection in CSF has a sensitivity of 74 to 92% and a specificity of 92 to 96%. Highly active antiretroviral therapy (HAART) and cidofovir have been used to treat this condition in patients also infected with HIV.

West Nile Virus

Please see Chapter 62 for information regarding West Nile Virus.

Arboviruses

Serology plays an important part in arbovirus diagnosis, but cross-reactivity among the arboviruses can limit the ability to make a specific diagnosis. IgM antibody capture enzyme immunoassay (EIA) tests run on serum or CSF may be helpful. Contacting the health department's state laboratory or commercial specialty laboratories may be useful in determining which tests are available to assist the clinician in making a diagnosis. Because nucleotide sequence data are available for some arboviruses, development of RNA reverse transcriptase (RT)-PCR techniques is promising for rapid, sensitive and specific detection of arboviruses.

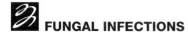

FUNGAL INFECTIONS

Coccidioides

Clinically this is seen as a chronic granulomatous meningitis, usually involving the basilar meninges. Initial CSF findings show a mononuclear cell pleocytosis, with a low glucose and elevated protein concentrations. Up to 70% of patients may have eosinophils in their CSF. The fungus grows on most culture media and may appear after incubation at most temperatures. It may grow relatively rapidly and be seen as early as 2 days after inoculation into media, although more often 5 days or longer are required. Culture of large volumes of CSF is recommended for the detection of all fungi causing meningitis.

Complement fixation (CF) antibodies also can be detected in the CSF of patients with meningitis and similarly can be used to monitor disease. The direct examination of CSF is rarely positive for characteristic spherules and endospores, and culture is positive only in one third of the cases. Antibodies against a 33-kDa antigen from *Coccidioides immitis* have been detected by enzyme-linked immunosorbent assay (ELISA) in patients' CSF. Measurement of anti–33-kDa antibodies is a sensitive indicator of coccidioidal meningitis and of its clinical course.

Histoplasmosis

Antibodies (CF) can be measured in the CSF but should be tested in parallel with serum titers. PCR testing is still investigational at this time. Antigen testing shows some promise in the diagnosis of meningitis as well, with a sensitivity approaching 70%. The specificity of the antigen test is lower because of cross-reactivity with other fungi. Cultures may take several weeks but are often negative in half of all cases of meningitis caused by this fastidious fungus.

Cryptococcosis

Abnormal CSF findings, such as pleocytosis, low glucose concentrations, and high protein concentrations, are seen in most patients with cryptococcal meningitis. HIV-infected patients may have very few abnormal CSF findings, so a normal fluid analysis does not rule out the disease in those patients. In fact, they may have a worse prognosis under those circumstances.

The CSF opening pressure is greater than 200 mm H_2O in 70% of patients with cryptococcal meningitis. Increased pressures are a marker for increased mortality in these patients and need to be aggressively managed.

Cultures often take several days to turn positive. It will more often be positive (75%) than the other endemic fungi. The India ink test offers a rapid means of detection but often requires an experienced observer. Cryptococcal antigen (CrAg) testing in CSF is sensitive (91%) and specific (95%) for the diagnosis. Very rarely, false-positive results can occur in the presence of rheumatoid factor but are usually of low titer. *Trichosporon beigelii* has been reported to cross-react as well.

In persons infected with HIV, the serum CrAg can be used to help screen for those with meningitis. A negative serum titer makes meningitis much less likely in these patients, but the initial or subsequent serum titers do not necessarily correlate with disease severity or treatment outcome in most patients. The capsule is a high-molecular-weight polysaccharide. This results in a slow clearance from the serum and CSF that can persist for many years. Changes in the CSF cryptococcal antigen titers have limited value in the management of cryptococcal meningitis, although it is expected that a decrease should be seen after 2 or more weeks of therapy. Baseline titers do not necessarily correlate with outcome. Studies have shown a significant difference in responders compared with nonresponders among those patients whose initial CSF cryptococcal antigen was higher than 1:8; specifically, 86% of responders had a decrease in titer, compared with 44% of nonresponders. Treatment decisions should be based on the patient's overall condition, and not just the value of their antigen test.

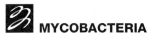 MYCOBACTERIA

The typical CSF findings consist of a lymphocytic pleocytosis (usually of 100 to 500 cells/mm^3), increased protein concentration, and low glucose levels in two-thirds of the patients on the initial lumbar puncture. Culture often requires several weeks to grow and may only be positive from 20 to 80% of the time. Multiple, large-volume cultures may be helpful to increase the yield of culture.

PMN cells may predominate during the first 7 to 10 days until the typical lymphocytic predominance occurs. Smears are often negative (10–20% positive). Sputum cultures may be positive in 15 to 50% of cases. Isolated tuberculous meningitis is not rare.

Most PCR assays for Mycobacterium tuberculosis (MTB) amplify the MPB64 gene or IS6110, an insertion element with multiple copies in the genome of members of the *Mycobacteria tuberculosis* complex. The sensitivity will range between 50 and 100%, but the specificity is close to 100%. The PCR assays can be more sensitive than CSF culture, but a negative test does not rule out the diagnosis. Prior antituberculous therapy can affect the results.

Adenosine deaminase (ADA) is a purine salvage pathway enzyme that catalyzes the irreversible deamination of adenosine into inosine and ammonia. Studies have shown that there are increased levels in some patients with tuberculous meningitis. ADA is released by T-lymphocytes. Increased CSF levels are found in those patients who have tuberculous meningitis in contrast to those with viral or bacterial etiologies. The normal value is less than 10.0 U/L in the CSF. ADA levels also are elevated in cases of tuberculosis peritonitis and pleuritis but may also be increased by a variety of other conditions (www.arup-lab.com/index.jsp).

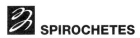 SPIROCHETES

Lyme disease

Typically patients will have a lymphocytic predominance with a normal to low glucose and a normal to high protein level. These findings are nonspecific. Serologic tests might be ordered as well. Intrathecal synthesis needs to be demonstrated to improve the diagnostic accuracy. The CSF/serum ratio of titers to *Borrelia burgdorferi* may be compared to the ratio of albumin in the CSF compared to serum. The sensitivity of intrathecal serologic tests is variable. CSF titers might remain elevated for a while even after treatment but other findings, such as pleocytosis, should improve sooner.

PCR testing has been studied as well. In one study, *B. burgdorferi* DNA was detected in CSF samples in six (38%) of 16 patients with acute neuroborreliosis, 11 (25%) of 44 with chronic neuroborreliosis, and none of 42 samples from patients with other illnesses. There was a significant correlation between PCR results and the duration of previous intravenous antibiotic therapy. PCR may assist the physician in establishing a diagnosis of neuroborreliosis; however, a negative result does not necessarily rule out neuroborreliosis. PCR is an adjunct, not a substitute for clinical judgment and serology in most patients. The role of PCR still needs to be better defined. (JWM)

Bibliography
Ahmed A, et al. Clinical utility of the polymerase chain reaction for diagnosis of enteroviral meningitis in infancy. *J Pediatr* 1997;131:393–397.
  Comparison of results of PCR assay of CSF with viral culture, the gold standard for diagnosis of enteroviral meningitis, demonstrated a sensitivity of 100% and a specificity of 90%.
Aurelius E, et al. Rapid diagnosis of herpes simplex encephalitis by nested polymerase chain reaction assay of cerebrospinal fluid. *Lancet* 1991;337:189–192.
  The PCR result remained positive in samples drawn up to 27 days after the onset of neurologic symptoms. This method is a rapid and noninvasive means to diagnose herpes simplex encephalitis; it is highly sensitive and specific.

Baty V, et al. Prospective validation of a diagnosis model as an aid to therapeutic decision-making in acute meningitis. *Eur J Clin Microbiol Infect Dis* 2000;19:422–426.

The aim of this study was to validate a diagnosis model that provides pABM, the probability of bacterial versus viral meningitis, based on four parameters collected at the time of first lumbar tap: cerebrospinal fluid protein level, cerebrospinal fluid PMN cell count, blood glucose level, and leucocyte count. The results confirm that the model evaluated is reliable and aids in the identification of patients in whom antibiotics can be safely avoided.

Bialek R, et al. Evaluation of two nested PCR assays for detection of Histoplasma capsulatum DNA in human tissue. *J Clin Microbiol* 2002;40:1644–1647.

To evaluate the diagnostic relevance of two nested PCR assays for diagnosis of histoplasmosis in clinical specimens, 100 paraffin-embedded biopsy specimens were examined. In this preliminary study, the novel 100-kDa–like protein gene nested PCR revealed a specificity of 100% without requiring sequencing, which was necessary for identification of the 18S ribosomal DNA-nested PCR products in order to avoid a high rate of false-positive results.

Bonsu BK, Harper MB. Differentiating acute bacterial meningitis from acute viral meningitis among children with cerebrospinal fluid pleocytosis: a multivariable regression model. *Pediatr Infect Dis J* 2004;23:511–517.

Among children with CSF pleocytosis, a prediction model based exclusively on age, CSF total protein and CSF neutrophils differentiate accurately between acute bacterial and viral meningitis.

Burke DG, et al. Polymerase chain reaction detection and clinical significance of varicella-zoster virus in cerebrospinal fluid from human immunodeficiency virus-infected patients. *J Infect Dis* 1997;176:1080–1084.

VZV causes ocular and other CNS disease in HIV-infected persons. VZV DNA was detected in the CSF of 7% of HIV-infected patients who had neurologic symptoms; the diagnosis of VZV-related CNS disease was facilitated by this assay. Improvement in association with antiviral therapy was observed in some patients.

Burke DG, et al. The utility of clinical and radiographic features in the diagnosis of cytomegalovirus central nervous system disease in AIDS patients. *Mol Diagn* 1999;4:37–43.

These clinical and radiographic features may serve as useful adjuncts toward the establishment of the diagnosis of CMV-associated neurologic disease in AIDS patients.

Caws M, et al. Role of IS6110-targeted PCR, culture, biochemical, clinical, and immunological criteria for diagnosis of tuberculous meningitis. *J Clin Microbiol* 2000;38:3150–3155.

The study showed IS6110-targeted PCR to be a rapid, sensitive, and specific test in routine use for the diagnosis of tuberculous meningitis.

De Luca A, et al. The effect of potent antiretroviral therapy and JC virus load in cerebrospinal fluid on clinical outcome of patients with AIDS-associated progressive multifocal leukoencephalopathy. *J Infect Dis* 2000;182:1077–1083.

Among HAART-treated patients, a baseline JCV DNA less than 4.7 log, and reaching undetectable levels after therapy predicted longer survival.

Galgiani JN, et al. Cerebrospinal fluid antibodies detected by ELISA against a 33-kDa antigen from spherules of *Coccidioides immitis* in patients with coccidioidal meningitis. The National Institute of Allergy and Infectious Diseases Mycoses Study Group. *J Infect Dis* 1996;173:499–502.

Antibodies against a 33-kDa antigen from C. immitis were detected by ELISA in patients' CSF. Measurement of anti–33-kDa antibodies is a sensitive indicator of coccidioidal meningitis and of its clinical course.

Gendrel D, et al. [Procalcitonin, C-reactive protein and interleukin 6 in bacterial and viral meningitis in children]. *Presse Med* 1998;27:1135–1139.

Procalcitonin (PCT) is a sensitive and specific marker for early diagnosis of viral meningitis versus bacterial meningitis in children.

Gerdes LU, et al. C-reactive protein and bacterial meningitis: a meta-analysis. *Scand J Clin Lab Invest* 1998;58:383–393.

The authors concluded that only a negative test is highly informative in a typical clinical setting. This, as well as the absence of analyses to show if CRP tests contribute independent diagnostic information relative to the information held in the traditionally used clinical and biochemical variables, makes it difficult to decide on the clinical usefulness of CRP tests in the management of patients suspected of having bacterial meningitis.

Gopal AK, et al. Cranial computed tomography before lumbar puncture: a prospective clinical evaluation. Arch Intern Med 1999;159:2681–2685.
Because of the low prevalence of lesions that contraindicate LP, screening cranial CT solely to establish the safety of performing an LP typically provides limited additional information. Physicians can use their overall clinical impression and three clinical predictors to identify patients with the greatest risk of having intracranial lesions that may contraindicate LP.

Grimley PM. The laboratory role in diagnosis of infections transmitted by arthropods. Clin Lab Med 2001;21:495–512, viii.
This article provides an overview of arbovirus diseases from the perspective of laboratory diagnosis and related responsibilities of health personnel.

Halperin JJ. Nervous system Lyme disease. Vector Borne Zoonotic Dis 2002;2:241–247.
Excellent review article.

Halperin JJ, et al. Central nervous system abnormalities in Lyme neuroborreliosis. Neurology 1991;41:1571–1582.
Concluded that (1) measurement of intrathecal antibody production is a reliable indicator of CNS infection, (2) North American neuroborreliosis includes the same spectrum of neurologic dysfunction as described in Europe, and (3) histocompatibility leukocyte antigen (HLA) typing may be useful in furthering our understanding of severe CNS involvement.

Hamilton MS, et al. Clinical utility of polymerase chain reaction testing for enteroviral meningitis. Pediatr Infect Dis J 1999;18:533–537.
PCR testing has clinical utility for diagnosis of enteroviral meningitis. Although the demands for daily testing make the test expensive, it appears to be cost effective with savings related to shorter hospital stays.

Ivers LC, et al. Predictive value of polymerase chain reaction of cerebrospinal fluid for detection of Epstein-Barr virus to establish the diagnosis of HIV-related primary central nervous system lymphoma. Clin Infect Dis 2004;38:1629–1632.
In a review of the operational characteristics of this test in our clinical practice, the positive predictive value of CSF PCR for EBV for establishing the diagnosis of primary central nervous system lymphoma (PCNSL) was only 29%. Of seven patients with CSF PCR positive for EBV, two had PCNSL, and five received alternative diagnoses (specificity, 79.1%).

Kaiser R, Lucking CH. Intrathecal synthesis of specific antibodies in neuroborreliosis. Comparison of different ELISA techniques and calculation methods. J Neurol Sci 1993;118:64–72.
In uncertain cases of neuroborreliosis, calculation of the Antibody Index (AI) from ELISA titers will be useful in clarifying the diagnosis.

Koskiniemi M, et al. Herpes encephalitis is a disease of middle aged and elderly people: polymerase chain reaction for detection of herpes simplex virus in the CSF of 516 patients with encephalitis. The Study Group. J Neurol Neurosurg Psychiatry 1996;60:174–178.
Samples taken 1 to 29 days from the onset of symptoms from 38 patients (7.4%) were positive, 32 (6.2%) for HSV-1 and six (1.2%) for HSV-2. At follow up, eight of 28 patients studied were still HSV-PCR positive.

Markoulatos P, et al. Laboratory diagnosis of common herpesvirus infections of the central nervous system by a multiplex PCR assay. J Clin Microbiol 2001;39:4426–4432.
The present multiplex PCR assay detects simultaneously five different herpesviruses and sample suitability for PCR in a single amplification round of 40 cycles with excellent sensitivity. It can, therefore, provide an early, rapid, reliable noninvasive diagnostic tool allowing the application of antiviral therapy on the basis of a specific viral diagnosis. The results of this preliminary study should prompt a more exhaustive analysis of the clinical value of the present multiplex PCR assay.

Mazor SS, et al. Interpretation of traumatic lumbar punctures: who can go home? *Pediatrics* 2003;111:525–528.

To determine whether a ratio of observed to predicted (O:P) cerebrospinal fluid (CSF) white blood cells (WBCs) after a traumatic lumbar puncture (LP) can be used to predict which patients do not have meningitis and can safely be discharged from the hospital. The predicted CSF WBC count was calculated using the formula CSF WBC (predicted) = CSF RBC × (blood WBC/blood RBC). The O:P ratio was obtained by dividing the observed CSF WBC by the predicted CSF WBC. The simple ratio of WBCs to RBCs was also calculated. A WBC:RBC ratio of 1:100 (0.01) or less and an O:P ratio of 0.01 or less identified a large group of patients without meningitis. Using these methods in children younger than age 1 month, the majority of patients without meningitis can be differentiated from those with meningitis despite the CSF abnormalities associated with a traumatic LP. However, the clinician should examine all clinical and laboratory information before opting not to treat a child after a traumatic LP.

Michelow IC, et al. Value of cerebrospinal fluid leukocyte aggregation in distinguishing the causes of meningitis in children. *Pediatr Infect Dis J* 2000;19:66–72.

The finding of leukocyte aggregation in CSF might be of value as a sensitive adjunctive screening tool for the timely diagnosis of bacterial meningitis, recognizing that it has low specificity and potential practical limitations.

Najioullah F, et al. Diagnosis and surveillance of herpes simplex virus infection of the central nervous system. *J Med Virol* 2000;61:468–473.

Four HSV encephalitis cases were monitored by PCR detection in CSF. Despite acyclovir therapy, PCR remained positive in CSF up to 20 days in two cases.

Samra Z, et al. Use of the NOW Streptococcus pneumoniae urinary antigen test in cerebrospinal fluid for rapid diagnosis of pneumococcal meningitis. *Diagn Microbiol Infect Dis* 2003;45:237–240.

The NOW S. pneumoniae antigen test in CSF yields a rapid and very reliable diagnosis of pneumococcal meningitis, enabling prompt and adequate treatment. Its low sensitivity in urine indicates that this mode of testing is not useful for the diagnosis of pneumococcal meningitis.

Sauerbrei A, et al. Virological diagnosis of herpes simplex encephalitis. *J Clin Virol* 2000; 17:31–36.

The detection of HSV-DNA by PCR is the method of choice for diagnosis of HSE in the early phase of the disease. During the later stage, it has to be diagnosed by the estimation of intrathecally synthesized antibodies.

Tarrago D, et al. Quantitation of cytomegalovirus DNA in cerebrospinal fluid and serum specimens from AIDS patients using a novel highly sensitive nested competitive PCR and the cobas amplicor CMV monitor. *J Med Virol* 2004;72:249–256.

The nQC-PCR assay described below is a very sensitive test for accurate quantitative detection of CMV DNA in different clinical specimens that avoids the need for high-cost instrumentation.

Thwaites GE, et al. Diagnosis of adult tuberculous meningitis by use of clinical and laboratory features. *Lancet* 2002;360:1287–1292.

Five features were predictive of a diagnosis of tuberculous meningitis: age, length of history, WBC count, total CSF white cell count, and CSF neutrophil proportion. A diagnostic rule developed from these features was 97% sensitive and 91% specific by resubstitution, and 86% sensitive and 79% specific when applied prospectively to a further 42 adults with tuberculous meningitis, and 33 with bacterial meningitis.

van de Beek D, et al. Clinical features and prognostic factors in adults with bacterial meningitis. *N Engl J Med* 2004;351:1849–1859.

In adults presenting with community-acquired acute bacterial meningitis, the sensitivity of the classic triad of fever, neck stiffness, and altered mental status is low, but almost all present with at least two of the four symptoms of headache, fever, neck stiffness, and altered mental status. The mortality associated with bacterial meningitis remains high, and the strongest risk factors for an unfavorable outcome are those that are indicative of systemic compromise, a low level of consciousness, and infection with S. pneumoniae.

Weinberg A, et al. Quantitative CSF PCR in Epstein-Barr virus infections of the central nervous system. *Ann Neurol* 2002;52:543–548.
These studies demonstrate the utility of quantitative CSF PCR and establish the presence of lytic cycle EBV mRNA in the CSF of patients with EBV-associated neurologic disease.
Wheat LJ, et al. Histoplasma capsulatum infections of the central nervous system. A clinical review. *Medicine (Baltimore)* 1990;69:244–260.
Review article.
Zunt JR, Marra CM. Cerebrospinal fluid testing for the diagnosis of central nervous system infection. *Neurol Clin* 1999;17:675–689.
Excellent review article that discusses how these CSF tests are performed and addresses the sensitivity and specificity of such tests for the diagnosis of selected CNS infections.

CENTRAL NERVOUS SYSTEM INFECTION IN IMMUNE SUPPRESSED HOSTS

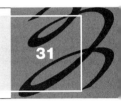

31

*I*mmune suppression may arise either from underlying disease (eg, leukemias, lymphoma, AIDS) or from therapy. More recently, therapies for rheumatologic disorders have been associated with risks of infection not heretofore noted. As a result, many physicians regularly encounter patients with some form of immune suppression. The development of neurologic signs and symptoms in these patients should alert the clinician to the possibility of an infectious etiology that may differ significantly from that which is seen in normal hosts. Excluding patients with AIDS, organ transplant recipients and persons with underlying malignancies are among the highest risk groups for potentially life-threatening CNS infections. In recent years, use of immunosuppressive agents such as cyclosporine, tacrolimus, azathioprine, mycophenolate mofetil, and prednisone, along with aggressive prevention and treatment of infections, have helped improve both patient and graft survival, especially in renal transplant patients. Nonetheless, CNS infections are still common and can have mortality rates of 42 to 77%. The part of the immune system suppressed by either disease or treatment helps target likely pathogens. CNS infection patients will present with combinations of altered consciousness, headache, and fever. Nuchal rigidity is present in one-third of patients. Seizures may occur, and focal neurologic findings may be present.

Diverse organisms that include selected bacteria, fungi, viruses, and protozoa may be involved in these infections, and are depicted in Tables 31-1 to 31-3. This is distinctly dissimilar to more normal hosts in which bacteria such *Streptococcus pneumoniae, and Neisseria meningitidis* predominate. The predilection for fungal infections in compromised hosts has been recently emphasized. A retrospective autopsy study found that in brain parenchymal infections in bone marrow transplant recipients, 60% had fungi isolated. Thirty percent of these isolates were *Aspergillus*, whereas 18% involved *Candida* spp. *Toxoplasma gondii* encephalitis was demonstrated in 30% of these patients whereas only 10% had bacterial abscesses. The majority of these patients died within 3 months of diagnosis, demonstrating that CNS infection in immunosuppressed bone marrow recipients is a highly fatal event. Other unusual organisms such as *Blastoschizomyces capitatus*, and viruses such as *Herpes zoster, Herpes simplex*, papovaviruses, and measles also have been found in some of these infections.

In the setting of rheumatologic diseases that include systemic lupus erythematosus (SLE), some authors have appreciated an increase in morbidity and mortality due in part to increased occurrence of secondary infections in the setting of increasingly effective immunosuppressive therapy. Patients with SLE are intrinsically at higher risk for infection—a risk that is augmented by many of the therapies used. Treatment with corticosteroids plus

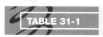

TABLE 31-1	Bacteria Associated With CNS Infection in Immunosuppressed Persons

Organism	Clinical Setting
Anaerobes	Focal CNS infection/mass in immunocompromised and in patients with malignancy
Enterococcus	Meningitis in liver transplantation, diabetes
Escherichia coli	Meningitis in newborn, elderly, immunosuppressed
Other Enterobacteriaceae	Acute meningitis/meningoencephalitis in patients with malignancy
Haemophilus influenzae, type B	Common meningitis cause in normal patients and in those with malignancy
Klebsiella pneumoniae	Meningitis in immunosuppressed from all causes and elderly
L. monocytogenes	Meningitis, may occur in normal patients, also may cause focal CNS infection/mass
M. avium complex	Meningitis in immunosuppressed/compromised
M. tuberculosis	Meningitis in immunosuppressed, including renal transplant recipients; travel to endemic tuberculous areas a risk
N. meningitidis	Recurrent meningitis, bacteremia especially in complement deficiency
Nocardia	Meningitis in setting of immunosuppressive drugs, malignancy, sarcoidosis, chronic granulomatous disease; also may cause localized cerebral deficit
Pseudomonas aeruginosa	Meningitis in immunosuppressed from all causes, elderly
S. aureus	Focal CNS infection/mass in immunocompromised, and in patients with malignancy
Streptococcus agalactiae	Meningitis in newborns, elderly, collagen vascular diseases, malignancy, diabetes, renal or liver failure, and in corticosteroid-treated
S. pneumoniae	Most common cause of meningitis in normal patients (in USA), also in those with alcoholism, diabetes, liver or renal disease, malignancy, and diabetes

cyclophosphamide poses the strongest risks. Differentiation between CNS infection and CNS involvement by SLE may be impossible on clinical grounds. MRI and laboratory findings, including cerebrospinal fluid analysis are rarely specific. Often a variety of investigation that may include organism-specific serologic tests and brain biopsy are necessary to make a definitive diagnosis. Recent data continue to demonstrate that no truly specific signs exist to differentiate between underlying disease and opportunistic infection; thus, the clinician must remain ever vigilant. Until infection is ruled out, it is generally inadvisable to enhance immunosuppression.

Renal transplant recipients had previously been thought to be at low risk for fungal infections compared with other transplant recipients. However, recent data suggest that they may have 80 to 90 times the annual rate of fungal infections compared with the general population. Up to 8% of all these infections represented meningitis, and approximately 80% of these occurred less than 2 months after transplantation. Most commonly implicated organisms were *Candida* spp. and *Aspergillus* spp. Use of tacrolimus appears to be particularly associated with fungal infections, perhaps in part due to drug interactions with fluconazole, which may be used prophylactically in this population.

Tuberculous meningitis can also rarely occur in renal transplant recipients. Unexplained fever should alert the clinician to the possibility of extrapulmonary manifestations of mycobacterial infections. Rapid diagnosis and treatment is essential to improve survival. Isoniazid prophylaxis has been suggested for immunocompromised patients traveling to endemic tuberculosis (TB) areas. Nontuberculous mycobacterial meningitis due to *Mycobacterium avium* also has been reported and is often fatal.

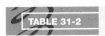

TABLE 31-2 Fungi Associated With CNS Infection in Immunosuppressed Persons

Organism	Clinical setting
Aspergillus fumigatus	Rhinocerebral involvement with a variety of CNS manifestations, especially in neutropenic patients and steroid-treated individuals
Blastomyces dermatitidis	Meningitis or focal abscess, in malignancy, AIDS
Candida species (especially *albicans*)	Meningitis, CNS abscesses, in trauma, neurosurgery, premature infants, and other immunocompromised states
Coccidioides immitis	Basilar meningitis, often chronic, exposure usually in southwestern US and Texas, in elderly and immunocompromised for other reasons
Cryptococcus neoformans	Classic meningitis or, rarely, mass lesions in the form of single or multiple cryptococcomata, usually in patients with lymphoproliferative diseases or steroid usage
Histoplasma capsulatum	Rare cause of chronic meningitis
Mucoraceae	Rhinocerebral involvement with a variety of CNS manifestations, some predilection for diabetics, rarely seen in hemodialysis patients getting deferoxamine therapy

Bacteremia, meningitis, and meningoencephalitis caused by *Listeria monocytogenes* have been described in bone marrow transplant recipients and tend to occur earlier in unrelated donor transplant recipients. In these patients, there is an increased need for immunosuppression, which may predict an increasing and earlier occurrence of listeriosis.

Patients with underlying malignancies present another group of commonly compromised patients at risk for CNS infections. Evaluation of this cohort should be guided by both acuity of presentation and anatomic distribution of neurologic findings. These infections may present as meningitis/meningoencephalitis, or as focal masses, or even strokelike illness with focal deficits. Meningitis associated with bacteria is most commonly an acute

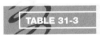

TABLE 31-3 Viruses and Protozoa Associated With CNS Infection in Immunosuppressed Persons

Virus	Clinical setting
Adenoviruses	Chronic meningoencephalitis in hypogammaglobulinemics
Arboviruses	Encephalitis
Cytomegalovirus	Acute meningitis and sometimes myelopathy or neuropathy
Herpes simplex types 1 and 2	Acute meningitis or meningoencephalitis and sometimes myelopathy
Human polyoma virus	Progressive multifocal leukoencephalopathy, usually focal defect, mimicking a mass
Poliovirus	Aseptic meningitis, myelitis, encephalomyelitis encephalitis
Varicella-zoster	Focal cerebral deficit/mass or acute meningitis sometimes myelopathy
Protozoa	
Strongyloides stercoralis	Meningitis in patients with altered cellular immunity
Toxoplasma gondii	CNS mass lesion/focal deficit or meningoencephalitis, especially in AIDS

Other protozoa that include *Plasmodium falciparum*, *Entamoeba histolytica*, and *Taenia solium* may also be noted but are more commonly seen in normal individuals.

event, whereas meningoencephalitis associated with fungi or mass lesions associated with abscess evolve more slowly.

Acute meningitis can be caused by *Listeria monocytogenes*, Enterobacteriaceae, *Haemophilus influenzae*, *S. pneumoniae*, or *Cryptococcus neoformans*. Focal lesions can be caused by abscesses with the etiologic agents including *Staphylococcus aureus*, anaerobes, *L. monocytogenes*, *Nocardia asteroides*, or fungi that include *Aspergillus fumigatus*, *C. neoformans* or *Mucoraceae*. Viruses including Human polyoma (JC), and varicella-zoster, and protozoa such as *Toxoplasma gondii* can also play a role. Other organisms and presentations can be seen in Tables 31-1 to 31-3.

Examination of cerebrospinal fluid is often helpful in establishing a diagnosis. However, lumbar puncture should not be performed in patients with a suspected cerebral mass lesion. An elevated pressure, pleocytosis, elevated protein, and low sugar may be found. However, the absence of cells in the CSF does not exclude an infection, and a Gram's stain, acid-fast stain, India ink preparation, serologic studies for *Cryptococcus* (latex agglutination test), and appropriate cultures are indicated. A differential cell count showing a predominance of mononuclear cells suggests *Listeria*, *Mycobacterium* spp. *or Toxoplasma*. An eosinophilic pleocytosis of the CSF rarely occurs and usually indicates a helminthic parasitic infection or lymphoma.

Because outcome depends on rapid diagnosis and treatment, much attention has been focused on development of techniques to meet these needs. Historically, techniques such as microscopy, histology, cultures and sensitivities of organisms, and serologic testing have been the standards. Bacterial and viral antigen testing have added additional tools. In the past decade, polymerase chain reaction (PCR) testing has become increasingly available. Positive results generally imply active infection. DNA chip and microarray technology are already being tested and described. This modality is also likely helping to identify new infectious agents. (RBB)

Bibliography

Abbott K, et al. Hospitalizations for fungal infections after renal transplantation in the United States. *Transpl Infect Dis* 2001;3:203–211.
> *This is a large retrospective study of patients hospitalized with fungal infections. Meningitis made up 7.6% of cases. Opportunistic infections accounted for more than 95% of infections. These infections occurred later than previously reported and were associated with greatly decreased patient survival.*

Blaschke S, et al. Tuberculous meningitis in a renal transplant recipient. *J Nephrol* 2002;15:93–95.
> *This is a case report of a transplant patient who traveled to an area endemic for tuberculosis and developed tuberculous meningitis, a rare and serious extrapulmonary complication of mycobacterial infection. This study underscores the need for careful epidemiologic history. Unexplained fever should raise concern in these patients, and isoniazid prophylaxis may be considered for those risking exposure in endemic areas.*

Cunha B. Central nervous system infections in the compromised host: a diagnostic approach. *Infect Dis Clin North Am* 2001;15:567–590.
> *The diagnostic approach to these infections depending upon the mode of their clinical expression is reviewed. The usual organisms involved, and both empiric and specific antimicrobial therapy, are reviewed.*

de Medeiros B, et al. Central nervous system infections following bone marrow transplantation: an autopsy report of 27 cases. *J Hematother Stem Cell Res* 2000;9:535–540.
> *The authors report that 60% of these cases had fungal isolates at autopsy and that most died within 3 months of transplantation, thus demonstrating the frequency of fungal infections in these patients and the high fatality rate.*

Flor A, et al. Nontuberculous mycobacterial meningitis: report of two cases and review. *Clin Infect Dis* 1996;23:1266–1273.
> *NTMM is frequently associated with immunosuppression. M. avium is the most commonly isolated species. Death rates approach 70%. Case report and review of 50 additional cases.*

Kang I, Park S. Infectious complications in SLE after immunosuppressive therapies. *Curr Opin Rheumatol* 2003;15:528–534.

SLE patients are at increased risk for infection. Steroids and cyclophosphamide are the strongest risk factors for infection. Mycophenolate mofetil usage results in less frequent infections in these patients than in those treated with cyclophosphamide.

Leedom J, Uderman A. Epidemiology of central nervous system infections. *Neuroimaging Clin N Am* 2000;10:297–308.

A detailed review of the bacterial, fungal, viral, and protozoal causes of various types of CNS infections, including meningitis, brain abscess and others.

Nissen M, Sloots T. Rapid diagnosis in pediatric infectious diseases: the past, the present and the future. *Pediatr Infect Dis J* 2002;21:605-12; discussion 613–614.

The current status of PCR testing is reviewed with specifics on the technique. Future techniques are discussed, including automated PCR testing, DNA chips, and microarray technology.

Pruitt A. Nervous system infections in patients with cancer. *Neurol Clin* 2003;21:193–219.

An excellent review. The author presents a detailed overview and approach to patients with these problems. Diagnostic clues, categories of presentation, classes of organisms involved, and noninfectious mimics are reviewed in some detail. Laboratory, neuroimaging, and other diagnostic tools are included. Treatment options are also presented.

Sindic C, van Antwerpen M, Goffette S. Clinical relevance of polymerase chain reaction (PCR) assays and antigen-driven immunoblots for the diagnosis of neurological infectious diseases. *Brain Res Bull* 2003;61:299–308.

The power of PCR testing as a tool for detecting these infections is reviewed. The authors describe their experience, using this approach, in a number of different infectious genomes.

Warnatz K, et al. Infectious CNS disease as a differential diagnosis in systemic rheumatic diseases: three case reports *Ann Rheum Dis* 2003;62:50–57.

Extended report of 20 cases of PML or cerebral nocardiosis in rheumatic patients on immunosuppressive agents. The morbidity and mortality of autoimmune diseases are increasingly related to secondary infection resulting from more effective immunosuppressive treatment. Clinical aspects of these infections, the role of brain imaging, CSF analysis, and brain biopsy are reviewed by the authors.

Zunt J. Central nervous system infection during immunosuppression. *Neurol Clin* 2002;20:1–22.

Diagnosis and treatment of selected CNS infections are reviewed. The level and type of immunosuppression also can help the clinician determine the etiology of the infection.

ACUTE PERIPHERAL FACIAL PALSY 32

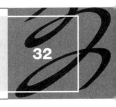

*T*he presentation of facial palsy (weakness of cranial nerve VII) can be acute or chronic, peripheral or central, mild (paresis) or complete (paralysis), unilateral or bilateral. Each of these clinical factors is important for diagnosis, prognosis, and management. The facial nerve is the most commonly injured cranial nerve. This is most likely explained by its prolonged course through the temporal bone (over 3 cm). The nerve's location within a narrow bony canal makes it very susceptible to injury from either trauma or inflammation. The majority of facial nerve disorders are acute, peripheral, or self limited, and they occur in otherwise healthy adults. Most of these cases are considered to be "idiopathic" (Bell's palsy)

and have an excellent prognosis. However, facial palsy can be the initial sign of a serious disorder. Therefore, a thorough history and physical and a logical diagnostic approach to each patient with facial palsy is warranted. A major goal of therapy in all patients with facial palsy is to prevent corneal ulceration caused by ineffective lacrimation, and to take necessary steps to avoid long-term morbidity. Pharmacologic therapy can decrease complications in many patients, and the choice of medication depends upon etiology. This chapter will focus on a practical approach to the patient with nontraumatic acute peripheral facial palsy.

 ## CLINICAL ANATOMY AND PHYSIOLOGY

The facial nerve arises by a somatic motor root and a visceral mixed sensory root (nervus intermedius) from the pons in the posterior cranial fossa. These two roots travel together with the vestibulocochlear nerve (CN VIII) on the cerebellopontine cistern (a tumor of the cerebellopontine angle can, therefore, affect both cranial nerves VII and VIII) before entering the internal acoustic meatus in the petrous temporal bone. Here the motor root and the nervus intermedius join to form the complete facial nerve, which enters the facial (fallopian or internal auditory) canal. This canal runs through the petrous portion of the temporal bone, is about 33 mm in length, and consists of four consecutive segments: labyrinthine, geniculate, tympanic, and mastoid. Thus, tumors or inflammatory processes related to the inner or middle ears or the mastoid air cells can injure the facial nerve. Because the labyrinthine is the narrowest segment (0.68 mm in diameter), and here the nerve is surrounded by bone with little connective tissue support, even minimal inflammation in this region can cause nerve injury. Most authors believe that this is usually, but not always, the site of injury in idiopathic (Bell's) facial palsy. Furthermore, it is the long interosseous course of this nerve that makes it so vulnerable to injury with basal skull fractures.

Upon exiting the labyrinthine segment, the facial nerve widens because of the sensory cell bodies of the geniculate ganglion. Here the nerve bifurcates and sends off the greater superficial petrosal nerve. It is this branch that carries the efferent axons to the lacrimal gland and the afferent taste fibers from the palate. After the geniculate ganglion, the larger fork retains the name *facial nerve*. Within the mastoid wall the facial nerve gives off two branches. The first branch is the nerve to the stapedius muscle which, when injured, often results in hyperacusis. The second branch is the chorda tympani, which passes into the tympanic cavity. In some patients the chorda tympani can be seen by otoscopy as it passes behind the upper posterior quadrant of the tympanic membrane. The chorda tympani consists of the efferent fibers supplying the submandibular and sublingual salivary glands and the afferent fibers from the tongue. The facial nerve exits the temporal bone via the stylomastoid foramen and quickly enters the parotid gland before dividing into many small branches that supply all the muscles of facial expression.

The facial nerve is a mixed nerve carrying at least four types of nerve fibers: (1) somatic motor fibers to the muscles of facial expression and the stapedius muscle; (2) parasympathetic visceral motor fibers to the lacrimal, submandibular, and sublingual salivary glands (but not the parotid glands); (3) special sensory (taste) afferent fibers from the anterior two-thirds of the tongue and palate; (4) somatic sensory afferent fibers from the external auditory canal and pinna.

A basic understanding of the anatomy and function of this complicated nerve is critical for the evaluation of patients with acute facial paralysis. A careful clinical evaluation may allow the clinician to identify the site of facial nerve dysfunction, and this may make an accurate diagnosis possible. For example, a diagnosis of varicella-zoster infection of the geniculate ganglion may be made because of vesicles on the external canal, the tongue, or the palate. Similarly, loss of lacrimation in the setting of facial palsy is evidence of facial nerve injury proximal to the geniculate ganglion. Therefore, a middle ear or mastoid process would not be a likely cause of facial palsy in this instance.

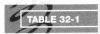

TABLE 32-1	Causes of Acute Peripheral Facial Palsy
Bell's palsy	51–78%
Ramsay Hunt syndrome	7–37%
Trauma	4–22%
Tumor	4–6%
Otitis media/cholesteatoma	3–4%
Neonatal conditions	3–6%
Hemifacial spasm	2–5%
CNS disease	1%

(Adapted from May M, Klein SR. Differential diagnosis of facial nerve palsy. *Otolaryngol Clin North Am* 1991;24:613–645.)

CAUSES OF ACUTE FACIAL PALSY

Table 32-1 presents the most common causes of acute peripheral facial palsy. The incidence of each disease is shown as a range based on several large published series of patients. Table 32-2 shows the most common disorders of the 13% of patients who were initially misdiagnosed with Bell's palsy in a series of 1675 patients. Recent evidence suggests that varicella-zoster virus (VZV; zoster sine herpete) causes 8 to 25% of cases initially diagnosed as Bell's palsy. Similarly, in regions endemic for Lyme disease, 10 to 25% of cases of Bell's palsy may actually be due to Lyme borreliosis.

APPROACH TO THE PATIENT WITH ACUTE FACIAL PALSY

The most important aspect of the history is the time course of the motor deficit. Bell's palsy and varicella-zoster infection occur suddenly, with maximal facial weakness developing within 48 hours. A subacute time course is suggestive of a more serious disorder, such as acoustic neuroma, cholesteatoma, or mastoiditis. Progressive hearing loss or vertigo suggests an internal auditory canal or cerebellopontine angle tumor. Pain behind the ear is common in many causes of facial palsy including Bell's palsy. However, severe aural, anterior facial, or radicular pain is highly suggestive of herpes zoster infection. A recent history of cold exposure is thought by some to suggest Bell's palsy, but a recent review of 171 cases found no association with weather conditions. A family history of idiopathic facial palsy is present in up to 14% of cases of Bell's palsy and those with Melkersson's syndrome, a familial

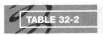

TABLE 32-2	Etiology of 224 Cases of Facial Palsy Misdiagnosed as Bell's Palsy
Tumor	38%
Herpes zoster ophthalmicus	23%
Infection	13%
Other	13%
Atypical Bell's palsy	4%
CNS	4%
Birth	3%
Trauma	1%
Hemifacial spasm	0.5%

(Adapted from May M, Klein SR. Differential diagnosis of facial nerve palsy. *Otolaryngol Clin North Am* 1991;24:613–645.)

disorder characterized by recurrent, alternating facial edema and facial palsy associated with a fissured tongue. A history of recent travel to an area endemic for Lyme disease should be sought. Recent vaccination may be associated with facial palsy. A careful sexual history may help identify the rare case of facial palsy due to syphilis or HIV.

Physical examination should initially focus on discriminating between a central (supranuclear) or peripheral cause of facial palsy. A lesion in the cerebral cortex or corticobulbar tract (central lesion) will affect only the lower face. That is, testing of the frontalis and orbicularis oculi will show no impairment. Alternatively, a lesion at or distal to the motor nucleus of the facial nerve will produce complete unilateral facial weakness. A central cause of facial paralysis should not impair lacrimation, salivation, or taste. Because facial palsy can be subtle, examination of facial muscles should include (1) observation for facial asymmetry, especially flattening of the nasolabial fold on the affected side; (2) assessment for symmetric wrinkling of the forehead as the patient raises her eyebrows; (3) attempt to open the patient's eyelids against maximal resistance; (4) instruction of the patient to show teeth and puff out cheeks. Asking the patient to close each eye individually may identify mild peripheral facial palsy. The patient with Bell's palsy will not be able to close one eye without also closing the other.

Once the presence of a peripheral facial lesion has been determined, the examiner should look for signs of serious disease. Even in the absence of known trauma, Battle's sign (bruise over the mastoid) is highly suggestive of a basal skull fracture. This examination is of particular importance in patients with alcoholism or epilepsy. Trauma is also suggested by hemotympanum. Granulation tissue or polyps in the ear canal may be associated with malignant otitis externa or cholesteatoma. A reddened chorda tympani has been noted by otoscopy in both Bell's palsy and varicella-zoster infection.

The ear canal, pinna, palate, and tongue should be examined for the vesicles of Ramsay Hunt syndrome. Fluorescein staining of the eye should be performed because of the high risk of corneal ulcers with peripheral facial paralysis. The parotid glands should be palpated for masses. Hearing loss, nystagmus and ataxia are evidence against idiopathic facial paralysis and, in the absence of zoster vesicles, suggest tumor. A thorough skin survey for erythema migrans should be performed.

The history and physical examination is usually sufficient to make a diagnosis of acute peripheral facial palsy. No laboratory or imaging studies are necessary in the setting of an acute-onset facial palsy in a young adult. Diabetes is associated with Bell's palsy, especially in the elderly. Therefore, a fasting blood sugar and urinalysis should be considered in older patients who have this condition. In any patient with particularly severe or atypical symptoms, gadolinium-enhanced magnetic resonance imaging (MRI) can rule out a posterior fossa or inner ear tumor. Electrodiagnostic testing may be indicated occasionally, in cases of complete facial paralysis with no clinical improvement after 2 weeks.

 IDIOPATHIC (BELL'S) FACIAL PALSY

Bell's palsy has traditionally been defined as a sudden, isolated, peripheral facial palsy or paralysis of unknown etiology. It accounts for the majority of cases (51–78%) of acute facial palsy in published series. Incidence is approximately 20 of 100,000 population in both the United States and United Kingdom and 30 of 100,000 in Japan. It is estimated that 1–2% of persons will be affected during their lifetime. Incidence increases to 45 of 100,000 women during the third trimester of pregnancy and the immediate postpartum period. In the nonpregnant population, men and women are affected equally. Mean age of onset is 40 years, with the lowest incidence in children younger than age 10. Facial paralysis may be incomplete (33–65%) or complete (35–66%) and is usually maximal on the second day of the illness. Commonly associated symptoms are listed in Table 32-3. Bell's palsy recurs on the same or opposite side in 8–12% of patients. A family history of Bell's palsy is present in 14% of patients; it is more common in patients with diabetes mellitus and hypertension.

Prognosis is generally very good, with 71% of patients demonstrating complete recovery. Patients with incomplete paralysis have a 94% chance of clinical resolution whereas only 60% of patients with complete paralysis return to normal function. Long-term sequelae include persistent weakness, contracture, hemifacial spasm, synkinesis (involuntary

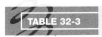

TABLE 32-3	Frequency of Early Symptoms and Signs of Bell's Palsy
Decreased stapes reflex	90%
Epiphora (excessive tearing)	68%
Pain	61%
Viral prodrome	60%
Ageusia	57%
Reddened chorda tympani	40%
Hyperacusis	29%
Decreased tearing, Schirmer test	17%
Decreased tearing, subjective	15%

(Adapted from Adour KK, Wingerd J. Idiopathic facial paralysis (Bell's palsy): factors affecting severity and outcome in 446 patients. *Neurology* 1974;24:1112–1116.)

movement of facial muscles accompanying voluntary movement, such as involuntary eye blink with a voluntary smile), and "crocodile tears"—tearing while eating. Poor prognostic indicators also include hyperacusis, decreased tearing demonstrated by the Schirmer test, diabetes, hypertension, psychoneurosis, and age older than 60. A recent study found that only 25% of diabetic patients with complete Bell's palsy recovered normal facial muscle function.

A viral or immune-mediated cause of Bell's palsy has been postulated for almost 40 years. Serologic evidence for an association between Bell's palsy and different viruses has been published, and includes Herpes simplex virus type 1 (HSV-1), VZV, cytomegalovirus, Epstein-Barr virus, adenovirus, rubella virus, mumps virus, influenza virus, and HIV. Additionally, postmortem examinations of the facial nerve in patients with Bell's palsy often suggest a viral etiology. Recent evidence strongly supports HSV-1 as a major factor in Bell's palsy. A study of endoneural fluid obtained during decompression surgery of the facial nerve found that 11 of 14 patients (79%) with Bell's palsy had detectable HSV-1 genomes. None of the 12 controls had such evidence. It is now widely accepted that most cases of "idiopathic" facial paralysis represent an HSV-1 facial nerve neuritis. This has important implications for therapy.

Management of patients with Bell's palsy includes counseling and reassurance. A favorable prognosis should be emphasized, but the patient should be instructed to return if no improvement is noted within 1 week. Some authorities advocate for electroneurography if complete facial paralysis persists after 1 week of medical treatment. Facial nerve decompression surgery may be considered if this test documents more than 90% nerve degeneration.

Therapy directed at prevention of corneal ulceration is always mandatory. Inability to close the eyelid, collection of tears in the lower conjunctival sac, and decreased lacrimation increase risk of corneal drying and injury. Methylcellulose solution should be applied hourly during the day. At night, a lubricating ointment can be used along with either taping of the eyelid or an eye patch. Patients should be instructed to return immediately for eye pain, discharge, or a change in vision.

Bell's palsy is commonly treated with glucocorticoids with or without the addition of antiviral medication. However, the evidence supporting this practice is highly controversial. Individual clinical trials have shown benefit with corticosteroids, whereas other trials have not. Three recent meta-analyses comparing glucocorticoids with placebo found a significant trend that glucocorticoids decrease the number of patients with incomplete facial recovery. A practice parameter published by the American Academy of Neurology concluded "steroids are safe and *probably* effective in improving facial functional outcomes in patients with Bell's palsy." A more recent systematic review published by the Cochrane Library found no significant benefit with corticosteroids in patients with Bell's palsy. It is noteworthy that one study found a significantly higher rate of recovery in diabetic patients with complete Bell's palsy treated with prednisolone (97%) versus no treatment (58%).

Several studies have shown that acyclovir is not as effective as prednisone in reducing complications in patients with Bell's palsy. However, a recent randomized trial found a significantly greater rate of recovery in the group treated with both prednisone and acyclovir versus prednisone alone (92% vs. 76%, confidence interval [CI] = 1.7–30.3%). A recent retrospective study of 480 patients with complete Bell's palsy found that early treatment with prednisone and acyclovir resulted in significantly better early (79% vs. 63%) and late (100% vs. 91%) recovery rates when compared with prednisone alone.

Most authorities now recommend the use of prednisone (60–80 mg per day) and an antiviral for 1 week in patients with moderate or severe (complete) Bell's palsy. Valacyclovir is often used because of ease of administration and better absorption when compared to acyclovir. In mild cases, the prognosis is excellent and treatment usually unnecessary. Recurrence of pain after stopping or tapering corticosteroids may be a sign of ongoing nerve degeneration and should prompt a return to the previous dose. Patients with diabetes and Bell's palsy have a worse prognosis than the general population, and combination therapy may be particularly beneficial in these individuals.

Use of acupuncture has resulted in enhanced outcome in three small studies, but their poor quality makes it impossible to draw firm conclusions. Physical therapy has not been shown to be of benefit in the setting of Bell's palsy, but "mime" therapy in patients with incomplete recovery at 9 months may be beneficial.

 RAMSAY HUNT SYNDROME

Ramsay Hunt syndrome is defined as acute peripheral facial nerve palsy associated with zosteriform vesicles on the ear (zoster oticus), tongue, or palate. Incidence is approximately 5 in 100,000. It is often accompanied by vestibulocochlear dysfunction, including nausea, vomiting, nystagmus, tinnitus, and hearing loss. Severe pain is common. Reactivation of VZV within the geniculate ganglion causes inflammation in the sensory branches of the facial nerve and the anatomically related vestibulocochlear nerve (VIII) by a "bystander effect." In one-third of patients, the characteristic herpetic eruption may not appear for 2 to 14 days after onset of facial paralysis. Vesiculation does not always appear despite confirmation of VZV by IgM seroconversion (zoster sine herpete). Thus, VZV-associated acute facial palsy may be clinically indistinguishable from Bell's palsy. Eight to 25% of Bell's palsy cases actually represent zoster sine herpete.

VZV infection is the second most common cause of acute peripheral facial palsy. Ramsay Hunt syndrome has a worse prognosis, as compared with Bell's palsy. Complete facial paralysis occurs initially in two-thirds of patients. In those with complete palsy, a minority show resolution of symptoms and most develop synkinesis. Permanent hearing loss rarely (5%) may result.

Treatment within 3 days of onset of facial palsy with acyclovir and prednisone has been shown to improve outcomes. In a retrospective study, patients treated within the first 72 hours had a significantly higher rate of complete motor recovery (75%, $P <.05$) than those treated between days 3 and 7 (48%) or after 7 days (30%). Previous studies have shown decreased hearing loss rates with early combination therapy. Thus, patients with Ramsay Hunt syndrome and those with Bell's palsy associated with severe ear pain (zoster sine herpete) should be treated early with prednisone (1 mg/kg per day for 5 days followed by a 10-day taper) and acyclovir (800 mg five times a day) or valacyclovir.

 LYME BORRELIOSIS

Acute peripheral facial palsy is the most common neurologic symptom of *Borrelia burgdorferi* infection (neuroborreliosis), and may be unilateral or bilateral. Other signs and symptoms of Lyme disease usually accompany this manifestation. However, in some patients, it may be the only manifestation. Most patients do not acknowledge a recent tick bite. Lyme disease is much more common in the spring and summer. In endemic areas, *Borrelia* infection occurs in approximately 100 cases per 100,000 population per year. Borrelial facial palsy usually resolves without treatment, but other complications may develop. A study in a hyperendemic area found that 10 to 25% of Bell's palsy cases was actually caused by Lyme disease.

Several studies demonstrate that corticosteroid treatment in *Borrelia* infection increases morbidity. Therefore in areas endemic for Lyme disease, corticosteroid therapy for Bell's palsy should be prescribed cautiously, and consideration should be given to doxycycline therapy. Isolated facial palsy owing to Lyme disease can be treated with a 21-day course of doxycycline (100 mg bid) and does not require parenteral treatment.

 OTHER INFECTIONS

Numerous viral, bacterial, and other infections are associated with peripheral facial palsy (Table 32-3). Proof of causality is generally lacking and treatment is supportive. Most are likely to represent reactivation of latent HSV-1 or VZV in the setting of another infection. However, Bell's palsy can be the initial manifestation of HIV infection or secondary syphilis. Therefore, it is prudent to encourage all patients at risk for sexually transmitted diseases to be screened for these. Epstein-Barr virus is found in up to 20% of patients diagnosed with Bell's palsy. Most of these patients have other manifestations of infectious mononucleosis. A recent study found seroconversion of *Mycoplasma pneumoniae* in 26% of patients with Bell's palsy. Serologic evidence of hepatitis B infection was found in 71% of patients with Bell's palsy, as compared with 32% of controls. The clinical significance of these findings is unclear.

 SUMMARY AND RECOMMENDATIONS

1. In patients presenting with acute facial palsy, the clinician must determine if the location of the lesion is central or peripheral.
2. A thorough history and physical is needed to identify a diagnosis in most patients with acute peripheral facial palsy.
3. Most cases of acute peripheral facial palsy are caused by HSV-1 (Bell's palsy) or VZV (Ramsay Hunt syndrome or zoster sine herpete).
4. Bell's palsy does not require treatment if the weakness is mild.
5. Patients with moderate or severe weakness owing to Bell's palsy should be treated with a 7-day course of prednisone (60–80 mg/day) and valacyclovir (1 g b.i.d. or t.i.d.). We recommend this treatment for presumed zoster sine herpete as well.
6. Patients with Ramsay Hunt syndrome also should be treated early with prednisone (1 mg/kg per day) and high-dose acyclovir (800 mg five times a day) or valacyclovir.
7. Bell's palsy caused by Lyme disease should be treated with doxycycline 100 mg b.i.d. for 21 days without prednisone.
8. Complete paralysis persisting after longer than 1 week of treatment in a patient with Bell's palsy should prompt a referral for electroneurography and an evaluation with a surgeon. (RBB)

Bibliography

Adour KK, et al. Bell's palsy treatment with acyclovir and prednisone compared with prednisone alone: a double-blind, randomized, controlled trial. *Ann Otol Rhinol Laryngol* 1996;105:371–378.
> Sophisticated testing was used to compare outcomes in two groups of patients with Bell's palsy treated with prednisone with and without acyclovir. Those who received acyclovir had more rapid return of function.

Benatar M, Edlow J. The spectrum of cranial neuropathy in patients with Bell's palsy. *Arch Intern Med* 2004;164:2383–2385.
> The authors assessed patients with Bell's palsy in an emergency department and found almost 10% had evidence of additional cranial neuropathies. These included glossopharyngeal nerve and probable trigeminal nerve involvement. The implications of these findings are uncertain, but the authors lead the reader to believe that outcomes were equally unremarkable in these individuals. The "Bell's palsy" syndrome may need to be expanded.

Geates GA. Facial paralysis. *Otolaryngol Clin North Am* 1987;20:113–131.

Excellent discussion of the anatomy and physiology of the facial nerve. Also provides a reasonable approach to the history, physical, and laboratory testing useful in differential diagnosis.

Gevers G, Lemkens P. Bilateral simultaneous facial paralysis-differential diagnosis and treatment options. A case report and review of the literature. *Acta Otolaryngol Belg* 2003;57:139–146.

The authors present a differential diagnosis of bilateral simultaneous facial paralysis, based on literature review. Lyme borreliosis is by far the most common etiology (>35%). Other important causes include Guillain-Barré syndrome, trauma, and HIV infection. A table of all causes and a flow chart for assessment are provided.

Gilden DH. Bell's palsy. *N Engl J Med* 2004;351:1323–1331.

Thorough review with excellent representations of patients with central and peripheral facial weakness. It represents a case-based approach to the patient who has a unilateral facial droop. Excellent diagrams and discussions are provided to distinguish central from peripheral disease. A framework for treatment is given regarding need for medications and work-up in addition to standard history and physical examination.

Jaamaa S, et al. *Varicella zoster* and *Borrelia burgdorferi* are the main agents associated with facial paresis, especially in children. *J Clin Virol* 2003;27:146–151.

The authors compared serologic/nucleic markers for infectious agents in 42 patients with acute facial palsy compared with a similar number with other neurologic conditions. VZV and B. burgdorferi were the most common etiologies in patients with acute facial palsy, especially notable in children. These were significantly less common in controls. Other etiologies found included Mycoplasma pneumoniae and Chlamydia pneumoniae.

May M, Klein SR. Differential diagnosis of facial nerve palsy. *Otolaryngol Clin North Am* 1991;24:613–645.

Excellent review of the varied causes of facial nerve paralysis that includes the large personal experience of one of the authors. Contains characteristic presentation of typical and atypical Bell's palsy and charts indicating probable causes based on the anatomic location of the lesion.

Morgan M, Nathwani D. Facial palsy and infection: The unfolding story. *Clin Infect Dis* 1992;14:263–271.

Reviews evidence of infectious causes of Bell's palsy. Has an excellent section on Lyme borreliosis as a cause of facial palsy.

Murakami S, et al. Treatment of Ramsay Hunt syndrome with acyclovir-prednisone: significance of early diagnosis and treatment. *Ann Neurol* 1997;41:353–357.

A retrospective analysis of acyclovir-prednisone treatment in 80 Ramsay Hunt patients. Early treatment (within 3 days) had significantly best outcome.

Murakami S. Bell palsy and herpes simplex virus: identification of viral DNA in endoneurial fluid and muscle. *Ann Intern Med* 1996;124:27–30.

Landmark study providing compelling evidence that HSV causes most cases of Bell's palsy.

Salinas RA, Alvarez G, Ferreira J. Corticosteroids for Bell's palsy (idiopathic facial paralysis). *Cochrane Database Syst Rev* 2002;1:CD001942.

Systematic review of the evidence for corticosteroid therapy in Bell's palsy. Only three trials were included in the analysis because of strict inclusion criteria. The authors conclude the available evidence from randomized controlled trials does not support a benefit from corticosteroids.

Sweeney CJ, Gilden DH. Ramsay Hunt syndrome. *J Neurol Neurosurg Psychiatry* 2001;71:149–154.

Excellent review. Concise and clear discussion of the virology and evidence for therapy in patients with this syndrome.

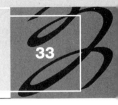

ACUTE INFECTIONS OF THE CENTRAL NERVOUS SYSTEM IN IMMUNOCOMPETENT PERSONS

33

*P*hysicians frequently care for patients who present with signs or symptoms that suggest central nervous system (CNS) dysfunction. The differential diagnosis is broad, as disease of any organ system, when sufficiently severe, can alter CNS function. Rapid diagnosis and treatment is often necessary to prevent morbidity or mortality. Primary factors that drive the brain's susceptibility to damage from infection are (1) inadequate room for expansion when inflammation is present; (2) poor immune function within the blood-brain barrier; (3) difficulty in achieving adequate antimicrobial concentrations in the cerebrospinal fluid (CSF) and parenchyma; and (4) inability of the brain to regenerate neural tissue once cell death has occurred.

 INITIAL EVALUATION

Patients with CNS infections can present with minimal signs and symptoms of CNS irritation or with obtundation and shock. Differential diagnosis is staggering in length and complexity, and the variety of serum, CSF, and radiographic tests that can be ordered is equally broad. Efficiency and economy, therefore, should be the rule. The purpose of this chapter is to outline such an approach without reviewing the entire gamut of organisms and tests that may ultimately apply to a given patient.

The first step is to ensure that patients are hemodynamically and neurologically stable. Selected individuals may require aggressive hydration and hemodynamic support. If suspicion for CNS infection is high, blood cultures are drawn and empiric antimicrobials are immediately administered, preferably within 1 hour of presentation. This may occur prior to lumbar puncture (LP) in some circumstances. Although the sensitivity of Gram's stain and culture is decreased when antibiotics are given before LP, the effect is small if LP is performed within 1 to 2 hours of antibiotics, and sensitivities as high as 38% have been reported when LP was delayed for 24 hours. Patients who have altered mental status or focal neurologic signs or seizures must undergo brain imaging prior to LP.

History and Physical Examination

A thorough history and physical examination is paramount. All subsequent radiographic and laboratory testing should be guided by the initial assessment. It is common to find a history of fever, headache, stiff neck, and confusion. These cardinal symptoms are frequently not all present, however, especially in the elderly or immunocompromised. The history helps determine whether the illness is acute or chronic, community acquired or nosocomial. It also helps to determine whether the suspected CNS infection is primary or metastatic. Review of symptoms helps determine where this source might be. Sinus pain, otorrhea, productive cough, abdominal pain, or dysuria may point to a primary focus of infection and help determine selection of initial antimicrobials. Exposure to individuals with known infections suggests a common pathogen. Past medical history alerts the clinician to underlying illnesses that may predispose to a particular CNS infection or organism. Regarding meningitis, important items in the medical history include prior CNS infections or neurosurgical procedures (*Staphylococcus* and aerobic gram-negative bacilli), immunosuppression (*Toxoplasma*, fungi, and mycobacteria), diabetes (fungi), head trauma (*Staphylococci* and *Streptococci*), and alcoholism (*Streptococcus pneumoniae* and *Listeria monocytogenes*). When

191

brain abscess or subdural empyema is considered, a history of chronic ear, sinus, and dental infections is supportive. The social history should determine homelessness, ethanol or drug abuse, animal or insect exposure, employment, and HIV risk factors. The medication list should be reviewed with special attention to new medications, as signs and symptoms of CNS infection can be mimicked by many medications. Alternatively some medications are associated with aseptic meningitis. A review of adverse reactions to medications may implicate an agent that was recently resumed. Recent antibiotics may suggest resistance patterns to be considered and may confound testing by reducing the sensitivity of Gram's stain and culture.

The physical exam helps confirm the hemodynamic and neurologic stability of the patient, and helps to target suspicions about a primary source of infection. Special attention is paid to the neurologic exam to determine if subtle alterations in cognitive function or focal neurologic signs exist. Classically, meningitis presents with fever and headache accompanied by meningeal signs such as Kernig's and Brudzinsky's signs. Encephalitis is much more likely to appear with cognitive dysfunction and personality changes. Sinus tenderness or otitis, or dental infection suggest intracranial extension from these sites. Focal findings on auscultation of the lungs suggest *pneumococcal* pneumonia and meningitis. A new murmur accompanied by peripheral stigmata suggests endocarditis with intracranial complications. Rash may suggest *meningococcal, rickettsial,* or viral etiologies, among others.

Laboratory Evaluation

Primary questions are whether to perform LP, and whether preprocedure brain imaging is necessary. Generally if there is any question of meningitis, LP is warranted. Computed tomography (CT) of the brain has been used to predict intracranial hypertension and the risk for brainstem herniation from LP. When focal neurologic signs, seizures, or signs of elevated intracranial pressure on physical examination are present, a CT scan of the brain is indicated. Otherwise, preprocedure radiography is generally not indicated and may increase time to appropriate antibiotic therapy and increase costs of care. A recent study reported that the absence of the following factors had a high negative predictive value for abnormalities on head CT: age older than 60, immunocompromised state, history of a CNS lesion such as a tumor, recent seizure, altered mental status/cognition, and focal neurologic findings. Of note, 56 patients had abnormal CT findings, but 52 of these underwent LP without complication.

The most common complication of LP is headache, which occurs in 10 to 30% of patients. Spinal hematoma occurs in less than 1% of procedures and is almost always associated with anticoagulation or a platelet count less than 50,000/mL. De novo infection resulting from LP is rare.

CSF pressure should be measured during every diagnostic LP. Generally four tubes of CSF are withdrawn. Tube #1 is sent for Gram's stain and culture; tube #2 for protein and glucose; tube #3 for cell count and differential; and at least one additional tube is set aside for further testing as indicated. Generally, 8 to 16 mL of CSF is removed initially. Much more fluid may be required, however, depending mostly on the number of cultures and DNA studies desired, and on whether cytology will be ordered. Forty milliliters can be removed safely during one procedure. One milliliter is adequate for both protein and glucose measurement and for cell count and differential. Each culture that is sent requires an additional 1 mL of fluid, whereas DNA studies (polymerase chain reaction [PCR]) require 1 to 2 mL, and each antibody test requires 1 mL. When mycobacteria or fungi infections are considerations, 10 to 20 mL may be required. In patients with potential AIDS-related diagnoses, CSF testing for cryptococcal antigen and VDRL should be considered. Each of these tests requires 1 mL of fluid.

The results of CSF testing are classically used to determine whether a septic or an aseptic process is operative (Table 33-1). Although there is much overlap, this model remains useful. Normal values include an opening pressure of less than 20 cm H_2O, less than 5 white blood cells (WBC)/mm^3 with approximately 85% of these being lymphocytes, a protein concentration of 15 to 45 mg/dL, and a glucose concentration of 45 to 90 mg/dL or more than 30% of the serum glucose concentration. Results suggesting septic inflammation include an elevated CSF opening pressure, several hundred to many thousands of mostly

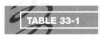

Parameter	Normal CSF	Acute bacterial	Viral
Opening pressure	6–20 cm H_2O	Elevated	Often normal
CSF WBCs/mm³	0–5 (lymphocytes)	Hundreds-thousands (PMNs predominate)	Few to several hundred* (lymphocytes predominate, but early on may see PMNs)
Protein (mg/dL)	18–45	100–500 (occasionally >1,000)	Often normal or only slightly elevated
Glucose (mg/dL)	45–80, or 0.6 × serum glucose	Often 5–40, or <0.3 × serum glucose	Usually normal; can be depressed in mumps and HSV
Miscellaneous	For traumatic LP, add one WBC and one mg/dL protein for each 1,000 RBCs	Gram's stain (+) in 60–80% cases, somewhat organism specific, and related to prior use of antimicrobials	Usually not necessary to identify specific etiology of viral meningitis

*Lymphocytes >5,000 commonly noted with lymphocytic choriomeningitis (LCM)
(Adapted from Choi CK. Bacterial meningitis in aging adults. *Clin Infect Dis* 2001;33:1380–1385.)

polymorphonuclear (PMN) WBCs, protein levels generally higher than 100 mg/dL, and glucose levels of 5 to 40 mg/dL or less than 30% of the serum glucose. An aseptic picture includes a normal or only slightly elevated opening pressure, several hundred cells mostly of mononuclear lineage, normal or slightly elevated protein, and a normal glucose concentration. The CSF profile of many patients will lie between the "classic" septic and aseptic profiles. This "mixed" category comprises a large group of diagnoses, including parameningeal foci, infective endocarditis, rheumatologic disorders, early aseptic meningitis, partially treated septic meningitis, medication-induced disease, and postsurgical inflammation.

 GENERAL ANTIBIOTIC CONSIDERATIONS

The ideal antibiotic for CNS infection would be cheap, cover a broad range of gram-positive and -negative bacteria, allow for once-daily dosing, achieve high concentrations in the CSF and brain parenchyma regardless of the presence of inflammation, have a high therapeutic index, be well tolerated, and be bactericidal. Unfortunately such an agent is not available, leaving the clinician to develop a regimen that satisfies as many criteria as possible. Perhaps the most difficult criterion to meet is that of achieving a high concentration in the CSF and parenchyma while remaining bactericidal against offending pathogens. Penicillins and cephalosporins penetrate the uninflamed meninges poorly. In the presence of inflammation, however, the percent concentration of selected β-lactams increase to levels that can effectively treat bacterial meningitis caused by sensitive pathogens, and they are bactericidal against most sensitive pathogens. Because of these qualities and because of their antimicrobial spectra, penicillin, ampicillin, and ceftriaxone are workhorses historically used to treat CNS infections. Penetration increases to clinically effective levels in the setting of acute inflammation. Because of its high molecular weight, vancomycin poorly penetrates the CSF, even when the meninges are inflamed. Its bacteriostatic effect in some instances also contributes to vancomycin's weakness as an agent for CNS infections. Unfortunately, no other agent has a sufficient record to replace it when coagulase-negative and methicillin-resistant *Staphylococcus aureus* or resistant *Streptococcus pneumoniae* are considerations. When broader coverage is required, agents that include ceftazidime, piperacillin, and meropenem can be used. Metronidazole is an effective anaerobic agent and achieves high concentrations within abscesses.

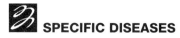 **SPECIFIC DISEASES**

Acute Bacterial Meningitis

Best current data for community-acquired acute bacterial meningitis suggest that almost 50% of cases are due to *S. pneumoniae*, 25% to *Neisseria meningitidis*, 13% to group B streptococci, 8% to *Listeria monocytogenes*, and 7% to *Haemophilus influenzae*. Nosocomially-acquired meningitis may also be associated with enteric gram-negative bacilli in up to 33% of cases. Mortality rates for bacterial meningitis in adults remain at approximately 20% but rise to at least 40% among those older than age 60.

The classic presentation of bacterial meningitis is fever, headache, and meningismus, with or without altered mental status. A recent evidence-based review demonstrated that one of three findings—fever, neck stiffness, or altered mental status—was present in nearly all patients with the disease. The presence of at least one of these three findings was 99% sensitive for acute bacterial meningitis. Therefore, the absence of all three signs has a high negative predictive value. It is uncommon for all these signs to be present simultaneously, especially in the elderly and immunocompromised. Kernig's and Brudzinski's signs are present in 50% of adults. (Table 33-2).

The decision to empirically treat patients who have suggestive signs and symptoms of meningitis is based on clinical suspicion, CSF profile, and severity of illness. A CSF WBC count of more than 3000/mL consisting predominately of PMN cells is highly suspicious for bacterial infection. The WBC count is higher than 2000/mL in 38% of bacterial cases. Whereas a low glucose is classic, this occurs in only 50% of cases. A CSF/serum glucose ratio of less than 0.4 is 80% sensitive and 96% specific for acute bacterial meningitis (as opposed to acute viral meningitis), and a ratio of less than 0.25 is found in less than 1% of cases of viral meningitis. A CSF protein level of more than 100 mg/dL is 82% sensitive and 98% specific for acute bacterial meningitis (as opposed to acute viral meningitis). Gram's stain is positive in up to 85% of cases of untreated bacterial meningitis. CSF culture is positive in up to 85% of cases, and blood culture identifies the causative organism in 80 to 95% of cases. CSF bacterial antigen testing is an additional option. This test is most useful when antibiotics have been given prior to LP. Negative tests are generally not helpful, but positive tests are considered diagnostic for a particular organism.

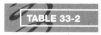 **TABLE 33-2** | **Initial Symptoms and Signs in Patients with Bacterial Meningitis**

Symptom/Sign	Relative frequency (%)
Headache	≥90
Fever	≥90
Meningismus	≥85
Altered sensorium	>80
Kernig's sign	≥50
Brudzinski's sign	≥50
Vomiting	35
Seizure	30
Focal findings	10–20
Papilledema	<1

(Adapted from Mandell G, Bennett J, Dolin R. *Mandell, Douglas, and Bennett's Principles and Practice of Infectious Diseases.* 5th ed. Philadelphia: Churchill Livingstone; 2000:973.)

Because penicillin-resistant *S. pneumoniae* has become more common, empiric treatment has changed. Current recommendations in immunocompetent hosts younger than age 50 includes ceftriaxone (2 g IV every 12 hours) or cefotaxime (2 g IV every 6 hours) plus vancomycin (1 g IV every 12 hours). This regimen covers sensitive and resistant *S. pneumoniae, N. meningitidis, H. influenzae,* group B streptococci, and many Enterobacteriaceae. Chloramphenicol (1 g IV every 6 hours) is an acceptable alternative to ceftriaxone for patients with *H. influenzae,* pneumococcal or meningococcal meningitis who cannot tolerate β-lactam antimicrobials. In the elderly or immunocompromised, ampicillin (2 g IV every 4 hours) is added for coverage of *L. monocytogenes.* In penicillin-allergic individuals, trimethoprim-sulfamethoxazole (10 mg/kg [trimethoprim component] IV every 12 hours) is recommended. If a specific organism is found, the regimen should be changed to a "best agent" based on sensitivities. Duration of therapy is generally 10 to 14 days for *S. pneumoniae,* and up to 21 days for *L. monocytogenes, S. agalactiae,* and Enterobacteriaceae. One week of antibiotics is sufficient for meningitis caused by *N. meningitidis;* most recent data suggest that 3 days is acceptable. Table 33-3 lists major pathogens that cause disease in various age groups and suggests appropriate empirical antimicrobial therapy. Table 33-4 presents a list of the antimicrobials mentioned in this chapter and appropriate dosing regimens for treating CNS infections.

Use of corticosteroids has historically been controversial. A meta-analysis of trials suggested that steroids were effective in reducing the incidence of severe hearing loss in children. In 2002 the largest study to date to test the use of steroids (dexamethasone) in patients with suspected acute bacterial meningitis was published. The use of dexamethasone (10 mg IV every 6 hours for 4 days) before or with the first dose of antibiotics was associated with a relative risk of death of 0.4, and a relative risk of neurologic sequelae of 0.6, when compared with patients who did not receive steroids. The effect was statistically significant only in the group with pneumococcal meningitis, but a favorable trend was noted for other pathogens. A subsequent meta-analysis confirmed this effect and suggested that there was no adverse effect of giving steroids in the manner studied. We recommend giving dexamethasone, before or concurrent with the first dose of antibiotics, to all patients in whom acute bacterial meningitis is suspected.

Tuberculous meningitis may have a CSF profile identical to that in "classic" acute septic meningitis in 25% of cases, particularly early in the course. Lymphocytic predominance is usual, however, and decreased CSF glucose (generally progressive on successive LPs) is often noted. Large volumes (10–20 mL) of CSF may need to be removed on up to four separate occasions to increase the sensitivity of staining and culture above 75%. PCR testing for *M. tuberculosis* DNA has become standard where available. Management is best left to an infectious disease specialist, but standard three- and four-drug regimens are usually used. In severely ill patients, problems may arise because few agents are available parenterally.

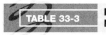 **TABLE 33-3**   **Recommended Empiric Antibiotic Therapy for Bacterial Meningitis Based on Age**

Age	Major pathogens	Antibiotic regimens	Alternatives
3 months–18 years	*N. meningitidis, S. pneumoniae, H. influenzae*	Ceftriaxone or cefotaxime plus vancomycin	Meropenem or chloramphenicol plus vancomycin
18–50 years	*S. pneumoniae, N. meningitidis, H. influenzae*	Same as above	Same as above
>50 years	*S. pneumoniae, L. monocytogenes,* enteric gram-negative bacilli	Ampicillin plus ceftriaxone or cefotaxime plus vancomycin	Ampicillin plus fluoroquinolones plus vancomycin

(Adapted from Spack D, Jackson L. Bacterial meningitis. *Neurol Clin* 1999;17:711–735.)

TABLE 33-4	Recommended Dosages of Antimicrobial Agents for Central Nervous System Infections in Adults*	

Agent	Daily dosage	Dosing interval (hours)
Ampicillin	12 g	4
Cefotaxime	8–12 g	4–6
Ceftazidime	6 g	8
Ceftriaxone	4 g	12
Chloramphenicol	4–6 g	6
Gentamicin	3–5 mg/kg	8
Imipenem	2 g	6
Metronidazole	30 mg/kg	6
Nafcillin	9–12 g	4
Penicillin	24 million units	4
Piperacillin/ Tazobactam	13.5 g	6
Pyrimethamine	50–75 mg (oral)	24
Sulfadiazine	4–6 g	6
Ticarcillin/clavulanate	12.4 g	6
Trimethoprim- sulfamethoxazole	10–20 mg/kg[†]	6–12
Vancomycin	2–3 g[‡]	8–12

*Patients with normal renal and hepatic function. All doses are intravenous.
[†] Dosage based on trimethoprim component.
[‡] Need to monitor trough serum concentrations.
(Adapted from Mandell G, Bennett J, Dolin R. *Mandell, Douglas, and Bennett's Principles and Practice of Infectious Diseases*. 5th ed. Philadelphia: Churchill Livingstone; 2000:973.)

Acute Aseptic Meningitis

Aseptic meningitis represents inflammation of the meninges with no bacterial cause identifiable on initial assessment. The annual number of cases is 8,300 to 12,700; most are caused by enteroviruses. Aseptic meningitis caused by such agents can present in a fashion identical to bacterial meningitis, causing great confusion when patients are first evaluated. Herpes simplex virus (HSV) accounts for 1 to 3% of all cases of aseptic meningitis, and HSV-2 is associated with meningitis in 11 to 33% of all primary genital infections. However most have a more protracted and subacute course than those with bacterial meningitis.

Regarding aseptic meningitis, one must consider etiologies other than viruses. Parameningeal foci (brain or epidural abscess) may need to be considered; consideration is given based on other findings. Partially treated bacterial meningitis may also present with a lymphocytic pleocytosis in the CSF, as may infection with HIV. In the proper setting, hematologic malignancies and metastatic solid cancers may be the cause. Treatable organisms that may present with an "aseptic" picture include *Mycobacterium tuberculosis, L. monocytogenes, M. pneumoniae, Rickettsia rickettsii, Ehrlichiae, Borrelia burgdorferi, Treponema pallidum, Leptospira* species, *Bartonella* species, *and Brucella* species. In the immunocompromised patient *M. tuberculosis*, fungal infections, *Toxoplasma gondii, T. pallidum*, Epstein-Barr virus (EBV), cytomegalovirus (CMV), varicella-zoster virus (VZV) or HSV should be considered. A variety of noninfectious diseases (e.g., collagen vascular and autoimmune diseases) and medications can also be implicated. Of medications, nonsteroidal anti-inflammatory drugs, antibiotics (particularly trimethoprim-sulfamethoxazole) and intravenous immunoglobulins are the most frequent offenders. Treatment is discontinuation of the agent. Table 33-5 lists infectious and noninfectious causes of meningitis that can present with CSF profiles that are consistent with "aseptic" meningitis. When cause of meningitis is uncertain, patients may

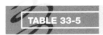

TABLE 33-5	Common Causes of Aseptic Meningitis

Infectious
Bacterial: M. tuberculosis, parameningeal infection, acute or subacute bacterial endocarditis,
   Brucella, Listeria
Fungal: C. albicans, C. immitis, C. neoformans, H. capsulatum
Mycoplasmal: M. pneumoniae, M. hominis (in neonates)
Protozoal: T. gondii, Plasmodium spp., amoebas, visceral larva migrans
Rickettsial: Rocky Mountain spotted fever, Q fever, typhus
Spirochetal: Syphilis, leptospirosis, Lyme disease
Viral: Enteroviruses, mumps virus, lymphocyte choriomeningitis agent,
   Epstein-Barr virus, arboviruses, cytomegalovirus, VZV, HSV, HIV
Malignant
Primary medulloblastoma, metastatic leukemia, lymphoma, Hodgkin's disease,
   metastatic carcinomatosis, craniopharyngioma
Noninfectious
Autoimmune disease: Guillain-Barré syndrome
Collagen-vascular disease: systemic lupus erythematosus, Sjögren's syndrome
Direct toxin exposure: Intrathecal injections of contrast media, spinal anesthesia
Granulomatous disease: Sarcoidosis
Poisoning: Lead, mercury
Trauma: Subarachnoid hemorrhage, traumatic lumbar puncture, neurosurgery
Medications
Sulfamethoxazole, trimethoprim, nonsteroidal anti-inflammatory agents,
   carbamazepine, isoniazid, penicillin
Vaccinations
Mumps, measles
Miscellaneous
Behçet's syndrome, Kawasaki's disease, Mollaret's meningitis, multiple sclerosis

(Adapted from Nelsen S, Sealy D, Schneider E. The aseptic meningitis syndrome. *Am Fam Phys* 1993; 48:809–815.)

be treated empirically initially. Alternatively, a second LP can be performed 12 to 24 hours later. Changes in CSF formula may help identify the likely cause.

Acute Encephalitis

Encephalitis implies brain inflammation and is virtually always associated with altered mental status. Two entities comprise acute encephalitis: acute viral encephalitis and acute postinfectious encephalomyelitis or acute disseminated encephalomyelitis (ADEM). The morbidity and mortality associated with acute viral encephalitis is the result of direct infection of neural cells, primarily in the gray matter, with subsequent cell edema, death, and brain necrosis. ADEM generally follows a nonspecific viral infection by 1 to 3 weeks, can mimic acute viral encephalitis in its presentation, and is characterized by the presence of multifocal gadolinium-enhancing white matter lesions on magnetic resonance imaging (MRI) that represent immune demyelination. ADEM probably accounts for 10 to 15% of cases of acute encephalitis in the United States. This section only addresses acute viral encephalitis.

Approximately 20,000 cases of acute viral encephalitis occur annually in the United States, mostly in children. The majority are caused by HSV-1 and arboviruses. Noninfectious causes that can mimic acute viral encephalitis include lupus cerebritis, vasculitis, carcinomatous meningitis, and paraneoplastic syndromes. Table 33-6 lists nonviral causes of encephalitis.

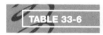

TABLE 33-6	Nonviral Causes of Encephalomyelitis

Rocky Mountain spotted fever	*Nocardia*
Typhus	Actinomycosis
Ehrlichia	Tuberculosis
Q fever	*Cryptococcus*
Chlamydia	*Histoplasma*
Mycoplasma	*Naegleria*
Legionella	*Acanthamoeba*
Brucellosis	*Balamuthia mandrillaris*
Subacute bacterial endocarditis	*Toxoplasma*
Listeria	*Plasmodium falciparum*
Whipple's disease	Trypanosomiasis
Cat-scratch disease	Behçet's disease
Syphilis (meningovascular)	Vasculitis
Relapsing fever	Carcinoma
Lyme disease	Drug reactions
Leptospirosis	

(Adapted from Mandell G, Bennett J, Dolin R. *Mandell, Douglas, and Bennett's Principles and Practice of Infectious Diseases.* 5th ed. Philadelphia: Churchill Livingstone; 2000:973.)

Encephalitis commonly presents with fever, headache, and meningismus. Neurologic signs are varied. Patients have altered mental status ranging from mild lethargy to coma. Focal neurologic signs and seizures are common. A plethora of other neurologic findings may occur, depending on the anatomic location affected.

HSV is the most common cause of sporadic encephalitis, representing approximately 20% of cases. It is caused by reactivation of latent virus in the trigeminal ganglion and is generally not associated with evidence of active herpetic infection elsewhere. Age distribution is biphasic, with most cases occurring between ages 5 and 30, or in those older than age 50, and presentation is generally acute. Localized temporal lobe symptoms and signs suggest HSV and include personality changes, episodes of terror, hallucinations, and bizarre behavior. Focal neurologic signs may include hemiparesis (30%), arm and facial weakness, and superior quadrant visual field defects. Up to half will present with seizures early in the course.

Early diagnosis of HSV encephalitis is important, as more than 70% of untreated patients die, and morbidity is related primarily to mental status at the time that antivirals are initiated and patient age. CSF analysis, MRI, and electroencephalogram (EEG) may assist in the diagnosis. The CSF profile is consistent with an "aseptic" picture. The presence of red blood cells and xanthochromia are useful clues, but are nonspecific. MRI is the imaging modality of choice when evaluating encephalitis, and in HSV disease characteristically shows high signal intensity on T_2-weighted imaging in the medial and inferior temporal lobe or lobes. The EEG may show the classic finding of periodic, stereotyped, sharp-and-slow wave complexes that occur every 2 to 3 seconds. Findings may be unilateral or bilateral and occur in two-thirds of biopsy-proven cases. PCR has replaced brain biopsy as the procedure of choice, with sensitivity and specificity of 97% and 100%, respectively, when samples are collected within 10 days of symptom onset. Sensitivity of PCR decreases to 30% when testing occurs between days 11 and 21, and to 19% when testing occurs between days 21 and 40. Intravenous acyclovir, 10 to 12 mg/kg every 8 hours for up to 3 weeks, should be begun empirically immediately while awaiting further results. It is reasonable to treat selected patients with fever, meningismus, and confusion with both empiric antibiotics and acyclovir while awaiting formal diagnosis.

Arboviral Encephalitis

Worldwide, the most common cause of arboviral encephalitis is Japanese encephalitis virus. This agent, transmitted by the culicine mosquito, causes epidemic disease in China, northern Southeast Asia, and parts of India and Sri Lanka. In the United States, the most important pathogens are West Nile, California encephalitis (LaCrosse strain), St. Louis encephalitis, western equine, and eastern equine encephalitis viruses, depending on location. Symptoms are generally those of an influenza-like syndrome with fever, malaise, headache and fatigue, with or without meningismus. With a sufficiently high viral load, invasion of the CNS ensues. The specific viruses differ with respect to vector, average age of the host, clinical severity, and geographic distribution among other factors. The peak incidence is in late summer and fall.

West Nile virus (WNV) encephalitis was little known in the United States until 1999, when it was associated with seven deaths in the New York City area. By 2002 it had spread to the West Coast, and in the same year caused the largest arboviral meningoencephalitis outbreak ever recorded in North America—4000 cases. Principle hosts are birds, such as American crows and house sparrows, which can suffer mass deaths. The primary vector is the Culex mosquito, but others may serve as vectors as well. In 2003 four patients were infected with WNV when they received organs from a single donor, who had contracted the virus during transfusion of blood, 1 day prior to organ recovery.

Most infected individuals are asymptomatic. Up to 20% of infected people develop West Nile fever, a flulike syndrome that may be accompanied by an erythematous maculopapular rash. However, only 1% of infected people develop encephalitis, meningitis, or acute flaccid paralysis (AFP); the latter is a poliomyelitis-like destruction of anterior horn cells that produces an asymmetric quadriparesis. Mortality from WNV encephalitis is up to 18%, and many patients do not return to their premorbid state. Diagnosis is made by finding anti-WNV IgM antibody in the CSF or serum or PCR. Convalescent serum may need to be collected and assayed for the presence of the antibody when the diagnosis is suspected but initial testing was negative. Treatment is supportive.

The diagnostic criteria for arboviral encephalitis in the United States have been defined by the Centers for Disease Control and Prevention. A confirmed case is defined as a febrile illness with signs suggestive of encephalitis that occurs during the summer or fall and is supported by one of the following criteria: (1) at least a fourfold rise in serum viral antibody titers, between the acute and convalescent (4–6 weeks) phases of the illness; (2) viral isolation from tissue, blood, or CSF; or (3) specific IgM antibody in the CSF during the acute presentation. Imaging is not likely to be helpful. Treatment is supportive.

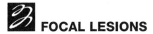 **FOCAL LESIONS**

Brain Abscess

Brain abscess is a focal intracerebral collection of pus that often presents as a mass lesion with localized neurologic defects related to the area involved. Up to 2,500 cases are treated in the United States annually. It affects males more often than females and occurs most commonly in those who are ages 30 to 40. Prior to antibiotics and refinement of surgical techniques, mortality approached 100%. The advent of antibiotics, enhanced brain imaging, and stereotactic drainage techniques has decreased the mortality to near zero when cases are optimally managed.

Although the primary source of abscess is often cryptogenic, 50% are caused by contiguous spread from the middle ear, paranasal sinuses, or dentition, and 25% of cases are thought to occur after hematogenous spread from heart or lung. Penetrating head trauma and immunosuppression are other predisposing conditions. The clinical presentation of brain abscess is variable. With virulent organisms such as *S. aureus*, initial headache or fever may be followed rapidly by deteriorating mental status and focal neurologic signs. Alternatively, patients may have an indolent course spanning more than 1 month, with only a headache as a complaint. Headache is the most common presenting complaint, occurring in approximately 70% of cases. Fever is noted in about 50% of patients. Other signs or symptoms include mental status changes, focal neurologic deficits, seizures, nausea, vomiting, and nuchal rigidity. Evaluating patients carefully for these signs and symptoms is important; mortality is highest in patients who report having more than 4 days of these signs and symptoms. Table 33-7 lists the most common signs and symptoms and their frequencies.

The diagnosis of brain abscess is based on a high index of suspicion plus brain imaging. Leukocytosis is frequently absent, so that absence of fever, leukocytosis, or other signs of inflammation should not deter evaluation when suspicion exists. Blood cultures are positive in only 10% of cases. Because intracranial pressure is elevated in many patients, LP is generally contraindicated when brain abscess is suspected. Results are nonspecific and up to 20% die of complications. The imaging modality of choice is gadolinium-enhanced MRI. Characteristic changes over time are often noted. During the first week (acute cerebritis stage), only mild edema or microhemorrhages may be seen. After 7 days, the late cerebritis stage begins, characterized by a focus or foci of necrotic tissue, separated from normal brain by a thin rim of vascular granulation tissue. Local mass effect is usually present. After approximately 2 weeks, a capsular stage characterized by a maturing collagenous capsule filled with liquefied debris occurs. It is here that drainage should be considered. Earlier drainage is unlikely to yield pus but more likely to result in bleeding. If allowed to become chronic and untreated, brain abscesses continue to enlarge, causing death from brainstem herniation or from rupture into the subarachnoid space or ventricular system.

Abscess location helps to indicate the primary infection. Temporal lobe and cerebellar lesions suggest chronic otitis media or mastoiditis, frontal lobe lesions suggest complications of paranasal sinusitis, and multiple lesions at the gray–white matter interface suggest hematogenous spread.

Once diagnosed, aspiration of one or more of the lesions is indicated, to both determine microbiology and to rule out alternative diagnoses, such as glioblastoma, metastasis, infarct, or demyelination. Generally, lesions larger than 2.5 cm in diameter should be aspirated. The microbiology of a brain abscess is dictated by the location of the primary source. The majority are bacterial and 60% of cases are polymicrobial. Streptococcal species are found in 70% of cases, most commonly *Streptococcus milleri* group. *S. aureus* is noted in up to 20% of cases, most commonly associated with hematogenous spread or penetrating or neurosurgical trauma. Enteric gram-negative bacilli and anaerobic bacteria are found in up to 20% and 50% of cases, respectively, with *Bacteroides* and *Fusobacterium* spp. the most common anaerobes.

After initial evaluation, antibiotics may be indicated. In nonemergent situations, aspiration of the abscess should occur before empiric antimicrobial therapy, and Gram's stain results may aid with an initial regimen. This should be based in part on the suspected primary source of infection. When thought a complication of otitis, metronidazole and an

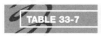 **TABLE 33-7**   **Common Signs and Symptoms of Brain Abscess**

Symptom or Sign	Frequency (%)
Headache	70
Altered mental status	70
Focal neurologic defect	>60
Fever	45–50
Seizures	25–35
Nausea, vomiting	25–50
Nuchal rigidity	25
Papilledema	25

(Adapted from Mandell G, Bennett J, Dolin R. *Mandell, Douglas, and Bennett's Principles and Practice of Infectious Diseases*. 5th ed. Philadelphia: Churchill Livingstone; 2000:973.)

antipseudomonal penicillin or advanced generation cephalosporin can be used. Metronidazole plus a third-generation cephalosporin is effective for a suspected source in the paranasal sinuses. Suspected dental sources can be covered with penicillin or a third-generation cephalosporin plus metronidazole; for patients who have undergone neurosurgical procedures or have sustained penetrating skull trauma, vancomycin can be added to an extended-spectrum penicillin or cephalosporin with antipseudomonal activity. When there is no history to guide therapy, vancomycin with metronidazole and a third-generation cephalosporin, or vancomycin with an extended-spectrum penicillin/β-lactamase inhibitor combination can generally be used. The duration of therapy is dictated by clinical and radiographic response but generally continues for 4 to 8 weeks, depending on the adequacy of initial drainage. Brain imaging should be repeated within several weeks after antibiotics have been initiated—and periodically thereafter—to gauge response.

A feared complication of brain abscess is rupture into the ventricular system with resultant bacterial meningitis. Focal neurologic findings are common and patients appear toxic. Because focal neurologic findings in acute meningitis are uncommon, their presence should cause the clinician to suspect a ruptured brain abscess or subdural empyema. Mortality approaches 100%. LP is frequently performed in these cases, especially when an antecedent brain abscess is not known to exist. Therapy consists of high-dose parenteral antimicrobials (based on Gram's stain results), intensive support, and, occasionally, neurosurgical intervention.

Subdural Empyema

Infection in this space is uncommon but associated with up to 20% mortality, even with prompt neurosurgical and antibiotic therapy. This infection is most common in young males and complicates paranasal sinus infections (60–70%) and middle ear infections (20%) most commonly. In 80% of cases, both hemispheres become involved. Most patients are toxic and febrile; 75% demonstrate focal neurologic signs and often have meningismus. Focal seizures occur in up 50% of cases. Presence of focal neurologic disturbances should prompt rapid imaging, as these are unusual in uncomplicated meningitis. Mortality is closely associated with mental status level at initiation of treatment. Contrast-enhanced MRI represents the best imaging modality. Osteomyelitis or epidural abscess is present in up to 50% of cases. LP should not be performed because intracranial pressure is frequently significantly elevated, and because CSF findings are generally not helpful. The bacteriology of subdural empyema is similar to that of brain abscess, and empiric antimicrobial therapy should follow the same guidelines. Urgent surgical drainage is mandatory. Most patients are treated with intravenous therapy for at least 4 weeks after drainage. (RBB)

Bibliography
Attia J, et al. Does this adult patient have acute meningitis? *JAMA* 1999;282:175–181.
   The authors explain the results of their evidence-based review of the clinical examination for identifying adults with meningitis. Ninety-nine percent of patients with meningitis will present with at least one of three findings: fever, nuchal rigidity, or altered mental status. Their absence excludes the diagnosis. Less than half of patients with meningitis presented with all three signs.
Choi CK. Bacterial meningitis in aging adults. *Clin Infect Dis* 2001;33:1380–1385.
Chowdhury MH, Tunkel AR. Antibacterial agents in infections of the central nervous system. *Infect Dis Clin North Am* 2000;14:391–408.
   The authors explain the principles that determine whether an antibacterial agent will penetrate the CNS and cause bacterial cell death. Individual antibiotics are reviewed with regard to these principles. Empiric and species-specific antimicrobial therapy is discussed.
Dill SR, et al. Subdural empyema: analysis of 32 cases and review. *Clin Infect Dis* 1995;20:372–386.
   The authors divide patients with subdural empyema into those resulting from sinusitis, trauma, or miscellaneous. Sinusitis was the most common cause and was generally associated with streptococci and anaerobes. Cases resulting from trauma (including neurosurgery) were more likely to harbor gram-negative bacilli or S. aureus. Surgical drainage plus at least 1 month of antibiotics is considered appropriate therapy.

Dominques RB, et al. Evaluation of the range of clinical presentations of herpes simplex encephalitis by using polymerase chain reaction assay of cerebrospinal fluid samples. *Clin Infect Dis* 1997:25:86–91.

Forty-nine patients with various neurologic presentations were studied with PCR for herpes simplex DNA. This study demonstrates that patients with more subtle forms of encephalitis may still have herpes simplex as the causative organism.

Ellis-Pegler R, et al. Three days of intravenous benzyl penicillin treatment of meningococcal disease in adults. *Clin Infect Dis* 2003;37:658–662.

The authors conducted a prospective observational study of 61 adults with meningococcal disease, most of which included meningitis and demonstrated that 3 days of treatment resulted in cures without relapse (five persons died). It has been long known that meningococcal disease can be treated for shorter durations than other organisms. This investigation "lowers" the bar still further.

Hasbun R, et al. Computed tomography of the head before lumbar puncture in adults with suspected meningitis. *N Engl J Med* 2001;345:1727–1733.

The authors prospectively studied 301 adults with suspected meningitis to determine the clinical characteristics that would predict abnormalities on head CT prior to lumbar puncture. The absence of all the following characteristics yielded a negative predictive value of 97%: age older than 60 years, immunocompromise, a history of CNS disease, a history of seizure less than 1 week, an abnormal level of consciousness, an alteration in cognition, and a focal neurologic exam. Even patients with mass effect on CT, but without any of these characteristics, could safely undergo lumbar puncture.

Heilpern KL, Lorber B. Focal intracranial infections. *Infect Dis Clin North Am* 1996; 10:879–898.

An excellent review of the clinical presentation, demographics, diagnosis, complications, and treatment of brain abscess, subdural empyema, cranial epidural abscess, and septic thrombosis of the dural venous sinuses.

Lindvall P, et al. Reducing intracranial pressure may increase survival among patients with bacterial meningitis. *Clin Infect Dis* 2004;38:384–390.

The authors identified 18 patients with bacterial meningitis and initially assessed and followed intracranial pressures (ICP). Identification of elevated ICP and its successful management was associated with decreased mortality. The authors feel that management of ICP is important and should be part of the strategy for all patients with bacterial meningitis. We feel that all patients undergoing LP for meningitis should have the initial ICP recorded, and managed if elevated.

Mandell G, Bennett J, Dolin R. *Mandell, Douglas, and Bennett's Principles and Practice of Infectious Diseases.* 5th ed. Philadelphia: Churchill Livingstone; 2000:973.

Motis G, Garcia-Monaco JC. The challenge of drug-induced aseptic meningitis. *Arch Intern Med* 1999;159:1185–1194.

An excellent systematic review, with160 references, that highlights the clinical characteristics, CSF profiles, related underlying conditions, differential diagnoses, and most common offending drugs. The authors note that the clinical presentation, CSF profile, and even the findings on contrast-enhanced MRI can be indistinguishable from those in acute bacterial meningitis. Outcome was always excellent with discontinuation of the offending agent.

Nelsen S, Sealy D, Schneider E. The aseptic meningitis syndrome. *Am Fam Phys* 1993; 48:809–815.

Petersen L, Marfin A, Gubler D. West Nile Virus. *JAMA* 2003;290:524–528.

The authors present an up-to-date, concise, yet complete review of West Nile virus and its manifestations in humans. West Nile fever, a mild viral syndrome, is the most common clinical manifestation of the disease. The overwhelming majority of infected patients, however, are asymptomatic. Less than 1% of infected patients present with meningitis, encephalitis, or acute flaccid paralysis.

Roos K. Encephalitis. *Neurol Clin* 1999;17:813–833.

Johnson R. Acute encephalitis. *Clin Infect Dis* 1996;23:219–226.

Two excellent reviews of encephalitis are noted that detail the demographics, presentations, diagnosis, complications, and treatments of the most common microbial causes of this disease. Both papers review HSV encephalitis in detail. The paper by Roos includes a nice section on encephalitis in the immunosuppressed patient.

Schuchat A, et al. Bacterial meningitis in the United States in 1995. *N Engl J Med* 1997;337:970.

The authors review the epidemiology of bacterial meningitis in the United States before and after the introduction of the H. influenzae *vaccine. They estimate that the total number of cases of bacterial meningitis have been halved, and the median age at diagnosis nearly doubled since the vaccine's introduction. This demographic shift was caused by a 94% decrease in* H. influenzae *meningitis.*

Spack D, Jackson L. Bacterial meningitis. *Neurol Clin* 1999;17:711–735.

Thomson RB Jr, Bertram H. Laboratory diagnosis of central nervous system infections. *Infect Dis Clin North Am* 2001;15:1047–1071.

A complete review of the various tests used to diagnose bacterial, viral, fungal, protozoal, and parasitic infections of the CNS. Information is included on the volume of CSF required for each test. The optimal methods of transport and assay are detailed.

Van de Beek D, et al. Steroids in adults with acute bacterial meningitis: a systematic review. *Lancet Infect Dis* 2004;4:139–143.

Relying heavily on their own study of dexamethasone in the treatment of suspected acute bacterial meningitis (N Engl J Med 2002;347:1549), the authors perform a systematic review of the benefits and risks of using dexamethasone for this disease. Compared with placebo, the relative risk (RR) for both death and neurologic sequelae was 0.6, (both statistically significant). When stratified by causative organism, a significant mortality benefit was found only for pneumococcal meningitis (RR 0.5). A reduction in neurologic sequelae was not significant for any specific organism. Dexamethasone was not associated with excessive adverse events. The authors recommend initiating dexamethasone (10 mg IV every 6 hours) before or concurrent with the first dose of parenteral antibiotics in all patients with suspected bacterial meningitis.

Wong J, Quint D. Imaging of central nervous system infections. *Semin Roentgenol* 1999;34:123–143.

The authors review this large topic and include multiple computed tomographic (CT) and MRI images, that display the "classic" cranial radiographic findings in meningitis, encephalitis, brain abscess, HIV-related CNS infections, and tuberculosis. Additional images of fungal, Actinomycetes, and parasitic CNS infections are included. MRI is more sensitive than CT for imaging all CNS inflammatory processes.

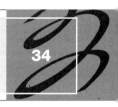

CHRONIC MENINGITIS 34

*C*hronic meningitis is defined as a symptom complex of insidious onset, usually lasting 4 weeks or more, that is characterized by headache, fever, and mental status changes in association with cerebrospinal fluid (CSF) pleocytosis. The CSF protein is usually elevated, and the CSF glucose is often low. This syndrome may be caused by viral, bacterial, fungal, or parasitic agents. Noninfectious causes include malignancy, sarcoidosis, Behçet's syndrome, and vasculitis. Diagnosis may be difficult, but extremely important, as therapy is often prolonged, relatively toxic, and specific.

APPROACH TO THE PATIENT WITH CHRONIC MENINGITIS

A history of exposure to infectious agents will be particularly important. Inquiry into exposure to tuberculosis should include symptoms of fever, cough, chills, night sweats, and weight loss. Occupations and family history may also suggest clues to tuberculosis.

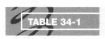

TABLE 34-1 **History in Evaluation of Chronic Meningitis**

1. Travel
2. Animal exposure
3. Family member with tuberculosis
4. High risk sexual activity
5. Symptoms outside CNS (rash, lymphadenopathy, vision, cough, etc.)

Travel history will define the likelihood of fungal and parasitic disease. Fungal infections, such as coccidioidomycoses (arid Southwest), blastomycoses (Mississippi valley and Southeast), and histoplasmosis (Ohio River Valley), will be suspected based on area of residence and travel history. Exposure to animals may also provide clues to the etiologic agent in chronic meningitis. For example, brucellosis may be acquired from exposure to farm animals; leptospirosis from rats or mice; tularemia, from rabbits.

Symptoms outside the central nervous system (CNS) might suggest a systemic disease as a cause of chronic meningitis. For example, the complaint of recurrent oral or genital ulcers will suggest Behçet's syndrome. The history should explore risk factors for underlying disease that would predispose to chronic meningitis, particularly HIV disease. Table 34-1 summarizes the important elements of the history in the diagnosis of chronic meningitis.

The physical exam may also provide clues to the specific cause of chronic meningitis. Skin lesions occur in such diseases as sarcoidosis, blastomycoses, and cryptococcosis. Skin biopsy will have a high diagnostic yield when skin lesions are present concomitantly with chronic meningitis. Eye examination also is extremely valuable as specific abnormalities may suggest tuberculosis (choroidal tubercles), sarcoidosis (granulomas), or Behçet's syndrome (uveitis). Neurologic exam should uncover cranial nerve palsies, peripheral neuropathy, and spinal cord processes that might narrow the spectrum of processes.

Although laboratory evaluation must be based on clinical clues, the laboratory tests shown in Table 34-2 are generally part of initial evaluation.

TUBERCULOSIS MENINGITIS

Tuberculosis remains the most common cause of the chronic meningitis syndrome; it is a treatable disease even in the immunosuppressed patient. Hence, the diagnosis must be made and, at times, empiric therapy may be initiated. The diagnosis of tuberculous meningitis continues to be a difficult one. The disease is usually the result of the breakdown of a long-standing granuloma. In about half of all patients, this breakdown is associated with some underlying condition, such as sarcoidosis, AIDS, malnutrition, or steroid therapy.

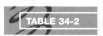

TABLE 34-2 **Initial Laboratory Evaluation of Chronic Meningitis**

1. Lumbar puncture with opening pressure, CSF WBCs, protein, glucose (with serum glucose). Cerebrospinal fluid cytology, VDRL, cryptococcal antigen, India ink, acid-fast stain and *Mycobacterium* TB PCR, large volume culture for TB and fungi. Prolonged incubation in 5% CO_2 for *Nocardia, Brucella, Actinomyces*
2. CBC, ESR, liver, and renal function tests
3. Blood and urine cultures including TB and fungi
4. Serology for syphilis, HIV, cryptococcal antigen, antinuclear antibody, rheumatoid factor
5. CT scan or MRI
6. PPD

TB, Tuberculosis; CBC, Complete blood count; ESR, Erythrocyte sedimentation rate; CT, Computed tomogram, MRI, Magnetic resonance imaging; PPD, Purified protein derivative

Clinical manifestations of tuberculous meningitis generally are similar to those of other chronic meningitides. A miliary picture on chest radiographs and inappropriate antidiuretic hormone secretion are the only features useful to distinguish between tuberculous and cryptococcal meningitis. In one study, symptoms of tuberculous meningitis included fever (99°F–103°F), lethargy, and headache. Duration of symptoms on presentation ranges from 2 days to 6 months. Hospitalization is often precipitated by complaints of headache. Meningeal signs are present in more than half of all cases. Peripheral white blood cell (WBC) counts range from low normal to very elevated (>20,000/mm^3).

Tuberculous meningitis is often a disease of the inner-city population in the United States. Mortality and morbidity in this group are high. The disease was similar in HIV-positive and HIV-negative patients in two different studies.

A variety of antigen and antibody tests have been developed for CSF studies. The amount of tubercular DNA in the CSF is relatively low; however, sensitivity of these tests is superior to culture. Rapid diagnosis has been successful with use of ligase chain reaction amplification. Adenosine deaminase levels in CSF are usually elevated.

 # CRYPTOCOCCAL MENINGITIS

The presentation of cryptococcal meningitis is very similar to that of tuberculosis. The disease has become much more common in the AIDS era and may be the first manifestation of AIDS. In addition, lymphoma, systemic lupus erythematosus, sarcoidosis, and renal transplantation are important predisposing conditions. From 20 to 50% of patients with cryptococcal meningitis have no underlying illness. Cultures of specimens from sputum, bone marrow, or skin lesions may be useful in some patients. Spinal fluid findings, as in tuberculous meningitis, usually show a CSF pleocytosis. An India ink preparation yields positive results in 50% of cases; cryptococcal antigen can be detected in 80 to 90% of cases by a rapid, simple latex fixation test. Computed tomography may be necessary to identify cryptococcomas or to rule out hydrocephalus. The poor prognostic signs in cryptococcal meningitis have been well defined: (1) high opening CSF pressure, (2) low CSF glucose, (3) fewer than 20 WBCs in CSF, (4) high titers of cryptococcal antigen and positive India ink stain, and (5) concomitant disease, such as lymphoma.

 # OTHER FUNGAL MENINGITIDES

Coccidioidomycosis is another common cause of chronic meningitis syndrome. A careful travel history may be an important clue to the disease. Residents of southern California, Nevada, Utah, Arizona, New Mexico, Texas, Mexico, and Central America are at risk for the disease by inhaling arthrospores of *Coccidioides immitis*. Visitors to these areas may also contract the disease. Two-thirds of patients who contract the disease have no risk factors. However, disseminated disease and meningitis are more likely to develop in blacks, Filipinos, and pregnant women after pulmonary infection. The symptoms of coccidioidomycosis meningitis cannot be distinguished from those of chronic meningitis due to other causes, but evaluation for lesions of skin, bone, and lung may provide critical information. CSF parameters are nonspecific. In some patients, a polymorphonuclear leukocyte predominance in CSF may be noted. Eosinophils are commonly seen in the CSF. CSF cultures are often negative.

Culture plates must be handled with care because they are infectious to laboratory personnel. Detection of complement-fixing antibody in the CSF is specific and 75 to 90% sensitive for diagnosis.

Blastomyces dermatitidis can also cause chronic meningitis. Meningitis occurs in about one-third of patients with disseminated disease. Diagnosis is usually made by concomitant culture of sputum, skin lesions, bone or joint fluid, and prostatic secretions. The organism is rarely cultured from CSF, and serologic tests are not reliable for extrapulmonary infection.

The presentation of histoplasmosis meningitis is similar to that of *B. dermatitidis* meningitis, and culture of other sites is often required for diagnosis. Half the patients have positive CSF cultures; 90% have CSF antibody.

BACTERIAL AGENTS SOMETIMES CAUSING CHRONIC MENINGITIS

Actinomycosis can be associated with many CNS lesions, including brain abscess, meningitis, subdural empyema, and epidural abscess. Brain abscesses appear with focal neurologic findings, and many patients have evidence of dental infection, mastoiditis, sinusitis, or skin infection. Actinomycosis may involve the meninges alone, producing a basilar meningitis that is indolent and manifested solely by a lymphocytic pleocytosis. In such cases, the disease is frequently misdiagnosed as tuberculous meningitis. *Actinomyces* organisms are fastidious, gram-positive, filamentous bacteria. They often grow slowly and have anaerobic or microaerophilic growth requirements. High-dose penicillin remains the drug of choice.

Nocardia asteroides infection may also appear as chronic meningitis without brain abscess, but this is unusual. Sulfonamides are the antimicrobials of choice.

 SPIROCHETAL MENINGITIS

Several spirochetes are neurotrophic and can cause a chronic meningitis syndrome. Syphilitic meningitis usually occurs within 2 years of acute infection. Fever is often absent, and headache may be the sole complaint. A CSF pleocytosis with high protein and low sugar may mimic the findings of other chronic meningitides. The diagnosis is suggested by a positive result on treponemal tests and CSF VDRL tests. Many investigators have reported a change in the clinical spectrum of neurosyphilis recently. Patients may complain of vague chronic symptoms, including headache. They tend not to have classic tertiary signs, such as tabes dorsalis or pupillary changes.

The CNS effects of Lyme disease have received increasing attention. *Borrelia burgdorferi* can cause chronic meningitis as a second stage of Lyme disease, months after tick exposure and initial infection. Bell's palsy and radiculopathic syndromes are most common. Meningitis patients often are seen without fever but with headache, photophobia, and stiff neck, and they may report long-standing symptoms. A CSF pleocytosis is found. Protein is elevated, and about 15% of patients have low CSF sugar. Results of a CSF VDRL test may be false-positive, but treponemal tests will be negative. Local CSF antibody production occurs, but serologic tests appear to lack sensitivity and specificity. Polymerase chain reaction (PCR) to detect *B. burgdorferi* in CSF is still not sensitive enough for routine use.

Other spirochetal diseases, including leptospirosis and relapsing fever, may present with meningitis in addition to other systemic symptoms. These meningitides are usually self-limited.

Other bacteria can cause a chronic meningitis syndrome. Brucellosis usually presents with night sweats, lymphadenopathy, and hepatosplenomegaly. CNS involvement is rare, but when it does occur, a chronic meningitis syndrome is common. Culture from blood or CSF requires special media and longer incubation (2–4 weeks). Blood or CSF agglutination titers may be needed for diagnosis. *Listeria monocytogenes* and *Neisseria meningitidis* infections, which are more likely to produce an acute meningitis, can also present as a more protracted, insidious disease. An underlying immunodeficiency state may be present in these cases.

Viral infections usually cause meningoencephalitis or aseptic meningitis, with CSF pleocytosis and normal CSF sugar in most cases. Chronic meningitis caused by echovirus or coxsackievirus occurs in patients with agammaglobulinemia or multiple myeloma. HIV infection itself or with concomitant progressive multifocal leukoencephalopathy may cause mental status abnormalities and a chronic CSF pleocytosis.

Noninfectious disease processes may mimic a chronic infectious meningitis syndrome. Metastatic carcinoma from an unsuspected primary carcinoma in the breast or lung can cause a chronic meningitis syndrome, as can lymphoma and melanoma. In many cases, back pain, radicular pain, and cranial nerve abnormalities also will be present. Most patients have a CSF pleocytosis. Cytology is positive for malignant cells in 50 to 80% of patients. CSF lactate dehydrogenase has recently been shown to be a useful test. Findings on computed tomography and magnetic resonance imaging usually will be positive.

Sarcoidosis presents with neurologic findings in 48% of patients. Cranial nerve abnormalities, peripheral neuropathy, and focal cerebral and intraspinal lesions are most common. Aseptic meningitis rarely occurs without other manifestations of sarcoidosis. In one study, CSF pleocytosis was noted in 43% of patients, and hypoglycorrhachia in only 10%. CSF angiotensin-converting enzyme levels are probably too nonspecific to be of value. When this disease is suspected, careful examination of optic and other cranial nerves, as well as evaluation of other systems, is crucial. Diagnosis is usually made outside the CNS, such as by biopsy of lymph node, liver, or parotid or other salivary gland. Specific CNS markers for sarcoid have not yet been developed.

Behçet's disease usually is recognized by the triad of oral or genital ulcers, skin lesions, and uveitis. Meningoencephalitis develops in 25% of patients, often in association with flare-up of other symptoms. CSF pleocytosis is present, with elevated protein and normal sugar. (SLB)

Bibliography

Anderson NE, Willoughby EW. Chronic meningitis without predisposing illness: a review of 83 cases. *Q J Med* 1987;63:283.
Tuberculosis was the most common cause of chronic meningitis.

Bouza E, et al. Coccidioidal meningitis. An analysis of 31 cases and review of the literature. *Medicine (Baltimore)* 1981;3:139.
Complement-fixing antibody is an important test in coccidioidal meningitis. Intrathecal administration of amphotericin is more effective than IV administration.

Bouza E, et al. Brucellar meningitis. *Rev Infect Dis* 1987;9:810.
Review of the neurologic manifestations of systemic brucellosis.

Buggy BP. *Nocardia asteroides* meningitis without brain abscess. *Rev Infect Dis* 1987;9:228.
Case reports of N. asteroides *meningitis without brain abscess or focal findings.*

Butler WT, et al. Diagnostic and prognostic value of clinical and laboratory findings in cryptococcal meningitis. A follow-up study of 40 patients. *N Engl J Med* 1964;270:59.
Variability in both clinical symptoms and CSF parameters in patients with cryptococcal meningitis.

Coyle PK. Central nervous system infection. *Neurol Clin* 1999;17:691.
Detailed overview of both acute and chronic meningitis.

Dube MP, Holton PD, Larsen RA. Tuberculous meningitis in patients with and without human immunodeficiency virus infection. *Am J Med* 1992;93:520.
HIV infection had little impact on the findings and on hospital mortality of patients with tuberculous meningitis. Intracerebral mass lesions were more common in AIDS patients.

Finkel MF. Lyme disease and its neurologic complications. *Arch Neurol* 1988;45:99.
Patients with CNS Lyme disease may present with long-standing headache and CSF pleocytosis. CSF IgG and IgM levels should be obtained when CNS Lyme disease is suspected.

Haas EJ, et al. Tuberculous meningitis in an urban general hospital. *Arch Intern Med* 1977;137:1518.
Acid-fast smears of CSF were positive in only 6 of 19 cases.

Harvey RI, Chandrasekar PH. Chronic meningitis caused by *Listeria* in a patient infected with human immunodeficiency virus. *J Infect Dis* 1988;157:1091.
L. monocytogenes *may cause a picture of chronic meningitis in the immunosuppressed patient.*

Hildebrand J, Aoun M. Chronic meningitis: still a diagnostic challenge. *J Neurol* 2003; 250:653.
An algorithm for differential diagnosis for both normal and immunocompromised patients will be very useful to clinicians.

Kadival GV, et al. Radioimmunoassay for detecting *Mycobacterium tuberculosis* antigen in cerebrospinal fluid of patients with tuberculous meningitis. *J Infect Dis* 1987; 155:608.
M. tuberculosis antigen can be detected in CSF by radioimmunoassay early in the course of disease.

Klein NC, Damsker B, Hirschman SZ. Mycobacterial meningitis. Retrospective analysis from 1970 to 1983. *Am J Med* 1985;79:29.

Reviews CNS presentation in 21 patients with mycobacterial meningitis. CSF findings are variable and may include predominance of polymorphonuclear leukocytes, normal protein, and normal sugar.

Kovacs JA, et al. Cryptococcosis in the acquired immunodeficiency syndrome. *Ann Intern Med* 1985;103:533.

In AIDS patients with cryptococcal meningitis, CSF WBC count, sugar, and protein were frequently normal. Relapse was very common.

Kravitz GR, et al. Chronic blastomycetic meningitis. *Am J Med* 1981;71:501.

CSF cultures are rarely positive in blastomycosis meningitis, and serologic tests are not specific.

Lecour H, Miranda M. Human leptospirosis. A review of 50 cases. *Infection* 1989;17:8.

Meningitis usually occurs concurrently with other symptoms in leptospirosis.

Lukehart SA, et al. Invasion of the central nervous system by *Treponema pallidum*: implications for diagnosis and treatment. *Ann Intern Med* 1988;109:855.

Discusses implications of CNS syphilis in patients with AIDS.

McKinney RE, Katz SL, Wilfert CM. Chronic enteroviral meningoencephalitis in agammaglobulinemic patients. *Rev Infect Dis* 1987;9:334.

Echovirus causes a culture-proven chronic meningitis in patients with agammaglobulinemia.

Meyers BR, Hirschman SZ. Unusual presentations of tuberculous meningitis. *Mt Sinai J Med* 1974;41:407.

Describes presentation of tuberculous meningitis. Fifty percent of patients have predisposing underlying disease.

Moosa MY, Coovadia YM. Cryptococcal meningitis in Durban, South Africa: a comparison of clinical features, laboratory findings, and outcome for human immunodeficiency virus-positive and -negative patients. *Clin Infect Dis* 1997;24:131.

Headache, fever, stiff neck, and neurologic findings were more common in HIV-infected patients.

Ogawa SK, et al. Tuberculous meningitis in an urban medical center. *Medicine (Baltimore)* 1987;66:371.

Detailed discussion of symptomatology. Fever is almost invariably present in tuberculous meningitis.

Porkert MT, et al. Tuberculous meningitis at a large inner-city medical center. *Am J Med Sci* 1997;13:325.

Thirty-four patients with tuberculous meningitis were studied at a public hospital in Atlanta. Tuberculous meningitis is a devastating disease in inner-city residents with a delay in diagnosis and has a high mortality rate. Whether a patient was HIV-positive did not affect the clinical presentation.

Rajo MC, et al. Rapid diagnosis of tuberculous meningitis by ligase chain reaction amplification. *Scand J Infect Dis* 2002;34:14.

PCR was reported to be rapid and specific, staying positive several weeks after treatment.

Reik L. Disorders that mimic CNS infection. *Neurol Clin* 1986;4:223.

When granulomatous involvement of basal meninges is the predominant pathology, disease will look like tuberculous meningitis.

Richardson EP. Progressive multifocal leukoencephalopathy 30 years later. *N Engl J Med* 1988;318:315.

Progressive multifocal leukoencephalopathy may occur in as many as 38% of AIDS patients. This article provides a good overview of this disease.

Rosen MS, Lorber B, Myer AR. Chronic meningococcal meningitis. An association with C5 deficiency. *Arch Intern Med* 1988;148:1441.

N. meningitidis may cause chronic meningitis in patients with complement deficiency.

Smego RA Jr. Actinomycosis of the central nervous system. *Rev Infect Dis* 1987;9:855.

Actinomycosis causes several types of CNS disease, particularly brain abscess. An isolated chronic meningitis picture can occur.

Southern PM, Sanford JP. Relapsing fever: a clinical and microbiological review. *Medicine (Baltimore)* 1969;48:129.

Relapsing fever is associated with CNS disease in 8% of tick-borne and 30% of louse-borne infections.

Steere AC. Lyme disease. *N Engl J Med* 2001;345:115.
  Chronic meningitis presents as demyelinating encephalitis with dementia, radicular symptoms.
Steere AC, Pachner AR, Malawista SE. Neurologic abnormalities of Lyme disease: successful treatment with high-dose intravenous penicillin. *Ann Intern Med* 1983;99:767.
  Chronic meningeal symptoms caused by Lyme disease resolve with high-dose penicillin therapy.
Stern BJ, et al. Sarcoidosis and its neurological manifestations. *Arch Neurol* 1985;42:909.
  Sarcoidosis presents with neurologic symptoms in 48% of cases. However, an isolated chronic meningitis syndrome is unusual.
Stockstill MT, Kauffman CA. Comparison of cryptococcal and tuberculous meningitis. *Arch Neurol* 1983;40:81.
  The clinical pictures of tuberculous and cryptococcal meningitis are similar. A miliary pattern on chest radiographs and inappropriate secretion of antidiuretic hormone support a diagnosis of tuberculous meningitis.
Tan TQ. Chronic meningitis. *Semin Pediatr Infect Dis* 2003;14:131.
  Provides an up-to-date, general approach to work-up of chronic meningitis.
Wasserstrom WR, Glass JP, Posner JB. Diagnosis and treatment of leptomeningeal metastases from solid tumors: experience with 90 patients. *Cancer* 1982;49:759.
  Metastatic carcinoma, particularly from primary carcinoma of lung and breast, can cause chronic meningitis syndrome.
Wheat J, et al. Cerebrospinal fluid *Histoplasma* antibodies in central nervous system histoplasmosis. *Arch Intern Med* 1985;145:1237.
  CSF antibodies in histoplasmosis meningitis are 90% sensitive. The disease is increasing in HIV-positive patients.
Yechoor VK, et al. Tuberculosis meningitis among adults with and without HIV infection. Experience in an urban public hospital. *Arch Intern Med* 1996;156:1710.
  Tuberculous meningitis was found to be a relatively common disease in urban nonwhites. Underlying HIV disease did not affect clinical or laboratory features of the disease or response to therapy.

GUILLAIN-BARRÉ SYNDROME 35

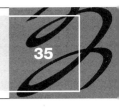

*G*uillain-Barré syndrome (GBS) is an acute inflammatory polyneuropathy. The eponym comes from a 1916 article by G. Guillain and J. A. Barré, who described a polyneuropathy in association with protein elevation in cerebrospinal fluid (CSF) but no inflammatory cells. GBS is an autoimmune disease triggered by an infectious or immunologic stimulus. Though usually presenting as a demyelinating neuropathy with ascending weakness, variants of the disease continue to be better defined. Infectious agents produce specific antibodies against gangliosides and glycolipids, such as ganglioside GM 1 and Gd1b. Both plasma exchange and immunoglobulin therapy have proved to be effective. Acute inflammatory demyelinating polyneuropathy has been frequently reported as a complication of HIV disease.

The clinical features of GBS have been well described; however, the initial presentation may be variable. In general, patients first experience paresthesia and numbness in the extremities. A symmetric weakness develops over several days, usually in the lower extremities, making climbing stairs or walking difficult. Weakness characteristically ascends to the trunk and arms. Muscle pain and sciatica are frequent additional complaints. Weakness may progress for several weeks, affecting respiration, swallowing, eye movements,

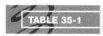

TABLE 35-1   **Symptoms of Guillain-Barré Syndrome**

Antecedent upper respiratory or gastrointestinal illness
Ascending, symmetrical weakness with lower limbs involved before upper limbs
Paresthesias or numbness, also ascending
Cranial nerve involvement in half of patients—diplopia, dysarthria, facial droop
Pain—back and leg. Burning nerve pain in half of patients
Shortness of breath may develop from respiratory muscle involvement

and autonomic nervous system function. Table 35-1 lists the common symptoms of the disease.

Table 35-2 describes physical exam findings that may occur, particularly as the disease progresses.

Several variations in this clinical picture may be noted. The ascending nature of the process may not be striking. Miller-Fisher syndrome, which represents about 5% of all GBS, is characterized by ophthalmoplegia, ataxia, and areflexia. A specific antiganglioside antibody against GQ1b is involved. An acute motor axonal neuropathy (AMAN) is another well-described variant. Cases are reported in children, usually outside of North America. The disease is a pure motor axonopathy and is usually related to *Campylobacter jejuni* infection and high titer of antibody to gangliosides GM1, GD1a, and GD1b. A pure sensory variant also has been reported. This variant presents with sensory loss and areflexia that is symmetric.

As noted, CSF findings confirm the diagnosis. The CSF will show few or no cells and a protein concentration greater than 0.55 g/L. Protein elevation occurs after about 1 week of illness. Abnormalities of nerve conduction reflect the demyelination process. Conduction block in motor nerves and spontaneous discharges in demyelinated sensory nerves make this study both sensitive and specific. Serum autoantibodies are available but are usually not necessary unless diagnosis is questionable. Evaluation for peripheral neuropathy, in general, may be advisable, depending on presentation. The differential diagnosis depends on the history and physical examination findings but may include spinal cord compression, transverse myelitis, myasthenia gravis, chronic meningitis, metabolic myopathies, paraneoplastic neuropathy, poliomyelitis, tick paralysis, botulism, and shellfish poisoning.

The list of infectious organisms that may trigger this process continues to grow. Viral agents such as herpes simplex virus, Epstein-Barr virus, cytomegalovirus, influenza virus, measles virus, mumps virus, respiratory syncytial virus, and hepatitis B virus have been implicated. GBS also occurred as a complication of swine flu vaccination in about 500 persons in 1977; however, no other cases of GBS have occurred in subsequent flu vaccination programs. However, *C. jejuni* is the most common agent, by far, to precipitate this process, occurring in 30 to 60% of cases.

The treatment of GBS is supportive and specific. Patients should be hospitalized, at least for observation. GBS is the most common neuromuscular disease requiring respiratory support. Paralysis of the respiratory muscles can occur suddenly, without clinical warning. Patients with vital capacities that are declining or below 18 mL/kg should be observed in an ICU setting.

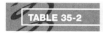

TABLE 35-2   **Physical Exam Findings**

Lower extremity, symmetrical weakness
  Variable upper extremity, facial, or oropharyngeal weakness
  Absent reflexes
  Cranial nerve weakness, particularly CN VII
The following do not suggest GBS:
  Asymmetric weakness, sensory level, Babinski reflex, fever

Specific treatment for GBS includes plasma exchange or infusion of gamma globulin. Corticosteroids have been used, but randomized controlled trials have not found them to be of benefit.

Plasma exchange has been shown to be beneficial in several randomized trials. The standard regimen appears to be five plasma exchanges (200 to 250 mL/kg in five sessions within 7–14 days). Plasma exchange decreased the time until patients could walk unassisted and decreased the need for mechanical ventilation. Benefit was less apparent if exchange was started after 2 weeks of illness. Because immune globulin has been used with beneficial effects in several autoimmune diseases, it was of interest to study its effects in GBS. The Dutch Guillain-Barré Study Group compared IV immune globulin with plasma exchange in 150 GBS patients who were unable to walk but had had the disease for less than 2 weeks. The incidence of improvement was higher in the immune globulin patients (53% vs. 34% in the exchange group) as measured by motor function grading. The median time to improvement by one grade was 41 days in the plasma exchange group and 27 days in the immune globulin group. The immune globulin patients had less need for artificial ventilation.

The Plasma Exchange/Sandoglobulin Guillain-Barré Syndrome Trial Group completed a randomized trial of plasma exchange versus intravenous immune globulin versus the combined treatments. The two treatments were equally efficacious, and the combination offered no advantage. Other studies have also concluded the two treatments to be equivalent. The optimal number of plasma exchanges also has been better defined. For mild disease, two plasma exchanges were better than none with respect to time to onset of motor recovery. For moderate disease, four exchanges were better than two. Six exchanges were no better than four, even in severe disease.

Physical therapy is necessary for some patients. Occupational therapy and speech therapy are assessed on a patient-by-patient basis. More than 80% of patients have a good recovery at the 2-year mark.

GBS has been associated with AIDS and HIV disease. GBS can occur in association with HIV seroconversion or may be a late manifestation of AIDS. As in other patients with GBS, patients with AIDS may report sudden or gradual onset of weakness. It may be particularly difficult in patients with AIDS to distinguish GBS from other causes of peripheral neuropathy. (SLB)

Bibliography

Allos BM. *Campylobacter jejuni* infection as a cause of Guillain-Barré syndrome. *Infect Dis Clin North Am* 1998;12:173.
Molecular mimicry between lipopolysaccharide of some Campylobacter *organisms and ganglioside antigens is the probable explanation for GBS as a sequela of* Campylobacter *infection. In 30 to 40% of cases, GBS is preceded by* C. jejuni *infection.*
Appropriate number of plasma exchanges in Guillain-Barré syndrome. The French Cooperative Group on Plasma Exchange in Guillain-Barré syndrome. *Ann Neurol* 1997;41:298.
In moderate and severe disease, four plasma exchanges were better than two; six exchanges were no more beneficial than four.
Berlit P, Rakicky J. The Miller-Fisher syndrome. Review of the literature. *J Clin Neuroophthalmol* 1992;12:57.
GBS variant of the Miller-Fisher syndrome, which presents with ataxia, areflexia, and ophthalmoplegia. Prognosis is good, with a mean recovery of 10 weeks.
Chio A, et al. Guillain-Barré syndrome: a prospective, population-based incidence and outcome survey. *Neurology* 2003;60:1146.
Prospective study evaluating incidence and long-term prognosis of the disease. Age older than 50 predicted poorer prognosis.
Dalakas MC, Pezeshkpour GH. Neuromuscular diseases associated with human immunodeficiency virus infection. *Ann Neurol* 1988;23:S38.
GBS is one of six subtypes of peripheral neuropathy commonly associated with AIDS. GBS may occur early or late in HIV disease.
French Cooperative Study Group on Plasma Exchange in Guillain-Barré Syndrome. Efficiency of plasma exchange in Guillain-Barré syndrome: role of replacement fluids. *Ann Neurol* 1987;22:753.

The French Cooperative Study found improvement in GBS patients who received plasma exchange. There was no improvement in comparison with controls in an albumin or fresh-frozen plasma group.

Green DM. Advances in the management of Guillain Barré syndrome. *Curr Neurol Neurosci Rep* 2002;6:541.
Evidence-based guidelines for intubation and admission to the intensive care unit.

Hartung HP. Immune-mediated demyelination. *Ann Neurol* 1993;33:563.
Describes the mechanism of the aberrant immune response responsible for GBS. Tumor necrosis factor may contribute to the inflammatory demyelinating process.

Hughes RA, Rees JH. Clinical and epidemiologic features of Guillain-Barré syndrome. *J Infect Dis* 1997;176(suppl 2):S92.
Updates signs and symptoms of the disease and describes worldwide incidence and predisposing factors, emphasizing C. jejuni *infection.*

Hund EF, et al. Intensive management and treatment of severe Guillain-Barré syndrome. *Crit Care Med* 1993;21:433.
Describes the expected complications and treatment of GBS in the intensive care unit. Prevention of thrombosis and pneumonia, psychologic support, and adequate nutrition are all important aspects of management.

Kieseier BC, Hartung HP. Therapeutic strategies in the Guillain-Barre syndrome. *Semin Neurol* 2003;23:159.
Describes how current treatment strategies target the immune system's effect on peripheral nerve.

Randomized trial of plasma exchange, intravenous immunoglobulin, and combined treatments in Guillain-Barré syndrome. Plasma Exchange/Sandoglobulin Guillain-Barré syndrome Trial Group. *Lancet* 1997;349:225.
Plasma exchange and IV globulin were equally effective in the treatment of severe GBS when given during the first 2 weeks after onset of neuropathic symptoms.

Ropper AH. The Guillain-Barré syndrome. *N Engl J Med* 1992;326:1130.
Comprehensive review that summarizes clinical features, pathophysiology, and results of treatment protocols.

Ropper AH, Wijdicks EFM, Shahani BT. Electrodiagnostic abnormalities in 113 consecutive patients with Guillain-Barré syndrome. *Arch Neurol* 1990;47:881.
Describes the types of electrodiagnostic abnormalities found in acute GBS. The types of abnormalities did not generally correlate with prognosis.

Shearn MA, Shearn L. A personal experience with Guillain-Barré syndrome: are the psychologic needs of patient and family being met? *South Med J* 1986;79:800.
Describes the personal and psychologic aspects of the disease by means of a patient and family diary.

van der Meche FGA, Schmitz PIM, Dutch Guillain-Barre Study Group. A randomized trial comparing intravenous immune globulin and plasma exchange in Guillain-Barré syndrome. *N Engl J Med* 1992;326:1123.
The Dutch Guillain-Barré Study Group found immune globulin superior to plasma exchange in the treatment of GBS. Patients improved faster on immune globulin and had fewer side effects.

Winer JB, Hughes RAC, Osmond C. A prospective study of acute idiopathic neuropathy. I. Clinical features and their prognostic value. *J Neurol Neurosurg Psychiatry* 1988; 51:605.
Prospective study gives details of clinical features and prognosis in 100 patients. Age and action potential of abductor pollicis brevis were prognostic factors.

Winer JB. Guillain Barré syndrome. *Mol Pathol* 2001;54:381.
Reviews clinical syndromes as they relate to specific antibodies that cause disease.

Yuki N, et al. Acute axonal polyneuropathy associated with anti-GM_1 antibodies following *Campylobacter* enteritis. *Neurology* 1990;40:1900.
Describes two cases of GBS after Campylobacter *enteritis. In both cases, high titers of IgF antibody against GM ganglioside were demonstrated.*

TREATMENT OF VARICELLA-ZOSTER VIRUS AND POSTHERPETIC NEURALGIA

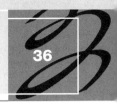

36

*U*nfortunately, the pain of zoster does not always resolve when the rash heals but continues for months to years and is termed *postherpetic neuralgia* (PHN) It affects the elderly the most. Possibly because the nerve cells conveying pain sensation are affected most or are extremely sensitized by the virus attack, pain is the principal persistent complication of shingles. PHN can last for months to years. It is extremely incapacitating and can result in insomnia, weight loss, and an inability to perform daily tasks of living.

The pathophysiology of PHN remains unclear. However, pathologic studies have demonstrated damage to the sensory nerves, the sensory dorsal root ganglia, and the dorsal horns of the spinal cord in patients with this condition. In essence, the pain of herpes zoster (HZ) results from a sequence of changes in neuronal sensitivity starting at the point of neural damage in the periphery and moving centrally to affect one cell after another within the pain pathway. Once central sensitization occurs, attempts to reduce the pain purely by influencing peripheral nociceptor function are unlikely to be successful. Furthermore, once established, such neuropathic pain is notoriously difficult to control. Treatment of the acute illness is thus chiefly directed at minimizing the risk of the prolonged pain. The cascades of responses that lead to pain after acute neuronal injury occur very rapidly: neurotransmitter release within seconds, wind-up and sensitization within minutes, sprouting and remodeling within hours, and structural responses over days to months.

Four placebo-controlled trials of oral acyclovir (ACV) with 692 patients provided marginal evidence for reduction in pain incidence at 1 to 3 months after zoster onset. Famciclovir significantly reduced duration but not incidence of PHN in one placebo-controlled trial of 419 patients. Valacyclovir significantly reduced duration but not incidence of PHN in one ACV-controlled trial of 1,141 patients. Steroids had no effect on PHN. Amitriptyline for 90 days reduced pain incidence at 6 months in one placebo-controlled trial of 80 patients. A single trial of percutaneous electrical nerve stimulation (PENS) in 50 patients suggested a decrease in pain incidence at 3 and 6 months compared with famciclovir. There is limited evidence that current interventions prevent or shorten PHN. See Tables 36-1 and 36-2 for more information.

The pain associated with HZ has three phases: an acute herpetic neuralgia that accompanies the rash and lasts for about 30 days after the onset of rash, a subacute herpetic neuralgia that lasts for 30 to 120 days after the onset of rash, and PHN, defined as pain that persists for 120 days or more after the onset of rash. The most debilitating aspect of the disease is often this phase of the illness, and not the acute phase.

Pharmacologic approaches can be classified into three groups: (1) drugs that act topically in the affected skin area; (2) drugs that act on nerve excitability and conduction in sensory axons; and (3) drugs that act on neural damage-related synaptic changes. Traditionally, tricyclic antidepressants (TCAs) have been considered the first-line treatment for patients with PHN. However, newer therapies may be more effective and could be considered the drugs of choice for PHN. This is because opioid analgesics and TCAs generally have poorer tolerability and require greater caution in patients with PHN (who are often elderly), and because gabapentin and lidocaine patch 5% have been approved by the U.S. Food and Drug Administration for the treatment of PHN.

Unfortunately, there are no data regarding the additive or synergistic benefits of combination treatment with the agents discussed in Tables 36-1 and 36-2.

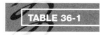

TABLE 36-1	Treatment Options for PHN
Medication	**Dosage**
Topical agents	
Capsaicin cream (Zostrix)	Apply to affected area three to five times daily
Lidocaine (Xylocaine) patch	Apply to affected area every 4–12 hours as needed (http://www.endo.com/PDF/lidoderm_pack_insert.pdf)
Tricyclic antidepressants	
Amitriptyline (Elavil)	25 mg orally at bedtime; increase dosage by 25 mg every 2–4 weeks until response is adequate, or to maximum dosage of 150 mg per day
Nortriptyline (Pamelor)	25 mg orally at bedtime; increase dosage by 25 mg every 2–4 weeks until response is adequate, or to maximum dosage of 125 mg per day
Desipramine (Norpramin)	25 mg orally at bedtime; increase dosage by 25 mg every 2–4 weeks until response is adequate, or to maximum dosage of 150 mg per day
Anticonvulsants	
Gabapentin (Neurontin)	100–300 mg orally at bedtime; increase dosage by 100–300 mg every 3 days until dosage is 300–900 mg three times daily or response is adequate (http://www.rxlist.com/cgi/generic/gabapent.htm)

(Adapted from Stankus SJ. et al. Management of herpes zoster (shingles) and postherpetic neuralgia. *Am Fam Physician* 2000;61:2437–2444, 2447–2448.)

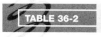

TABLE 36-2	Antiviral Therapy of Zoster	
Medication	**Dose**	
ACV	800 mg orally five times daily for 7–10 days 10 mg per kg IV every 8 hours for 7–10 days	Antiviral therapy has been shown to be beneficial only when patients are treated within 72 hours of onset of the HZ rash
Famciclovir	500 mg orally three times daily for 7 days	
Valacyclovir	1,000 mg orally three times daily for 7 days	
Prednisone	30 mg orally twice daily on days 1 through 7; then 15 mg twice daily on days 8 through 14; then 7.5 mg twice daily on days 15 through 21	Prednisone used in conjunction with ACV has been shown to reduce the pain associated with HZ but probably is ineffective for PHN. Probably more useful for those patients older than age 50

GABAPENTIN

Gabapentin is structurally related to the neurotransmitter GABA (gamma-aminobutyric acid). However, it does not modify $GABA_A$ or $GABA_B$ radioligand binding, it is not converted metabolically into GABA or a GABA agonist, and it is not an inhibitor of GABA uptake or degradation. The mechanism by which gabapentin exerts its analgesic action is unknown. This second-generation anticonvulsant was recently demonstrated to provide significant benefits when compared with placebo. Gabapentin was evaluated for the management of PHN in two randomized, double-blind, placebo-controlled multicenter studies that included 563 patients in the intent-to-treat (ITT) population. Patients were enrolled if they continued to have pain for more than 3 months after healing of the HZ skin rash. In these trials, treatment with gabapentin at daily doses of 1800 to 3600 mg was associated with a statistically significant reduction in daily pain ratings as well as improvements in sleep, mood, and quality of life.

Gabapentin is eliminated from the systemic circulation by renal excretion as unchanged drug. Patients should be advised that gabapentin may cause dizziness, somnolence, and other symptoms and signs of CNS depression. Accordingly, they should be advised neither to drive a car nor to operate other complex machinery until they have gained sufficient experience on gabapentin to gauge whether it affects their mental or motor performance adversely. Gabapentin may cause or exacerbate gait and balance problems and cognitive impairment in elderly patients.

To reduce side effects and increase patient compliance with treatment, gabapentin should be initiated at low dosages (100–300 mg in a single dose taken at bedtime or 100 mg taken three times per day) and then titrated by 100 mg three times per day, as tolerated. The target dosages studied in the two controlled trials ranged from 1800 to 3600 mg per day. Dosing information can also be found on the internet at (www.rxlist.com/cgi/generic/gabapent.htm).

 OPIOID ANALGESICS

In one study, patients with PHN of at least moderate intensity were randomized to controlled-release oxycodone 10 mg or placebo every 12 hours, each for 4 weeks, using a double-blind, crossover design. The dose was increased weekly up to a possible maximum of 30 mg every 12 hours. Pain intensity and pain relief were assessed daily, and steady (ongoing) pain, brief (paroxysmal) pain, skin pain (allodynia), and pain relief were recorded at weekly visits. Clinical effectiveness, disability, and treatment preference were also assessed. Compared with placebo, oxycodone resulted in pain relief and reductions in steady pain, allodynia, and paroxysmal spontaneous pain. Global effectiveness, disability, and masked patient preference all showed superior scores with oxycodone relative to placebo.

To compare the analgesic and cognitive effects of opioids with those of TCA and placebo in the treatment of PHN, 76 patients with PHN were randomized in a double-blind, placebo-controlled, crossover trial. Fifty patients completed two periods, and 44 patients completed all three. Treatment with opioids and TCA resulted in greater pain relief (38% and 32%) compared with placebo, but more patients completing all three treatments preferred opioids than TCA. More people dropped out of the study while taking opioids (n = 20) than TCAs (n = 6) or placebo (n = 1). Response to one drug did not predict response to the other. Although there is no maximum dosage of opioid analgesics with careful titration and monitoring, evaluation by a pain specialist may be considered when morphine equianalgesic dosages exceeding 120 mg per day are contemplated.

 LIDOCAINE PATCH 5%

Topical local anesthetics have shown promise in both uncontrolled and controlled studies. Thirty-five subjects with established PHN affecting the torso or extremities completed a four-session, random order, double-blind, vehicle-controlled study of the analgesic effects of topically applied 5% lidocaine in the form of a nonwoven polyethylene adhesive patch. Lidocaine-containing patches significantly reduced pain intensity at all time points 30 minutes to 12 hours, compared with no-treatment observation, and at all time points 4 to 12 hours compared with vehicle patches. The highest blood lidocaine level measured was 0.1 mcg/mL, indicating minimal systemic absorption of lidocaine. Patch application was without systemic side effects and well tolerated when applied on allodynic skin for 12 hours. Treatment with the lidocaine patch 5% consists of the application of a maximum of three patches per day for a maximum of 12 hours applied directly to the area of maximal PHN-associated pain and allodynia, which typically overlaps the primary affected dermatome. It should not be used for patients with open lesions, because the available formulation is not sterile. It is important to note that the patient's obtaining satisfactory relief from lidocaine patch 5% usually will be apparent within 2 weeks, and time-consuming dose escalation is not required. Further dosing information can be found on the Internet at www.endo.com/healthcare/products/lidoderm.html and www.endo.com/PDF/lidoderm_pack_insert.pdf.

 TRICYCLIC ANTIDEPRESSANTS

These agents most likely lessen pain by inhibiting the reuptake of serotonin and norepinephrine neurotransmitters. These drugs are best tolerated when they are started in a low dosage and given at bedtime. The dosage is increased every 2 to 4 weeks to achieve an effective dose. Amitriptyline (AT) is a standard therapy for PHN. Other agents might be just as effective. A randomized, double-blind, crossover trial of AT versus nortriptyline (NT) was conducted in 33 patients. Twenty-one of 31 (67.7%) had at least a good response to AT or NT, or both. Intolerable side effects were more common with AT. We concluded that this study provides a scientific basis for an analgesic action of NT in PHN because pain relief occurred without an antidepressant effect, and because although there were fewer side effects with NT, AT and NT appear to have a similar analgesic action for most individuals. Patients at risk of increased toxicity with this class of drugs include those with a history of cardiovascular disease, glaucoma, urinary retention, and autonomic neuropathy.

Desipramine has the least anticholinergic and sedative effects of the first generation tricyclic antidepressant agents, but its pain-relieving potential has received little study. In a randomized double-blind crossover design, 26 PHN patients were given 6 weeks of treatment with desipramine (mean dose, 167 mg/day) and placebo. Pain relief with desipramine was statistically significant from weeks 3 to 6. These drugs should be titrated for effect and the patient should understand that he or she need not be depressed for these agents to work. Because tricyclic antidepressants do not act quickly, a clinical trial of at least 3 months is required to judge a patient's response.

Tricyclic antidepressant drugs inhibit the reuptake of noradrenaline (norepinephrine) and serotonin in the CNS and are thought to increase the inhibition of nociceptive signals within the dorsal horn of the spinal cord. The onset of pain relief using tricyclic antidepressants may be enhanced by beginning treatment early in the course of HZ infection in conjunction with antiviral medications. (JWM)

Bibliography

Ali NM. Does sympathetic ganglionic block prevent postherpetic neuralgia? Literature review. *Reg Anesth* 1995;20:227–233.
Considering the degree of uncertainty and the seriousness of PHN, sympathetic block in addition to treatment with ACV should be considered early during acute HZ. Large controlled trials are needed to provide the necessary scientific evidence.
Alper BS, Lewis PR. Does treatment of acute herpes zoster prevent or shorten postherpetic neuralgia? *J Fam Pract* 2000;49:255–264.
There is limited evidence that current interventions prevent or shorten PHN. Famciclovir and valacyclovir have been shown to reduce the duration of PHN in single published trials.

Alper BS, Lewis PR. Treatment of postherpetic neuralgia: a systematic review of the literature. *J Fam Pract* 2002;51:121–128.

No single best treatment for PHN is known. Tricyclic antidepressants, topical capsaicin, gabapentin, and oxycodone are effective for alleviating PHN; however, long-term, clinically meaningful benefits are uncertain and side effects are common. Patients with PHN refractory to these therapies may benefit from intrathecal methylprednisolone. Little evidence is available regarding treatment of PHN of less than 6 months' duration.

Backonja M, Glanzman RL. Gabapentin dosing for neuropathic pain: evidence from randomized, placebo-controlled clinical trials. *Clin Ther* 2003;25:81–104.

Based on available data, it appears that treatment should be started at a dose of 900 mg/day (300 mg/day on day 1,600 mg/day on day 2, and 900 mg/day on day 3). Additional titration to 1,800 mg/day is recommended for greater efficacy. Doses up to 3,600 mg/day may be needed in some patients. The effective dose should be individualized according to patient response and tolerance.

Bernstein JE, et al. Topical capsaicin treatment of chronic postherpetic neuralgia. *J Am Acad Dermatol* 1989;21:265–270.

After 6 weeks, almost 80% of capsaicin-treated patients experienced some relief from their pain.

Bowsher D. The management of postherpetic neuralgia. *Postgrad Med J* 1997;73:623–629.

Effective treatment of acute shingles by systemic antivirals at the appropriate time may have some effect in reducing the incidence of PHN, making it easier to treat with tricyclics and greatly reducing scarring (25% of all cases affect the face). Preemptive treatment with low-dose tricyclics (AT or NT 10–25 mg nocte) from the time of diagnosis of acute shingles reduces the incidence of PHN by about 50%.

Bowsher D. Factors influencing the features of postherpetic neuralgia and outcome when treated with tricyclics. *Eur J Pain* 2003;7:1–7.

This paper retrospectively reviews features of PHN in up to 279 personal patients in relation to treatment outcome when treated with tricyclic antidepressants. Factors affecting characteristics of PHN: (1) Patients with allodynia (89%) and/or burning pain (56%) have a much higher visual analogue pain intensity score than those without; (2) ACV given for acute shingles (HZ) does not reduce the incidence of subsequent PHN, but reduces the pain intensity in PHN patients with allodynia; (3) ACV given for acute HZ reduces the incidence of burning pain in subsequent PHN, but not of allodynia; (4) ACV given for acute HZ reduces the incidence of clinically detectable sensory deficit in subsequent PHN. Factors affecting outcome of tricyclic antidepressant-treated PHN: (1) The point in time at which TCA treatment is commenced is by far the most critical factor: started between 3 and 12 months after acute HZ onset, more than two-thirds obtain pain relief (NNT = 1.8); between 13 and 24 months, two-fifths (41%) (NNT = 3.6); and more than 2 years, one-third (NNT = 8.3). Background and paroxysmal pain disappears earlier and is more susceptible of relief than allodynia. (2) Twice as many (86%) of PHN patients without allodynia obtain pain relief with TCA treatment than those with (42%); (3) The use of ACV for acute HZ more than halves the time-to-relief of PHN patients by tricyclic antidepressants; (4) PHN patients with burning pain are significantly less likely to obtain pain relief with tricyclic antidepressants than those without (P <.0001).

Curran MP, Wagstaff AJ. Gabapentin: in postherpetic neuralgia. *CNS Drugs* 2003;17:975–982.

Adverse events associated with gabapentin in patients with PHN were usually mild to moderate in intensity, with dizziness, somnolence, and peripheral edema being commonly reported.

Dworkin, RH, et al. Postherpetic neuralgia: impact of famciclovir, age, rash severity, and acute pain in herpes zoster patients. *J Infect Dis* 1998;178(suppl 1):S76–S80.

The results of these analyses indicated that greater age, rash severity, and acute pain severity are risk factors for prolonged PHN. In addition, they demonstrated that treatment of acute HZ patients with famciclovir significantly reduces both the duration and prevalence of PHN.

Ernst ME, et al. Oral corticosteroids for pain associated with herpes zoster. *Ann Pharmacother* 1998;32:1099–1103.
  It is apparent from published studies that corticosteroids do not prevent the development of PHN. In more recent larger and well-designed studies, similar rates of PHN were observed in the corticosteroid and control groups. As a result of these findings, corticosteroids should not be recommended for the prevention of PHN. Despite lack of efficacy in preventing PHN, limited studies suggest corticosteroids, such as prednisone (40–60 mg/day tapered over 3 weeks), are well tolerated and may confer slightly significant benefits in reducing the duration of acute neuralgia and improving quality-of-life measures. Until the results of these studies are repeated in more diverse patient populations, corticosteroids appear to have a limited role in the management of acute neuralgia associated with HZ.

Fields HL, et al. Postherpetic neuralgia: irritable nociceptors and deafferentation. *Neurobiol Dis* 1998;5:209–227.
  It is clear that both peripheral and central pathophysiologic mechanisms contribute to PHN pain. Some PHN patients have abnormal sensitization of unmyelinated cutaneous nociceptors (irritable nociceptors). Such patients characteristically have minimal sensory loss. Other patients have pain associated with small fiber deafferentation. In these patients, pain and temperature sensation are profoundly impaired but light moving mechanical stimuli can often produce severe pain (allodynia). In these patients, allodynia may be due to the formation of new connections between nonnociceptive large diameter primary afferents and central pain transmission neurons. Other deafferentation patients have severe spontaneous pain without hyperalgesia or allodynia and presumably have lost both large-and small-diameter fibers. In this group the pain is likely the result of increased spontaneous activity in deafferented central neurons and/or reorganization of central connections. These three types of mechanisms may coexist in individual patients, and each offers the possibility for developing new therapeutic interventions.

Gammaitoni AR, et al. Safety and tolerability of the lidocaine patch 5%, a targeted peripheral analgesic: a review of the literature. *J Clin Pharmacol* 2003;43:111–117.
  The safety, tolerability, and efficacy of the lidocaine patch 5% (Lidoderm), a targeted peripheral analgesic with a Food and Drug Administration (FDA)-approved indication for the treatment of PHN, has been well established. The lidocaine patch provides a treatment option that carries a relatively low systemic adverse event and drug-drug interaction risk burden, even with continuous application of up to four patches per day.

Harke HP, et al. Spinal cord stimulation in postherpetic neuralgia and in acute herpes zoster pain. *Anesth Analg* 2002;94:694–700; table of contents.
  In many patients with PHN and acute HZ, pain is not satisfactorily alleviated with pharmacologic approaches. We report on 23 of 28 patients with PHN and four of four with acute HZ whose chronic pain was improved by electrical spinal cord stimulation.

Herr H. Prognostic factors of postherpetic neuralgia. *J Korean Med Sci* 2002;175:655–659.
  The investigation was aimed to determine prognostic factors related to PHN and treatment options for preventing PHN. The age (50 years and older), surface area involved (9% or more), and duration of severe pain (4 weeks or more) might be the main factors that lead to PHN. On the other hand, gender, dermatomal distribution, accompaning systemic conditions, and interval between initial pain and initiation of treatment might not be implicated in PHN.

Kishore-Kumar R, et al. Desipramine relieves postherpetic neuralgia. *Clin Pharmacol Ther* 1990;47:305–312.
  These authors concluded that desipramine administration relieves PHN and that pain relief is not mediated by mood elevation. Blockade of norepinephrine reuptake, an action shared by desipramine, amitriptyline, and other antidepressant agents that have relieved neuropathic pain, may be involved in relief of PHN.

Kotani N, et al. Intrathecal methylprednisolone for intractable postherpetic neuralgia. *N Engl J Med* 2000;343:1514–1519.
  There is no effective treatment for intractable PHN. In the patients who received methylprednisolone, interleukin-8 concentrations decreased by 50%, and this decrease correlated with the duration of neuralgia and the extent of global pain relief (P <.001 for

both comparisons). The results of this trial indicate that the intrathecal administration of methylprednisolone is an effective treatment for PHN.

Meglio M, et al. Spinal cord stimulation (SCS) in the treatment of postherpetic pain. *Acta Neurochir Suppl (Wien)* 1989;46:65–66.

Spinal cord stimulation is considered to be of poor value in treating postherpetic pain. The results of spinal cord stimulation in our patients, although positive in only 60% of them, are remarkably stable with time. We therefore recommend a percutaneous test trial of spinal cord stimulation in every case of PHN resistant to medical treatment.

Raja SN, et al. Opioids versus antidepressants in postherpetic neuralgia: a randomized, placebo-controlled trial. *Neurology* 2002;59:1015–1021.

Opioids effectively treat PHN without impairing cognition. Opioids and tricyclic antidepressants act through independent mechanisms and with varied individual effect.

Rowbotham M, et al. Gabapentin for the treatment of postherpetic neuralgia: a randomized controlled trial. *JAMA* 1998;280:1837–1842.

Gabapentin is effective in the treatment of pain and sleep interference associated with PHN. Mood and quality of life also improve with gabapentin therapy.

Rowbotham MC, et al. Lidocaine patch: double-blind controlled study of a new treatment method for post-herpetic neuralgia. *Pain* 1996;65:39–44.

This study demonstrates that topical 5% lidocaine in patch form is easy to use and relieves PHN.

Santee JA. Corticosteroids for herpes zoster: what do they accomplish? *Am J Clin Dermatol* 2002;3:517–524.

Oral corticosteroids may confer a slight benefit for initial symptoms as long as the patient is not at risk for complications resulting from corticosteroid therapy. Two controlled, blinded trials investigating the use of intrathecal corticosteroid administration for intractable PHN suggest that corticosteroid administration results in a significant improvement in pain. Despite this, several authors have voiced concern over possible serious adverse events with the intrathecal administration of corticosteroids. Intrathecal corticosteroids may provide a benefit for intractable PHN, but because of risks of serious complications, this is a last-line option and should only be administered by experienced personnel.

Stankus SJ, et al. Management of herpes zoster (shingles) and postherpetic neuralgia. *Am Fam Physician* 2000;61:2437–2444, 2447–2448.

Good overall review article with useful references.

Watson CP, Babul N. Efficacy of oxycodone in neuropathic pain: a randomized trial in postherpetic neuralgia. *Neurology* 1998;50:1837–1841.

Controlled-release oxycodone is an effective analgesic for the management of steady pain, paroxysmal spontaneous pain, and allodynia, which frequently characterize PHN.

Watson CP, et al. Nortriptyline versus amitriptyline in postherpetic neuralgia: a randomized trial. *Neurology* 1998;51:1166–1171.

AT is a standard therapy for PHN. Our hypothesis was that NT, a noradrenergic metabolite of AT, may be more effective. We concluded that this study provides a scientific basis for an analgesic action of NT in PHN because pain relief occurred without an antidepressant effect, and that although there were fewer side effects with NT, AT and NT appear to have a similar analgesic action for most individuals.

Wood MJ, et al. A randomized trial of acyclovir for 7 days or 21 days with and without prednisolone for treatment of acute herpes zoster. *N Engl J Med* 1994;330:896–900.

In acute HZ, treatment with ACV for 21 days or the addition of prednisolone to ACV therapy confers only slight benefits over standard 7-day treatment with ACV. Neither additional treatment reduces the frequency of PHN.

Wood M. Understanding pain in herpes zoster: an essential for optimizing treatment. *J Infect Dis* 2002;186(suppl 1):S78–S82.

There is no clear consensus regarding the optimal means of determining the benefits of antiviral therapy in the management of pain of HZ. A novel statistical approach using rates of disappearance of pain of differing pathophysiologic mechanisms is proposed.

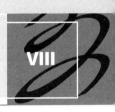

Bones and Joints VIII

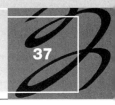

$\mathcal{V}$ertebral osteomyelitis, which represents 2 to 4% of all bone infections, is an uncommon but increasingly recognized process that may be difficult to diagnose and can be complicated by potentially devastating neurologic or vascular complications. In adults, hematogenous dissemination is the most common method of spread. Recent data suggest that its risk as a complication of *Staphylococcus aureus* bacteremia is increasing. Other modes of acquisition include complications of orthopedic/neurosurgery, trauma, and complication of epidural catheter placement.

EPIDEMIOLOGY

Reasons for the increased recognition of this disease include higher prevalence of parenteral drug use and nosocomial infection (primarily related to use of intravenous catheters), prevalence of diabetes and an aging population, better imaging techniques, and greater appreciation for this illness. The disease is more common in adults than children. A recent investigation demonstrated that 95% of cases were in men. Most cases occur in persons older than age 50, which may be explained in part by the increased frequency of urinary tract infections in the elderly and the presence of Batson's plexus, a low-pressure, valveless venous plexus that drains blood from the pelvis toward the vertebral column and potentially allows passage of infection into this area. Thus, it differs from other forms of osteomyelitis by having a higher male:female ratio, occurring in an older population, and being more closely associated with diabetes mellitus. With regard to pyogenic vertebral osteomyelitis, at least 50% of cases involve the lumbar spine (possibly related to the noted anatomic considerations). The thoracic spine (approximately 30%) and cervical spine are involved in decreasing order of frequency. Tuberculous vertebral osteomyelitis most commonly involves lower thoracic vertebrae (Pott's disease).

CLINICAL PRESENTATION

Clinical presentation is often subtle, and the physician must have a high index of suspicion to make an early diagnosis. Although about 10% of cases occur acutely, with positive blood cultures substantiating the diagnosis, subacute or chronic back pain is the most common presentation and is noted in more than 90% of cases. Duration of complaints is frequently longer than 3 months. Unusual clinical presentations may occur as a result of extension into surrounding tissues. Pleural empyema and retropharyngeal abscess have been described recently as initial presentations of pyogenic vertebral osteomyelitis. Neurologic complaints often imply the presence of spinal epidural abscess. These may include root pain and root weakness, and may progress rapidly to frank paralysis. Intravenous substance abusers with vertebral osteomyelitis tend to have a more abbreviated course. Additionally, two cases of gas-forming osteomyelitis caused by enteric gram-negative bacilli have been reported. Both involved diabetic patients and both ran fulminant courses. Fever is present in up to 90% of cases, but is usually low grade. Rigors are unusual.

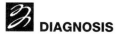

DIAGNOSIS

Initial assessment must include a careful history to evaluate for a primary focus of infection. Clinical conditions predisposing to vertebral osteomyelitis include intravenous substance abuse, diabetes mellitus, trauma to the back (including surgery), distant skin or soft tissue infection, and history of urinary tract infection or instrumentation. In patients with current or recent hospitalization, the intravenous catheter must be strongly considered. History should also include an epidemiologic assessment for unusual pathogens, such as *Myobacterium tuberculosis*, fungi, and *Brucella* species. A recent investigation demonstrated that approximately 33% of patients with vertebral osteomyelitis had *M. tuberculosis* as the pathogen; all came from endemic areas. However, in at least 33% of cases, the etiology of vertebral osteomyelitis remains obscure (Table 37-1).

Physical examination should include an assessment for localized tenderness over vertebral bodies and a search for feeding foci, such as infected intravenous lines, stigmata of intravenous substance abuse, and signs of urinary tract infection. Examination should also assess for neurologic complications. Initial laboratory data are generally nonspecific. Leukocytosis is seen in less than 50% of cases. The erythrocyte sedimentation rate (ESR) is elevated in more than 80% of cases but is nonspecific. However, decline of this parameter by 33 to 50% during antimicrobial therapy may help to predict cure.

Radiographic assessment of the suspected area is mandatory. Plain films may not turn positive for 2 to 8 weeks after clinical presentation. Initial findings are often nonspecific and may include paravertebral swelling or sclerosis of the vertebral endplates. However, more advanced cases may involve both a disk and adjacent vertebrae. The finding of disk space narrowing with adjacent changes should prompt consideration of this disease. This is in contradistinction to metastatic tumor, which is characteristically confined to the vertebral body with sparing of the disk. The clinician must have a high index of suspicion when the course of metastatic cancer is different than expected and must consider additional diagnoses.

Magnetic resonance imaging (MRI) has proven especially useful in this regard. Recent observations also have noted patients with confirmed vertebral osteomyelitis (in the setting of underlying osteoporosis) who had localized vertebral disease with resultant collapse that mimicked compression fracture and resulted in diagnostic delay. Gallium, indium-111–labeled leukocyte, and technetium bone scanning are more sensitive than standard radiographs and may turn positive in less than 7 days. Gallium and indium-111–labeled leukocyte scanning have the capacity to demonstrate complications within adjacent tissues. However, none is specific. MRI remains the best test for making the diagnosis of vertebral osteomyelitis in a timely fashion, and it should be used early in management. MRI changes suggestive of vertebral osteomyelitis are noted in 90% of patients with symptoms for less than 2 weeks and rise to 96% in patients with symptoms longer than 2 weeks. It may prove to be particularly

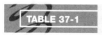
TABLE 37-1 Likely Pathogens in Vertebral Osteomyelitis

Risk factor	Pathogen
Intravenous drug use	*S. aureus* (including MRSA), viridans streptococci, *P. aeruginosa*, Enteric gram-negative bacilli
Urinary tract disease	Enteric gram-negative bacilli *P. aeruginosa*, Enterococci
Skin/skin structure infections	*S. aureus* (including MRSA), streptococci, *Staphylococcus* spp.
Orthopedic/neurosurgery	*S. aureus* (including MRSA), *Staphylococcus* spp., enteric gram-negative bacilli, *P. aeruginosa*
Travel/epidemiologic exposure	*Brucella* spp., *M. tuberculosis*, environmental fungi

useful in diagnosing vertebral osteomyelitis in the known setting of metastatic tumor to a vertebral body. Changes considered diagnostic of vertebral osteomyelitis included erosion of endplates and occult paravertebral swelling. Similarly, MRI can provide timely information concerning complications of the spinal canal or aorta. Thus, in cases of patients with obscure back, chest, or abdominal pain or in the evaluation of fevers of unknown origin, a computed tomographic (CT) scan or MRI can provide invaluable information concerning diagnosis and potential complications and should be performed early in the diagnostic evaluation.

MRI also may suggest differences between pyogenic and tuberculous osteomyelitis. The former is associated with involvement of fewer vertebral bodies, smaller paravertebral abscesses, and a more homogenous magnetic intensity of vertebral bodies. The authors recommend initial plain films and then MRI as the sequence for diagnosis of vertebral osteomyelitis. If emergent (e.g., neurologic signs), MRI should be used as the initial imaging modality.

Once osteomyelitis is suspected, bacteriologic confirmation should be sought before initiation of antibiotics. Although blood and urine cultures should be performed, they are unlikely to provide confirmatory data. The best approach is to perform percutaneous bone aspiration of the involved site under CT guidance. This approach may also allow simultaneous drainage of any paravertebral abscesses. Material obtained should be sent for (1) Gram's stain and acid-fast stain; (2) routine (aerobic and anaerobic), mycobacterial, and fungal cultures; and (3) histopathologic analysis. If initial assessment proves negative, routine cultures should be held for several weeks, so that pathogens such as *Brucella* species are not overlooked. Yield from percutaneous bone aspiration will decrease if the anterior portion of the bone is involved. In these circumstances, a decision will be needed regarding more aggressive surgery or empiric therapy.

 BACTERIOLOGY

Bacteriology is variable and relates to the underlying cause of disease. A recent investigation demonstrated that the presence of HIV/AIDS did not affect bacteriology of vertebral osteomyelitis. Most cases involve single isolates. Occasionally, cultures remain sterile, perhaps because of previous antimicrobial therapy or sampling error. *S. aureus* is the most commonly identified pathogen and may involve methicillin-resistant *S. aureus* (MRSA). Gram-negative enteric bacilli, especially *Escherichia coli* and *Salmonella* spp., account for about 30% of cases. The latter are especially noted in patients with sickle cell disease and in those whose illness is complicated by aortic mycotic aneurysm. *Pseudomonas aeruginosa* has been commonly identified in patients whose vertebral osteomyelitis is associated with intravenous substance abuse, and may occur in clusters. Infections caused by species of *Brucella* should be suspected in persons from selected areas of the world. Tuberculous vertebral osteomyelitis usually involves thoracic or upper lumbar vertebrae and often is associated with evidence of pulmonary tuberculosis. Duration of symptoms is longer in patients with *M. tuberculosis* than in those with pyogenic vertebral osteomyelitis. A history of active tuberculosis at other sites should be sought. In some series it has accounted for almost 40% of cases of vertebral osteomyelitis. Failure to identify a bacterial pathogen should intensify a search for unusual organisms.

 TREATMENT

Normally, systemic antimicrobial therapy active against the offending pathogen is the cornerstone of therapy for uncomplicated pyogenic vertebral osteomyelitis. In most instances, therapy can be withheld until a pathogen is identified. Treatment is usually continued for at least 4 weeks; the ESR and response of back pain may be used to gauge response to therapy. A recent review has favored up to 6 months of treatment, with duration being individualized on parameters that include those mentioned above. However, the need for oral versus intravenous treatment will depend to a great extent on the pathogen identified and the agents available for therapy. As an example, several agents that include the fluorinated quinolones, trimethoprim/sulfamethoxazole, linezolid, and rifampin result in systemic blood levels orally that are virtually identical to those resulting from intravenous dosing. For gram-positive infections not caused by MRSA or vancomycin-resistant enterococcus (VRE), a single intravenous β-lactam agent usually suffices. It is important to monitor for adverse reactions, such as interstitial nephritis, toxic hepatitis, or neutropenia or thrombocytopenia that can occasionally be observed with prolonged β-lactam therapy. Infections caused by MRSA or VRE may respond to linezolid, vancomycin, or daptomycin, among others. Patients infected with methicillin-sensitive *S. aureus* may have at least some of their therapy given orally with a combination of a fluoroquinolone and rifampin, if the organism is susceptible to both of these agents.

Treatment of infections caused by gram-negative bacilli should be guided by susceptibility data. It is the opinion of the authors that many cases can be treated with full doses of oral fluoroquinolones as monotherapy, when the pathogen is sensitive to this class. Such treatment has been successfully used with other forms of osteomyelitis. In occasional cases empiric therapy has been required, as a specific etiologic diagnosis may not be made. In these instances, the authors have had success with a fluoroquinolone plus rifampin, given orally for at least 4 weeks. Uncomplicated cases of vertebral osteomyelitis are usually managed medically. Drainage, most commonly performed percutaneously, is generally indicated for spinal epidural abscess and other neurologic or vascular complications or if frank paravertebral abscess is demonstrated by imaging. Immobilization also has generally been recommended; this is currently interpreted to mean modest bed rest early in treatment.

 PROGNOSIS

Recent data suggest that almost 90% of patients recover from pyogenic vertebral osteomyelitis, although approximately one-third will have neurologic or painful sequelae. Risk factors for these complications include (1) delayed diagnosis, (2) neurologic compromise at clinical presentation, and (3) infection acquired within the hospital. However, with appropriate diagnosis and treatment, mortality and neurologic sequelae should be limited. The major challenge for the clinician remains the diagnosis of vertebral osteomyelitis, as presentation may mimic numerous other infectious and noninfectious conditions. (RBB)

Bibliography

An HS, et al. Differentiation between spinal tumors and infections with magnetic resonance imaging. *Spine* 1991;16(suppl 8):S334–S338.
The authors studied 30 patients with proven spinal tumors or infections. MRI correctly diagnosed 29 of 30 processes. Involvement of disk spaces was seen only with infectious processes, as was involvement of contiguous vertebrae. The authors believe MRI to be the best imaging modality to differentiate infection from tumor.

Arnold PM, et al. Surgical management of nontuberculous thoracic and lumbar vertebral osteomyelitis: report of 33 cases. *Surg Neurol* 1997;47:551–561.
Indications for surgery were either neurologic deficit or failure of antibiotic therapy. Long-term outcomes after surgery were good.

Carragee EJ. The clinical use of magnetic resonance imaging in pyogenic vertebral osteomyelitis. *Spine* 1997;22:780–785.
One hundred three cases of vertebral osteomyelitis were reviewed by the author. Within the first 2 weeks of symptoms, MRI was either positive or suggestive of the diagnosis in about 90% of cases. After 2 weeks, this number rose to about 96%. The author feels that MRI is valuable for the initial diagnosis of vertebral osteomyelitis. However its role in follow-up is uncertain, as often the MRI demonstrates worsening disease while clinical improvement has been noted.

McHenry MC, Easley KA, Locker GA. Vertebral osteomyelitis: long-term outcome for 253 patients from 7 Cleveland-area hospitals. *Clin Infect Dis* 2002;34:1342–1350.
The authors present a retrospective analysis of many patients followed for a mean of more than 6 years. Among other parameters investigated, they noted a relapse rate of

almost 15%, and sequelae in more than 33% of survivors. Mortality was 11%. The authors also noted that initial MRI interpretations were incorrect in more than 25% of patients, and often suggested noninfectious etiologies. Antibiotic therapy should be continued for a minimum of 4 to 6 weeks, but the authors feel that treatment as long as 6 months may be indicated in selected patients and should be guided by individual factors that include residual pain and the ESR response.

Patzakis MJ, et al. Analysis of 61 cases of vertebral osteomyelitis. *Clin Orthop Rel Res* 1991;264:178–183.

The authors compared diagnostic imaging techniques in 61 patients with confirmed vertebral osteomyelitis and conclude that MRI is the most sensitive technique for making the diagnosis.

Perronne C, et al. Pyogenic and tuberculous spondylodiskitis (vertebral osteomyelitis) in 80 adult patients. *Clin Infect Dis* 1994;19:746–750.

This retrospective study demonstrated that almost 40% of patients had tuberculous disease, based primarily on the population that was studied. This investigation establishes need for a careful epidemiologic history. Cases caused by both tuberculosis and S. aureus were associated with histories of prior active infection, which could help the clinician in making the diagnosis. In this study, more than 50% of patients with pyogenic disease had positive blood cultures, whereas about 75% had positive bone aspirate cultures.

Sapico RL, Montgomerie JZ. Vertebral osteomyelitis. *Infect Dis Clin North Am* 1990;4:539–550.

The authors review data on the diagnosis, bacteriology, and management of vertebral osteomyelitis. They rightfully conclude that diagnosis may be subtle, and all attempts should be made to isolate a pathogen rather than treat empirically.

Torda AJ, Gottlieb T, Bradbury R. Pyogenic vertebral osteomyelitis: analysis of 20 cases and review. *Clin Infect Dis* 1995;20:320–328.

This investigation demonstrated that most patients were elderly, and only 30% reported with fever. Nosocomial infection, often associated with intravenous cannula use and MRSA, was common. MRI and CT scan were the most useful radiographic modalities.

Turner DPJ, Weston VC, Ispahani P. Streptococcus pneumoniae spinal infection in Nottingham, United Kingdom: not a rare event. *Clin Infect Dis* 1999;28:873–881.

The authors identified eight cases of Streptococcus pneumoniae *back infection in 8 years, three of which were vertebral osteomyelitis. Literature review revealed an additional 20 patients with spinal infection, most of whom had vertebral osteomyelitis. A variety of predispositions were identified; presentation was often acute and was associated with infective endocarditis or meningitis. Unusual organisms occasionally may be noted in vertebral osteomyelitis.*

INFECTIONS OF PROSTHETIC JOINTS

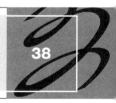

38

$\mathcal{T}$otal hip and knee replacements are frequent orthopedic procedures, with about 600,000 arthroplasties performed each year in the United States. Infection is the most dreaded complication of joint replacement operations. For most series, the overall infection rate after total hip or shoulder replacement is 1%. The rate of infection after knee replacement is higher—2%. The rate of infection is still higher for certain types of prostheses, such as a metal-hinged knee (11%). Infection is more likely to develop after total joint arthroplasty in patients with rheumatoid arthritis or who have had prior surgery than in those who have underlying osteoarthritis or are undergoing a primary operation. Although the overall infection rate after hip replacement is low (approximately 1%), more than 1,000 infected patients are seen annually in the United States.

Prosthetic joint infections can be classified as early (within the first 3 months after replacement), delayed (after 3 months to 2 years), and late (after 2 years). In the early category, most of the infections occur within the first month after operation. The majority (67%) of prosthetic infections are detected within the first 2 years after replacement, and about one-third of patients are seen with late infections after 2 years. Underreporting of late infections may occur; moreover, the potential for late infections persists indefinitely. Infections that develop within the first 2 years are largely the result of contamination of the prosthetic joint or wound at the time of replacement or of other nosocomial events, such as undetected line-related bacteremias. Infections that occur after 2 years are the result of hematogenous seeding from an infected focus, such as a distant cellulitis, a urinary tract infection, or, rarely, from a transient bacteremia related to a minor dental or surgical procedure. Late infections also can develop from very-low-grade infections initiated at the time of replacement or during the perioperative period. The proportion of late infections attributed to a hematogenous source compared with that of infections from other sources is debatable.

Early prosthetic joint infections often result from the contiguous spread of bacteria from a local wound infection to the prosthesis. The patient may have an obviously infected wound early in the postoperative period. Whether the infection is superficial and does not involve the prosthesis or is deep and does affect the joint replacement is often unclear. Surgical exploration of the wound may be required to establish the correct diagnosis. The patient also may have a painful hematoma that proves to be infected after it is aspirated. Frequently, joint pain is the prominent symptom, and the wound may appear entirely normal (no warmth, erythema, tenderness, or inflammation) or only slightly inflamed. Pain usually occurs with active and passive motion of the affected joint. Another clue to deep infection is persistent wound drainage. Fever is usually present.

The clinical presentation of delayed infection is more insidious, key findings being pain on bearing weight and motion of the joint. Clues that usually indicate infection, such as inflammation, drainage, and fever, are often absent. Late infection is usually characterized by the acute onset of joint pain and fever after a long asymptomatic period after the initial surgery. The history may reveal an earlier distant focus of infection that may have been untreated. The diagnosis of an infected joint is frequently difficult to make and may be established only at reoperation. Pain, usually constant, is the hallmark of joint infection. The pain caused by mechanical loosening of the prosthesis is generally related to motion and weight bearing and is not present at rest.

A number of laboratory studies are used to support the clinical diagnosis of an infected prosthetic joint: WBC count, erythrocyte sedimentation rate (ESR), plain radiographs, sinogram, arthrogram, joint aspiration, technetium bone scan, and gallium and indium 111 scans. The WBC count in patients with infection is variable. An elevated ESR (>20 mm/hour) suggests infection if no other explanation for the increase, such as underlying rheumatoid arthritis, can be found. A normal ESR makes infection unlikely (3–11% of cases) but does not exclude it entirely. The ESR usually falls to 20 mm/hour at 6 months after an uncomplicated joint replacement. Serial plain radiographs are helpful in assessing the presence of infection. Deep infections may produce radiolucencies at the prosthesis–cement–bone interface. These changes of bone resorption may result from mechanical loosening of the prosthesis. Arthrography and sinography may provide useful information to establish the diagnosis of infection.

Aspiration of the joint is the most reliable test to diagnose infection. A Gram's stain should be performed, and the aspirate should be cultured aerobically and anaerobically, along with fungi and mycobacteria in selected cases. Positive results on technetium bone, gallium, and indium 111 scans suggest infection; however, with mechanical loosening of the prosthesis, results of the gallium scan are normal, and the technetium bone scan result is abnormal.

Another approach to differentiate infection from mechanical loosening of the prosthesis is to obtain five biopsy samples for culture. Bacterial growth in one or two cultures indicates contamination, and growth in all five samples suggests infection. Growth in both solid and broth media indicates infection; growth only in broth medium indicates contamination.

Staphylococci are the most common cause of prosthetic joint infections, accounting for at least 30 to 40% of all infections. The most common infecting organism is *Staphylococcus coagulase* negative (30 to 43%) followed by *S. aureus* (12 to 23%). *S. epidermidis* infection usually appears as an indolent infection, causing minimal symptoms and signs. The symptoms and signs of *S. aureus* infection can vary from fulminant sepsis to an indolent infection. Because *S. epidermidis* also is a frequent cause of contamination of culture specimens, more than one isolate is needed to confirm this as the etiologic agent.

After staphylococci, streptococci (10%) and gram-negative bacilli, such as *Escherichia coli*, *Proteus* species, *Enterobacter* species, and *Pseudomonas aeruginosa*, account for 3 to 6% of infections. Gram-negative bacilli are more common in the early-onset period than in late-onset infections. Genitourinary and gastrointestinal tract procedures or infections are associated with gram-negative prosthetic infections. Other organisms that are implicated less often include anaerobic streptococci, *Propionibacterium acnes*, and, rarely, fungi or mycobacteria. Anaerobes account for about 4% of cases, and in about 10% of patients, all cultures are negative despite clinical evidence of infection. Cultures can be negative because of prior administration of antimicrobials and, occasionally, inadequate bacteriologic techniques. Polymicrobial infections can also occur.

A number of studies address the problems of treating prosthetic joint infections. If the patient has an early-onset infection, the prosthesis can be left in place if, during surgical procedures, there is no evidence of loosening of the device. Adequate debridement should be performed, and appropriate antimicrobials, depending on the results of culture and sensitivity testing, must be given parenterally for 6 weeks. Most studies report better results with gram-positive than with gram-negative bacilli.

A loose hip prosthesis can be replaced with a new one even when infection is present. This procedure is limited to gram-positive infections, and a favorable outcome is reported in up to 85% of selected patients. Appropriate antimicrobials should then be continued for 6 weeks. Some authorities favor surgical debridement of the wound, removal of the prosthesis, a subsequent 6-week course of parenteral antimicrobials, and then reimplantation of another joint. If reimplantation is not possible, an excision arthroplasty and prolonged antimicrobial suppression can be attempted. In delayed infections, salvage of the prosthetic hip is rare, and the prosthesis should be removed at the time of the debridement. An attempt can be made to save the hip prosthesis in patients with acute hematogenous joint infection. Some patients (30%) can be cured with debridement and prolonged parenteral antimicrobials. In the majority of these patients, however, either removal and a reimplantation procedure or an excision arthroplasty is required.

The management of prosthetic knee infections is similar to that of hip infections. If the prosthesis is not loose and the etiologic agent is a gram-positive organism, then debridement and parenteral antimicrobials may be adequate. More often, however, the prosthesis must be removed.

Administering antimicrobials to prevent late-onset joint infection in patients who undergo procedures involving dental or genitourinary tract manipulation, which causes a transient bacteremia, is controversial. Most late-onset infections in patients with rheumatoid arthritis result from hematogenous seeding of a joint from established distant foci of infection. Examples of these infections are skin abscesses and urinary tract infections. Prompt treatment of these infections with appropriate antimicrobials prevents hematogenous seeding and subsequent joint infection. The risk for hematogenous seeding of a prosthetic joint from a transient bacteremia, such as that caused by a dental cleaning, appears to be extremely low. In one report, the risk associated with dental procedures was 0.05%, so low that the cost to prevent a single case of joint infection would be high. Legal issues must also be considered in such situations. Because most late-onset infections result from established infections, patients should be treated promptly when infections are present.

An advisory committee of the American Dental Association and American Academy of Orthopaedic Surgeons has formulated guidelines to determine the need for antibiotic prophylaxis to prevent hematogenous prosthetic joint infections in patients undergoing a procedure such as a dental extraction. The panel of experts has suggested that antibiotics are not necessary for patients undergoing a dental procedure if they have a pin, plate, or screw, or for most patients with a total joint replacement. Patients who are at increased risk for hematogenous joint infection and who should receive antibiotic prophylaxis include those who are immunosuppressed (e.g., rheumatoid arthritis or systemic lupus erythematosus), have had a joint replacement within the previous 2 years, have had previous prosthetic joint infections, or have diabetes and are receiving insulin. These patients should receive a single dose of amoxicillin, or a cephalosporin such as cephalexin or cefazolin, or clindamycin if they are allergic to penicillin. In addition to antibiotic prophylaxis to prevent hematogenous seeding of a prosthetic joint, maintenance of good oral health is critical. (NMG)

Bibliography

Ainscow DAP, Denham RA. The risk of hematogenous infection in total joint replacement. *J Bone Joint Surg Br* 1984;66:580.
  Patients with rheumatoid arthritis are at increased risk for development of hematogenous infection of a prosthetic joint.
American Academy of Orthopaedic Surgeons. Antibiotic prophylaxis for dental patients with total joint replacements. Document no 1014. Available at: http://www.aaos.org/wordhtml/papers/advistmt/1014.htm. Accessed September 17, 2004.
  Guidelines for prophylaxis.
Anonymous. Advisory statement. Antibiotic prophylaxis for dental patients with total joint replacements. American Dental Association; American Academy of Orthopaedic Surgeons. *J Am Dent Assoc* 1997;128:1004–1008.
  Antibiotic prophylaxis is not indicated for patients with pins, plates, and screws or for most patients with total joint replacements who are undergoing a dental procedure, such as an extraction.
Bernard L, Lübbeke A, Stern R. Value of preoperative investigations in diagnosing prosthetic joint infection: retrospective cohort study and literature review. *Scand J Infect Dis* 2004;36:410–416.
  An elevated C-reactive protein (≥10 mg/L) and joint aspiration were the best tests to diagnose infection.
Booth RE Jr, Lotke PA. The results of spacer block technique in revision of infected total knee arthroplasty. *Clin Orthop* 1989;248:57.
  Describes use of a tobramycin-impregnated polymethylmethacrylate spacer block to treat infection locally during the exchange interval.
Bose WJ, et al. Long-term outcome of 42 knees with chronic infection after total knee arthroplasty. *Clin Orthop* 1995;319:285–296.
  The overall success rate was 74%. Use of a two-stage reimplantation procedure was most effective.
Brandt CM, et al. *Staphylococcus aureus* prosthetic joint infection treated with debridement and prosthesis retention. *Clin Infect Dis* 1997;24:914–919.
  Debridement of an infected prosthetic joint without replacement has a high failure rate (69%).
Buechel FF, Femino FP, D'Alessio J. Primary exchange revision arthroplasty for infected total knee replacement: a long-term study. *Am J Orthop* 2004;33:190–198.
  Favors a single stage procedure followed by prolonged antibiotic therapy orally for 6 to 12 months.
Darouiche RO. Treatment of infections associated with surgical implants. *N Engl J Med* 2004;350:1422–1429.
  Review. Four surgical approaches include joint debridement plus retention of the prosthesis, removal of the prosthesis without replacement, one-stage replacement, and two-stage replacement.
Forster IW, Crawford R. Sedimentation rate in infected and uninfected total hip arthroplasty. *Clin Orthop* 1982;168:48.
  An elevated sedimentation rate suggests infection rather than aseptic loosening of the prosthesis.
Goksan SB, Freeman MAR. One-stage reimplantation for infected total knee arthroplasty. *J Bone Joint Surg Br* 1992;74-B:78.

In a small series of infected knee prostheses caused by gram-positive organisms, a one-stage exchange procedure was effective in eradicating the infection.

Goldman RT, Scuderi GR, Insall JN. Two-stage reimplantation for infected total knee replacement. *Clin Orthop* 1996;331:118–124.

Infected prosthetic knees responded (77%) to an approach with three phases: (a) removal of the prosthesis and debridement, (b) 6 weeks of antibiotics, and (c) reimplantation with a new knee.

Giulieri SG, Graber P, Ochsner PE. Management of infection associated with total hip arthroplasty according to a treatment algorithm. *Infection* 2004;32:222–228.

Treatment guidelines.

Hanssen AD, Spangehl MJ. Treatment of the infected hip replacement. *Clin Orthop* 2004;420:63–71.

Review of management.

Inman RD, et al. Clinical and microbial features of prosthetic joint infection. *Am J Med* 1984;77:47.

Presenting symptoms included pain (95%), fever (43%), swelling (38%), and drainage (32%).

Kamme C, Lindberg L. Aerobic and anaerobic bacteria in deep infections after total hip arthroplasty. *Clin Orthop* 1981;154:201.

A normal sedimentation rate does not exclude infection.

Lachiewicz PF, Rogers GD, Thomason HC. Aspiration of the hip joint before revision total hip arthroplasty. Clinical and laboratory factors influencing attainment of a positive culture. *J Bone Joint Surg Am* 1996;78-A;749–754.

In patients with a high sedimentation rate (mean of 80 mm/hour), aspiration of the hip joint was helpful in predicting infection (sensitivity of 92%).

Levine BR, Evans BG. Use of blood culture vial specimens in intraoperative detection of infection. *Clin Orthop Rel Res* 2001;382:222–231.

Favors injecting joint aspirates into blood culture bottles rather than submitting swabs to diagnose infection.

McDonald DJ, Fitzgerald RH Jr, Ilstrup DM. Two-stage reconstruction of a total hip arthroplasty because of infection. *J Bone Joint Surg Am* 1989;71-A:828.

The rate of recurrence was lower for patients who had a reimplantation more than 1 year after the resection arthroplasty. For gram-negative bacilli and enterococci, antimicrobial therapy should be given for at least 28 days.

Pagnano MW, Trousdale RT, Hanssen AD. Outcome after reinfection following reimplantation hip arthroplasty. *Clin Orthop* 1997;338:192–204.

Patients in whom infection develops after reimplantation of a new prosthesis are candidates for an attempt at a third prosthesis in which a two-stage approach is used (success rate of 27%).

Pellegrini VD Jr. Management of the patient with an infected knee arthroplasty. *Instr Course Lect* 1997;46:215–219.

Review. Factors that predispose patients to infection include use of steroids, rheumatoid disease, prior knee surgery, and the presence of open skin lesions on the affected leg.

Rao N, et al. Long-term suppression of infection in total joint arthroplasty. *Clin Orthop Rel Res* 2003;414:55–60.

Long-term antibiotic suppression is useful for patients with an infected prosthesis when joint removal is not feasible.

Salvati EA, et al. Infection rates after 3,175 total hip and knee replacements performed with and without a horizontal unidirectional filtered air-flow system. *J Bone Joint Surg Am* 1982;64:525.

Infection rates were 0.9% after total hip replacement and 3.9% after total knee replacement.

Scher DM, et al. The predictive value of Indium-111 leukocyte scans in the diagnosis of infected total hip, knee, or resection arthroplasties. *J Arthroplasty* 2000;15:295–300.

Sensitivity of Indium-111 scan was 77% and specificity 86% in diagnosing infection.

Somme D, et al. Contribution of routine joint aspiration to the diagnosis of infection before hip revision surgery. *Joint Bone Spine* 2003;70:489–495.
Routine hip aspiration before surgery had a sensitivity of 83% and specificity of 100% in diagnosing infection.

Tsukayama DT, Goldberg VM, Kyle R. Diagnosis and management of infection after total knee arthroplasty. *J Bone Joint Surg* 2003;85-A:75–80.
Biofilms produced by bacteria are a major factor in pathogenesis.

Wilson MG, Kelley K, Thornhill TS. Infection as a complication of total knee-replacement arthroplasty. *J Bone Joint Surg Am* 1990;72:878–883.
Infection occurred in 1.6% of patients after knee replacement arthroplasty. Risk factors associated with infection included underlying rheumatoid arthritis, presence of skin ulcers, and prior surgery.

Zimmerli W, Trampuz A, Ochsner PE. Prosthetic-joint infections. *N Engl J Med* 2004; 351:1645–1654.
Review.

Zimmerli W, et al. Role of rifampin for treatment of orthopedic implant-related staphylococcal infections: a randomized controlled trial. Foreign-Body Infection (FBI) Study Group. *JAMA* 1998;279:1537–1541.
In selected patients with staphylococcal infections and early-onset infection, rifampin plus ciprofloxacin for 3 to 6 months after an initial debridement was effective without removal of the implant.

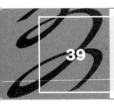

39   FEVER AND JOINT PAIN

Joint effusion is a common problem and a diagnostic challenge because septic arthritis is a medical emergency. Failure to establish an early diagnosis and administer appropriate therapy may lead to loss of joint function or death. The differential diagnosis in a patient with one or more warm, swollen joints is extensive and includes both infectious and noninfectious causes. Bacteria (including mycobacteria), viruses, and fungi are all among the infectious causes.

Bacterial arthritis can be classified as gonococcal or nongonococcal. The frequency distribution of organisms depends on differences in the population studied, such as location (city hospital vs. suburban community hospital), patient age, and the presence of an underlying illness. At one city hospital, approximately 60% of the patients with septic arthritis had gonococcal infection. This finding contrasts with the distribution in a community hospital, where nongonococcal disease predominates. In recent years, there appears to have been a decrease in the incidence of gonococcal arthritis. Of the nongonococcal causes, *Staphylococcus aureus* is seen most often and accounts for 30 to 50% of cases. This is followed by various species of streptococci (25%), including groups A, B, and G. Gram-negative bacilli have emerged as an important cause (20%) and are responsible for disease, particularly in IV drug users and immunosuppressed patients. *Pseudomonas aeruginosa* tends to affect drug users and often attacks the sternoclavicular joint. *Streptococcus pneumoniae* is an infrequent cause of septic arthritis and accounts for 5% of cases. Pneumococcal arthritis usually results from bacteremic seeding of a joint in a patient with pneumococcal pneumonia or another focus of infection. *Haemophilus influenzae* was formerly a common cause of septic arthritis in infants and young children but only infrequently produces disease in children and adults (<1%).

A number of viruses are associated with arthritis, the most frequent causes being hepatitis B virus, hepatitis C virus, rubella virus, mumps virus, parvovirus B19, HIV, and arbovirus. A painful, subacute, oligoarthritic syndrome involving the knees and ankles has been described in patients with AIDS. The pathogenesis is unknown. Other musculoskeletal disorders that have been reported in association with HIV infection include Reiter's syndrome, psoriatic arthritis, and avascular necrosis of bone.

Fungal and tuberculous causes of joint pain are rarer. Lyme disease, rheumatic fever, subacute bacterial endocarditis, Whipple's disease, and *Yersinia enterocolitica* infection are other infectious causes. Lyme disease is possible in a patient with a sudden onset of monoarthritis or oligoarthritis. Joint pains are usually preceded by the characteristic skin lesion, erythema chronicum migrans, in 60 to 70% of patients. The interval between appearance of the skin lesion and start of the joint symptoms is approximately 4 weeks, with a range of 0.6 to 24 weeks. The knee is the joint most often affected, followed by the shoulder. The arthritis usually lasts 1 week, but attacks recur frequently. A chronic arthritis, usually of the knees, is reported in 10% of patients. Serologic testing is an invaluable aid in the diagnosis, as most patients will have an increased IgG antibody titer to *Borrelia burgdorferi*. The synovial fluid is inflamed, with a median white blood cell (WBC) count of $25,000/mm^3$. Most of the cells are polymorphonuclear leukocytes. Oral doxycycline or amoxicillin for 1 month is recommended for Lyme arthritis. Two grams of ceftriaxone per day given intravenously or high-dose penicillin administered intravenously for 2 to 3 weeks is also effective. Intra-articular steroid injections should be avoided because they may increase the risk for antimicrobial failure.

Joint pain of noninfectious causes, such as the inflammatory diseases (gout, pseudogout, rheumatoid arthritis, Reiter's syndrome, psoriatic arthritis, collagen diseases), and the arthritis of ulcerative colitis, or regional enteritis, can mimic septic arthritis. Hemarthrosis, secondary to hemophilia or other hemorrhagic disorders, and trauma, such as an auto accident, should also be considered.

Organisms reach the synovium and joint space by one of three routes: direct introduction, extension from a contiguous focus, or hematogenous spread. Direct involvement can occur after trauma, surgery, or, rarely, the intra-articular injection of steroids. Spread from an overlying cellulitis or from an adjacent osteomyelitis is an example of a contiguous focus as the source. Hematogenous seeding of the synovium occurs most often. With a hematogenous origin, an extra-articular focus may be present. For example, a patient with pneumococcal arthritis may have pneumonia, or the organism may be found in the cervix or pharynx of a woman with disseminated gonococcal arthritis. A careful search for a bacterial source is often rewarding.

Factors that predispose the host to septic arthritis include damaged joints from prior rheumatoid arthritis, diabetes mellitus, cirrhosis, neoplasms, immunosuppressive therapy, and extra-articular foci of infection. The factors that permit an organism such as the gonococcus to infect a joint space during dissemination are unknown. The joint symptoms in patients with gonococcal disease often appear as a result of immune system processes.

Clinically, the onset of bacterial arthritis is usually abrupt. The symptoms include chills, fever, and monoarthritis with warmth, redness, swelling, and tenderness. Polyarthritis occurs in about 10% of patients. Any joint can be affected, but the large joints are the main targets, especially the knees, ankles, and wrists. The sternoclavicular joint may be infected in IV drug users or as a rare complication of subclavian venous catheterization, and the hip or sacroiliac joints can become infected in patients with inflammatory bowel disease; however, these joints are less commonly involved. The presentation can be cryptic in patients with rheumatoid arthritis and in infants, who may show only irritability and immobility. Patients with bacterial arthritis of the hip may have only knee pain.

The gonococcus is a common cause of septic arthritis in adults. Two forms are known, although overlap can occur. The disease usually occurs in young, healthy women, and it typically begins during the menses, pregnancy, or early postpartum period. An asymptomatic genital, pharyngeal, or rectal infection is the usual source. In one form, symptoms are chills, fever, migratory polyarthritis, and characteristic skin lesions. Tenosynovitis may occur and strongly suggests a gonococcal origin. Blood cultures are positive in 20% of patients, but little synovial fluid is present, and the results of a joint culture are often negative.

Monoarthritis occurs in the other form, and the gonococcus is usually isolated from the joint fluid.

Synovial fluid analysis is the critical test for establishing the cause of an arthritis. Typical results of this analysis of a pyogenic joint infection are a WBC count of 50,000 to 100,000/mm^3 with 90% neutrophils, a poor mucin clot, and a sugar concentration at least 50 mg/dL below that of the blood sugar; occasionally, the joint fluid WBC count may be as low as 10,000/mm^3. A Gram's stain of a sediment is necessary for a diagnosis. The use of polymerase chain reaction may yield a diagnosis. Blood cultures, Gram's stains, and cultures for the gonococcus or meningococcus from other sites of infection, particularly the throat, cervix, rectum, and skin pustules, may be helpful. Synovial fluid should be plated on blood and chocolate agar and immediately incubated in 10% carbon dioxide for both aerobes and anaerobes. Thayer-Martin medium is not used, as it inhibits bacteria other than the gonococcus. Acid-fast stains, synovial biopsy, and cultures are performed if mycobacteria and fungi are suspected. Results of joint roentgenography are negative in septic arthritis unless an associated osteomyelitis is present.

Treatment consists of drainage and administration of antimicrobials directed toward the specific organism. The initial antimicrobial therapy should be guided by the patient's age and underlying disease, as well as the results of the synovial fluid Gram's stain. Needle aspirations must be repeated whenever the effusions reaccumulate to prevent cartilage destruction by leukocytic enzymes and debris. Open drainage is indicated for all hip joint infections, often for the shoulder joint, and when closed drainage does not permit adequate removal of the fluid because of adhesions and loculation. Arthroscopic techniques may be used for debridement as an alternative to the open arthrotomy. Intra-articular antimicrobial injections are unnecessary and may result in chemical synovitis.

The effectiveness of therapy can be judged by the clinical response and serial synovial fluid analyses. Physical therapy is instituted to maintain joint function. The joint fluid should become sterile after a few days, the WBC count should decrease progressively, and the sugar concentration should rise. The outcome depends on the duration of symptoms before treatment, the infecting organism, and the nature of the patient's underlying illness. The prognosis is poor in patients whose symptoms have been present for more than 5 days before initiation of antimicrobial therapy and in those with infections caused by gram-negative bacilli or staphylococci. Rapid improvement without sequelae can be expected in patients with gonococcal arthritis after 24 to 48 hours of therapy. Any warm, swollen joint should be considered infected until proved otherwise, and it should be treated as a medical emergency to avoid complications. (NMG)

Bibliography

Amirault JD. Septic arthritis in the elderly. *Clin Orthop* 1990;215:241.
Most patients were afebrile and had a normal WBC count.

Bayer AS, et al. Gram-negative bacillary septic arthritis: clinical, radiographic, therapeutic, and prognostic features. *Semin Arthritis Rheum* 1977;7:123.
Sternoclavicular joint involvement in heroin addicts was caused by P. aeruginosa.

Black J, et al. Oral antimicrobial therapy for adults with osteomyelitis or septic arthritis. *J Infect Dis* 1987;155:968.
A small series reporting the successful use of oral antimicrobials to treat osteomyelitis or septic arthritis in adults while monitoring trough serum bactericidal titers.

Borenstein DG, Simon GL. *Haemophilus influenzae* septic arthritis in adults: a report of four cases and a review of the literature. *Medicine (Baltimore)* 1986;65:191.
Although uncommon, septic arthritis is suspect in an immunocompromised host with an extra-articular focus of H. influenzae *infection.*

Bronze MS, Whitby S, Schaberg DR. Group G streptococcal arthritis: case report and review of the literature. *Am J Med Sci* 1997;313:239–243.
A rare cause of septic arthritis.

Ellis LC, et al. Joint infections due to *Listeria monocytogenes*: case report and review. *Clin Infect Dis* 1995;20:1548–1550.
A rare cause of septic arthritis, usually seen in renal transplant recipients or patients with rheumatoid arthritis.

García-De La Torre I. Advances in the management of septic arthritis. *Rheum Dis Clin N Am* 2003;29:61–75.
Review.

Gardner GC, Weisman MH. Pyarthrosis in patients with rheumatoid arthritis: a report of 13 cases and a review of the literature from the past 40 years. *Am J Med* 1990;88: 503.
S. aureus is the most common infecting organism, and the skin is often the source.

Garrido G, et al. A review of peripheral tuberculous arthritis. *Semin Arthritis Rheum* 1988;18:142.
Review.

Goldenberg DL. Infectious arthritis complicating rheumatoid arthritis and other chronic rheumatic disorders. *Arthritis Rheum* 1989;32:496.
Diagnosis is often delayed. Twenty percent of patients had polyarticular septic arthritis.

Hansen BL, Andersen K. Fungal arthritis. A review. *Scand J Rheumatol* 1995;24: 248–250.
Candida is the most frequent fungal cause of septic arthritis.

Hirsch R, et al. Human immunodeficiency virus-associated atypical mycobacterial skeletal infections. *Semin Arthritis Rheum* 1996;25:347–356.
Consider atypical mycobacteria in HIV patients with septic arthritis and a CD4 cell count below 100/mm³.

Hollander JL. Examination of synovial fluid as a diagnostic aid in arthritis. *Med Clin North Am* 1966;50:1281.
A discussion of synovial fluid analysis.

Krey PR, Bailen DA. Synovial fluid leukocytosis: a study of extremes. *Am J Med* 1979; 67:436.
Search for crystals in synovial fluid with high as well as low cell counts.

Laster AJ, Michels ML. Group B streptococcal arthritis in adults. *Am J Med* 1984; 76:910.
A rare cause of septic arthritis.

Lawson JP, Rahn DW. Lyme disease and radiologic findings in Lyme arthritis. *AJR Am J Roentgenol* 1992;158:1065.
Joint effusion involving the knee is the most common radiologic manifestation of Lyme arthritis.

Nade S. Septic arthritis. *Best Pract Res Clin Rheumatol* 2003;17:183–200.
Review. Staphylococcus aureus is the most common infecting organism in all age groups.

Nelson JD. Antibiotic concentrations in septic joint effusions. *N Engl J Med* 1971;284:349.
The penicillins and cephalothin penetrate into joint fluid.

O'Brien JP, Goldenberg DL, Rice PA. Disseminated gonococcal infection: a prospective analysis of 49 patients and a review of pathophysiology and immune mechanisms. *Medicine (Baltimore)* 1983;62:395.
More than 60% of patients had tenosynovitis and more than 70% had skin lesions. N. gonorrhoeae was isolated in half the joint effusions.

Phillips PE. Viral arthritis. *Curr Opin Rheumatol* 1997;9:337–344.
Update on viruses, particularly parvovirus B19, rubella virus, and hepatitis viruses B and C as causes of acute arthritis.

Rahman MU, Shenberger KN, Schumacher HR Jr. Initially unrecognized calcium pyrophosphate dihydrate deposition disease as a cause of fever. *Am J Med* 1990; 89:115.
Pseudogout can mimic septic arthritis when fever is present.

Rahn DW, Malawista SE. Lyme disease: recommendations for diagnosis and treatment. *Ann Intern Med* 1991;114:472.
Reviews diagnostic methods and therapy.

Rompalo AM, et al. The acute arthritis-dermatitis syndrome: the changing importance of *Neisseria gonorrhoeae* and *Neisseria meningitidis*. *Arch Intern Med* 1987;147:281.
Consider N. meningitidis as well as N. gonorrhoeae as a cause of the acute arthritis-dermatitis syndrome. A decrease in the incidence of disseminated gonococcal infection was noted.

Ross JJ, Hu LT. Septic arthritis of the pubic symphysis. *Medicine* 2003;82:340-345.
Most patients also had osteomyelitis of the symphysis pubis.

Ross JJ, Saltzman CL, Carling P. Pneumococcal septic arthritis: review of 190 cases. *Clin Infect Dis* 2003;36:319–327.

Only 50% of adults with pneumococcal septic arthritis had another focus such as pneumonia.

Ross JJ, Shamsuddin H. Sternoclavicular septic arthritis review of 180 cases. *Medicine* 2004;83:139–148.
Staphylococcus aureus was the cause of half the infections and the major pathogen in intravenous drug users.

Sack K. Monoarthritis: differential diagnosis. *Am J Med* 1997;102:30S–34S.
Review. Acute monoarthritis should be regarded as infectious until an arthrocentesis excludes the diagnosis.

Sapico FL, Liquete JA, Sarma RJ. Bone and joint infections in patients with infective endocarditis: review of a 4-year experience. *Clin Infect Dis* 1996;22:783–787.
About half (44%) the patients with endocarditis will have musculoskeletal complaints.

Shirtliff ME, Mader JT. Acute septic arthritis. *Clin Microbiol Rev* 2002;15:527–544.
Review of pathogenesis, diagnosis, and treatment. Most infections result from hematogenous seeding of a joint.

Steere AC. Diagnosis and treatment of Lyme arthritis. *Med Clin North Am* 1997;81:179–194.
Lyme arthritis usually involves the knee and responds to a 2-month course of oral doxycycline or amoxicillin.

Steere AC, Schoen RT, Taylor E. The clinical evolution of Lyme arthritis. *Ann Intern Med* 1987;107:725.
In approximately 10% of patients with untreated Lyme arthritis, chronic synovitis develops later in the illness.

Steere AC, et al. Erythema chronicum migrans and Lyme arthritis. The enlarging clinical spectrum. *Ann Intern Med* 1977;86:685.
Onset is usually in the summer, with the characteristic skin lesion.

Syrogiannopoulos GA, Nelson JD. Duration of antimicrobial therapy for acute suppurative osteoarticular infections. *Lancet* 1988;1:37.
In children, a shorter duration of therapy is often effective.

Taillandier J, et al. *Aspergillus* osteomyelitis after heart-lung transplantation. *J Heart Lung Transplant* 1997;16:436–438.
A rare complication of solid-organ transplantation.

Vyskocil JJ, et al. Pyogenic infection of the sacroiliac joint: case reports and review of the literature. *Medicine (Baltimore)* 1991;70:188.
Pyogenic sacroiliitis is usually unilateral, and diagnosis depends on fine-needle aspiration of the joint under fluoroscopic guidance or during open biopsy.

Yagupsky P. *Kingella kingae*: from medical rarity to an emerging paediatric pathogen. *Lancet Infect Dis* 2004;4:358–367.
A short gram-negative rod, which is a cause of septic arthritis in children.

Zimmermann B 3rd, Mikolich DJ, Lally EV. Septic sacroiliitis. *Semin Arthritis Rheum* 1996;26:592–604.
MRI is useful in diagnosing septic sacroiliac joint arthritis.

Skin and Soft Tissue

IX

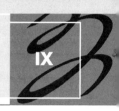

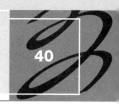

*L*yme disease is a multisystem disease with protean manifestations. The illness was brought to attention in 1977 when it was thought that the "juvenile rheumatoid arthritis" of a group of children in Lyme, Connecticut, had an infectious cause. Subsequent studies identified *Ixodes* ticks as vectors of the disease, and in 1982, a spirochete, now called *Borrelia burgdorferi*, was isolated from *Ixodes scapularis* (formerly *Ixodes dammini*). Features of the illness were recognized in Europe early in this century.

Lyme disease is the most commonly reported tick-borne disease in the United States. Cases have been reported from all states except Montana, although the disease is regional, with more than 90% of cases reported from the northeastern states, Maryland, Wisconsin, Missouri, and California. The disorder has also been noted in Europe, China, Japan, Australia, and the former Soviet Union. Cases have been reported worldwide except in the Antarctic.

Although the disorder is not rare, confusion exists for most clinicians regarding the diagnosis. For every case of Lyme disease that is diagnosed, it is estimated that 50 to 100 serologic tests for Lyme disease are performed. A number of factors have contributed to the diagnostic dilemma for clinicians and confusion for patients. First, unlike most bacterial infections, Lyme disease is not diagnosed by isolation of the etiologic agent or demonstration of the antigen or organism by special stains in tissue. Second, the clinical features are protean and may mimic those of several other diseases. The pathognomonic skin lesion, erythema migrans, which develops at the site of the tick bite, is absent in one-third of patients. Third, confusion exists regarding the interpretation of a positive or negative result of the serologic test for Lyme disease antibody. Clinicians believe that a positive Lyme disease test result alone confirms the diagnosis. A positive Lyme serology may be a false-positive because of cross-reacting antibodies; alternatively, it may indicate past infection with *B. burgdorferi* or suggest active infection. Elevated antibody titers may persist for years with or without therapy and do not indicate the presence of an active infection that requires antimicrobial therapy. A false-negative serologic test result may be seen early in the illness because the antibody response may not appear until 3 to 6 weeks after the tick bite. Antimicrobial therapy also can diminish the antibody response, resulting in a false-negative serologic test result. Finally, confusion exists regarding how to manage a patient who reports a tick bite and is concerned about the development of Lyme disease.

Lyme disease can be classified into early and late infection. Early infection can be further subdivided into localized infection (stage 1) or disseminated infection (stage 2). Erythema migrans is the hallmark of early localized disease. The rash usually occurs 3 to 32 days (median, 7 days) after the initial tick bite. The rash is described as an annular, expanding, erythematous lesion with central clearing that is at least 5 cm in diameter. The center of the lesion may become vesicular and necrotic or remain erythematous. Secondary annular skin lesions occur in half the patients. These lesions resemble those of erythema migrans. The skin lesions usually fade within 3 to 4 weeks, even if untreated. Fever and minor constitutional symptoms, such as malaise and fatigue or regional lymphadenopathy, may accompany the classic skin rash. It is extremely difficult to diagnose Lyme disease in a patient with flulike symptoms alone without a rash because the serology is usually negative at this time.

Manifestations of early disseminated disease may involve the nervous, cardiovascular, or musculoskeletal system. The spectrum of neurologic disease includes lymphocytic meningitis; cranial neuritis, such as Bell's palsy; radiculoneuropathy; or, rarely, encephalomyelitis.

Bell's palsy is the most common cranial neuropathy. Headache, paresthesia, and a mild stiff neck alone are not accepted as criteria for the diagnosis of neurologic disease. Symptoms of musculoskeletal involvement can include migratory arthralgias, muscle and bone pain, and transient arthritis affecting the large joints, such as the knees. The arthritis usually begins 6 months after onset. Cardiac manifestations begin about 2 to 6 weeks after onset and include atrioventricular block and, less often, myocarditis or pericarditis. Syncope caused by cardiac conduction abnormality may be the presenting complaint. Late or persistent infection is manifested as a chronic arthritis, lasting a year or more, involving the knees; neurologic disorders, such as an encephalomyelitis; and a localized cutaneous disorder, acrodermatitis chronica atrophicans. Ocular abnormalities may occur as part of early disseminated disease.

Because it is difficult to culture the spirochete from most patients with Lyme disease, the diagnosis must rely heavily on the clinical presentation and epidemiologic clues. The diagnosis is often a challenge because laboratory support depends on detection of an immune response to the organism, which has the limitations already noted. Current methods of testing use mainly an enzyme-linked immunosorbent assay (ELISA) and Western blot (immunoblot) test. Specific IgM antibodies against the organism appear about 1 month after the onset, peak at 2 months, and then decline. Specific IgG antibodies are detectable in the second month and may remain elevated for life. Antibody levels decline with treatment but usually persist indefinitely. Antibody levels should not be monitored to indicate success or failure of therapy. Similarly, the presence of antibodies may indicate a previous infection, with the patient's acute symptoms having another cause. Serologic testing is not helpful to diagnose recurrent disease.

Immunoblot testing (Western blot) can support the diagnosis of Lyme disease, but a negative test result does not exclude the disorder. In early disease, an antibody response to a flagellar protein (flagellin) and to a fragment of this protein, designated as 41G, develops in some patients. In late disease, the antibody response is directed to outer-surface proteins A and B in addition to the flagellar proteins. Again, cross-reacting antibodies directed against other spirochetes can confuse the picture, and the clinician should discuss with the laboratory personnel the criteria used to classify a Western blot test as positive. Some laboratories require the presence of four or five bands on the Western blot to consider the result positive. Serologic tests for Lyme disease can easily be misinterpreted. A two-step approach is advised. The first step is to perform an ELISA or indirect immunofluorescence test. A positive or equivocal result should be followed by a Western blot assay. This second test is supplemental rather than confirmatory, because of suboptimal specificity. A negative test result does not exclude the diagnosis, and another sample should be obtained 1 month later.

In addition to antibody responses to infection, specific cellular immune responses occur. Other laboratory methods, such as the polymerase chain reaction (PCR), are still experimental. In one report in which material obtained by 2-mm skin biopsy was used, the sensitivity of the PCR was about 60%. These new methods may prove to be invaluable, considering the limitations of making the diagnosis by means of the various antibody tests.

The topic of Lyme disease has generated numerous questions from both clinicians and patients:

1. *How long must a tick be attached to transmit the disease?* In experimental studies, it is unlikely for ticks attached for less than 48 hours to transmit disease. It is important to prevent tick bites by using appropriate insect repellents and protective clothing. Ticks should be removed with a forceps.

2. *How would you interpret a positive ELISA or a positive immunoblot test?* A positive test result indicates possible exposure to *B. burgdorferi* but does not confirm active infection. The diagnosis of Lyme disease is a clinical one supported by laboratory studies.

3. *Does a negative serologic test result for Lyme disease exclude the diagnosis?* No. False-negative results occur mainly during the first several weeks of the illness. Late infection is usually associated with a positive serologic test result. Rarely, patients will have a negative serologic test for Lyme antibody with late infection.

4. *What are the causes of a false-positive serologic test result for Lyme antibody?* Causes of a false-positive Lyme serology include systemic lupus erythematosus, rheumatoid

arthritis, Rocky Mountain spotted fever, infectious mononucleosis, and various spirochetal diseases, such as syphilis, relapsing fever, and periodontal disease. Patients with Lyme disease will have a negative result on a nontreponemal test for syphilis, such as the VDRL test or rapid plasma reagin circle card test (RPR-CT), and may have a false-positive result on the fluorescent treponemal antibody absorption test (FTA-ABS) test. Another problem that should always be considered is the patient with an asymptomatic *B. burgdorferi* infection and a positive Lyme serologic test. In this situation, the patient's symptoms may be falsely attributed to Lyme disease because of the positive antibody test result, and the correct diagnosis is missed.

5. *Does Lyme disease cause chronic fatigue syndrome?* The diagnosis of chronic fatigue syndrome depends on excluding other diseases. The diagnosis of Lyme disease should not be searched for as a cause of fatigue unless a patient has epidemiologic evidence to suggest infection with *B. burgdorferi,* plus other clinical manifestations of Lyme disease. Rarely, chronic fatigue syndrome or fibromyalgia may develop in patients with treated Lyme disease. In patients with fibromyalgia triggered by prior Lyme disease, there is no evidence that antimicrobial therapy alters the course of the illness.

6. *Is there a role for prolonged antimicrobial therapy in a patient with Lyme disease?* Although the optimal therapy for Lyme disease is unknown, it appears that antimicrobials usually should be administered for 3 weeks to eradicate the organism. There is no evidence that antimicrobial therapy for longer than 30 days, even for patients with Lyme arthritis, provides any advantage. After therapy is started, patient symptoms may worsen because of a Jarisch-Herxheimer reaction. Oral therapy should be adequate for most infections, and IV therapy should be reserved for patients with well-documented chronic disease, such as Lyme arthritis, or disseminated disease with major organ involvement, such as Lyme carditis or Lyme meningitis.

7. *How should you manage someone in an endemic area who is asymptomatic and has a positive Lyme serology?* In endemic areas, rates of Lyme seropositivity may be as high as 22.5%. No data are available to indicate whether late complications of Lyme disease will develop in patients who are asymptomatic. The role of antimicrobials in this setting is unclear.

8. *What is the role for prophylactic antimicrobials to prevent Lyme disease after the bite of a deer tick?* The risk for acquiring Lyme disease, even in an endemic area, after a deer tick bite is low. Therefore, prophylactic antimicrobials usually are not indicated, but a single dose of doxycycline may be effective. One exception might be a pregnant patient, but this issue has not been studied.

9. *Is there a risk for transmitting* B. burgdorferi *infection to the fetus during pregnancy?* Although there is a potential for maternal-to-fetal transmission of *B. burgdorferi* during pregnancy, the risk appears to be extremely low. There is no need to screen for Lyme antibodies in asymptomatic women during pregnancy. However, suspected or documented cases of Lyme disease should be treated during pregnancy. Controlled studies are needed to assess the risk to the fetus associated with maternal Lyme disease.

10. *After a patient with Lyme disease is treated, should antibody titers be monitored to assess cure?* Antimicrobial therapy usually causes a decline in antibody levels against *B. burgdorferi.* However, the patient usually remains seropositive indefinitely, and repeated serologic testing is not indicated.

Despite a tremendous increase in our understanding of Lyme disease, controversies and confusion still exist regarding this illness. It is hoped that better answers to many questions concerning Lyme disease will be forthcoming. (NMG)

Bibliography

Agger W, et al. Lyme disease: clinical features, classification, and epidemiology in the upper Midwest. *Medicine (Baltimore)* 1991;70:83.
  Half the early cases and about 10% of the late cases recalled a tick bite. In the Midwest, onset of early disease occurred mainly from June through November.
Bunikis J, Barbour AG. Laboratory testing for suspected lyme disease. *Med Clin North Am* 2002;86:311–340.

A review of testing. The urine antigen assay has frequent false-positives.

Cox J, Krajden M. Cardiovascular manifestations of Lyme disease. *Am Heart J* 1991; 122:1449.
Atrioventricular block usually resolves within 6 weeks with antimicrobial therapy.

Coyle PK. *Borrelia burgdorferi* infection: clinical diagnostic techniques. *Immunol Invest* 1997;26:117–128.
Use a two-test approach for serologic diagnosis. If results of the enzyme immunoassay are positive, then obtain a Western immunoblot. (Order IgM immunoblot if the illness has been present less than 1 month; otherwise obtain an IgG immunoblot.)

Dinerman H, Steere AC. Lyme disease associated with fibromyalgia. *Ann Intern Med* 1992;117:281.
Fibromyalgia may develop in treated patients with Lyme disease; antimicrobials are not indicated for these patients.

Dressler F, et al. Western blotting in the serodiagnosis of Lyme disease. *J Infect Dis* 1993;167:392.
With the Western blot test, the sensitivity varied between 32 and 83%, and the specificity was 95 to 100%.

Dumler JS. Is human granulocytic ehrlichiosis a new Lyme disease? Review and comparison of clinical, laboratory, epidemiological, and some biological features. *Clin Infect Dis* 1997;25(suppl 1):S43–S47.
Although ehrlichiosis and Lyme disease are both transmitted by deer ticks (Ixodes scapularis), *leukopenia, thrombocytopenia, and abnormal hepatic transaminases occur with the former and are usually absent in Lyme disease.*

Feder HM Jr, Whitaker DL. Misdiagnosis of erythema migrans. *Am J Med* 1995;99:412–419.
A typical lesion of erythema migrans is annular, erythematous, and at least 5 cm in diameter, and it begins to develop 3 to 30 days after a tick bite.

Fikrig E, et al. Serologic diagnosis of Lyme disease using recombinant outer surface proteins A and B and flagellin. *J Infect Dis* 1992;165:1127.
Measurement of antibodies to outer-surface proteins A and B, flagellin, and region of flagellin (41G) from B. burgdorferi with an immunoblot and ELISA was useful in the serodiagnosis of Lyme disease.

Gerber MA, Shapiro ED. Diagnosis of Lyme disease in children. *J Pediatr* 1992;121:157.
A skin lesion that appears immediately after a tick bite, resolves within 1 to 2 days without appropriate antimicrobial therapy, and is less than 5 cm is unlikely to be erythema migrans.

Keller TL, Halperin JJ, Whitman M. PCR detection of *Borrelia burgdorferi* DNA in cerebrospinal fluid of Lyme neuroborreliosis patients. *Neurology* 1992;42:32.
PCR on cerebrospinal fluid is a useful method to detect B. burgdorferi. This test appears to be an alternative to the measurement of intrathecal production of specific Lyme antibody.

Klempner MS, et al. Two controlled trials of antibiotic treatment in patients with persistent symptoms and a history of lyme disease. *N Engl J Med* 2001;345:85–92.
Chronic Lyme disease is similar to chronic fatigue syndrome or fibromyalgia. Prolonged antibiotics had no effect on reducing symptoms.

Krause PJ, et al. Disease-specific diagnosis of coinfecting tickborne zoonoses: babesiosis, human granulocytic ehrlichiosis, and lyme disease. *Clin Infect Dis* 2002;34:1184–1191.
Consider a coinfection with Babesia or ehrlichia the cause of human granulocytic ehrlichiosis in a patient with treated Lyme disease and persistent symptoms.

Kuiper H, et al. Absence of Lyme borreliosis among patients with presumed Bell's palsy. *Arch Neurol* 1992;49:940.
Lyme disease was identified in 6% of patients with peripheral facial palsy, compared with a rate of 4.5% in controls. Screening for Lyme disease is not indicated in this setting unless other evidence suggests the diagnosis.

Lawson JP, Rahn DW. Lyme disease and radiologic findings in Lyme arthritis. *AJR Am J Roentgenol* 1992;58:1065.
The most frequent abnormality is a joint effusion involving the knee. Loss of cartilage occurs in about 25% of patients with chronic Lyme arthritis.

Luft BJ, et al. Invasion of the central nervous system by *Borrelia burgdorferi* in acute disseminated infection. *JAMA* 1992;267:1364.

In a small study, B. burgdorferi was identified in the cerebrospinal fluid of 67% of patients with early disseminated disease when a PCR assay was used.

Malane MS, et al. Diagnosis of Lyme disease based on dermatologic manifestations. *Ann Intern Med* 1991;114:490.

A review of the cutaneous lesions. Erythema migrans occurs in about 75% of patients with Lyme disease.

Nadelman RB, et al. Comparison of cefuroxime axetil and doxycycline in the treatment of early Lyme disease. *Ann Intern Med* 1992;117:273.

A 20-day course of cefuroxime axetil (500 mg twice daily) or doxycycline (100 mg three times daily) was effective in patients with early Lyme disease.

Nadelman RB, et al. Prophylaxis with single dose doxycycline for the prevention of Lyme disease after *Ixodes scapularis* tick bite. *N Engl J Med* 2001;348:2424–2430.

One dose (200 mg) of doxycycline, if given within 72 hours of a tick bite, will prevent Lyme disease in 87% of persons.

Pachner AR, Ricalton NS. Western blotting in evaluating Lyme seropositivity and the utility of a gel densitometric approach. *Neurology* 1992;42:2185.

Use of a quantitative Western blot test was helpful in establishing the diagnosis. Patients with secondary syphilis had positive results on immunoblots.

Rahn DW, Malawista SE. Lyme disease: recommendations for diagnosis and treatment. *Ann Intern Med* 1991;114:472.

A review of the national surveillance case definition for diagnosis and treatment guidelines.

Reid MC, et al. The consequences of overdiagnosis and overtreatment of Lyme disease: an observational study. *Ann Intern Med* 1998;128:354–362.

Of a group of referred patients with presumptive Lyme disease, only 21% met criteria for active Lyme disease. Most positive results on serologic tests for Lyme disease are false positives.

Schwartz I, et al. Diagnosis of early Lyme disease by polymerase chain reaction amplification and culture of skin biopsies from erythema migrans lesions. *J Clin Microbiol* 1992;30:3082.

The sensitivity of PCR for the detection of B. burgdorferi in skin biopsy specimens was about 60%. The yield was similar when culture was used.

Shapiro ED, et al. A controlled trial of antimicrobial prophylaxis for Lyme disease after deer tick bites. *N Engl J Med* 1992;327:1769.

In an endemic area, prophylactic amoxicillin is not indicated to prevent Lyme disease after a deer tick bite.

Sigal LH. Summary of the first 100 patients seen at a Lyme disease referral center. *Am J Med* 1990;88:577.

Lyme disease was diagnosed in only 37% of patients referred for evaluation. Fibromyalgia was common.

Smith RP, et al. Clinical characteristics and treatment outcome of early Lyme disease in patients with microbiologically confirmed erythema migrans. *Ann Intern Med* 2002;136:421–428.

Fifty nine percent of patients with erythema migrans presented with a rash that consisted of homogeneous erythema and less than ten (32%) with the classic bull's-eye rashes.

Stanek G, Strle F. Lyme borreliosis. *Lancet* 2003;362:1639–1647.

Review. Persistence of symptoms after treatment is not equated with bacteriologic failure.

Steere AC. Lyme disease. *N Engl J Med* 2001;345:115–125.

Review.

Steere AC. Musculoskeletal manifestations of Lyme disease. *Am J Med* 1995;98(suppl 4A);44S–51S.

Lyme arthritis usually responds to a 1-month course of antibiotics—doxycycline, amoxicillin, or ceftriaxone (see also Steere AC. Diagnosis and treatment of Lyme arthritis. Med Clin North Am 1997;81:179–194).

Steere AC, Schoen RT, Taylor E. The clinical evolution of Lyme arthritis. *Ann Intern Med* 1987;107:725.

The spectrum of disease in untreated patients with Lyme arthritis includes intermittent episodes of arthritis (64%), arthralgias alone (23%), and chronic arthritis (14%).

Steere AC, et al. Treatment of the early manifestations of Lyme disease. *Ann Intern Med* 1983;99:22.

Erythema migrans responded to antimicrobial therapy in 5 days with and in 10 days without treatment. Major late complications did not occur in patients who were treated with tetracycline.

Treatment of Lyme disease. *Med Lett Drugs Ther* 2000;42:37–39.

For erythema migrans, doxycycline, amoxicillin, or cefuroxime axetil is recommended.

Tugwell P, et al. Laboratory evaluation in the diagnosis of Lyme disease. *Ann Intern Med* 1997;127:1109–1123.

Although Lyme disease is the most common tick-borne disease in North America, laboratory testing is indicated only if the pretest probability is .20 or higher (see also American College of Physicians. Guidelines for laboratory evaluation in the diagnosis of Lyme disease. Ann Intern Med *1997;127:1106–1108).*

Wormser GP. Treatment and prevention of Lyme disease, with emphasis on antimicrobial therapy for neuroborreliosis and vaccination. *Semin Neurol* 1997;17:45–52.

Ceftriaxone is the drug of choice for neuroborreliosis.

Wormser GP, et al. Use of a novel technique of cutaneous lavage for diagnosis of Lyme disease associated with erythema migrans. *JAMA* 1992;268:1311.

Culture of material obtained by a 2-mm skin biopsy and fluid from a technique called cutaneous needle lavage yielded B. burgdorferi. *Skin biopsy culture was more sensitive than lavage culture (74% vs. 40%).*

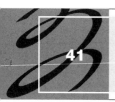

41   CELLULITIS AND OTHER SKIN AND SOFT-TISSUE INFECTIONS

*C*ellulitis is an acute infectious disease process that results in inflammation of the skin and subcutaneous tissues. Although streptococci and staphylococci cause the majority of cases of cellulitis, there are many potential sites of infections. Clinical clues to the etiologic agent include the anatomic site and the patient's medical and exposure history. Animal or human bites, exposure to soil or water, previous trauma, drug abuse, or history of surgery all predispose to certain types of cellulitis.

Erysipelas remains a common cause of cellulitis. A sharply demarcated, advancing, and palpable border suggests this infection. The etiologic agent is almost always group A β-hemolytic streptococci. *Staphylococcus aureus* can rarely cause the same clinical picture. However, the lesions of *S. aureus* cellulitis usually have less distinct borders and may be associated with bullae, pustules, or other primary localized areas of infection. Other hemolytic streptococci, such as groups C and G, also may cause cellulitis, often in patients with underlying malignancy.

An erysipeloid cellulitis, particularly around the fingers or on the hand, has been associated with the occupations of fishermen, butchers, and other persons handling raw fish and poultry. The organism causing this cellulitis is *Erysipelothrix rhusiopathiae*. The cellulitis often has a violet hue. There is local tenderness but little systemic reaction. Penicillin G is the antimicrobial of choice. More recently, cellulitis caused by a fish pathogen, *Streptococcus iniae,* has been described in association with an outbreak in Canada. All the patients had handled live or freshly killed fish. *Aeromonas hydrophilia* is an organism reported to cause cellulitis after exposure to fresh water. Cellulitis occurs at the site of an abrasion or laceration. Aeromonas cellulitis also has been reported after therapeutic application of leeches. Ciprofloxacin or imipenem-cilastin has been used in therapy.

Vibrio vulnificus has caused a spectrum of skin infections in saltwater wounds. Immunocompromised patients and patients with liver disease are prone to life-threatening infection. A cellulitis may be acquired from the exposure of abraded skin to seawater. Bites, fishing injuries, or puncture by a fin or spine may be the predisposing event. Cellulitis, bullous disease, necrotizing fasciitis, and myositis have all been well described.

V. vulnificus bacteremia may develop in immunocompromised patients after ingestion of shellfish. Metastatic skin lesions, particularly vesicles and bullae, may be associated with this bacteremia. Antimicrobial therapy (tetracyclines and aminoglycosides have been most commonly used), blood pressure support, and often wound debridement are required because the disease is rapidly progressive.

Pseudomonas aeruginosa folliculitis has been described, almost exclusively in association with the use of hot tubs and whirlpools. Papules or nodules that are red or violaceous appear on the abdomen or trunk. The neck and face are usually spared. Patients may have low-grade fever but do not become bacteremic or systemically ill. Avoidance of the source of infection is usually sufficient therapy because the rash is self-limited.

Cellulitis caused by Enterobacteriaceae can occur in association with trauma and diabetes or after surgery. *Escherichia coli* and *Klebsiella* sp. can cause a gas-forming gangrene that must be distinguished from purely anaerobic soft-tissue infection. Necrotizing fasciitis is a potentially life-threatening infection because of the virulence of the causative organism and the depth of involvement to the fascia. Bacteremia is common, and mortality from the disease is high. Toxic strains of hemolytic streptococci have made the disease more common. Necrotizing fasciitis requires rapid diagnosis and early antibiotic therapy and surgical intervention. Although definitive diagnosis is difficult, clues to deeper infection include bullae formation, anesthesia over the infected area, dusky discoloration, and failure to respond to antibiotics. Recently, a laboratory risk indicator has been used to distinguish necrotizing fasciitis from severe cellulitis using white blood cell count, hemoglobin, creatinine, and C-reactive protein. Deep-tissue infection may be the result of mixed anaerobic and gram-negative infection.

 ## CELLULITIS AFTER BREAST SURGERY

Breast cellulitis has been reported recently as a complication of breast-conservation therapy. More than 80% of patients had radiologically demonstrated fluid collections at the site of lumpectomy. Episodes of cellulitis developed, on average, 4.9 months after the end of radiotherapy for stage I or II breast carcinoma.

Cellulitis in the ipsilateral arm occurs after mastectomy and is associated with lymphedema. Non-group A β-hemolytic streptococci frequently have been implicated in breast surgery infections.

 ## ANIMAL BITES

Animal bites are a common cause of soft-tissue infection, with more than half a million bites, mostly from dogs and cats, occurring in the United States each year. Several factors are important in developing a diagnostic and therapeutic plan: the animal involved, severity and location of the wound, circumstances of the attack, and interval between injury and presentation. A plan for treatment must include (1) local care, with thorough cleaning of the wound with soap and water and adequate irrigation; (2) tetanus prophylaxis; (3) rabies prophylaxis, depending on the animal involved and the epidemiology of rabies in the specific locale; and (4) antimicrobials. Prophylactic antimicrobial therapy is controversial; however, routine prophylaxis for dog bites is becoming increasingly recommended. Patients with deep wounds or wounds of the face, and patients with wounds who are immunocompromised or have liver disease probably should receive prophylaxis (prospective studies are lacking). The antimicrobial of choice is controversial. A broad-spectrum agent, such as amoxicillin-clavulanate, is often recommended.

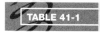

TABLE 41-1	Etiologic Agents in Cellulitis With Site or Cause of Infection
Mastectomy or lumpectomy	Non-group A β streptococci
Salt water abrasion	*V. vulnificus*
Fresh water abrasion	*A. hydrophilia*, *S. iniae*
Hot tub cellulitis	*P. aeruginosa*
Dog and cat bites	*P. multocida*, *Neisseria canis*, *C. canimorsus*, staphylococci, streptococci
In fisherman, butcher	*E. rhusiopathiae*
Liposuction	Group A β-hemolytic streptococci
Complicated body piercing	Group A β-hemolytic streptococci *S. aureus*
Diabetic foot	Gram-negative bacilli, anaerobes, *S. aureus*
After saphenous vein stripping	Hemolytic streptococci

Treatment of animal bite soft-tissue infection should be directed against the etiologic agent. *Pasteurella multocida,* the most common organism in dog and cat bites, is a small, gram-negative rod (appearing much like *Haemophilus* species organisms on Gram's stain). Penicillin is the drug of choice; tetracycline is an effective alternative.

Dysgonic fermenter 2 (DF-2), now called *Capnocytophaga canimorsus,* recently has been recognized to cause soft-tissue infection and overwhelming sepsis after dog bites. The disease also has occurred after cat bite. Patients with cirrhosis and splenectomized patients are at high risk for septic shock and disseminated intravascular coagulation. Penicillin in high doses is the drug of choice. *Bacteroides* and *Prevotella* species are commonly isolated from bite wounds and are now better characterized.

Table 41-1 lists anatomic sites or predispositions to infection with the likely etiologic agent.

 DIAGNOSIS

The likely etiologic agent in cellulitis usually can be determined clinically by careful history and physical exam. Bacteria can, at times, be cultured by needle aspiration of the affected skin. There is extensive literature on this subject that suggests that an agent can be isolated in about 25% of patients. Nevertheless, aspiration is not recommended in routine evaluation. Similarly, some studies have had good results with punch biopsy of the skin to evaluate the etiologic agent by smear and culture. Biopsy may be used to evaluate unusual presentations or cellulitis that is not responding to therapy. Blood cultures are positive in only 4% of patients with cellulitis. They are considered unlikely to be cost effective. However, decisions on the use of blood cultures should be made on a case-by-case basis. Blood cultures should be obtained in those who have high fever, shaking chills, or elevated white blood cell counts. Patients who have cellulitis superimposed on lymphedema are more likely to have positive blood cultures.

Plain film radiographs and computed tomographic (CT) scans are rarely necessary in the evaluation of cellulitis. They may be used to assess the possibility of underlying osteomyelitis. Magnetic resonance imaging can be used to distinguish cellulitis from necrotizing fasciitis.

 TREATMENT

β-Lactam antibiotics with activity against both staphylococci and streptococci will be the mainstay of therapy for cellulitis in the great majority of cases. Clinical data from history and physical exam will determine other specific organisms and their concomitant treatment as appropriate. Hospitalization with intravenous antibiotics or therapy at home with oral antibiotics will depend on an assessment of the patient's severity of illness and evaluation of the cellulitis itself with respect to location and rapidity of spread. Chills, fever, and temperature above 100.5°F would be indications for hospitalization. Periorbital cellulitis or cellulitis of the face also would be more appropriate for hospitalization. Immunosuppressed patients would require closer follow-up and intravenous antibiotics. If methicillin-resistant staphylococci are suspected, admission and treatment with vancomycin will be indicated. Spread of community-acquired methicillin-resistant staphylococci is increasing and represented 55% of all isolates in one Native American community. This spread will make empirical therapy more difficult. Decisions on initial treatment of cellulitis may be based on monitoring local susceptibility data on community-acquired staphylococci.

Initial treatment for the hospitalized patient with the usual type of cellulitis would include intravenous nafcillin, 1 g every 4 to 6 hours, or cefazolin, 1 g every 6 to 8 hours, or ceftriaxone, 1 g each day. Vancomycin or linezolid would be reserved for those with anaphylaxis to penicillin, suspicion of methicillin-resistance, or high incidence of methicillin-resistance in the community. For oral therapy of methicillin-sensitive organisms, quinolones have been shown to be as effective as oral cephalexin or oxacillin. (SLB)

Bibliography

Alexander CJ, et al. Characterization of saccharolytic *Bacteroides* and *Prevotella* isolates from infected dog and cat bite wounds in humans. *J Clin Microbiol* 1997; 35:406.
Many species of Bacteroides *and* Prevotella *can be isolated from human bites. Clinical laboratories need to be aware of these species.*

Auerbach PS. Natural microbiologic hazards of the aquatic environment. *Clin Dermatol* 1987;5:52.
Describes risk for Erysipelothrix *infection in fish handlers.*

Brenner DJ, et al. *Capnocytophaga canimorsus* sp. nov. (formerly CDC group DF-2), a cause of septicemia following dog bite, and *C. cynodegmi* sp. nov., a cause of localized wound infection following dog bite. *J Clin Microbiol* 1989;27:231.
Capnocytophaga *may cause sepsis after dog bite, particularly in the splenectomized or cirrhotic patient.*

Chuang YC, et al. *Vibrio vulnificus* infection in Taiwan: report of 28 cases and review of clinical manifestations and treatment. *Clin Infect Dis* 1992;15:271.
Summary of 28 episodes of V. vulnificus *infection. Twenty-three of 27 patients had skin involvement.*

Eady Ea, Cove JH. Staphylococcus resistance revisited: community-acquired methicillin resistant Staphylococcus aureus—an emerging problem for the management of skin and soft tissue infection. *Curr Opin Infect Dis* 2003;16:103.
Describes increasing pattern of resistance to β-lactam antibiotics among community-acquired strains of staphylococci. This pattern will require more empirical therapy with vancomycin.

Graham DR, et. al. Once-daily high-dose levofloxacin versus ticarcillin-clavulanate alone or followed by amoxicillin-clavulanate for complicated skin and skin structure infections: a randomized, open label trial. *Clin Infect Dis* 2002;35:381.
Both regimens had success rates of about 80%.

Gustafson TL. *Pseudomonas* folliculitis: an outbreak and review. *Rev Infect Dis* 1983; 3:1.
Clinical description of hot-tub folliculitis.

Merz KR, et al. Breast cellulitis following breast conservation therapy: a novel complication of medical progress. *Clin Infect Dis* 1998;26:481.
Cellulitis, which is sometimes recurrent, is now more commonly seen after breast-sparing surgery, often after radiation therapy. Most episodes occur less than 3 months after treatment.

Miller SR, et al. Delayed cellulitis associated with conservative therapy for breast cancer. *J Surg Oncol* 1998;67:242.
Delayed occurrence of cellulitis in the ipsilateral breast is now more common owing to local lymphedema.

Stevens DL, et al. Linezolid versus vancomycin for the treatment of methicillin-resistant Staphylococcus aureus infection. *Clin Infect Dis* 2002;34:1481.

Included many cases of cellulitis and soft tissue infection. Cure rate was about the same for both drugs.

Swartz MN. Cellulitis. N Engl J Med 2004;350:904.
Succinct, up-to-date review of the diagnosis and treatment of cellulitis.

Weber DJ, Hansen AR. Infections resulting from animal bites. *Infect Dis Clin North Am* 1991;5:663.
Review of epidemiology and treatment of animal bites, including infections with Pasteurella multocida and C. canimorsus.

Weinstein MR, et al. Invasive infections due to a fish pathogen, *Streptococcus iniae*. N Engl J Med 1997;337:589.
Describes nine patients with invasive skin infections caused by this organism after they handled fresh fish.

Weiss HB, Friedman DI, Coben JH. Incidence of dog-bite injuries treated in the emergency departments. *JAMA* 1998;278:51.
There are 12.9 dog-bite injuries per 10,000 population. Most occur in children ages 5 to 9.

Wong CH, et. al. The LRINEC score: a tool for distinguishing necrotizing fasciitis from other soft tissue infection. *Crit Care Med* 2004;32:1535.
Uses laboratory tests, such as white count, C-reactive protein, creatinine, to predict necrotizing fasciitis likelihood.

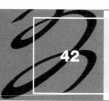

42   PARVOVIRUS INFECTIONS

*H*uman parvovirus B19 is a single-stranded DNA virus that usually infects rapidly dividing cell lines, such as erythroid progenitor cells. Most persons with parvovirus B19 infection remain asymptomatic. In the normal host, parvovirus infection can be symptomatic, resulting in erythema infectiosum or arthropathy.

B19 is found worldwide and occurs as both sporadic cases and in recurrent epidemics. Parvovirus B19 is the only parvovirus clearly linked with human disease. Canine parvovirus cannot be transmitted to humans. The virus belongs to the family Parvoviridae and the genus *Erythrovirus*. It is a nonenveloped, single-stranded DNA virus and is typically resistant to heat and detergent because of its small genome and lack of a membrane. Epidemics can occur every 3 to 4 years. During these outbreaks, about 10% of cases occur among children younger than age 5, 70% of cases occur in children ages 5 to 15, and 20% of cases occur among patients older than age 15. The peak incidence of erythema infectiosum is found in the late winter and early spring. In school or household settings the secondary attack rate during epidemics of erythema infectiosum is about 50% in susceptible children and 20 to 30% in susceptible teachers. Day care workers are at an increased risk as well.

PATHOGENESIS

The virus is composed of three proteins in association with a DNA molecule. These proteins include one nonstructural protein, NS1, and two structural proteins, VP1 and VP2. The cellular receptor for B19 is a globoside, also known as blood group P antigen. Viral replication causes maturation arrest at the giant pronormoblast stage of erythroid development.

Transmission of infection occurs through the respiratory route, through blood-derived products administered parenterally, and vertically from mother to fetus. Respiratory spread appears to be the most common route of transmission.

Viremia occurs during the first week of infection, accompanied by constitutional symptoms of fever and malaise, and by erythroid progenitor cell depletion in the bone marrow. Parvovirus B19 infects the bone marrow; therefore, patients who have underlying hematologic abnormalities are much more likely to have a cessation of red blood cell production. Individuals with chronic hemolytic anemia, such as sickle cell disease or hereditary spherocytosis, develop transient aplastic crisis during the areticulocytosis phase of the infection. Of note, the reduction in the reticulocyte count is occasionally accompanied by leukopenia and thrombocytopenia.

The appearance of IgM antibodies in the second week corresponds with clearance of the viremia. They may persist in the serum for 3 months. IgG antibody will usually appear at 2 to 3 weeks after inoculation. After IgG antibodies appear in the serum, the rash of erythema infectiosum and arthropathy will develop. Approximately 50% of adults are anti-B19 IgG seropositive, indicating past infection. IgG antibody is considered to be a protective antibody and persists for life.

 CLINICAL MANIFESTATIONS

Most persons with parvovirus B19 infection remain asymptomatic. However, several classic clinical syndromes described below may occur.

Fifth Disease

The most common presentation in children (usually infected between the ages of 4 and 10) is the exanthema erythema infectiosum, also known as "fifth disease." This eruption spreads from the trunk to the extremities in a centrifugal progression, often appearing blotchy or even fishnet-like. Classically, heat or sun exposure will exacerbate the rash. Because this exanthem most commonly involves the malar eminences and spares the nasal bridge and perioral areas, a so-called "slapped-cheek" appearance becomes evident. In this stage, erythema of the cheeks is associated with relative circumoral pallor. See Table 42-1 for the typical clinical manifestations.

Several types of purpuric manifestations have been described, including nonspecific vascular petechiae and purpura. Case reports of TTP, ITP have also been described. Other specific syndromes manifesting purpura have been described, including the "gloves-and-socks" syndrome, leukocytoclastic vasculitis, and Henoch-Schönlein purpura.

Arthropathy

As opposed to children, most adults do not develop a rash, but instead they have a sudden onset of a symmetric rheumatoid-like polyarthritis. Most patients usually improve within 2 weeks, but in some adults (20%) complaints may persist for months to years. Joints involved include the hands, wrists, ankles, and knees.

Although parvovirus infections in adults are most commonly asymptomatic, an estimated 60% of women with symptomatic disease manifest arthropathy. Men appear to be affected much less frequently. The presence of fever is rare, but some patients will have an associated generalized rash, and about 15% have the typical facial exanthem.

Parvovirus infection has been linked to several chronic rheumatologic disorders. Several investigators have studied a possible link to systemic lupus erythematosus. A number of investigators also have examined the role that parvovirus may play in the pathogenesis of rheumatoid arthritis and juvenile idiopathic arthritis (Still's disease). A smaller body of evidence has proposed a role for B19 in the pathogenesis of scleroderma and dermatomyositis.

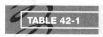

	Classic Course of Parvovirus B19 Infection and Erythema Infectiosum

Stage 1 (Incubation period of 4–14 days)	Stage 2 (3–7 days after prodrome)	Stage 3 (1–4 days after the facial exanthema)
*Period of transmissibility**	Facial exanthem, or "slapped cheek" appearance	Lacy, erythematous maculopapular exanthem on trunk and extremities
Mild prodromal illness	Clearance of viremia	Evanescent course of exanthem over 1–3 weeks
Viremia	Development of parvovirus B19-specific IgG antibodies	Arthropathy
Erythroid progenitor cell depletion		
Development of parvovirus B19-specific IgM antibodies	*Note: patient is not contagious*	*Note: patient is not contagious*

*Patients should be considered infectious from 7 days post exposure until either 18 days post exposure or 24 hours after onset of rash or arthritis.
(Adapted from http://www.aafp.org/afp/991001ap/1455.html)

Erythrocyte Aplasia

Immunocompromised individuals may develop chronic or recurrent episodes of anemia, leukopenia, or thrombocytopenia. Rarely, isolated anemia, leukopenia, or thrombocytopenia may occur in an immunocompetent patient. Infection can result in a transient aplastic crisis, which may occur in persons with chronic hemolytic anemia and conditions of bone marrow stress. These patients will often have a viral prodrome followed by anemia, with hemoglobin concentrations falling below 5.0 g per dL (50 g per L) and reticulocytosis. Administration of intravenous immune globulin also may be beneficial. In immunocompromised patients with persistent B19 infection and chronic or recurrent bone marrow suppression because of failure to make neutralizing anti-VP1 antibody, intravenous immunoglobulin may allow clearing of apparent infection and resolution of bone marrow suppression. Transfusions may be needed as well. Likewise, fetal hydrops may require intrauterine transfusion for anemia.

Other manifestations include hepatitis, acute fulminant liver failure, myocarditis, vasculitis, Henoch-Schönlein purpura, vesicular skin eruptions, "socks and gloves" acral rash, purpura with or without thrombocytopenia, benign acute lymphadenopathy, hemophagocytic syndrome, peripheral neuropathy, sensorineural hearing loss, aseptic meningitis and, rarely, encephalopathy have all been described in association with B19 infection. B19 is the leading cause of pure red cell aplasia in AIDS patients.

Hydrops Fetalis

The diagnosis of parvovirus B19 in any individual requires a history of potential exposures to pregnant women. B19 is not considered a cause of congenital anomalies. However, parvovirus infection can lead to fetal infection, possibly resulting in miscarriage or nonimmune hydrops fetalis. Because most pregnant women who become infected with this virus are asymptomatic, it has been difficult to determine the risk of fetal infection, fetal wastage, and nonimmune hydrops. In infected pregnant women, parvovirus B19 is believed to affect the fetus approximately 30% of the time; however, only 2 to 10 % of infected fetuses experience poor outcomes. Fetal outcomes range from hydrops fetalis to congenital anemia to death.

Approximately 50% of women are seropositive for the virus before pregnancy, and the likelihood of infection ranges from 30 to 50% after a close exposure. Hydrops fetalis

TABLE 42-2	Useful Web Sites

Web site	Internet address
CDC Fifth Disease	http://www.cdc.gov/ncidod/diseases/parvovirus/B19.htm
NEJM B19 Review	http://content.nejm.org/cgi/content/short/350/6/586
e Medicine B19	http://www.emedicine.com/ped/topic192.htm
Dermatology images	http://dermatlas.med.jhmi.edu/derm/IndexDisplay.cfm?ImageID=192334097

is manifested at birth by severe anemia, high-output cardiac failure, and extramedullary hematopoiesis. Parvovirus B19 has been shown to cause a congenital infection syndrome, manifested by rash, anemia, hepatomegaly, and cardiomegaly.

 ## DIAGNOSIS

Detection of IgG antibody is not very helpful. In contrast, the detection of IgM may be more useful clinically, because it may be present for as long as 2 to 3 months after acute infection.

The presence of giant pronormoblasts should suggest the diagnosis. Patients with aplastic crisis have hemoglobin that is significantly decreased compared with baseline values. At that time, few or no reticulocytes will be present in the peripheral blood smear. Mild thrombocytopenia and leukopenia are occasionally seen as well. Early in the course, bone marrow examination shows a marked erythroid hypoplasia, and among the few erythroid precursors seen may be the characteristic giant forms. Later during the recovery phase, the reticulocytes will be increased in the peripheral blood smear and there will be a rebound erythroid hyperplasia in the bone marrow.

Some studies have shown that polymerase chain reaction can amplify and identify B19 DNA in tissue samples, such as synovium or skin. Also, electron microscopy may demonstrate viral particles in suspected tissues.

 ## INFECTION CONTROL ISSUES

Because the appearance of the rash corresponds with the development of IgG antibodies and occurs after the viremia has cleared, the rash of erythema infectiosum signifies that the virus can no longer be transmitted.

Patients should be considered infectious from 7 days post exposure until either 18 days post exposure or 24 hours after onset of rash or arthritis. B19 is not removed from blood by current solvent detergent-based methods of blood decontamination (lacks a lipid envelope) and, therefore, pooled blood products may contain infectious B19. Transmission by way of bone marrow also has been demonstrated.

Given the high prevalence of parvovirus B19 in the community, the routine exclusion of pregnant women from the workplace where erythema infectiosum is present is not recommended. Nevertheless pregnant healthcare employees should be informed of the preventive measures they can take to lower the risk of transmission, such as not caring for immunocompromised patients with acute or chronic parvovirus infection (Table 42-2). (JWM)

Bibliography

Al-Khan A, et al. Parvovirus B-19 infection during pregnancy. *Infect Dis Obstet Gynecol* 2003;11:175–179.

In view of this, a pregnant woman who is antibody negative should try to avoid contact with large groups of young children in order to decrease contact with potential vectors.

Barah F, et al. Neurological manifestations of human parvovirus B19 infection. *Rev Med Virol* 2003;13:185–199.

The purpose of this review is to summarize present knowledge of B19, its known and potential pathogenic mechanisms, and its association with human diseases, particularly those with neurologic manifestations.

Cavallo R, et al. B19 virus infection in renal transplant recipients. *J Clin Virol* 2003;263:361–368.

In conclusion, the relatively high occurrence (23%) of B19 virus infection in patients presenting with anemia, suggests that it should be considered in the differential diagnosis of persistent anemia in renal transplant recipients.

Chen S, Howard O. Images in clinical medicine. Parvovirus B19 infection. *N Engl J Med* 2004;350:598.

Crane J. Parvovirus B19 infection in pregnancy. *J Obstet Gynaecol Can* 2002;24:727–743; quiz 744–746.

Good review article.

Crowcroft NS, et al. Guidance for control of parvovirus B19 infection in healthcare settings and the community. *J Public Health Med* 1999;21:439–446.

This guidance aims to assist the local decision-making process to be as evidence based as the available evidence allows.

Dowell SF, et al. Parvovirus B19 infection in hospital workers: community or hospital acquisition? *J Infect Dis* 1995;172:1076–1079.

A suspected nosocomial outbreak of parvovirus B19 infection in a maternity ward was investigated in February 1994.

Erdman DD, et al. Human parvovirus B19 specific IgG, IgA, and IgM antibodies and DNA in serum specimens from persons with erythema infectiosum. *J Med Virol* 1991;352: 110–115.

Their data indicate that (1) Specific IgA antibodies are too persistent to be a useful indicator of recent B19 infection; (2) Specific IgM antibodies are the most sensitive indicator of acute B19 infection in immunologically normal persons but can persist up to 6 months; and (3) B19 DNA can often be detected up to 2 months after onset of illness even in immunologically normal hosts and might be a useful adjunct test for diagnosis of acute B19 infection.

Gallinella G, et al. Calibrated real-time PCR for evaluation of parvovirus b19 viral load. *Clin Chem* 2004;50:759–762.

Gallinella G, et al. Relevance of B19 markers in serum samples for a diagnosis of parvovirus B19-correlated diseases. *J Med Virol* 2003;71:135–139.

The contemporaneous determination of B19 DNA by polymerase chain reaction and specific IgM appears to be the most appropriate diagnostic protocol for the correct laboratory diagnosis of B19 infection.

Garewal G, et al. Parvovirus B19 infection-associated red-cell aplasia in renal-transplant recipients: clues from the bone marrow. *Transplantation* 2004;77:320–321.

Heegaard ED, Brown KE. Human Parvovirus B19. *Clin Microbiol Rev* 2002;15:485–505.

Good review article.

Katta R. Parvovirus B19: a review. *Dermatol Clin* 2002;20:333–342.

Infection with parvovirus B19 may result in a wide range of dermatologic manifestations.

Kerr JR, et al. Parvovirus B19 infection in AIDS patients. *Int J STD AIDS* 1997;8:184–186.

Bone marrow of 61 HIV-1–infected patients and 23 control patients was examined to determine the incidence of B19 infection and its clinical impact in HIV-1–infected persons. In conclusion, B19 persistence may be common and frequently subclinical in AIDS patients.

Lennerz C, et al. Parvovirus B19-related chronic monoarthritis: immunohistochemical detection of virus-positive lymphocytes within the synovial tissue compartment: two reported cases. *Clin Rheumatol* 2004;23:59–62.

The pathology of B19 arthropathy seems to be to the result of direct virus infection of cells within the synovia.

Mareschal-Desandes R, et al. Successful treatment of chronic parvovirus B19 infection by high-dose immunoglobulin. *Clin Nephrol* 2003;59:311–312.

Messina MF, et al. Purpuric gloves and socks syndrome caused by parvovirus B19 infection. *Pediatr Infect Dis J* 2003;22:755–756.

Miyamoto K, et al. Outbreak of human parvovirus B19 in hospital workers. *J Hosp Infect* 2000;45:238–241.

We report an outbreak of human parvovirus B19 (HPV B19) infection affecting five nursing staff, four hospital office workers and one physiotherapist and its possible transmission among hospital staff. Our findings suggest that transmission of HPV B19 among hospital staff members occurred.

Morgan-Capner P, Crowcroft NS. Guidelines on the management of, and exposure to, rash illness in pregnancy (including consideration of relevant antibody screening programmes in pregnancy). *Commun Dis Public Health* 2002;5:59–71.

These guidelines, produced by the Public Health Laboratory Service (PHLS), aim to help decision making in the investigation and management of pregnant women who have 'a rash compatible with a systemic viral illness,' or who have contact with a person with such an illness. They address particularly rubella, parvovirus B19, and varicella-zoster virus infection, but consider other infective causes of rash illness in the United Kingdom.

Naides SJ. Infection control measures for human parvovirus B19 in the hospital setting. *Infect Control Hosp Epidemiol* 1989;10:326–329.

Sabella C, Goldfarb J. Parvovirus B19 infections. *Am Fam Physician* 1999;60:1455–1460.

Infections caused by human parvovirus B19 can result in a wide spectrum of manifestations, which are usually influenced by the patient's immunologic and hematologic status.

Trotta M, et al. Intrauterine parvovirus B19 infection: early prenatal diagnosis is possible. *Int J Infect Dis* 2004;8:130–131.

Young NS, Brown KE. Parvovirus B19. *N Engl J Med* 2004;350:586–597.

Good review article.

Bacteremia

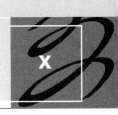

X

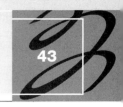

*H*ospital mortality from sepsis has ranged from 25 to 80% over the last few decades. Although mortality may be lower in recent years, sepsis is clearly still a very serious condition. There are three recognized stages of the inflammatory response, with progressively increased risk of end-organ failure and death: sepsis, severe sepsis, and septic shock. Patients with infection plus two or more elements of the systemic inflammatory response syndrome meet the criteria for *sepsis*; those who also have end-organ failure are considered to have *severe sepsis*; and those who also have refractory hypotension are considered to be in *septic shock*.

Microorganisms stimulate macrophages to elaborate a variety of cytokines which stimulate proteins located on small vessels and thereby alter the normally anti-inflammatory and anticoagulant ecology by causing inflammation and clotting. In sepsis and septic shock, levels of an important regulatory protein, activated protein C, are often reduced. This leads to procoagulation, failure of normal fibrinolysis, leaky capillaries, and other correlates of inflammation. Infectious agents and inflammatory cytokines such as tumor necrosis factor-alpha (TNF-α) and interleukin-1 activate coagulation by causing the release of tissue factor from monocytes and the endothelium, which leads to the formation of thrombin and a fibrin clot. Inflammatory cytokines and thrombin can both impair the endogenous fibrinolytic potential by stimulating the release of plasminogen-activator inhibitor 1 (PAI-1) from platelets and the endothelium. PAI-1 is a potent inhibitor of tissue plasminogen activator, the endogenous pathway for lysing a fibrin clot. In addition, the procoagulant thrombin is capable of stimulating multiple inflammatory pathways and further suppressing the endogenous fibrinolytic system by activating thrombin-activatable fibrinolysis inhibitor (TAFI). The conversion of protein C, by thrombin bound to thrombomodulin, to the serine protease activated protein C is impaired by the inflammatory response. Endothelial injury results in decreased thrombomodulin levels.

Activated protein C exerts an anti-inflammatory effect by inhibiting the production of inflammatory cytokines (TNF-α, interleukin-1, and interleukin-6) by monocytes and limiting the rolling of monocytes and neutrophils on injured endothelium by binding selectins. Activated protein C indirectly increases the fibrinolytic response by inhibiting PAI-1 and exerts an antithrombotic effect by inactivating factors Va and VIIIa, limiting the generation of thrombin. As a result of decreased thrombin levels, the inflammatory, procoagulant, and antifibrinolytic response induced by thrombin is reduced.

C5a also plays an important role. The location of C5a may be critical in terms of its potential to protect or harm. Local generation of C5a is essential for early control of infection, but an excess of intravascular C5a cripples neutrophils, allowing unrestrained proliferation of bacteria. In the sepsis syndrome, C3a and C5a may have opposite effects. Thus, it has been proposed that C3a receptors have an anti-inflammatory effect, and evidence suggests that the effect of C5a in the sepsis syndrome is mediated by cellular C5a receptors and that blockade of these G-protein–coupled receptors may be helpful.

There is increasing recognition that *apoptosis* plays a central role in the complex balance between the invading pathogen and host defense. Certain intracellular pathogens depend on host cells to survive and propagate. Apoptosis of infected cells may function as a defense mechanism to limit the spread of these intracellular organisms. As a consequence of this, some viruses and bacteria have acquired techniques to inhibit the host's apoptotic machinery in the cells that they infect. In contrast, other pathogens are able to induce apoptosis in the host's cells to enhance their pathogenic effects. Thus, depending on the type of pathogen, apoptosis of host cells may be either beneficial or detrimental to host survival. Animal models of sepsis (peritonitis) demonstrate that two types of cells—lymphocytes and gastrointestinal epithelial cells—undergo accelerated apoptosis. Apoptotic and necrotic cells are eliminated by specialized phagocytic cells, and the type of cell death (i.e., apoptotic or necrotic) may be the critical factor that links tissue damage to the appropriate immune response.

Attempts to understand the role of inflammation in sepsis have prompted studies of the impact of cytokines on outcome. However, because the ranges of cytokine levels from survivors and nonsurvivors typically overlap, such tests are of poor discriminative value.

Three agents that block coagulation at different stages have been evaluated in large, multicenter trials as adjunctive therapy for sepsis. Neither antithrombin III nor tissue factor-pathway inhibitor was effective in patients with severe sepsis or septic shock. This supports the view that the beneficial effect of activated protein C in patients with sepsis is not caused solely by its antithrombotic activity.

Activated protein C has been studied in patients with sepsis. In March 2001, Bernard presented data from a study showing a reduction in 28-day mortality among patients with severe sepsis and septic shock who received recombinant human activated protein C. Of note, the death rate was 30.8% among controls and 24.7% in the group receiving activated protein C ($P = .005$). Interestingly, 10 members of an advisory panel of the Food and Drug Administration (FDA) voted for approval of the drug and 10 voted against it, but drotrecogin was licensed in November 2001. Several letters and editorials have commented on the controversy that surrounds both the study and the FDA approval process. The cost of the drug, approximately $7,000 per treatment course, adds to the controversy.

In the second half of the study, the sponsor not only modified the eligibility criteria, but also used a different cell line for the production of human recombinant activated protein C. In terms of outcomes, the absolute difference in mortality—6.1%—seemed small to some, and there was an increased risk of serious bleeding (an absolute difference of 1.4%) associated

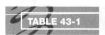 **TABLE 43-1**   Candidates for Drotrecogin Therapy*

Eligible	Probably not indicated
Has a reasonable expectation of survival exclusive of sepsis. Not a DNR.	Mild-to-moderate sepsis without evidence of end-organ dysfunction (*Apache II score less than 25*).
Three or more of the systemic inflammatory response criteria are met	Patients with uncorrectable coagulation disorders that would increase the risk of bleeding
Evidence of sepsis-induced end organ dysfunction in two or more systems within 24 hours	Bone marrow, small bowel, liver, lung, or pancreas transplantation. Use in these patients should be on a case-by-case basis.
Reasonably good evidence of infection such as:	
Positive culture(s)	
White blood cells in normally sterile body fluid	
Radiographic evidence of pneumonia with production of purulent sputum	

*The usual dose is 24 mcg/kg per hour for 96 hours. Infusions greater than 96 hours in duration have not been studied. No dose adjustment is recommended for renal or hepatic impairment.
Platelets and INR should be obtained at baseline and daily during therapy. Drotrecogin may variably prolong aPTT. Therefore, aPTT should not be used to monitor coagulopathy during drotrecogin infusion. See http://www.xigris.com/dose_tools.shtml for assistance with dosing.
DNR, Do not resuscitate.

with activated protein C therapy. A post hoc analysis of the data found that activated protein C benefited primarily the most seriously ill patients—those with scores of 25 or more on the Acute Physiology and Chronic Health Evaluation (APACHE II). In a later issue of the New England Journal of Medicine, three articles and a letter to the editor framed the issues of the debate over the value of activated protein C. Siegel, from the Center for Biologics Evaluation and Research, argued that the changes in eligibility criteria created inconsistencies over time only in the lower risk population (patients with APACHE II scores of 24 or less). Conversely, Warren and colleagues argued that the results of post hoc analyses require confirmation in a new study, and that the existing data fail to support the use of Xigris (activated protein C) as the standard of care. Manns and colleagues created mathematical models of the economic value of activated protein C. They estimate that the cost of a life-year gained with the use of the drug would be about $28,000. However, in patients with an APACHE II score of less than 25, the cost could exceed $500,000 per life-year gained. Further research is needed to determine the cost effectiveness of activated protein C for patients with sepsis and less severe illness, and its overall role in the management of patients with this devastating condition. Tables 43-1 to 43-2 provide additional information regarding the use of activated protein C.

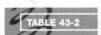

TABLE 43-2   Considerations for Therapy With Drotrecogin Alfa

Warnings—on a case-by-case basis	Contraindications
Concurrent *therapeutic* heparin	Active internal bleeding
Platelet count <30,000 × 10⁶/L, even if the platelet count is increased after transfusions	Recent (within 3 months) hemorrhagic stroke
Prothrombin time-INR >3.0	Recent (within 2 months) intracranial or intraspinal surgery, or severe head trauma
Recent (within 6 weeks) gastrointestinal bleeding	Trauma with an increased risk of life-threatening bleeding
Recent administration (within 3 days) of thrombolytic therapy	Presence of an epidural catheter
Recent administration (within 7 days) of oral anticoagulants or glycoprotein IIb/IIIa inhibitors	Intracranial neoplasm or mass lesion or evidence of cerebral herniation
Recent administration (within 7 days) of aspirin >650 mg per day or other platelet inhibitors	Also contraindicated in patients with known hypersensitivity
Recent (within 3 months) ischemic stroke	
Intracranial arteriovenous malformation or aneurysm	
Known bleeding diathesis	
Chronic severe hepatic disease	
Any other condition in which bleeding constitutes a significant hazard or would be particularly difficult to manage because of its location	
If a patient is receiving drotrecogin and needs surgery or an invasive procedure, the infusion should be stopped for at least 2 hours before the procedure and not resumed until at least 12 hours after major invasive procedures. Drotrecogin may be restarted immediately after less invasive procedures.	

See http://www.xigris.com/safety.shtml for more details.

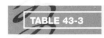 **TABLE 43-3   Useful Internet Sites for Sepsis**

Site Description	Address
Apache II scores	http://www.sfar.org/scores2/apache22.html
SCCM guidelines	http://www.sccm.org/professional_resources/guidelines/ table_of_contents/Documents/FINAL.pdf
Xigris information	http://www.xigris.com/index.shtml
IDSA-Candidiasis	http://www.journals.uchicago.edu/CID/journal/issues/v38n2/32301/ 32301.html
IDSA-Fever	http://www.journals.uchicago.edu/CID/journal/issues/v26n5/ my56_1042/my56_1042.web.pdf
IDSA-CAP	http://www.journals.uchicago.edu/CID/journal/issues/v37n11/32441/ 32441.html
IDSA-Catheter Rx	http://www.journals.uchicago.edu/CID/journal/issues/v35n11/ 021078/021078.html
IDSA-Catheter prevention	http://www.journals.uchicago.edu/CID/journal/issues/v32n9/001689/ 001689.html
International Sepsis Forum	http://www.sepsisforum.org/
University of Pennsylvania	http://www.uphs.upenn.edu/bugdrug/antibiotic_manual/sepsis.htm
Perspectives on Xigris	http://www.formkit.com/ptjournal/fulltext/PT_sepsis_suppl_0210.pdf
Steroids and sepsis	http://www.annals.org/cgi/content/full/141/1/I-64
Medline Plus	http://www.nlm.nih.gov/medlineplus/sepsis.html
Annals Steroids Meta-analysis	http://www.annals.org/cgi/content/full/141/1/47

SCCM, Society of Critical Care Medicine; IDSA, Infectious Diseases Society of America; CAP, Community-acquired pneumonia.

Many genetic polymorphisms have been identified in genes coding for key inflammatory molecules, and a number of investigators have examined the contribution of genetic predisposition to the incidence and the severity of sepsis. In particular, the presence of the TNF2 polymorphism in the promoter region of the gene for TNF was associated with a greater risk of death in septic populations.

The use of steroids in sepsis remains controversial, but recent studies have resurrected interest in this approach (Table 43-3). (JWM)

Bibliography

Aird WC. Vascular bed-specific hemostasis: role of endothelium in sepsis pathogenesis. *Crit Care Med* 2001;29(7 suppl):S28–S34; discussion S34–S5.
In sepsis, coagulation is initiated by the extrinsic pathway and is amplified through the intrinsic pathway. In addition, the body's natural anticoagulant mechanisms are significantly dampened. Together, these changes result in a net imbalance of hemostasis.
Angus DC, et al. Cost-effectiveness of drotrecogin alfa (activated) in the treatment of severe sepsis. *Crit Care Med* 2003;31:1–11.
Over the first 28 days (short-term base case), drotrecogin alfa (activated) increased the costs of care by $9,800 and survival by 0.061 lives saved per treated patient. Thus, drotrecogin alfa (activated) cost $160,000 per life saved (with 84.7% probability, that ratio is < $250,000 per life saved). Drotrecogin alfa (activated) cost $27,400 per quality-adjusted life-year when limited to patients with an APACHE II score of 25 or higher and was cost-ineffective when limited to patients with a score lower than 25. CONCLUSIONS: Drotrecogin alfa has a cost-effectiveness profile similar to that of many well-accepted healthcare strategies and below commonly quoted thresholds.

Banks SM, et al. Long-term cost effectiveness of drotrecogin alfa (activated): an unanswered question. *Crit Care Med* 2003;31:308–309.

Bernard GR. Drotrecogin alfa (activated) (recombinant human activated protein C) for the treatment of severe sepsis. *Crit Care Med* 2003;31(1 suppl):S85–S93.
Coagulopathy and systemic inflammation are almost universal in patients with severe sepsis. Treatment of this disorder with drotrecogin alfa (activated) directly addresses these derangements and substantially reduces morbidity and mortality rates with potential for bleeding during infusion as the only known risk.

Bhole D, Stahl GL. Therapeutic potential of targeting the complement cascade in critical care medicine. *Crit Care Med* 2003;31(1 suppl):S97–S104.
The advancement of this novel area of therapeutics may one day aid the clinician by providing several different complement inhibitors/antagonists for controlling complement activation or its biologically active mediators.

Bollaert PE, et al. Baseline cortisol levels, cortisol response to corticotropin, and prognosis in late septic shock. *Shock* 2003;19:13–15.
A high basal cortisol and low increase in corticotropin stimulation are predictors of a poor outcome in late septic shock. The underlying mechanisms of these prognostic patterns remain to be elucidated.

Chalfin DB, et al. A price for cost-effectiveness: implications for recombinant human activated protein C (rhAPC). *Crit Care Med* 2003;31:306–308.

Dellinger RP, et al. Surviving Sepsis Campaign guidelines for management of severe sepsis and septic shock. *Crit Care Med* 2004;32:858–873.
Comprehensive overview. In 2003, critical care and infectious disease experts representing 11 international organizations developed management guidelines for severe sepsis and septic shock that would be of practical use for the bedside clinician, under the auspices of the Surviving Sepsis Campaign, an international effort to increase awareness and improve outcome in severe sepsis. Evidence-based recommendations can be made regarding many aspects of the acute management of sepsis and septic shock that are hoped to translate into improved outcomes for the critically ill patient. The impact of these guidelines will be formally tested and guidelines updated annually, and even more rapidly as some important new knowledge becomes as available.

Eichacker PQ, Natanson C. Recombinant human activated protein C in sepsis: inconsistent trial results, an unclear mechanism of action, and safety concerns resulted in labeling restrictions and the need for phase IV trials. *Crit Care Med* 2003;31(1 suppl):S94–S96.

Ely EW, et al. Activated protein C for severe sepsis. *N Engl J Med* 2002;347:1035–1036.

Gerard C. Complement c5a in the sepsis syndrome—too much of a good thing? *N Engl J Med* 2003;348:167–169.

Hack CE, Zeerleder S. The endothelium in sepsis: source of and a target for inflammation. *Crit Care Med* 2001;29(7 suppl):S21–S27.
The endothelium is a key organ involved in the pathogenesis of sepsis. Dysfunction of or injury to the endothelium may be involved in the pathogenesis of multiple organ failure and should be discriminated from activation resulting from stimulation with inflammatory stimuli. Identification of the molecular mechanisms that contribute to endothelial dysfunction or damage is likely to provide novel targets for the treatment of sepsis.

Hotchkiss RS, Karl IE. The pathophysiology and treatment of sepsis. *N Engl J Med* 2003;348:138–150.

Hotchkiss RS, et al. Endothelial cell apoptosis in sepsis. *Crit Care Med* 2002;30 (5 suppl):S225–S228.
Apoptosis is an important mechanism of lymphocyte and gastrointestinal epithelial cell death in sepsis. The impact of endothelial cell apoptosis in sepsis may either be detrimental or beneficial to host survival, depending on the particular pathogen.

Klaitman V, Almog Y. Corticosteroids in sepsis: a new concept for an old drug. *Isr Med Assoc J* 2003;5:51–55.
Recently, a new concept has emerged with more promising results: low-dose, long-term hydrocortisone therapy, and this approach is now being evaluated in the treatment of

septic shock. It is supported by the observation that many sepsis patients have relative adrenal insufficiency.

Luce JM. Physicians should administer low-dose corticosteroids selectively to septic patients until an ongoing trial is completed. *Ann Intern Med* 2004;141:70–72.
The role of steroids remains to be firmly defined.

Mahidhara R, Billiar TR. Apoptosis in sepsis. *Crit Care Med* 2000;28(4 suppl):N105–N113.
Apoptosis is an evolutionarily conserved, energy-dependent mode of cell death requiring the initiation and regulation of complex genetic programs. It is the body's main method of getting rid of cells that are in excess, damaged, or no longer needed in a controlled manner. Much work has demonstrated that dysregulation of apoptosis does occur in immune and nonimmune cells in in vitro and in vivo models of sepsis.

Manns BJ, et al. An economic evaluation of activated protein C treatment for severe sepsis. *N Engl J Med* 2002;347:993–1000.
For patients with an APACHE II score of 25 or more, the cost per life-year gained increased with age ($16,309 for patients younger than age 40; $28,100 for those aged 80 or older). Further research is needed to determine the cost effectiveness of activated protein C for patients with sepsis and less severe illness.

Marik PE, Zaloga GP. Adrenal insufficiency during septic shock. *Crit Care Med* 2003;31: 141–145.
Adrenal insufficiency is common in patients with septic shock, the incidence depending largely on the diagnostic tests and criteria used to make the diagnosis. There is clearly no absolute serum cortisol concentration that distinguishes an adequate from an insufficient adrenal response. However, the authors believe that a random cortisol concentration of less than 25 mcg/dL in a highly stressed patient is a useful diagnostic threshold for the diagnosis of adrenal insufficiency.

Mathiak G, et al. Targeting the coagulation cascade in sepsis: did we find the "magic bullet?" *Crit Care Med* 2003;31:310–311.

Minneci PC, et al. Meta-analysis: the effect of steroids on survival and shock during sepsis depends on the dose. *Ann Intern Med* 2004;141:47–56.
Although short courses of high-dose glucocorticoids decreased survival during sepsis, a 5- to 7-day course of physiologic hydrocortisone doses with subsequent tapering increases survival rate and shock reversal in patients with vasopressor-dependent septic shock.

Opal SM, Gluck T. Endotoxin as a drug target. *Crit Care Med* 2003;31(1 suppl):S57–S64.
Despite compelling evidence of the critical importance of endotoxin in the pathogenesis of gram-negative bacterial sepsis in preclinical investigations and numerous clinical interventional trials, the utility of antiendotoxin approaches to reduce significantly the mortality rate in human septic shock remains unproven.

Pinsky MR, et al. Serum cytokine levels in human septic shock. Relation to multiple-system organ failure and mortality. *Chest* 1993;103:565–575.
TNF and interleukin-6 serum levels are higher in septic than in nonseptic shock, but the persistence of TNF and interleukin-6 in the serum rather than peak levels of cytokines predicts a poor outcome in patients with shock.

Rangel-Frausto MS. The epidemiology of bacterial sepsis. *Infect Dis Clin North Am* 1999; 13:299–312, vii.
The mortality and morbidity of each of the systemic inflammatory response syndrome stages have been described; our ability to understand better and predict these stages will help us to make better therapeutic decisions.

Root RK, et al. Multicenter, double-blind, placebo-controlled study of the use of filgrastim in patients hospitalized with pneumonia and severe sepsis. *Crit Care Med* 2003;31:367–373.
The addition of filgrastim to the antibiotic and supportive care treatment of patients with pneumonia complicated by severe sepsis appeared to be safe but not efficacious in reducing mortality rates or complications from this infection.

Sharma VK, Dellinger RP. Recent developments in the treatment of sepsis. *Expert Opin Investig Drugs* 2003;12:139–152.
Review article.

Sollet JP, Garber GE. Selecting patients with severe sepsis for drotrecogin alfa (activated) therapy. *Am J Surg* 2002;184(6 suppl): S11–S18.
Proper clinical judgment and use of the these inclusion criteria as a guide will help clinicians select and treat sepsis patients with drotrecogin alfa (activated).

Szabo G, et al. Liver in sepsis and systemic inflammatory response syndrome. *Clin Liver Dis* 2002;6:1045–1066, x.
In patients with sepsis and systemic inflammatory response syndrome, the liver has two opposing roles: a source of inflammatory mediators and a target organ for the effects of the inflammatory mediators. This article summarizes the functional changes that take place in the liver during sepsis and systemic inflammatory response syndrome and discusses the cellular and molecular mechanisms that underlie clinical outcomes.

Takala A, et al. Markers of inflammation in sepsis. *Ann Med* 2002;34:614–623.
The present review summarizes the studies on markers of inflammation and immune suppression used, first, as predictors of organ dysfunction in patients with systemic inflammation, and second, as indicators of infection in adults and neonates.

Toh CH, et al. Early identification of sepsis and mortality risks through simple, rapid clot-waveform analysis. Implications of lipoprotein-complexed C reactive protein formation. *Intensive Care Med* 2003;29:55–61.
To determine if the rapid waveform profile of the activated partial thromboplastin time (aPTT) assay, which detects lipoprotein-complexed C reactive protein (LCCRP) formation, predicts sepsis and mortality in critically ill patients. Waveform analysis within the first hour of ICU admission is a single, simple, and rapid method of identifying the risks of mortality and sepsis.

Warren HS, et al. Risks and benefits of activated protein C treatment for severe sepsis. *N Engl J Med* 2002;347:1027–1030.

Wenzel RP. Treating sepsis. *N Engl J Med* 2002;347:966–967.

Zingarelli B, et al. Nuclear factor-kappaB as a therapeutic target in critical care medicine. *Crit Care Med* 2003;31(1 suppl):S105–S111.
Nuclear factor-kappaB is a transcriptional factor required for the gene expression of many inflammatory mediators. Inappropriate and prolonged activation of nuclear factor-kappaB has been linked to several diseases associated with inflammatory events, including septic shock, acute respiratory distress syndrome, ischemia, and reperfusion injury. The purpose of our review is to describe these novel therapeutic approaches and their potential efficacy.

METHICILLIN-RESISTANT *STAPHYLOCOCCUS AUREUS*   44

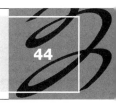

*A*fter its introduction into clinical practice in the 1940s, penicillin became the treatment of choice for infections caused by *Staphylococcus aureus;* however, penicillin-resistant strains of *S. aureus* rapidly emerged. The problem of resistant staphylococci appeared to have been eliminated with the development of the semisynthetic penicillins, such as methicillin and oxacillin, in the early 1960s. However, in 1961, strains of *S. aureus* resistant to the semisynthetic penicillins were isolated in England, and within 10 years, outbreaks of hospital-associated infections became common throughout Europe.

Before 1976, only sporadic outbreaks of nosocomial infection with methicillin-resistant *S. aureus* (MRSA) were reported in the United States. Since that time, hospital-acquired disease caused by MRSA has reached epidemic proportions. Although the initial outbreaks were confined to university medical centers, by 1979, more than 30% of community hospitals had patients with MRSA bacteremia, and by 1989, more than 90% of all acute-care hospitals reported having patients infected with this microbe. The fact that few antimicrobials are available to treat infected patients and the observation that the organism can be difficult to eliminate from an institution contribute to the concern about MRSA as a nosocomial pathogen. That concern has been dramatically accentuated since strains with reduced susceptibility to vancomycin (vancomycin-intermediate *S. aureus* [VISA]) have been described throughout the world. Many of the VISA isolates occurred in patients on hemodialysis after prolonged courses of vancomycin. Many of these isolates are susceptible to trimethoprim–sulfamethoxazole, linezolid, and quinupristin-dalfopristin. In 2002, the Centers for Disease Control and Prevention (CDC) reported the first isolate of vancomycin-resistant *S. aureus* (VRSA) in a patient on hemodialysis after a prolonged exposure to vancomycin. Fortunately, the isolate was susceptible to linezolid, quinupristin–dalfopristin, tetracycline, and trimethoprim–sulfamethoxazole.

Since 1997, when four pediatric deaths were reported from community-acquired MRSA infections, there has been an increasing number of community-acquired MRSA isolates. The source of these isolates is unknown, but it does not appear to be from the hospital. Community-acquired isolates of *S. aureus* differ from hospital isolates in that they are not multiresistant and are often susceptible to clindamycin, tetracycline, and trimethoprim–sulfamethoxazole. Both hospital-acquired and community-acquired MRSA isolates are usually susceptible to linezolid. The use of pulse field gel electrophoresis may help determine the relatedness of the various isolates. Infection control measures, such as hand washing, are critical to prevent outbreaks of community-acquired *S. aureus* infections.

The resistance of *S. aureus* to penicillin is mediated by a β-lactamase, which is an enzyme usually produced under the control of extrachromosomal DNA (plasmid). The β-lactamase is capable of hydrolyzing the β-lactam ring and thus chemically inactivating penicillin. In contrast, resistance to methicillin and related drugs is chromosomally linked, and it does not involve the inactivation of the antimicrobial. Rather, methicillin-resistant staphylococci express a penicillin-binding protein that possesses a greatly reduced affinity for β-lactam antimicrobials, including the semisynthetic penicillins; this protein is referred to as penicillin-binding protein 2a. The phenotypic expression of this intrinsic resistance can be modified by a number of factors; for example, raising the pH of the culture media or lowering the incubation temperature below 35°C increases the expression of methicillin resistance. The heterogeneity in the phenotypic expression of resistance is clinically relevant; if an intrinsically resistant strain is incubated at 37°C, only 1 in 10^5 or 10^6 bacteria will express resistance, and the isolate may be incorrectly characterized as methicillin susceptible. Of note, MRSA often contains plasmids that convey resistance to other antimicrobials. Finally, methicillin-resistant strains possess all the virulence factors found in methicillin-susceptible staphylococci, and so the organism is capable of producing life-threatening disease in humans.

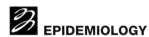

EPIDEMIOLOGY

MRSA is usually introduced into a hospital by patients who are transferred from other institutions, especially nursing homes, in which the organisms are endemic. Physicians also have been implicated as the source of interhospital spread. On occasion, spouses of patients have been found to be reservoirs of MRSA. Once introduced into a hospital, MRSA can disseminate rapidly and colonize patients and personnel, who then serve as sources of continued transmission. Diseases of the skin, including decubitus ulcers, burns, surgical wounds, and chronic dermatitis, increase the probability of colonization. In addition, colonization of the anterior nares of patients and hospital employees can occur and contribute to the spread of MRSA.

The risk for development of infection with MRSA is increased among colonized patients who are aged and debilitated, who have received prior antimicrobial therapy, who reside in intensive care units (ICUs), who undergo chronic hemodialysis, or who are hospitalized for prolonged periods. Resistant staphylococci can produce a number of potentially life-threatening diseases, including endocarditis, pneumonia, bacteremia, osteomyelitis, and septic thrombophlebitis. Because of the prevalence of serious underlying illnesses among patients infected with MRSA, case fatality rates are high; among patients with bronchopneumonia, for example, mortality rates above 50% have been reported.

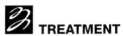 **TREATMENT**

The management of patients with infections caused by MRSA remains problematic, in part because of the limited number of useful antimicrobials. These organisms are invariably resistant to all penicillins. Some strains are susceptible in vitro to the cephalosporins; however, clinical experience indicates that patients infected with MRSA and treated with cephalosporins respond poorly, and MRSA must be considered resistant to this class of antimicrobials. Virtually all strains of MRSA exhibit susceptibility to vancomycin, and clinical studies have confirmed that vancomycin is an effective drug in the management of patients with serious infections. Vancomycin is the treatment of choice for patients with potentially life-threatening disease caused by MRSA, but it is not an ideal agent; some strains of MRSA are only inhibited by the drug, not killed, and treatment failures can occur in patients infected with these tolerant strains.

Linezolid, quinupristin-dalfopristin and daptomycin are alternative agents for patients who fail or cannot tolerate vancomycin. In one report, linezolid may be more effective than vancomycin.

Some strains of *S. aureus* resistant to the β-lactam antimicrobials are sensitive to trimethoprim–sulfamethoxazole, and the drug can be used to treat patients infected with MRSA. Ciprofloxacin also has been used with success on occasion. Of note, patients cured of MRSA infection often remain colonized by the pathogen.

Vancomycin is usually administered at a dosage of 1 g every 12 hours. Because the drug is excreted by the kidneys, dosage adjustments are mandatory in patients with renal dysfunction. Serum levels should be monitored, and peak concentrations of 30 to 40 mcg/mL and trough levels of 5 to 10 mcg/mL should be maintained. Vancomycin alone rarely produces nephrotoxicity; however, the potential for renal injury is substantially augmented in patients also receiving aminoglycosides. In general, renal function should be assessed twice weekly, and the use of other nephrotoxic drugs should be avoided. Vancomycin has been reported to cause hearing loss, although this complication is very rare. If the patient fails to respond to therapy with vancomycin, the addition of rifampin or an aminoglycoside should be considered; in general, the combination of vancomycin with rifampin or an aminoglycoside may produce synergistic killing. Vancomycin is dialyzed in patients receiving hemodialysis and another dose should be administered if the trough level is less than 15 mcg/mL.

 INFECTION CONTROL

To control the spread of MRSA within a hospital, patients known to be infected with the organism should be isolated. Stringent adherence to the isolation techniques is mandatory, and scrupulous attention must be paid to handwashing and the use of gloves, gowns, and masks.

If standard infection control measures fail to arrest an outbreak of MRSA disease, surveillance cultures should be obtained to identify colonized patients who may be the source of continuous person-to-person transmission. Physicians, nursing personnel, and other persons in contact with patients who are infected or colonized with MRSA should be screened for carriage by culturing the anterior nares and cutaneous lesions. If the survey of personnel fails to detect MRSA carriage but the outbreak continues, additional cultures of the healthcare workers' nares, throat, hands, axillae, rectums, and inguinal regions should be considered. Occasionally, ICUs must be closed to new admissions to control an outbreak of infection (Table 44-1).

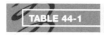

TABLE 44-1	Guidelines to Control Transmission of MRSA

- Surveillance cultures (nares, axillae, groin, rectum) weekly
- Culture high risk patients
- Emphasize hand hygiene using alcohol-based products
- Use gloves, gowns, and mask upon entering the room of a patient with MRSA

(Modified from Muto CA, et al. SHEA guideline for preventing nosocomial transmission of multidrug–resistant strains of *Staphylococcus aureus* and *Enterococcus*. *Infect Control Hosp Epidemiol* 2003;24:362–386.)

In the setting of outbreaks of infection, the use of antimicrobials in the management of patients and healthcare workers who are carriers of MRSA in concert with other infection control measures has proved effective in controlling epidemics. In particular, studies have shown that treatment of carriers is frequently associated with eradication of colonizing MRSA and control of epidemics. Thus, antimicrobials should be used if an outbreak of MRSA disease is not terminated by alternate infection control procedures.

Data from a number of studies have shown that topical 2% mupirocin applied to the anterior nares two to three times daily for 5 to 7 days may be an effective means of eliminating the nasal carrier state. Minocycline (100 mg twice daily) together with mupirocin and rifampin also has been highly effective in eradicating the nasal carrier state.

Patients with MRSA at sites that contain copious secretions, such as decubitus ulcers and tracheostomy wounds, often fail treatment. Further, the use of topical or systemic antimicrobials in the setting of foreign bodies, such as nasogastric or percutaneous gastrostomy tubes, will usually be unsuccessful in eliminating colonization, and the intervention may lead to the development of drug resistance. Finally, after the completion of a course of antimicrobials directed at the carrier state, follow-up cultures are necessary to ensure that the methicillin-resistant staphylococci have been eradicated from colonized patients and healthcare workers. (NMG)

Bibliography

Bradley SF, et al. Methicillin-resistant *Staphylococcus aureus:* colonization and infection in a long-term care facility. *Ann Intern Med* 1991;115:417.
Even in a chronic care facility with endemic MRSA, in 65% of the residents colonization never developed, and only 3% of the colonized patients experienced an infection.

Boyce JM, et al. Do infection control measures work for methicillin-resistant *Staphylococcus aureus?* *Infect Control Hosp Epidemiol* 2004;25:395–401.
Almost 40% of hospitalized patients are colonized with MRSA.

Centers for Disease Control and Prevention. *Staphylococcus aureus* resistant to vancomycin—United States, 2002. *MMWR Morb Mortal Wkly Rep* 2002;51:565–567.
First description of an S. aureus *isolate with a minimum inhibitory concentration of vancomycin ≥ 32 mcg/mL.*

Centers for Disease Control. Update: *Staphylococcus aureus* with reduced susceptibility to vancomycin—1997. *MMWR Morb Mortal Wkly Rep* 1997;46:765.
In 1997, the first U.S. isolate of S. aureus *intermittently susceptible to vancomycin (minimum inhibitory concentration, 8 μg/mL) was isolated in Michigan.*

Cooper BS, et al. Isolation measures in the hospital management of methicillin resistant *Staphylococcus aureus* (MRSA): systematic review of the literature. *BMJ* 2004;329:1–8.
A review of the effectiveness of isolation measures for MRSA.

Crossley K. Long-term care facilities as sources of antibiotic-resistant nosocomial pathogens. *Curr Opin Infect Dis* 2001;14:455–459.
Patients admitted to an acute care hospital from a nursing home may be a source of resistant organisms.

D'Agata EMC. Antimicrobial-resistant, gram-positive bacteria among patients undergoing chronic hemodialysis. *CID* 2002;35:1212–1218.
Hemodialysis and prolonged exposure to vancomycin may promote the development of resistant pathogens.

Darouiche R, et al. Eradication of colonization by methicillin-resistant *Staphylococcus aureus* by using oral minocycline-rifampin and topical mupirocin. *Antimicrob Agents Chemother* 1991;35:1612.
By using a combination of systemic (minocycline and rifampin) and topical (mupirocin) antimicrobial therapy, the authors eradicated MRSA colonization from 91% of the patients and 95% of the sites.

Doebbeling BN, et al. Elimination of *Staphylococcus aureus* nasal carriage in health care workers: analysis of six clinical trials with calcium mupirocin ointment. *Clin Infect Dis* 1993;17:466.
After analyzing the data from double-blinded studies performed at six institutions that involved 339 healthcare workers with stable nasal carriage of S. aureus, the authors concluded that calcium mupirocin ointment administered intranasally for 5 days was safe and effective in eliminating the organism.

Eady EA, Cove JH. Staphylococcal resistance revisited: community-acquired methicillin resistant *Staphylococcus aureus*—an emerging problem for the management of skin and soft tissue infections. *Curr Opin Infect Dis* 2003;16:103–124.
A comprehensive review of the genetics of community-acquired MRSA isolates.

Eliopoulos GM. Quinupristin-dalfopristin and linezolid: evidence and opinion. *Clin Infect Dis* 2003;36:473–481.
Review.

Farr BM. Prevention and control of methicillin-resistant *Staphylococcus aureus* infections. *Curr Opinion in Infect Dis* 2004;17:317–322.
Only vigorous infection control efforts can reduce rates of MRSA infection and colonization.

Fridkin SK. Vancomycin-intermediate and -resistant *Staphylococcus aureus*: what the infectious disease specialist needs to know. *Clin Infect Dis* 2001;32:108–115.
Emergence of VISA isolates.

Fung-Tomac J, et al. Emergence of homogeneously methicillin-resistant *Staphylococcus aureus*. *J Clin Microbiol* 1991;29:2880.
In a study of 47 clinical isolates, the authors note that 100% of the strains recovered before 1987 were inhibited in vitro by ciprofloxacin but that only 60% of the strains obtained after 1987 were susceptible to the drug.

Haley RW, et al. The emergence of methicillin-resistant *Staphylococcus aureus* infections in United States hospitals. *Ann Intern Med* 1982;97:297.
Describes the onset of the problem of MRSA in U.S. hospitals and implicates "the house staff-patient transfer circuit" as contributing to the interhospital spread of the microbe.

Harbarth S, et al. Impact of methicillin resistance on the outcome of patients with bacteremia caused by *Staphylococcus aureus*. *Arch Intern Med* 1998;158:182.
In a retrospective study of almost 200 patients with staphylococcal bacteremia, the authors concluded that methicillin resistance alone exerted no significant impact on mortality rates.

Hicks NR, Moore EP, Williams EW. Carriage and community treatment of methicillin-resistant *Staphylococcus aureus*: what happens to colonized patients after discharge? *J Hosp Infect* 1991;19:17.
The majority of infants and mothers colonized with MRSA at discharge had persistent carriage after 4 weeks; the most common site of colonization was the perineum in mothers and the throat in infants.

Howden BP, et al. Treatment outcomes for serious infections caused by methicillin-resistant *Staphylococcus aureus* with reduced vancomycin susceptibility. *Clin Infect Dis* 2004;38:521–528.
Use of linezolid with or without rifampicin and fusidic acid was effective for infections caused by MRSA with reduced susceptibility to vancomycin.

Hsu CC. Serial survey of methicillin-resistant *Staphylococcus aureus* nasal carriage among residents in a nursing home. *Infect Control Hosp Epidemiol* 1991;12:416.
In this prospective study of nursing home patients, the authors found that MRSA colonization was present in 70 to 80% of the residents who were bedridden or had decubitus ulcers or foreign bodies, and that the presence of the organism within the facility was perpetuated by persistently or intermittently colonized residents.

Kauffman CA, et al. Attempts to eradicate methicillin-resistant *Staphylococcus aureus* from a long-term care facility with the use of mupirocin ointment. *Am J Med* 1993;94: 371.
Although mupirocin ointment was effective in eliminating MRSA from the nares and wounds of colonized patients in a long-term care institution, recurrence rates were high and long-term use selected for resistant strains; these observations led the authors to conclude that mupirocin should be used only in the setting of an outbreak of infection with MRSA.

Kim S, et al. Outcome of inappropriate initial antimicrobial treatment in patients with methicillin-resistant *Staphylococcus aureus* bacteremia. *J Antimicrob Chemother* 2004; 54:489–497.
Delay of 2 days in appropriate therapy for MRSA bacteremia did not adversely affect the outcome.

Melzer M, et al. Is methicillin-resistant *Staphylococcus aureus* more virulent than methicillin-susceptible *S. aureus*? A comparative cohort study of British patients with nosocomial infection and bacteremia. *Clin Infect Dis* 2003;37:1453–1460.
Higher mortality in patients with nosocomial S. aureus *bacteremia compared with those with methicillin-susceptible* S. aureus.

Mulhausen PL, et al. Contrasting methicillin-resistant *Staphylococcus aureus* colonization in Veterans Affairs and community nursing homes. *Am J Med* 1996;100:24.
In this prospective survey of more than 200 nursing home patients, the authors found that the prevalence of colonization was about 30% in Veterans Affairs nursing homes and 10% in community facilities.

Muto CA, et al. SHEA guideline for preventing nosocomial transmission of multidrug-resistant strains of *Staphylococcus aureus* and *Enterococcus*. *Infect Control Hosp Epidemiol* 2003;24:362–386.
Surveillance cultures are useful to prevent the spread of MRSA and VRE.

Palavecino E. Community-acquired methicillin-resistant *Staphylococcus aureus* infections. *Clin Lab Med* 2004;24:403–418.
Review.

Sakoulas G, et al. Relationship of MIC and bactericidal activity to efficacy of vancomycin for treatment of methicillin-resistant *Staphylococcus aureus* bacteremia. *J Clin Microbiol* 2004;42:2398–2402.
Decreased efficacy of vancomycin against MRSA isolates reported as susceptible with a MIC of 1 to 2 mcg/mL.

Sheretz RJ, et al. A cloud adult: the *Staphylococcus aureus*-virus interaction revisited. *Ann Intern Med* 1996;124:539.
The importance of the colonized anterior nares as a potential reservoir for epidemics of MRSA infection is highlighted by this report.

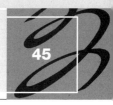

A report from the microbiology laboratory that a blood culture is positive for gram-positive cocci in grapelike clusters suggests that the organism most likely is *Staphylococcus aureus* or *Staphylococcus epidermidis*. Rarely, the organism will be identified as a *Micrococcus* or a *Peptococcus* (an anaerobic gram-positive coccus) species. Staphylococci are catalase-positive organisms that belong to the family Micrococcaceae. The staphylococci that produce coagulase are *S. aureus*, and those that are coagulase negative are designated as coagulase-negative staphylococci or *Staphylococcus* not *aureus*. There are multiple species of coagulase-negative staphylococci, but *S. epidermidis* is the most common. A coagulase-negative *staphylococcus*, called *Staphylococcus lugdunensis*, can produce valvular dehiscence, perforation, and abscess formation resembling infection caused by *S. aureus*. Another pathogenic coagulase-negative staphylococcal organism is *S. saprophyticus*, a well-recognized cause of urinary tract infections, especially in women. Resistance to novobiocin is the characteristic used most often to distinguish *S. saprophyticus* from other species of coagulase-negative staphylococci. All the factors that determine the virulence of *S. epidermidis* are unknown. The organism can adhere to and proliferate on prosthetic devices. Coagulase-negative staphylococci produce a slimelike substance biofilm that covers the organism but is not a true capsule. This substance interferes with phagocytosis.

Most (85%) coagulase-negative staphylococci isolated from a blood culture are contaminants, as the organisms colonize human skin and mucosal surfaces. In the other 15% of cases, the organisms are considered pathogens, especially in patients with indwelling medical devices such as prosthetic valves, central venous catheters, central nervous system shunts, vascular grafts, and pacemakers. *S. epidermidis* can also cause bacteremia in neutropenic patients with malignancy, neonatal bacteremia in low-birth-weight infants, and native valve endocarditis. To be able to interpret the meaning of a positive blood culture for a gram-positive coccus in clusters, the clinician must ask the following questions:

1. *How many blood cultures are positive?* A single positive culture suggests contamination unless the patient has an indwelling prosthetic device; if that is the case, repeated blood cultures are indicated, depending on the clinical situation. Obtaining a single set of blood cultures in an adult with a prosthetic device poses a dilemma for the clinician if the culture becomes positive. To avoid this problem, three sets of blood cultures should be obtained in the setting of suspected infection in a patient with an indwelling medical device.
2. *What if there are multiple positive blood cultures?* The finding of multiple positive blood cultures for coagulase-negative staphylococci suggests true invasive disease. The clinician should compare the antibiograms of the staphylococci isolated from the different blood culture bottles to determine if they are the same or different strains. The advantage of using the antimicrobial susceptibility test results to compare the strains is that the antibiograms are readily available. However, the technique is limited by the resistance of most nosocomial staphylococci to multiple antimicrobials, and the resistance may be unstable. Other methods of epidemiologic analysis are phage typing, biotyping, plasmid profile analysis, and restriction endonuclease analysis. The various techniques used to determine strain uniqueness are costly and may not be readily available, so that it is imperative to obtain blood cultures with the utmost care to avoid contamination.

269

3. *Does the patient have a persistent bacteremia?* Persistent recovery of a unique organism from the blood is powerful evidence that the coagulase-negative staphylococcal organism is a real pathogen and not a contaminant.
4. *Were the positive blood cultures obtained in a patient with intravascular lines?* Intravascular lines are often the source of *S. epidermidis* and should be inspected, removed, and cultured. If there is no obvious primary focus, such as an IV line, and the patient has persistent bacteremia, infective endocarditis must be suspected.
5. *Does the patient have cardiac valve involvement?* Transesophageal echocardiography may be of value in documenting a vegetation on a cardiac valve, which supports the diagnosis of infective endocarditis.

If the interpretation of the blood culture reports supports the diagnosis of a real bacteremia rather than contamination, therapy should be selected based on the results of antimicrobial susceptibility testing. Several caveats must be considered when therapy is selected for a coagulase-negative staphylococcal infection.

1. If the organism is β–lactamase-negative, penicillin can be used. However, this rarely occurs.
2. If the organism is β–lactamase-positive and susceptible to methicillin, nafcillin can be selected. However, these organisms can be heteroresistant—that is, a culture can comprise two populations, one susceptible to methicillin and the other resistant. This resistance can be overlooked unless testing is performed with a large inoculum on salt-containing media and the culture is incubated at 30 to 35°C. Unfortunately, methicillin resistance can be seen in as many as 40 to 80% of strains, depending on the hospital.
3. If an organism is resistant to methicillin, it must be assumed that it is resistant to all the cephalosporins, even if it is found to be susceptible by testing.
4. Vancomycin susceptibility testing is reliable.
5. Prospective studies to determine the optimal therapy of *S. epidermidis* native valve infection are lacking. Retrospective studies favor the use of a β-lactam antimicrobial (e.g., nafcillin or oxacillin), or vancomycin plus gentamicin. The dosage of gentamicin is that used for synergy (1 mg/kg every 8 hours) in a patient with normal renal function. The duration of gentamicin administration varied between 3 and 42 days in different studies. Rifampin can be substituted for gentamicin and given with nafcillin or vancomycin for the duration of therapy (4 weeks). I favor using gentamicin only for the initial 5 days, unless the patient is doing poorly, and then using a single drug for the remainder of the therapy.
6. If the patient has a prosthetic device and an infection caused by a methicillin-susceptible *S. epidermidis*, then nafcillin or oxacillin plus rifampin should be selected for a 6-week course. Antimicrobial susceptibility testing of the *S. epidermidis* must be appropriate to detect the presence of heteroresistance. If the organism is susceptible to gentamicin, administer gentamicin in doses to achieve a peak serum concentration of 3 g/mL. Gentamicin should be given only for the initial 2 weeks of therapy. In patients with infection caused by a methicillin-resistant *S. epidermidis*, use vancomycin plus rifampin along with gentamicin for the first 2 weeks, then continue vancomycin plus rifampin for the remaining 4 weeks of therapy. The role of linezolid, daptomycin, a lipopeptide, and quinupristin-dalfopristin in patients unable to tolerate vancomycin remains to be determined. A number of drugs for resistant gram-positive organisms are currently under evaluation. These include oritavancin and dalbavancin, glycopeptides, and tigecycline, a tetracycline derivative.
7. The mortality rate for native valve *S. epidermidis* endocarditis ranges from 13 to 36%.
8. The mortality rate for *S. epidermidis* prosthetic valve endocarditis is about 20%. However, a cure rate of 80% usually requires a combination of surgery plus 6 weeks of antimicrobial therapy. (NMG)

Bibliography

Boyce JM, et al. A common-source outbreak of *Staphylococcus epidermidis* infections among patients undergoing cardiac surgery. *J Infect Dis* 1990;161:493.

The hands of a cardiac surgeon were identified as the source of infection. The authors used plasmid profiles and restriction endonuclease digest analysis to determine that the strains were identical.

Caputo GM, et al. Native valve endocarditis due to coagulase-negative staphylococci. *Am J Med* 1987;83:619.

Although the presentation is usually subacute, complications such as arterial emboli, conduction system abnormalities, congestive heart failure, myocardial abscesses, and valve leaflet disruption occur frequently.

Garcia P, et al. Coagulase-negative staphylococci: clinical microbiological and molecular features to predict true bacteraemia. *J Med Microbiol* 2004;53:67–72.

A shorter time for blood cultures to become positive and slime production were features of true bacteremia.

Haimi-Cohen, et al. Use of incubation time to detection in BACTEC 9240 to distinguish coagulase-negative staphylococcal contamination from infection in pediatric blood cultures. *Pediatr Infect Dis J* 2003;22:968–973.

A longer time to blood culture positivity suggests contamination.

Hedin G. A comparison of methods to determine whether clinical isolates of *Staphylococcus epidermidis* from the same patient are related. *J Hosp Infect* 1996;34:31–42.

Biotyping and antibiotic resistance testing were helpful in determining whether the strains isolated were causing infection or were contaminants.

Herwaldt LA, et al. The positive predictive value of isolating coagulase-negative staphylococci from blood cultures. *Clin Infect Dis* 1996;22:14–20.

Twenty-six percent of coagulase-negative staphylococci isolated represented infections. Clues to infection-associated isolates included identification of the species as S. epidermidis in one of five biotype, and demonstration of resistance to at least five antibiotics.

Karchmer AW. Staphylococcal endocarditis: laboratory and clinical basis for antibiotic therapy. *Am J Med* 1985;78(suppl 6B):116.

Outline of guidelines for therapy.

Karchmer AW, Archer GL, Dismukes WE. *Staphylococcus epidermidis* causing prosthetic valve endocarditis: microbiologic and clinical observations as guides to therapy. *Ann Intern Med* 1983;98:447.

Surgery is indicated for patients on appropriate therapy who have persistent fever for more than 9 days or evidence of prosthetic valve dysfunction.

Lowy FD, Hammer SM. *Staphylococcus epidermidis* infections. *Ann Intern Med* 1983;99:834.

S. epidermidis is an important cause of infection in patients with a prosthetic valve, prosthetic hip, central nervous system shunt, vascular graft, or peritoneal dialysis catheter.

Mirrett S, et al. Relevance of the number of positive bottles in determining clinical significance of coagulase-negative staphylococci in blood cultures. *J Clin Microbiol* 2001;39:3279–3281.

The number of positive blood cultures in a set is not helpful in separating true infection from contamination.

Raad I, et al. Differential time to positivity: a useful method for diagnosing catheter-related bloodstream infections. *Ann Intern Med* 2004;140:18–25.

In patients with catheter infections, catheter-drawn cultures turn positive 2 or more hours before cultures drawn from a peripheral vein. See also the editorial in Farr BM. Ann Intern Med 2004;140:62–64.

Ruhe J, et al. Non-epidermidis coagulase-negative staphylococcal bacteremia: clinical predictors of true bacteremia. *Eur J Clin Microbiol Infect Dis* 2004;23:495–498.

Factors associated with a true bacteremia included (1) more than one positive blood culture, (2) presence of a central venous catheter, and (3) methicillin resistance.

Rupp ME. Coagulase-negative staphylococcal infections: an update regarding recognition and management. In: Remington JS, Swartz MN, eds. *Current Clinical Topics in Infectious Diseases.* Boston, Mass: Blackwell Science; 1997:17:51–87.

Review.

Seenivasan MH, Yu VL. Staphylococcus lugdunensis—the hidden peril of coagulase-negative staphylococcus in blood cultures. *Eur J Clin Microbiol Infect Dis* 2003;22:489–491.

May be mistaken for S. epidermidis.

Tacconelli E, et. al. Epidemiological comparison of true methicillin-resistant and methicillin-susceptible coagulase-negative staphylococcal bacteremia at hospital admission. *Clin Infect Dis* 2003;37:644–649.

The rate of methicillin-resistant strains of coagulase-negative staphylococcus were 62% for community-acquired isolates and 84% for patients admitted from long-term care facilities or who were recently hospitalized.

Tenover FC, Arbeit RD, Goering RV. How to select and interpret molecular strain typing methods for epidemiological studies of bacterial infections: a review for health care epidemiologists. *Infect Control Hosp Epidemiol* 1997;18:426–439.

A review of strain typing methods. For coagulase-negative staphylococci, pulse-field gel electrophoresis is preferred.

von Eiff C, Peters G, Heilmann C. Pathogenesis of infections due to coagulase-negative staphylococci. *Lancet Infect Dis* 2002;2:677–685

A key in pathogenesis is the formation of biofilms.

Winston DJ, et al. Coagulase-negative staphylococcal bacteremia in patients receiving immunosuppressive therapy. *Arch Intern Med* 1983;143:32.

An important pathogen in the patient with granulocytopenia and an IV catheter.

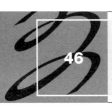

46 VANCOMYCIN-RESISTANT ENTEROCOCCI

ancomycin, a glycopeptide, was discovered in the mid 1950s. The drug inhibits peptidoglycan synthesis. Vancomycin has been the mainstay of therapy for infection with gram-positive organisms, including methicillin-resistant *Staphylococcus aureus*, coagulase-negative staphylococci, penicillin-resistant *Streptococcus pneumoniae*, and enterococci. The two most important enterococcal species are *Enterococcus faecalis* and *Enterococcus faecium*, with the former accounting for 80% of clinical isolates. Among vancomycin-resistant enterococci (VRE), 90% of the isolates are *E. faecium*.

In the late 1980s, the first clinical isolate of VRE was identified first in Europe and then in the United States. From 1989 through 1993, the percentage of nosocomial VRE isolates reported to the surveillance system of the Centers for Disease Control increased from 0.3 to 7.9%. In patients in intensive care units (ICUs), the increase in VRE was more dramatic, with almost 14% of isolates being resistant. Rates of resistance of enterococci to vancomycin in the non-ICU setting have increased and are now similar to rates in the ICU. Most hospitals in the United States have encountered at least one strain of VRE. VRE in the community has not been a problem in the United States, but the risk exists for transmission of strains of VRE from colonized patients after they leave the hospital.

Resistance of vancomycin can be classified as three phenotypes. Strains with van A resistance show a high level of resistance to vancomycin (minimum inhibitory concentrations [MICs] ≥ 64 μg/mL) and resistance to another glycopeptide, teicoplanin (MICs ≥16 μg/mL). Van A resistance occurs in both *E. faecalis* and *E. faecium*. Isolates with van B resistance are resistant to vancomycin (MICs from 4 μg/mL–1,000 μg/mL or higher) but remain susceptible to teicoplanin. Strains with van C resistance have a low level of resistance to vancomycin (MICs of 4–32 μg/mL) and are susceptible to teicoplanin. Van C resistance occurs in all isolates of *Enterococcus gallinarum*, an organism found in stool that does not appear to cause disease. VRE would not be such a serious problem if it were not for the fact that they are also resistant to ampicillin, oxacillin, cephalosporins, aminoglycosides, sulfa–trimethoprim, clindamycin, and the fluoroquinolones.

Enterococci, which are gram-positive cocci, are part of the normal gastrointestinal flora and are also found in small numbers in the mouth, vaginal secretions, and perineal skin. Enterococci rank second or third in frequency as causes of nosocomial infections in the United States. The sources of enterococci, which can either infect or colonize patients, are the patient's own normal flora (endogenous) and the hands of hospital personnel (exogenous). Enterococci also have been isolated in the hospital environment from bed rails, blood pressure cuffs, electronic thermometers, telephone handsets, and the surfaces of stethoscopes. Cultures of the surface environment yielded VRE in 7 to 46% of samples. Use of the usual disinfectants should be adequate to eradicate VRE from environmental surfaces. However, one report found that 8% of cultures after terminal cleaning still showed VRE.

Risk factors for acquiring VRE include serious underlying illness, advanced age, immunosuppression, ICU residence, prior surgery, renal insufficiency, long hospital stay (7 days or more), presence of a urinary or vascular catheter, and use of antibiotics, especially third-generation cephalosporins, vancomycin, and drugs for anaerobes. Once colonized with VRE, patients may remain so for years. When patients are not taking antibiotics, VRE counts in the stool may decrease, resulting in false-negative stool cultures for VRE. Cultures may again become positive when the patient is given an antibiotic.

Once a patient is identified as being either colonized or infected with VRE, contact precautions as recommended by the Hospital Infection Control Practices Advisory Committee (HICPAC) are instituted (Table 46-1).

Prudent use of vancomycin has been reported to decrease the risk for colonization and infection with VRE. Hospitals should adopt the guidelines recommended by HICPAC, which list the situations in which vancomycin use is appropriate and those in which its use should be discouraged (Tables 46-2 and 46-3). In addition to the prudent use of vancomycin and institution of barrier precautions, a decreased use of cefotaxime, ceftazidime, and clindamycin was noted in one report to result in a significant decrease (from 47 to 15%) in stools positive for VRE. Contamination of the environment and equipment for patient care with VRE is a problem, especially when patients have diarrhea. Because many patients may have both VRE and *Clostridium difficile*, measures to reduce the incidence of *C. difficile* may decrease the environmental contamination with VRE.

Treatment of infections caused by VRE remains a major problem. Chloramphenicol shows activity in vitro against many strains and has been used with modest success. Oral chloramphenicol is not available; the drug must be given intravenously. Surgical debridement with drainage of an abscess and removal of a Foley catheter or IV catheter without any specific antibiotic treatment also were effective prior to the availability of drugs to treat VRE. Dalfopristin–quinupristin, a streptogramin antibiotic, may be effective against some strains of *E. faecium*, but not *E. faecalis*. Linezolid, an oxazolidinone, has become the drug of choice

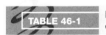 **Precautions to Prevent Patient-to-Patient Transmission of Vancomycin-Resistant Enterococci**

1. Place VRE-infected or VRE-colonized patient in a private room, or cohort two patients with VRE in the same room.
2. Wear gloves when entering the room. Change gloves after contact with stool, which may contain high colony counts of VRE.
3. Wear a gown if there will be contact with the patient or environment.
4. Remove gloves and gown before leaving room and wash hands with antiseptic soap.
5. Designate equipment, such as the stethoscope, blood pressure cuff, or thermometer, to a single patient with VRE or a cohort of VRE patients.
6. Continue VRE isolation until three stool or other cultures obtained at weekly intervals are negative.
7. Establish a system to identify patients with VRE so that they can be placed in isolation on readmission to the hospital.

(Modified from Centers for Disease Control and Prevention. Recommendations for preventing the spread of vancomycin resistance: recommendations of the Hospital Infection Control Practices Advisory Committee [HICPAC]. *MMWR Morb Mortal Wkly Rep* 1995;44:7–9.)

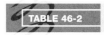

TABLE 46-2	Indications for Vancomycin Treatment

1. Treatment of infections caused by MRSA, *S. epidermidis* and enterococci in a penicillin-allergic patient.
2. Treatment of infections caused by gram-positive organisms in patients with a life-threatening penicillin allergy.
3. Treatment of antibiotic-associated colitis when metronidazole fails.
4. Prophylaxis for endocarditis in patients at high risk for infection.
5. Surgical prophylaxis in patients with a history of life-threatening penicillin allergy.

MRSA, Methicillin-resistant *S. aureus.*
(Modified from Centers for Disease Control and Prevention. Recommendations for preventing the spread of vancomycin resistance: recommendations of the Hospital Infection Control Practices Advisory Committee [HICPAC]. *MMWR Morb Mortal Wkly Rep* 1995;44:3–4.)

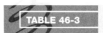

TABLE 46-3	Situations in Which the Use of Vancomycin Should Be Discouraged

1. Surgical prophylaxis other than in a patient with life-threatening allergy to β-lactam antibiotics.
2. Empiric antimicrobial therapy for a febrile neutropenic patient, unless there is strong evidence that the patient has an infection caused by a gram-positive microorganism.
3. Treatment of a single blood culture positive for coagulase-negative *Staphylococcus,* if other blood cultures drawn in the same time frame are negative.
4. Selective decontamination of the digestive tract.
5. Eradication of MRSA colonization.
6. Routine prophylaxis for patients on continuous ambulatory peritoneal dialysis or hemodialysis.
7. As a vancomycin solution for topical application or irrigation.
8. Initial treatment of *C. difficile* colitis.

MRSA, Methicillin-resistant *S. aureus.*
(Modified from Centers for Disease Control and Prevention. Recommendations for preventing the spread of vancomycin resistance: recommendations of the Hospital Infection Control Practices Advisory Committee [HICPAC]. *MMWR Morb Mortal Wkly Rep* 1995;44:4.)

for many VRE infections. It is active against both *E. faecium* and *E. faecalis,* but resistant strains have been identified. The drug is bacteriostatic and available for use intravenously and orally with almost 100% bioavailability. Bone marrow suppression and thrombocytopenia can occur in as many as 32% of patients receiving the drug. The drug should be avoided if the platelet count initially is less than 50,000. Daptomycin, a lipopeptide, is bactericidal for VRE but not yet approved for treatment of VRE infections. Other experimental drugs, such as tigecycline and oritavancin, may have a future role in treating VRE infections. Another experimental agent for gastrointestinal tract colonization of VRE is ramoplanin, a drug that is not absorbed when taken orally. For lower urinary tract infections resulting from VRE, nitrofurantoin or fosfomycin may have a role in therapy. Approaches to better control VRE are clearly needed. (NMG)

Bibliography

Anderson RL, et al. Susceptibility of vancomycin-resistant enterococci to environmental disinfectants. *Infect Control Hosp Epidemiol* 1997;18:195–199.
  No special disinfectants or procedures are needed to eradicate VRE from environmental surfaces.
Beezhold DW, et al. Skin colonization with vancomycin-resistant enterococci among hospitalized patients with bacteremia. *Clin Infect Dis* 1997;24:704–706.

Skin colonization (inguinal area and/or antecubital fossa) was common (86%) among patients with bacteremia and may be the source of catheter-related sepsis.

Bonilla HF, et al. Colonization with vancomycin-resistant *Enterococcus faecium*: comparison of a long-term-care unit with an acute-care hospital. *Infect Control Hosp Epidemiol* 1997;18:333–339.
VRE was found frequently (13 to 41%) on the hands of healthcare workers.

Centers for Disease Control and Prevention. Recommendations for preventing the spread of vancomycin resistance: recommendations of the Hospital Infection Control Practices Advisory Committee (HICPAC). *MMWR Morb Mortal Wkly Rep* 1995; 44:1–13.
Control of VRE will require (1) appropriate use of vancomycin, (2) staff education regarding VRE, (3) detection of VRE, and (4) implementation of infection control measures.

Edmond MB, et al. Vancomycin-resistant enterococcal bacteremia: natural history and attributable mortality. *Clin Infect Dis* 1996;23:1234–1239.
The mortality rate for patients with VRE bacteremia was 67%, which was twice that for matched controls.

Evans ME, Kortas KJ. Vancomycin use in a university medical center: comparison with Hospital Infection Control Practices Advisory Committee guidelines. *Infect Control Hosp Epidemiol* 1996;17:356–359.
Only 35% of the vancomycin orders were consistent with HICPAC guidelines.

Harbath S, Cosgrove S, Carmeli Y. Effects of antibiotics on nosocomial epidemiology of vancomycin-resistant enterococci. *Antimicrob Agents Chemother* 2002;46:1619–1628.
A discussion of the role of antibiotic usage and VRE epidemiology.

Kauffman CA. Therapeutic and preventative options for the management of vancomycin-resistant enterococcal infections. *J Antimicrob Chemo* 2003;51(suppl S3):iii23–iii30.
Treatment reviewed.

Lai KK, et al. The epidemiology of fecal carriage of vancomycin-resistant enterococci. *Infect Control Hosp Epidemiol* 1997;18:762–765.
VRE carriage is often prolonged (19–303 days).

McGowan JE. Debate—Guidelines for control of glycopeptide-resistant enterococci (GRE) have not yet worked. *J Hosp Infect* 2004;57:281–284.
A plea for better efforts to control glycopeptide-resistant enterococci (GRE).

Meka VG, Gold HS. Antimicrobial resistance to linezolid. *Clin Infect Dis* 2004;39:1010–1015.
Resistance to linezolid seen in isolates of VRE and S. aureus.

Montecalvo MA, et al. Natural history of colonization with vancomycin-resistant *Enterococcus faecium*. *Infect Control Hosp Epidemiol* 1995;16:680–685.
The rate of VRE colonization was 10 times the rate of infection among oncology patients and often persists for a year.

Murray BE. Vancomycin-resistant enterococcal infections. *N Engl J Med* 2000;342:710–721.
Review.

Muto CA, et al. SHEA guideline for preventing nosocomial transmission of multidrug-resistant strains of *Staphylococcus aureus* and *enterococcus*. *Infect Control Hosp Epidemiol* 2003;24:362–386.
Guidelines. Active surveillance recommended for patients at high risk for colonization.

Noskin GA, et al. Recovery of vancomycin-resistant enterococcus on fingertips and environmental surfaces. *Infect Control Hosp Epidemiol* 1995;16:577–581.
E. faecalis survived for 5 days and E. faecium *for 7 days on countertops.*

Perincevich EN, et al. Projected benefits of active surveillance for vancomycin-resistant enterococci in intensive care units. *Clin Infect Dis* 2004;38:1108–1115.
Active surveillance cultures and contact isolation can decrease the transmission of VRE in an ICU.

Porwancher R, et al. Epidemiological study of hospital-acquired infection with vancomycin-resistant *Enterococcus faecium*: possible transmission by an electronic ear probe thermometer. *Infect Control Hosp Epidemiol* 1997;18:1771–1773.
VRE transmitted by an electronic ear probe.

Quale J, et al. Manipulation of a hospital antimicrobial formulary to control an outbreak of vancomycin-resistant enterococci. *Clin Infect Dis* 1996;23:1020–1025.
Decreased use of cefotaxime, ceftazidime, and clindamycin was associated with a decrease in stool colonization with VRE.

Rafferty ME, et al. Vancomycin-resistant enterococci in stool specimens submitted for *Clostridium difficile* cytotoxin assay. *Infect Control Hosp Epidemiol* 1997;18:342–344.
Seventeen percent of stools submitted for C. difficile testing were positive for VRE.

Rice LB. Emergence of vancomycin-resistant enterococci. *Emerg Infect Dis* 2001;7:183–187.
Spread of VRE is promoted by poor infection control techniques and use of broad-spectrum cephalosporins and drugs with potent activity against anaerobes such as clindamycin.

Saurina G, Landman D, Quale JM. Activity of disinfectants against vancomycin-resistant *Enterococcus faecium. Infect Control Hosp Epidemiol* 1997;18:345–347.
Except for 3% hydrogen peroxide, phenolic and quaternary ammonium compounds were effective in eradicating VRE after a 10-minute exposure.

Slaughter S, et al. A comparison of the effect of universal use of gloves and gowns with that of glove use alone on acquisition of vancomycin-resistant enterococci in a medical intensive care unit. *Ann Intern Med* 1996;125:448–456.
Use of gloves and gowns was no better than gloves alone in preventing rectal colonization by VRE.

Stroud L, et al. Risk factors for mortality associated with enterococcal bloodstream infections. *Infect Control Hosp Epidemiol* 1996;17:576–580.
The mortality rate was 69% for patients with VRE bacteremia. The high mortality caused by bacteremia occurred in a cohort of severely ill patients.

Tacconelli E, et al. Preventing the influx of vancomycin-resistant enterococci into health care institutions, by use of a simple validated prediction rule. *Clin Infect Dis* 2004;39:964–970.
Risk factors for VRE included previous recovery of methicillin-resistant S. aureus, long-term hemodialysis, transfer from a long-term care facility, exposure to two or more antibiotics within the past month, prior hospitalization, and age older than 60.

Tornieporth NG, et al. Risk factors associated with vancomycin-resistant *Enterococcus faecium* infection or colonization in 145 matched case patients and control patients. *Clin Infect Dis* 1996;23:767–772.
Prolonged hospitalization (≥7 days), intrahospital transfers, and use of vancomycin or third-generation cephalosporins were associated with an increased risk for VRE infection or colonization.

Weber DJ, Rutala WA. Role of environmental contamination in the transmission of vancomycin-resistant enterococci. *Infect Control Hosp Epidemiol* 1997;18:306–309.
Environmental contamination in patients with VRE ranges from 7 to 46%.

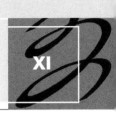

Fever XI

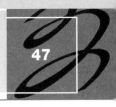

*I*ndividuals who have fever represent a complex group that may manifest a myriad of other symptoms, the diagnosis of which may be associated with infectious and noninfectious etiologies. Examples of noninfectious causes of fever include connective tissue disease, malignancy, medications, and myocardial or pulmonary infarction. In addition to a broad differential diagnosis, the issue of fever may be further confounded because sometimes it is absent in individuals with significant infections. This consideration is especially important in the elderly and in those with immune deficiency. Moreover, neither height of fever nor "fever curve" correlates with etiology or severity of disease. Finally, numerous important infections may not initially be associated with an obvious source. The history and physical examination findings in patients with fever may offer important clues to cause.

The likelihood that the acute onset of fever is due to bacterial infection is statistically associated with advanced age, presence of indwelling catheter, nursing home residency, and leukocytosis. Additionally elevated erythrocyte sedimentation rate and presence of diabetes mellitus may point toward fever being associated with bacterial infection. A scoring system to assess these has been developed. Examples of diseases in which acute onset of fever may be unaccompanied by focal complaints or significant physical findings are given in Table 47-1. Identification of the source of acute fever may be complicated if history and physical examination are difficult to obtain from the patient (e.g., elderly individuals, severely debilitated or noncompliant patients, those with overwhelming illness, or patients with language barriers). Thus, the clinician must have a sound understanding of potential causes of fever, as well as a studied approach to the patient who presents with this complaint. This chapter describes an initial assessment for the patient who reports with fever.

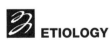 ## ETIOLOGY

The expanded history is a critical diagnostic tool. The clinician must inquire about travel, pets, occupation, recreational activities, medications, etc. As an example, an in-depth travel history may provide initial clues about illnesses that could include malaria, dengue, or yellow fever. Febrile patients returning from areas with malaria should be considered to have this illness until the diagnosis is excluded. Fever duration may be important and a comprehensive review of systems may elicit further clues. As with many diagnostics, the clinician must watch "the company that symptoms keep." These, in turn must be placed into the context of the "larger picture," which includes age, functional status, comorbidities, and general appearance on presentation. Immunosuppression from either underlying disease or treatment also enters into the paradigm.

In general, fevers that are of longer duration and unassociated with hemodynamic instability may be evaluated in a more relaxed fashion. In patients with HIV/AIDS, fever almost always accompanies the acute retroviral syndrome, and otherwise is generally noted as a component of opportunistic disease. In end-stage AIDS, fever may be the manifestation of disseminated infection with *Mycobacterium avium-complex*. It is also noted as an adverse effect of drugs (e.g., trimethoprim/sulfamethoxazole) and may accompany lymphoma, tuberculosis, or pneumonia caused by *Pneumocystis carinii*.

The presence of foreign bodies, such as joint implants and prosthetic heart valves, also should be noted. A history of rigors is generally sought but does not provide information

279

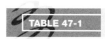

| TABLE 47-1 | Common Acute Febrile Diseases That May Be Nonfocal |

All hosts	Elderly/debilitated
Viral influenza	Pneumonia
Acute HIV Syndrome	
Malaria	Genitourinary infection
Primary bacteremia (meningococcemia,	Cholecystitis/cholangitis
S. aureus, typhoid fever, Capnocytophaga (DF-1)	
Rocky Mountain Spotted Fever	Myocardial/pulmonary infarction
Occult abscess	Apathetic hyperthyroidism
Hypoadrenalism	Drug fever (β-lactams, sulfonamides,
	procainamide, hydralazine)
	Cerebrovascular accident

beyond the fact that temperature became rapidly elevated; it does not imply a specific etiology.

A complete physical examination should be performed. General appearance and vital signs provide an important initial clue to severity of illness and may help with the decision to hospitalize. Vital signs should be sought from recent records that could include the ambulance and nursing home. Generally, height of fever does not correlate with etiology. Nevertheless, fever higher than 103°F generally is of greater concern and often points to infection. Recent data suggest that for some infections, such as shigellosis, degree of temperature elevation may correlate with severity of illness. Adults with fevers higher than 105.6°F should be hospitalized for fever reduction, as temperatures of this level may cause tissue damage. Contrary to classic dictum, many patients with temperature elevations of this level have treatable bacterial disease and should be treated empirically with antimicrobials.

Hypothermia is associated with impending sepsis, hypothyroidism, environmental exposure, and diabetes mellitus with autonomic instability. Hypothermia associated with infection is likely to be associated with a statistically lower systemic vascular resistance and higher cardiac index than that associated with the noninfectious etiologies already listed.

The respiratory rate may be an especially important and often overlooked sign. Older patients with rates higher than 25/minute often have lower respiratory infection, even in the absence of initial physical findings. These patients may have reduced functional status, may be dehydrated, and often have depressed cough. In the setting of community-acquired pneumonia, rates higher than 30/minute are associated with enhanced mortality. Low or unstable blood pressure may suggest impending septic shock and is an important reason for hospitalization. Elevated pulse of 10 to 15 beats/minute is anticipated with each degree of temperature elevation.

Temperature–pulse dissociation is associated with beta blockade and intrinsic coronary disease. Infectious reasons include viral influenza, Legionnaires' disease, yellow fever, typhoid fever (or, less commonly, other gram-negative bacteremias), and other viral syndromes. Rash should be sought in all body areas; even if subtle, it can provide useful information both etiologically and diagnostically. Careful attention must be paid to physical examination of the mouth, ears, genitalia, and rectum.

 MANAGEMENT

Initial decision-making focuses on the need for hospitalization, empiric or targeted antimicrobial therapy, and further testing. Hospitalization is indicated primarily for persons who are clinically unstable, believed to be at risk for rapid deterioration, or who may represent (through spread) a threat to others. Criteria are best determined for patients with community-acquired pneumonia, but exist for other infections that include cellulitis.

Advanced age and leukocytosis ($>15,000/mm^3$), altered vital signs, and presence of major comorbidities correlate with a likelihood of serious disease and can help determine the need for hospitalization. Other reasons need to be individualized and can include the need for intravenous antimicrobials or other fluids, the need for rapid evaluation likely to require sophisticated testing, and intense monitoring. The person with known major alterations of immunity should be hospitalized if significant infection cannot be rapidly ruled out. Alternatively, the younger, fit individual is more likely to be treated as an outpatient.

Management of the febrile patient without an obvious focus of infection will vary depending on the need for hospitalization. Basic laboratory data should be obtained from the hospitalized individual, including complete blood count (CBC), urinalysis, and (generally) several sets of blood cultures. Decisions regarding other tests, for example, chest radiograph, further blood tests, and cultures from sites other than blood will depend on clinical presentation and subtle clues obtained from the history and physical examination. The urgency of testing is dependent on clinical status. Generally, acutely febrile patients, especially those who have high-grade fevers or are unstable, require more intensive evaluation. If hospitalization is not felt to be warranted, testing is generally more relaxed and based on symptoms and signs.

Management of fever itself is based primarily on host factors and height of temperature. Under normal circumstances, elevated temperature is felt to be beneficial to the host, and thus attempts to lower it are often overzealous. Fever is known to stimulate immune function and to decrease serum iron felt necessary for survival of some pathogens. Furthermore, artificial regulation of temperature may result in an inability to follow this important parameter of response. Data suggest that physical cooling, with resultant decline in skin temperature, may actually elevate peak temperature. Additionally, investigations demonstrate that this form of fever management is associated with substantial patient misery and increased oxygen consumption and blood pressure. Reasons to lower fever include: (1) temperature higher than $105.6°F$ (potential tissue damage) and (2) metabolic stress of fever (e.g., acute coronary syndrome. Acetaminophen or nonsteroidals can generally be used if needed; salicylates should be avoided as they have been occasionally associated with severe hypothermia and death (especially in management of typhoid fever and lymphoma), and may be associated with Reye's syndrome if given for some febrile syndromes.

Antimicrobial needs are determined by the likelihood of treatable infection. Table 47-2 depicts conditions that usually warrant empiric antimicrobial therapy. This management strategy should be reserved for inpatients believed to have either a high likelihood of treatable infection or significant adverse outcome if untreated. Antimicrobials should always be initiated *after* obtaining cultures from appropriate sites; need should be reassessed after 2 to 3 days when more information is available and clinical response has been assessed. The choice of empiric antimicrobials is based on the presumed site of infection and likely microbe(s) from that site. As an example, *Pseudomonas aeruginosa* is an unlikely pathogen in most patients with community-acquired infection. Alternatively, *Staphylococcus aureus*

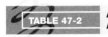 **TABLE 47-2** | **Acute Febrile Conditions Often Warranting Empiric Antimicrobials**

Fever $>105.6°F$
Immunosuppression
Neutropenia/granulocytopenia
Asplenia
Hypogammaglobulinemia
Cirrhosis
Elderly
Unstable vital signs
Presence of prosthetic device/foreign body
Epidemiologic evidence suggestive of infection
Recent bite
Recent travel

is a common community-acquired pathogen, and resistance to β-lactams has become sufficiently common in many areas to warrant an altered paradigm of care. For most hospitalized patients requiring antimicrobials, therapy is initiated intravenously to ensure uniform absorption and to reach high systemic levels quickly. In febrile patients not sufficiently ill to be hospitalized, antimicrobials should not be overused, especially for those with subacute or chronic onset. Overuse of oral antibiotics for viral infections has been identified as a major problem in the United States and one that may be associated with emerging antibiotic resistance of common bacteria. Persons with neither focal abnormalities nor significant underlying disease may often be observed. However, all patients should be followed regularly for changes in clinical status that point either to improvement or a more focused process.

The need for further testing is based on the presence of ongoing fever. Although no clear guidelines exist, blood tests that include CBC (with differential), liver function, sedimentation rate, antinuclear antibody, and renal function are often warranted. Early in the evaluation, posteroanterior and lateral chest radiographs should be obtained. The need for other blood, radiographic, microbiologic, and invasive tests for tissue must be individualized. (RBB)

Bibliography

Aronoff DM, Neilson EG. Antipyretics: mechanisms of action and clinical use in fever suppression. *Am J Med* 2001;111:304–315.

This manuscript reviews fever and the mechanisms of action by which antipyretics influence it. The authors conclude that adverse effects from attempts to lower fever occur, including patient discomfort and inability to judge response to therapies. Little data exist to judge the true benefits of antipyretics when they could be indicated; thus further studies are needed.

Gallagher EJ, Brooks F, Gennis P. Identification of serious illness in febrile adults. *Am J Emerg Med* 1994;12:129–133.

The authors conducted a prospective observational study within a cohort of approximately 600 adults who presented to an emergency department with fever higher than 100° F. Serious disease was defined as that (a) need for emergency surgery, (b) intubation, (c) hypotension necessitating treatment, (d) bacteremia, (e) death. Twelve percent of febrile individuals met criteria for serious illness. By regression analysis, only advanced age (50 years) and leukocytosis (>15,000/mm³) were associated with the presence of serious illness. The authors conclude that approximately one-third of adults with both parameters will be seriously ill. However, the absence of both parameters will not preclude serious disease as defined.

Leibovici L, Cohen O, Wysenbeek AJ. Occult bacterial infection in adults with unexplained fever. *Arch Intern Med* 1990;150:1270–1272.

This investigation of more than 100 patients admitted to a hospital with unexplained fever depicted a strategy to determine likelihood of bacterial infection. Patients with advanced age, selected underlying comorbidities, and elevated white blood cell (WBC) counts and erythrocyte sedimentation rates were more likely to harbor bacterial infection and be bacteremic.

Lenhardt R, et al. The effects of physical treatment on induced fever in humans. *Am J Med* 1999;106:550–555.

The authors investigated the effects of physical cooling (ice blanket) on volunteers with induced fever caused by injected interleukin-2. Cooling was associated with significant patient discomfort and increased metabolic load to the patients. No definitive benefits to this treatment could be noted. They did not, however, assess medicinal lowering of temperature, likely to work by other mechanisms.

Mackowiak PA, Bartlett JG, Borden EC, et al. Concepts of fever: recent advanced and lingering dogma. *Clin Infect Dis* 1997;25:119–138.

This is a round table discussion on a variety of issues related to fever. Those covered include pathogenesis, fever patterns, and fever in the HIV/AIDS population. Dr. Bartlett depicts those situations likely to be associated with fever and selected tests of value. Fever is most commonly noted during the acute retroviral syndrome (mononucleosis-like) and accompanies many opportunistic processes. Fever is unlikely to resolve spontaneously in advanced disease.

McFadden JP, et al. Raised respiratory rate in elderly patients: a valuable physical sign. *Br Med J* 1982;284:626–627.

Normal respiratory rate in elderly patients was 16 to 25/minute. Those with acute lower respiratory infections had higher rates. Observation of increased rate preceded diagnosis. Elevation of respiratory rate was not noted with other infections.

Pinson AG, et al. Fever in the clinical diagnosis of acute pyelonephritis. *Am J Emerg Med* 1997;15:148–151.

Adult women with pyuria with or without fever were studied as two groups to determine the presence of acute pyelonephritis. They were further stratified by need for hospitalization. Among both hospitalized and outpatient-treated women, lack of fever predicted alternative diagnoses that included pelvic inflammatory disease and cholecystitis. The authors conclude that fever is associated with pyelonephritis in patients with pyuria.

Sioson PB, Brown RB. Hyperpyrexia in a large community hospital: Etiologies, features, and outcomes. *South Med J* 1993;86:773–776.

Within a defined population of 39 patients with fever higher than 105.6° F, potentially treatable bacterial infections were commonly noted. This observation differs from that noted in earlier literature and has important implications for management. The authors feel that most patients with hyperpyrexia warrant empiric antibiotic therapy, pending results of cultures and other assessments for treatable infection.

FEVER AND PROSTHETIC HEART VALVES   48

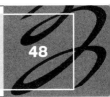

$\mathcal{F}$ ever occurring in a patient with a prosthetic heart valve may signal infective endocarditis or numerous other conditions. It is estimated that an infection will develop in 1 to 4% of patients with prosthetic devices during the life span of the device.

In diagnosis, it is helpful to note how long after the operation the fever developed. Any major surgical procedure can be associated with a low-grade fever (100°F [37.8°C]) for a few days. Possibilities during the initial 24-hour period include a transfusion reaction, atelectasis, aspiration pneumonia, or wound infection, especially with group A hemolytic streptococci or *Clostridium* spp. Fever developing after the first 24 hours may be caused by an anesthetic. Fever with lymphadenopathy and atypical lymphocytes, called the postperfusion syndrome, usually occurs 2 to 4 weeks after surgery. It is caused by the transfusion of fresh blood with cytomegalovirus or Epstein-Barr virus. Malaria may occur rarely after a blood transfusion. Other infectious complications to consider are phlebitis related to numerous IV lines, infusion of contaminated fluids, drug fever, abscesses secondary to intramuscular (IM) injections, bacterial pneumonia, pulmonary infarction, urinary tract infection, wound infection, deep vein thrombophlebitis, sternal osteomyelitis, and mediastinitis. A syndrome of unknown etiology, the postcardiotomy syndrome, occurs 10 days to 3 months after surgery and is characterized by fever, chest pain, and often a pericardial friction rub. Reactivation of rheumatic fever also may be responsible for fever.

It is important to obtain blood cultures from patients with fever and a prosthetic heart valve. Infective endocarditis occurring within 60 days after valve insertion is called *early endocarditis;* infection that occurs more than 12 months after surgery is called *late endocarditis.* Infections occurring between 2 and 12 months after surgery are called *intermediate onset* and consist of a mixture of hospital-acquired and community-acquired cases. The source of organisms responsible for early-onset infections may be contamination of the prosthetic valve or bloodstream at the time of operation or an infectious complication developing during the postoperative period, such as a sternal wound infection, pneumonia, or an infected IV line. The same organism often can be isolated from a peripheral site (a wound), sputum, or the blood. The prosthetic valve, like any other foreign body, is at high risk for becoming infected as a consequence of bacteremia. Late-onset infections may be caused by a transient bacteremia associated with either a dental, skin, or genitourinary tract procedure or an infection. Other organisms responsible for late-onset infections may be acquired at the time of operation and have a long incubation period.

The organisms causing prosthetic valve infections differ from those producing classic endocarditis. Certain bacteria, such as diphtheroids and, especially, coagulase-negative staphylococci, usually considered blood culture contaminants, account for about one-third of all infections in these patients. Of the early-onset cases, half are caused by *Staphylococcus aureus* or *Staphylococcus epidermidis*, 20% are caused by gram-negative bacilli, and 10% are produced by fungi such as *Candida* or, rarely, *Aspergillus*. The major causative organisms in late-onset infections are streptococci (36%), staphylococci (38%), gram-negative bacilli (10%), and other pathogens (10%). However, any organism can infect a prosthetic valve, and when blood cultures are positive for unusual pathogens or so-called nonpathogens, these should not be dismissed as contaminants. Approximately 5 to 10% of patients have culture-negative endocarditis.

The clinical features of early-onset infections are often dominated by other, concomitant infectious complications, such as pneumonia, wound infection, suppurative phlebitis, or urinary tract infection. Symptoms and signs include fever (90 to 100%), new insufficiency murmurs (60%), splenomegaly (20%), and shock (33%). The presence of petechiae, hematuria, or anemia is difficult to interpret during the early postoperative period, as these conditions may relate to the operation. A more fulminant clinical course often occurs in patients with early-onset prosthetic valve endocarditis (PVE). The manifestations of late-onset infection caused by streptococci are similar to those in patients without a prosthetic heart valve. Fever, a new aortic or mitral insufficiency murmur, splenomegaly, anemia, and peripheral stigmata, such as petechiae and splinter hemorrhages, are often present in late-onset infections.

Sustained bacteremia is characteristic of endocarditis, and blood cultures are positive in 95% of patients with prosthetic valve infections. Blood cultures may be negative in patients with *Candida* or *Aspergillus* endocarditis. Emboli occluding major arteries are common in fungal endocarditis. Culture and histologic examination of the clot may be useful for establishing the cause. Fastidious microorganisms such as members of the HACEK group (*Haemophilus, Actinobacillus, Cardiobacterium, Eikenella, Kingella*) and *Legionella* should be considered. Noninvasive cardiac procedures, such as transesophageal echocardiography, cinefluoroscopy, and electrocardiography, may be helpful. Cardiac cinefluoroscopy, although used less often now than in the past, may show an abnormal rocking motion of the prosthesis. A new murmur of aortic insufficiency or large vegetations on a valve may be detected on an echocardiogram. Selective cardiac catheterization with quantitative blood cultures may be useful for determining the site of infection if the patient has more than one prosthetic valve.

A diagnostic dilemma occurs in the interpretation of positive blood cultures during the postoperative period. Although the presence of a sustained bacteremia may indicate bacterial endocarditis, it is important not to assume that the positive blood cultures confirm the diagnosis of endocarditis. Other criteria that help to establish the diagnosis are the presence of a new or changing heart murmur or of embolic phenomena, and the absence of an extracardiac source for the bacteremia. However, no criterion will absolutely distinguish bacterial endocarditis from a sustained bacteremia without endocarditis. If the blood cultures are positive during this period, remove the IV and arterial lines, drain any focus of pus, and begin antimicrobials. If during the next 2 to 3 weeks no new murmur develops, the peripheral stigmata of endocarditis are absent, and the repeated blood cultures are sterile, discontinue therapy. If a new murmur develops, peripheral manifestations of endocarditis appear, or the blood cultures remain positive after the source has been eliminated, continue therapy for 4 to 6 weeks.

A bactericidal antimicrobial given in high doses parenterally is the cornerstone of therapy for prosthetic valve infections. Peak serum bactericidal levels should be present at a dilution of at least 1:8. Commonly accepted indications for surgery along with high-dose antimicrobial agents include a significant valvular leak or congestive heart failure, or both; persistent or recurrent bacteremia after 1 to 2 weeks of optimal treatment; multiple peripheral emboli; new-onset conduction abnormalities; and usually endocarditis caused by fungi. Recurrent emboli are a controversial indication for surgery. Surgery combined with antimicrobials may be indicated for infections caused by *S. aureus* and *S. epidermidis*, as well as for early-onset prosthetic valve infections caused by gram-negative bacilli. Late-onset infections caused by streptococci usually respond to antimicrobial therapy alone and do not require valve replacement.

The mortality in early-onset infection is 60 to 80%, and in late-onset endocarditis it is 40%. Congestive heart failure secondary to valve dehiscence or myocardial abscesses and cerebral arterial emboli are the leading causes of death. Because the effects of a prosthetic valve infection can be devastating, prevention is important. A prophylactic antistaphylococcal agent should be administered just before operation and during the perioperative period while the long lines are present (usually for 2–3 days postoperatively). Prophylaxis is indicated as well for procedures associated with transient bacteremias, such as dental work, genitourinary manipulations, or any surgery through a contaminated area. Antimicrobial prophylaxis for other procedures, such as upper gastrointestinal endoscopy or colonoscopy, is controversial. (NMG)

Bibliography

Akowual EF, et al. Prosthetic valve endocarditis: early and late outcome following medical or surgical treatment. *Heart* 2003;89:269–272.
Recurrence of endocarditis is more likely in medically treated patients.

Alsip SG, et al. Indications for cardiac surgery in patients with infective endocarditis. *Am J Med* 1985;78(suppl 6B):138.
Use a point system to determine the need for surgery. Surgery is indicated for moderate-to-severe heart failure, fungal etiology, persistent bacteremia, or unstable prosthesis.

Baddour LM, and the Infectious Diseases Society of America's Emerging Infections Network. Long-term suppressive antimicrobial therapy for intravascular device-related infections. *Am J Med Sci* 2001;322:209–212.
May be effective in patients who are not surgical candidates.

Blumberg EA, et al. Persistent fever in association with infective endocarditis. *Clin Infect Dis* 1992;15:983.
Causes of fever in patients with endocarditis and persistent fever included myocardial abscess (27%), drug fever (19%), other nosocomial infections (19%), persistent infection (24%), other (8%), and unknown (15%).

Calderwood SD. Risk factors for the development of prosthetic valve endocarditis. *Circulation* 1985;72:31.
One-third of the cases had an early onset, and two-thirds occurred late.

Chen TT, Schapiro JM, Loutit J. Prosthetic valve endocarditis due to *Legionella pneumophila. J Cardiovasc Surg* 1996;37:631–633.
A rare cause of culture-negative endocarditis.

Daniel WG, et al. Improvement in the diagnosis of abscesses associated with endocarditis by transesophageal echocardiography. *N Engl J Med* 1991;324:795.
The transesophageal approach was superior to transthoracic echocardiography, but a negative study result does not exclude a complication in a patient with a prosthetic valve.

Darouiche RO. Treatment of infections associated with surgical implants. *N Engl J Med* 2004;350:1422–1429.
Review of implanted device infections.

Dismukes WE, et al. Prosthetic valve endocarditis: analysis of 38 cases. *Circulation* 1973;48:365.
Staphylococci (both S. aureus *and* S. epidermidis*) are the most common organisms causing early-onset infections; streptococci are the leading causes among late-onset cases.*

Durack DT, Lukes AS, Bright DK, Duke Endocarditis Service. Criteria for diagnosis of infective endocarditis: utilization of specific echocardiographic findings. *Am J Med* 1994;96:200–209.
Criteria to improve accuracy of diagnosis.

Everett ED, Hirschmann JV. Transient bacteremia and endocarditis prophylaxis. A review. *Medicine (Baltimore)* 1977;56:61.

An extensive review of the incidence of and organisms associated with bacteremia secondary to various procedures or manipulations. The authors favor prophylactic antimicrobials for patients with prosthetic valves who undergo dental procedures, urologic manipulations, upper gastrointestinal endoscopy, sigmoidoscopy, liver biopsy, or barium enema.

Fang G, et al. Bacteremia in patients with prosthetic cardiac valves. *Ann Intern Med* 1993;119:560.

The most frequent source of bacteremia for a patient with nosocomial endocarditis was an intravascular catheter, wound, or skin infection.

Gibot S, et al. Soluble triggering receptor expressed on myeloid cells and the diagnosis of pneumonia. *N Engl J Med* 2004;350:451–458.

Assessing bronchoalveolar lavage fluid for soluble triggering receptor expressed on myeloid cells (TREM-1) was a marker for nosocomial pneumonia.

Giladi M, et al. Microbiological cultures of heart valves and valve tags are not valuable for patients without infective endocarditis who are undergoing valve replacement. *Clin Infect Dis* 1997;24:884–888.

When endocarditis is not suspected, cultures of heart valves or prosthetic valve tags are not indicated.

John MDV, et al. *Staphylococcus aureus* prosthetic valve endocarditis: optimal management and risk factors for death. *Clin Infect Dis* 1998;26:1302–1309.

In patients with S. aureus *infection, valve replacement during the treatment of infection was associated with reduced mortality.*

Karchmer AW, Archer GL, Dismukes WE. *Staphylococcus epidermidis* causing prosthetic valve endocarditis: microbiologic and clinical observations as guides to therapy. *Ann Intern Med* 1983;98:447.

Most (87%) isolates of S. epidermidis *were methicillin resistant. Therapy of choice consists of vancomycin, plus rifampin with or without an aminoglycoside.*

Karchmer AW, Longworth DL. Infections of intracardiac devices. *Cardiol Clin* 2003;21:253–271.

Review.

Karchmer AW, et al. Late prosthetic valve endocarditis. Clinical features influencing therapy. *Am J Med* 1978;64:199.

The occurrence of any two of three features (nonstreptococcal etiology, a new regurgitant murmur, and moderate-to-severe congestive heart failure) carried a high mortality. Surgery should be strongly considered.

Kluge RM, et al. Sources of contamination in open heart surgery. *JAMA* 1974;230:1415.

A variety of organisms, including diphtheroids and S. epidermidis, *were frequently (71%) isolated in cultures obtained from the operative sites.*

Lytle BW, et al. Surgery for acquired heart disease. Surgical treatment of prosthetic valve endocarditis. *J Thorac Cardiovasc Surg* 1996;111:198–210.

The risk for prosthetic valve endocarditis is about 3% after the first year and 1% per year thereafter. Mortality with surgery for prosthetic valve endocarditis has declined, with a survival rate of 82% at 5 years and 60% at 10 postoperative years.

Melgar GR, et al. Fungal prosthetic valve endocarditis in 16 patients. *Medicine* 1997;76:94–103.

Amphotericin B plus surgery resulted in a 67% survival rate, but relapse may occur that requires long-term suppression therapy.

Meyer DJ, Gerding DN. Favorable prognosis of patients with prosthetic valve endocarditis caused by gram-negative bacilli of the HACEK group. *Am J Med* 1988;85:104.

A group of fastidious gram-negative rods that includes Haemophilus *spp.,* Actinobacillus actinomycetemcomitans, Cardiobacterium hominis, Eikenella corrodens, *and* Kingella *species.*

Mullany CJ, et al. Early and late survival after surgical treatment of culture-positive active endocarditis. *Mayo Clin Proc* 1995;70:517–525.

Overall mortality was 26%. A higher mortality was seen in patients with an abscess at surgery (40%) and with an increased serum creatinine (40%).

Mylonakis E, Calderwood SB. Infective endocarditis in adults. *N Engl J Med* 2001;345: 1318–1330.

Review. The mortality rate for both native valve and prosthetic valve endocarditis is 20 to 25% owing to central nervous system embolic events and homodynamic deterioration.

Nasser RM, et al. Incidence and risk of developing fungal prosthetic valve endocarditis after nosocomial candidemia. *Am J Med* 1997;103:25–32.

Among patients with candidemia and a prosthetic heart valve, evidence of prosthetic valve endocarditis never developed in 75%, 16% had endocarditis at the time of the fungemia, and 9% had a late onset of endocarditis.

Nettles RE, et al. An evaluation of the Duke criteria in 25 pathologically confirmed cases of prosthetic valve endocarditis. *Clin Infect Dis* 1997;25:1401–1403.

The Duke diagnostic criteria had a sensitivity of 76% in cases of endocarditis that were confirmed pathologically.

Nguyen MH, et al. *Candida* prosthetic valve endocarditis: prospective study of six cases and review of the literature. *Clin Infect Dis* 1996;22:262–267.

In patients unable to tolerate surgery, antifungal therapy followed by chronic suppression may be effective (46%).

Sande MA, et al. Sustained bacteremia in patients with prosthetic cardiac valves. *N Engl J Med* 1972;286:1067.

Discusses the diagnostic dilemma of sustained bacteremia without endocarditis versus endocarditis.

Tornos P, et al. Clinical outcome and long-term prognosis of late prosthetic valve endocarditis: a 20-year experience. *Clin Infect Dis* 1997;24:381–386.

Staphylococcus aureus *infection had a mortality rate of 67%; streptococcal infection, 6%; other causes, 23%.*

Weinstein L, Rubin RH. Infective endocarditis 1973. *Prog Cardiovasc Dis* 1973;16:239.

Classic review.

Wilson WR, et al. Prosthetic valve endocarditis. *Ann Intern Med* 1975;82:751.

The incidence of prosthetic valve infections was low. In this series, most infections occurred more than 2 months after surgery.

Wilson WR, et al. Antibiotic treatment of adults with infective endocarditis due to streptococci, enterococci, staphylococci, and HACEK microorganisms. *JAMA* 1995;274:1706–1713.

Guidelines for therapy.

Wolff M, et al. Prosthetic valve endocarditis in the ICU. Prognostic factors of overall survival in a series of 122 cases and consequences for treatment decision. *Chest* 1995;108:688–694.

In patients with S. aureus *prosthetic valve endocarditis, survival was higher (45%) in those who received medical-surgical therapy compared with only antibiotics (0).*

PROLONGED FEVER AND GENERALIZED LYMPHADENOPATHY

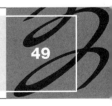

49

Prolonged fever with generalized lymphadenopathy is a symptom complex common to many different disease entities. Distinct categories of illness, such as infection, autoimmune disorders, malignancy, and drug hypersensitivity, may all present with fever and lymph node enlargement.

Table 49-1 lists infectious diseases that have been associated with generalized lymphadenopathy.

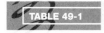

TABLE 49-1	Infectious Causes of Generalized Lymphadenopathy

Streptococcal and staphylococcal infection
Bartonella spp. (cat scratch fever and bacillary angiomatosis)
Secondary syphilis
Tuberculosis
Brucellosis
Tularemia
Tropheryma whippelii (Whipple's disease)
HIV disease—acute retroviral syndrome, persistent, generalized lymphadenopathy
CMV
Infectious mononucleosis

The range of infectious diseases that can cause generalized lymphadenopathy is extensive. Initial evaluation of the patient will require a detailed history. Clinical clues may be found in the symptoms themselves, an epidemiology system review, or the social or occupational history. Fungal diseases, such as histoplasmosis and coccidioidomycosis may be suggested by exposure history and geographic setting. A history of contact with sheep or employment in a slaughterhouse, or drinking unpasteurized milk requires that brucellosis be considered. Contact with ticks or rodents suggests the possibility of tularemia. Contact with cats might be a clue to cat scratch disease or toxoplasmosis. The patient should be asked about exposure to tuberculosis or travel to areas where trypanosomal or leishmanial organisms are endemic.

A detailed history of sexual activities and risk factors for AIDS needs to be obtained. HIV disease may present with lymphadenopathy in association with acute retroviral syndrome. Persistent generalized lymphadenopathy is defined as two or more extrainguinal sites lasting for 3 to 6 months with no other cause. Generalized lymphadenopathy may occur in HIV disease in association with non-Hodgkin's lymphoma. Secondary syphilis and lymphogranuloma venereum can also cause fever and diffuse lymphadenopathy with or without HIV disease.

AUTOIMMUNE DISORDERS

Rheumatoid arthritis, systemic lupus erythematosus (SLE), and Sjögren's syndrome are the most common autoimmune disorders to cause lymphadenopathy. Lymphadenopathy is present in 75% of rheumatoid arthritis patients at one time or another in the illness. Enlarged nodes may or may not occur in association with inflamed joints. Fever is also common. Pathology will show reactive lymphoid hyperplasia. Lymphadenopathy occurs in 25 to 70% of patients with SLE. Fever and lymphadenopathy can be the initial symptoms. Sjögren's syndrome will cause dry eyes and dry mouth with lymphocytic infiltration of salivary and lacrimal glands. Fever is less commonly associated with this syndrome. In the evaluation of the patient with fever and lymphadenopathy, a history of joint pain, rash, other lupus clinical signs and symptoms, dry mouth, and dry eyes, should be obtained.

DRUG HYPERSENSITIVITY

Hypersensitivity reactions to drugs are an increasingly common cause of diffuse lymphadenopathy. Fever, rash, or eosinophilia may be part of the syndrome. Phenytoin, carbamazepine, sulfa drugs and other antibiotics are most commonly implicated but many different drugs can produce this syndrome. Reactions occur within weeks to months of initiation of the medication. A wide range of pathology, from reactive hyperplasia to malignancy, may be seen.

Sarcoidosis is a systemic disease of unknown cause that usually affects middle-aged adults. The disease usually presents with bilateral hilar adenopathy, skin lesions, pulmonary infiltrates and ocular symptoms. The liver, spleen, salivary glands, kidneys, and central nervous system also may be involved. Histology shows noncaseating epithelioid granulomas. Fever and generalized lymphadenopathy would be an unusual presentation.

Whipple's disease is a systemic infectious disease presenting with fever, weight loss, arthralgia, and gastrointestinal symptoms of diarrhea and abdominal pain. The disease is caused by *Tropheryma whippelii*, an actinomycete, which can be seen on small-bowel biopsy with periodic-acid Schiff stain and can now be propagated in vitro. Peripheral lymphadenopathy as the sole clinical manifestation is rare but has been reported. The disease can mimic sarcoidosis or tuberculosis.

 LYMPHOPROLIFERATIVE DISORDERS

Benign and malignant lymphoproliferative disorders may present with fever and lymphadenopathy. Lymphoproliferative disorders that are benign, clonal, and malignant must be included in the differential diagnosis. As an example of benign reactive lymphoproliferative disorder, Kikuchi's disease is a histiocytic lymphadenitis characterized by fever, leukopenia, and lymphadenopathy, which can be cervical or generalized. It resolves spontaneously after several months. Atypical lymphoproliferative disorders have potential for, or have already acquired, a malignant phenotype. These include diseases such as angioimmunoblastic lymphadenopathy with dysproteinemia (AILD). AILD presents with a several-week history of fever, night sweats, weight loss, and generalized lymphadenopathy. Coombs' positive hemolytic anemia, and polyclonal hypergammaglobulinemia are usually present. Lymph nodes are characterized by destruction of nodal architecture and a pleomorphic cellular infiltrate. The most likely lymphoproliferative disorders to present with fever and lymphadenopathy are non-Hodgkin's and Hodgkin's lymphoma

On physical examination, it must be determined whether lymph node enlargement is localized or generalized. Localized adenopathy in the neck suggests pharyngitis or intraoral infection. Careful examination of the face, ears, throat, and mouth will follow. Hodgkin's disease may present as cervical adenopathy. Enlarged posterior cervical nodes may be caused by scalp infection or systemic disease, such as toxoplasmosis. If axillary adenopathy is the finding, examination of the breast and arms is most important. Cat scratch fever, staphylococcal and streptococcal infection, sporotrichosis, and lymphoma can cause isolated axillary adenopathy. Isolated inguinal adenopathy is not uncommon in the general population but may be caused by infections of the genitalia or perineum.

Generalized adenopathy, particularly when accompanied by night sweats and weight loss, should suggest the diagnosis of AIDS in any high-risk patient. Lymphoma may present as generalized adenopathy, but only at an advanced stage. As noted, many infectious processes, including infectious mononucleosis, toxoplasmosis, and cat scratch fever, present with generalized lymphadenopathy.

The laboratory evaluation of fever and generalized adenopathy proceeds according to clinical clues. All patients should have a complete blood count (CBC), with review of a blood smear for atypical lymphocytes and other abnormal cells. If the patient appears toxic, blood cultures should be obtained to rule out subacute endocarditis, tularemia, or brucellosis. A serologic test for Epstein-Barr virus (EBV), VDRL test for syphilis, IgM determination for toxoplasmosis, and HIV serology for AIDS will be indicated. A complement fixation test for cytomegalovirus (CMV) should be drawn, and titers greater than 128 are suggestive of infection with this agent. Some authors have recommended that EBV, HIV, and CMV infection and toxoplasmosis be ruled out first, with the investigation then proceeding to diseases caused by other agents. Agglutinin tests for brucellosis and tularemia and serology for histoplasmosis and coccidioidomycosis are obtained based on the index of suspicion for these processes. Antinuclear antibody and rheumatoid factors may be supportive of a diagnosis of systemic lupus erythematosus or Still's disease. A chest radiograph showing hilar adenopathy will require evaluation for tuberculosis, sarcoidosis, or lymphoma.

Definitive diagnosis may require lymph node biopsy. Slap et al. studied 123 young patients who had undergone biopsy of enlarged peripheral lymph nodes. In 42% of the cases, biopsy results led to specific treatment. Patients found to have granuloma or tumor were more likely to have abnormal findings on chest radiograph, lymph node greater than 2 cm in diameter, a history of night sweats or weight loss, and a hemoglobin level of less than 10 g/dL. Patients with a recent history of ear, nose, and throat symptoms were less likely to have a biopsy result that led to specific therapy.

When a lymph node biopsy is performed in a patient with generalized adenopathy, the node should be selected with care. Excisional biopsy is generally preferred; however, for fluctuant nodes, needle aspiration may be sufficient for diagnosis. Inguinal nodes should be avoided for biopsy because they frequently show nonspecific reactive hyperplasia. Supraclavicular nodes and scalene nodes have the highest yield. The node itself should be divided between the pathology and microbiology laboratories.

About 20% of patients in one series were given a specific diagnosis based on the results of subsequent biopsy. In patients subsequently found to have lymphoma, 90% had a diagnosis made within 8 months of the first biopsy. When a definitive diagnosis cannot be made by biopsy, careful follow-up is required. If the patient is anemic, bone marrow biopsy may be considered. If the patient has an associated hepatitis, liver biopsy is indicated. (SLB)

Bibliography

Alkan S, Beals TF, Schnitzer B. Primary diagnosis of Whipple disease manifesting as lymphadenopathy: use of polymerase chain reaction for detection of Tropheryma whippelii. *Am J Clin Pathol* 2001;116:898.
Describes two patients whose initial presentation was lymphadenopathy. The diagnosis is made by histopathology and molecular-based assays.

Brown JR, Skarin AT. Clinical mimics of lymphoma. *Oncologist* 2004;9:406.
Comprehensive review of conditions that must be differentiated from lymphoma, including differential for lymphadenopathy and fever.

Bujak JS, et al. Juvenile rheumatoid arthritis presenting in the adult as fever of unknown origin. *Medicine (Baltimore)* 1973;52:431.
Generalized significant lymphadenopathy may occur in febrile adults with Still's disease (juvenile rheumatoid arthritis).

Case records of the Massachusetts General Hospital. Weekly clinicopathological exercises. Case 30-1977. *N Engl J Med* 1977;297:206.
A discussion of the pathology of Hodgkin's disease, toxoplasmosis, angioimmunoblastic lymphadenopathy, and Lennert's lesion.

Chau I et. al. Rapid access multidisciplinary lymph node diagnostic clinic: analysis of 550 patients. *Br J Cancer* 2003;88:354.
Most patients with diffuse lymphadenopathy had toxoplasmosis, tuberculosis, HIV disease, or EBV infection.

De Vriese AS, et al. Carbamazepine hypersensitivity syndrome: report of four cases and review of the literature. *Medicine* 1995;74:144.
A syndrome of fever, rash, and lymphadenopathy occurs between 1 week and 3 months after the drug is taken. A patch test and lymphocyte transformation tests have been used to confirm the diagnosis.

Greenfield S, Jordan MC. The clinical investigation of lymphadenopathy in primary care practice. *JAMA* 1978;240:1388.
Provides an algorithm for the investigation of lymphadenopathy. Recommends serology for toxoplasmosis, EBV, and CMV before extensive workup.

Hjalgrim H, et. al. Characteristics of Hodgkin's lymphoma after infectious mononucleosis. *N Engl J Med* 2003;349:1324.
EBV infection is associated with a clinical spectrum of lymphoproliferative disease from infectious mononucleosis to transplant lymphoproliferation to Hodgkin's disease.

Holmes GP, et al. A cluster of patients with a chronic mononucleosis-like syndrome: is Epstein-Barr virus the cause? *JAMA* 1987;257:2297.

Describes an outbreak of 134 cases of fever, lymphadenopathy, and fatigue. The relationship of symptoms to EBV was unclear.

Horwitz CA, et al. Heterophil-negative infectious mononucleosis and mononucleosis-like illnesses. *Am J Med* 1977;63:947.
A diagnosis of mononucleosis-like syndrome was made in 43 patients. Thirty cases were caused by CMV based on serology findings.

Lamp LW, Scott MA. Cat scratch disease: historical, clinical, and pathologic perspective. *Am J Clin Path* 2004;121:S71.
Update of cat scratch disease with description of subacute regional lymphadenitis and other symptoms and signs.

Murakami, et al. Cat scratch disease: analysis of 130 seropositive cases. *J Infect Chemo* 2002;8:349.
Lymphadenopathy was present in 84% of cases.

Montoya JG, Remington JS. Studies on the serodiagnosis of toxoplasmic lymphadenitis. *Clin Infect Dis* 1995;20:781.
Compares the newer serologic tests with traditional tests in the diagnosis of toxoplasmic lymphadenopathy. The ELISA result was positive for IgM antibodies in the first 3 months of illness.

Relman DA, et al. Identification of the uncultured bacillus of Whipple's disease. *N Engl J Med* 1992;327:293.
T. whippelii is described as the etiologic agent of Whipple's disease, which can present as generalized adenopathy.

Rosenfeld S, et al. Syndrome simulating lymphosarcoma induced by diphenylhydantoin sodium. *JAMA* 1961;176:491.
A syndrome consisting of fever, joint swelling, facial edema, generalized aches and pains, and adenopathy was associated with phenytoin sodium therapy.

Saltzstein SL, Ackerman IV. Lymphadenopathy induced by anticonvulsant drugs and mimicking clinically and pathologically malignant lymphomas. *Cancer* 1959;12:164.
Phenytoin may cause prolonged fever and lymphadenopathy.

Sinclair S, Beckman E, Ellman L. Biopsy of enlarged superficial lymph nodes. *JAMA* 1974;228:602.
Thirty-seven percent of patients had lymphoma, 10% had carcinoma, and 5% had tuberculosis.

Slap GB, Brooks JSJ, Schwartz JS. When to perform biopsies of enlarged peripheral lymph nodes in young patients. *JAMA* 1984;252:1321.
Reviews records of 123 young patients to determine which had biopsy results that led to specific therapy. Those with abnormal findings on chest x-ray films, a node greater than 2 cm, night sweats, or weight loss benefited from biopsy diagnosis.

Wear DJ, et al. Cat scratch disease: a bacterial infection. *Science* 1983;221:1403.
Demonstration of organisms in lymph node biopsy by Warthin-Starry stain.

Weinstein L, Weinstein AJ. The pathophysiology and pathoanatomy of reactions to antimicrobial agents. *Adv Intern Med* 1974;19:109.
A clinical picture resembling infectious mononucleosis (sore throat, generalized lymphadenopathy, splenomegaly, lymphocytosis, and the presence of cells resembling typical Downey cells) is an uncommon manifestation of an allergic response to paraaminosalicylic acid.

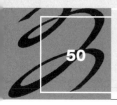

50   FEVER AND SKIN RASH

$\mathcal{T}$he acutely ill, febrile patient with a generalized skin rash presents a diagnostic challenge; the list of disorders in the differential diagnosis is extensive and includes both infectious and noninfectious causes. The skin is capable of reacting only in a limited way, and disease may be manifested by macules or papules; vesicles, bullae, or pustules; or purpuric macules, papules, or vesicles. The clinical features of the various disorders causing a skin rash are similar, and one infection may readily mimic another. Misdiagnosis and delay in starting specific therapy can be disastrous in patients with Rocky Mountain spotted fever, toxic shock syndrome (TSS), or meningococcal or staphylococcal bacteremia. It is critical to make a presumptive etiologic diagnosis rapidly and identify treatable infections for which immediate therapy is required to prevent death.

 ## DIAGNOSTIC PROCEDURES

Certain diagnostic procedures can be used to obtain a diagnosis in the acutely ill, febrile patient with a rash. Skin lesions can be aspirated, and the material obtained should be examined with Gram's stain. Gram-positive organisms in clusters are staphylococci, and gram-negative diplococci are either meningococci or gonococci. Organisms can sometimes be seen by Gram's-staining a smear of the buffy coat. Meningococci also can be identified by latex particle agglutination tests of the serum, cerebrospinal fluid, or other body fluids. A Tzanck preparation is useful in the diagnosis of a number of vesiculobullous disorders. This test consists of several steps: (1) selecting an intact vesicle, (2) swabbing the lesion with 70% isopropyl alcohol, (3) opening the vesicle with a scalpel blade, (4) scraping the base very gently to avoid bleeding, (5) placing the specimen on a glass slide, and (6) staining it with Giemsa or Wright's stain. Multinucleated, syncytial giant cells are present with varicella-zoster viral infection and herpes simplex but are absent in vaccinia and variola. A dark-field examination of material from a mucous membrane or skin lesion may reveal spirochetes. A cutaneous biopsy can be helpful in identifying rickettsiae; it provides material for an immunofluorescence technique that produces results before the results of serologic tests are positive. A vasculitis secondary to a noninfectious cause also can be identified by a cutaneous punch biopsy. Acute serum (at the time of presentation and 2 weeks later) should be drawn and frozen for various serologic tests. In addition, several sets of blood cultures are prepared, as well as cultures of throat, urine, and other tissues and fluids as indicated. Table 50-1 lists some of the conditions in which fever and a generalized rash may be prominent symptoms.

 ## TOXIC SHOCK SYNDROME

In 1978, an illness was described in seven children ages 8 to 17. It was characterized by high fever, generalized erythroderma, hypotension, and conjunctival hyperemia, with involvement of the kidneys, liver, and gastrointestinal system. This disease was called *toxic shock syndrome* and was attributed to toxins produced by *Staphylococcus aureus*. The illness was similar to staphylococcal scarlet fever, which had been described in 1927. Not until late in 1979 and 1980, however, did the syndrome attract widespread attention when studies demonstrated a statistically significant association between use of tampons and the

292

TABLE 50-1	Conditions in Which Rash and Fever are Prominent
Type of lesion	**Microbial agents and related diseases**
Maculopapular lesions	Viruses: measles, rubeola, rubella, enterovirus (echovirus, coxsackievirus), arbovirus, infectious hepatitis, infectious mononucleosis (cytomegalovirus, Epstein-Barr virus), human herpesvirus 6, parvovirus B19, HIV, West Nile virus
	Bacteria: scarlet fever, typhoid fever, secondary syphilis, rat-bite fever, leptospirosis, erysipeloid, toxic shock syndrome, Lyme disease, ehrlichiosis
	Rickettsiae: Rocky Mountain spotted fever (early), murine (endemic) typhus, scrub typhus
	Other: drug reactions, pityriasis rosea, collagen diseases (e.g., systemic lupus erythematosus), toxoplasmosis, trichinosis, rheumatic fever, mucocutaneous lymph node syndrome, acute graft-versus-host disease
Vesicles, bullae, or pustules	Viruses: varicella, herpes zoster, herpes simplex, variola, enterovirus (coxsackie-virus), smallpox, monkey pox
Petechial or purpuric lesions	Viruses: atypical measles
	Bacteria: bacteremia (meningococcal, gonococcal, streptococcal, or staphylococcal)
	Rickettsiae: Rocky Mountain spotted fever, epidemic typhus
	Other: drug reactions, allergic vasculitis, malaria

development of TSS. The peak incidence to date occurred in August 1980, when 135 cases were reported to the Centers for Disease Control (CDC). The number of new cases reported to the CDC has declined to approximately 20 per month. The majority of cases are nonmenstrual and occur in patients with staphylococcal infections associated with wounds, vaginal delivery, or cesarean section. In addition to patients with staphylococcal skin and soft-tissue infections, patients with primary staphylococcal bacteremia are at risk for TSS. Rarely, cases are associated with the use of vaginal contraceptive diaphragms.

Diagnosis

The diagnosis of TSS still requires use of the CDC case definition because no laboratory test has been developed to confirm the diagnosis. The initial CDC case definition has been modified to include orthostatic dizziness as evidence of hypotension and staphylococcal bacteremia. *S. aureus* isolated from patients with TSS can be studied for the production of toxic shock syndrome toxin 1 (TSST-1) and staphylococcal enterotoxins A and B. The absence of antibody to the toxin indicates susceptibility to the development of TSS. These toxins appear to activate T cells, resulting in the production of macrophage-derived mediators, such as interleukin-1 and tumor necrosis factor, which cause shocklike symptoms. The toxins interact with cells of the immune system and act as superantigens.

The diagnosis of TSS should be considered in any patient, particularly a postoperative or postpartum patient, and any menstruating woman who has unexplained fever, hypotension, and a diffuse rash resembling sunburn. Initially, the rash may be absent in patients with hypotension and may appear only after fluid replacement, or it may go unnoticed or be attributed to the flush of fever. The surgical wound infection often appears clinically trivial, and the patient may be discharged from the hospital before the onset of toxic shock symptoms. The menstrually related disease typically begins abruptly during the menstrual period. Sore throat or vomiting and diarrhea may be prominent complaints and suggest other diagnoses, such as group A streptococcal pharyngitis or gastrointestinal infection.

Criteria to establish a diagnosis of TSS are listed in Table 50-2. Neurologic examination usually reveals a confused, disoriented patient without focal symptoms. Until a specific

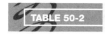

TABLE 50-2	Case Criteria for Toxic Shock Syndrome

Fever: temperature >38.9°C (102°F)

Rash: diffuse macular erythroderma; desquamation 1 to 2 weeks after onset of illness, particularly of palms and soles

Hypotension: systolic blood pressure <90 mm Hg for adults or below fifth percentile by age for children less than 16 years of age; orthostatic drop in diastolic blood pressure >15mm Hg from lying to sitting; orthostatic syncope or orthostatic dizziness

Multisystem involvement with three or more of the following:
Gastrointestinal: vomiting or diarrhea at onset of illness
Muscular: severe myalgia or creatine phosphokinase level at least twice the upper limit of normal
Mucous membrane: vaginal, oropharyngeal, or conjunctival hyperemia
Renal: blood urea nitrogen (BUN) or creatinine level at least twice the upper limit of normal, or urinary sediment with pyuria (>5 leukocytes per high-power field) in the absence of urinary tract infection
Hepatic: total billirubin, AST, ALT levels twice the upper the limit of normal
Hematologic: platelets <100,000/μL
Central nervous system: disorientation or alteration in consciousness without focal neurologic signs when fever and hypotension are absent

Negative results for the following tests, if performed:
Blood, throat, or cerebrospinal fluid cultures (blood culture may be positive for *Staphylococcus aureus*)
Rise in titer in Rocky Mountain spotted fever, leptospirosis, or rubeola

AST, serum aspartate transaminase; ALT, serum alanine transaminase.

laboratory test is developed, cases of mild toxic shock are excluded by the strict case definition. A vaginal examination should be performed to remove any tampon and obtain cultures for *S. aureus*. Normally, 10% of women have vaginal cultures positive for *S. aureus*, but 98% of vaginal cultures are positive in patients with menstrually associated TSS.

Treatment

Acute management of a patient with TSS requires aggressive treatment for shock with massive IV fluids (up to 12 L/day) and vasopressors to maintain blood pressure and renal output. In a retrospective study, use of high-dose corticosteroids for 3 days reduced the severity of illness and duration of fever if they were administered within 2 to 3 days of TSS onset, but there was no difference in mortality. High doses (400 mg/kg) of IV immune globulin given as a single dose may be useful, as high levels of TSST-1 antibody are present in commercial sera. Immune globulin is preferred to corticosteroids. A β-lactamase–resistant penicillin, such as nafcillin, should be administered to eradicate staphylococci and lessen the chance of recurrence. Rifampin, which may be useful to eradicate the staphylococcal carrier state, is given in combination with nafcillin or dicloxacillin if nafcillin administration alone fails to eliminate the organism. The recurrence rate is 2 to 30%, depending on the study and criteria for TSS. The case-fatality rate is about 5%. Women who have had TSS should not resume using tampons until more is known about the disease. Recurrent disease is more common with menstrual than nonmenstrual cases.

Numerous reports have described a life-threatening illness caused by group A streptococci that mimics TSS. Several streptococcal exotoxins (including streptococcal pyrogenic exotoxins A, B, and C) activate T cells, resulting in the production of various cytokines, such as tumor necrosis factor and interleukin-6. Various clinical manifestations include bacteremia, hypotension, pneumonia, myositis, and fasciitis. Patients may have renal failure, adult respiratory distress syndrome, and delirium or confusion; they lack the typical rash of scarlet fever or staphylococcal TSS. Petechial or maculopapular rashes may occur. Penicillin is the drug of choice, and clindamycin should be used in the penicillin-allergic patient. Clindamycin often is given in combination with penicillin. Clindamycin decreases toxin production by group A streptococci.

 ROCKY MOUNTAIN SPOTTED FEVER

Diagnosis

Several life-threatening illnesses are included in the differential diagnosis of patients with fever and a petechial or purpuric rash. Rocky Mountain spotted fever should be suspected in any patient living where this disease is endemic. A seasonal variation—most cases are seen from April to October—corresponds to the tick season and recreational exposure. In states with a warmer climate, the disease can occur throughout the year. The history of a tick bite can be elicited in about 75% of patients. The incubation period is 3 to 12 days. The illness begins with a nonspecific syndrome of headache, malaise, myalgias, and fever. The rash, which is the most characteristic feature, is usually delayed until the fourth day of fever (but ranges from the second to sixth day). The initial lesions are on the wrists, ankles, palms, and soles. After 6 to 12 hours, the rash spreads centripetally to the trunk and face. At first, the rash is macular and blanches with pressure, but it becomes maculopapular and petechial or purpuric after 2 to 3 days.

The pathologic changes, such as thrombus formation, are a result of rickettsial invasion of the endothelial cells of blood vessels. Disseminated intravascular coagulation and thrombocytopenia also account for the clinical observations. In addition to the rash, which occurs in 90% of patients, nonpitting edema is common, especially in the periorbital area. Other features are intense headache, myalgias with muscle tenderness, nausea, vomiting, constipation, and sometimes splenomegaly or hepatomegaly. Neurologic complications (stiff neck, mental confusion, seizures, hemiplegia, coma) may occur. Myocarditis, hepatitis, and interstitial pneumonitis are occasionally seen. The white blood cell (WBC) count and differential are normal, in contrast to the findings of leukocytosis in meningococcal infection. Thrombocytopenia is common.

A presumptive diagnosis must be made and specific antimicrobial therapy started based solely on the clinical observations, as the results of complement fixation and the Weil-Felix test usually are not positive until the eighth to the twelfth day of the illness. With an immunofluorescence test, rickettsiae can be identified in a skin biopsy specimen as early as the fourth day of illness.

Treatment

Therapy with tetracycline or parenteral chloramphenicol is started and continued until improvement occurs (usually for 5 afebrile days). A response is seen in 24 to 48 hours if treatment is begun before the sixth day of illness. Sulfonamides can make the illness worse. Usually, by the end of the second week of illness, rickettsial antibodies can be detected by complement fixation or the more sensitive indirect fluorescent antibody and microagglutination tests. Polymerase chain reaction may be used to identify the organism, but this procedure is not readily available at most centers.

 KAWASAKI DISEASE

Kawasaki disease, or mucocutaneous lymph node syndrome, is an illness of unknown cause. High fever lasting at least 5 days and an erythematous rash are prominent symptoms. The disease occurs predominantly in children younger than age 5, with a peak incidence between ages 1 and 2. The disease rarely occurs in persons older than age 8. Outbreaks continue to occur in the United States, particularly in the winter and spring. Person-to-person transmission has not been demonstrated. The case-fatality rate is 1 to 2%. Therapy consists of aspirin, other antiplatelet drugs (e.g., dipyridamole), and IV immunoglobulin.

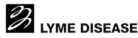

LYME DISEASE

Lyme disease is caused by a spirochete, *Borrelia burgdorferi,* which is transmitted by various ixodid ticks. In the United States, the disease occurs most frequently in areas where *Ixodes scapularis* or *I. pacificus* can be found. The disease has been described in many other countries around the world. After an incubation period of about 1 week, with a range of 3 to 32 days, the characteristic skin lesion, erythema migrans, appears. Fever is usually low grade and intermittent and is reported in half the patients. The fever may be high (up to 40°C) and persistent in children. Multiple skin lesions can develop, and erythema migrans usually lasts 2 to 3 weeks. Intense headache, malaise, fatigue, and regional lymphadenopathy are frequent early clinical features. Weeks to months later, neurologic manifestations, including meningoencephalitis, cranial nerve palsies (particularly of the facial nerve), and motor and sensor radiculoneuropathy, develop in 10% of patients. Neurologic abnormalities may persist for months but usually resolve completely. Weeks after onset, cardiac symptoms develop in 8% of patients, most commonly various degrees of atrioventricular block. Still later, weeks to several years after onset, migratory arthritis develops in some patients. Arthritis usually begins months after the onset of Lyme disease, affects primarily the large joints, such as the knees, and in 10% of patients becomes chronic, with destruction of cartilage and bone. (The diagnosis of Lyme disease is discussed in Chapter 40.)

DIFFERENTIAL DIAGNOSIS

A guide to the differential diagnosis of fever and a skin rash is given in Table 50-1; it includes treatable infectious disease emergencies (e.g., Rocky Mountain spotted fever, meningococcal or staphylococcal septicemia, and TSS). Failure to institute appropriate therapy based on the epidemiologic history and results of rapid diagnostic tests, such as Gram's stain, can be disastrous. (NMG)

Bibliography

Ackerman AB, Miller RC, Shapiro L. Gonococcemia and its cutaneous manifestations. *Arch Dermatol* 1965;91:227.
Illustrates lesions.
Anderson LJ, Torok TJ. The clinical spectrum of human parvovirus B19 infections. In: Remington JS, Swartz MN, eds. *Current Clinical Topics in Infectious Diseases.* Cambridge, Mass: Blackwell Science; 1991.
In adults, rash and arthralgias often occur. The arthritis can be present without a rash.
Baker RC, et al. Fever and petechiae in children. *Pediatrics* 1989;84:1051.
Of children with fever and petechiae, 7% had meningococcal disease.
Bergman SJ, Kundin WD. Scrub typhus in South Vietnam. *Ann Intern Med* 1973;79:26.
The characteristic features are fever (100%), adenopathy (85%), eschar (46%), and maculopapular eruption (34%).
Bodey GP. Dermatologic manifestations of infections in neutropenic patients. *Infect Dis Clin North Am* 1994;8:655–675.
Review. Sweet's syndrome, or acute febrile neutrophilic dermatosis, is often misdiagnosed as cellulitis.
Burns JC, Glode MP. Kawasaki syndrome. *Lancet* 2004;364:533–544.
The etiology remains unknown and misdiagnosis is a problem.
Cale DF, McCarthy MW. Treatment of Rocky Mountain spotted fever in children. *Ann Pharmacol* 1997;31:492–494.
Doxycycline can be given safely to children younger than 9 for Rocky Mountain spotted fever.
Carrol ED, et al. Procalcitonin as a diagnostic marker of meningococcal disease in children presenting with fever and a rash. *Arch Dis Child* 2002;86:282–285.
An elevated procalcitonin level is a marker for sepsis.

Case records of the Massachusetts General Hospital (case 26-1973). *N Engl J Med* 1973; 288:1400.
Discusses the differential diagnosis of an acutely ill patient with a rash and fever.

Case records of the Massachusetts General Hospital (case 16-1978). *N Engl J Med* 1978; 298:957.
Presentation of the case of a fish cutter with fever and a skin rash caused by Erysipelothrix rhusiopathiae *(erysipeloid).*

Case records of the Massachusetts General Hospital (case 27-1985). *N Engl J Med* 1985; 313:36.
Discussion of fever, rash, and pulmonary infiltrates in a veterinarian with tularemia.

Case records of the Massachusetts General Hospital (case 30-1990). *N Engl J Med* 1990; 323:254.
Discussion of a patient with fever and pustular skin lesions (neutrophilic dermatosis, or Sweet's syndrome).

Case records of the Massachusetts General Hospital (case 32-1997). *N Engl J Med* 1997; 337:1149–1156.
A fatal case of Rocky Mountain spotted fever.

Caumes E, et al. Dermatoses associated with travel to tropical countries: a prospective study of the diagnosis and management of 269 patients presenting to a tropical disease unit. *Clin Infect Dis* 1995;20:542–548.
Cutaneous larva migrans and cellulitis owing to S. aureus *and Group A streptococcus were the most common diagnoses.*

Centers for Disease Control. Case definition for public health surveillance. *MMWR* 1990;39:38.
Case definition revised.

Chambers HF, Korzoniowski OM, Sande MA. *Staphylococcus aureus* endocarditis: clinical manifestations in addicts and nonaddicts. *Medicine (Baltimore)* 1983;62:170.
A murmur was absent in about 25% of addicts on the initial presentation.

Cherry JD. Contemporary infectious exanthems. *Clin Infect Dis* 1993;16:199–207.
Pictures of classic exanthems. Epidemiologic clues (e.g., season) are key to diagnosis.

Clinicopathological Conference. A 54-year-old woman with fevers, arthralgias, myalgias, and rash. *Am J Med* 1988;85:84.
A discussion of leukocytoclastic vasculitis (allergic).

Clinicopathologic Conference. Abdominal pain, fever, and rash in a 39-year-old male. *Am J Med* 1994;97:300–306.
Diagnosis of Henoch-Schönlein purpura by skin biopsy in an adult with fever, abdominal pain, and rash.

Duma RJ, et al. Epidemic typhus in the United States associated with flying squirrels. *JAMA* 1981;245:2318.
Clinical features include headache, fever, myalgias, and rash.

Dumler JS, Bakken JS. Human ehrlichioses: newly recognized infections transmitted by ticks. *Annu Rev Med* 1998;49:201–213.
In this tick-borne disease, rash is present in up to one-third of patients. Treatment with doxycycline usually results in cure.

Dumler JS, Bakken JS. Ehrlichial diseases of humans: emerging tick-borne infections. *Clin Infect Dis* 1995;20:1102–1110.
Human granulocytic ehrlichiosis occurs most commonly in the northeastern or midwestern parts of the United States.

Dumler JS, Taylor JP, Walker DH. Clinical and laboratory features of murine typhus in south Texas, 1980 through 1987. *JAMA* 1991;266:1365.
The features often include fever, headache, chills, myalgias, and rash.

Fichtenbaum CJ, Peterson LR, Weil GJ. Ehrlichiosis presenting as a life-threatening illness with features of the toxic shock syndrome. *Am J Med* 1987;95:351.
Patients with ehrlichiosis may fulfill the criteria for TSS, including a rash and conjunctival hemorrhage or erythema.

Gentry LO, Zeluff B, Kielhofner MA. Dermatologic manifestations of infectious diseases in cardiac transplant patients. *Infect Dis Clin North Am* 1994;8:637–654.

A skin lesion in a transplant recipient may be a primary infection site or indicate another, occult focus of infection.

Greenberg RN, et al. Urticaria, exanthems, and other benign dermatologic reactions to smallpox vaccination in adults. *Clin Infect Dis* 2004;38:958–965.
Rash may complicate smallpox vaccination.

Haynes RE, Sanders DV, Cramblett HG. Rocky Mountain spotted fever in children. *J Pediatr* 1970;76:685.
Classic. A clinical diagnosis requiring empiric therapy.

Hill WR, Kinney TD. The cutaneous lesions in acute meningococcemia. *JAMA* 1947;134:513.
Discusses the clinical and pathologic features of meningococcal skin lesions.

Kain KC, Schulzer M, Chow AW. Clinical spectrum of nonmenstrual toxic shock syndrome (TSS): comparison with menstrual TSS by multivariate discriminant analyses. *Clin Infect Dis* 1993;16:100.
S. aureus from patients with nonmenstrual TSS produced TSST-1 with a frequency comparable with that of strains from patients with menstrual TSS (62% vs. 84%). Nonmenstrual TSS was often nosocomial.

Kahn JO, Walker BD. Acute human immunodeficiency virus type 1 infection. *N Engl J Med* 1998;339:33–39.
Consider HIV in a patient with fever, fatigue, rash, and thrombocytopenia.

Kassutto S, Wolf MA. A wrinkle in time. *N Engl J Med* 2003;349:597–601.
Consider the diagnosis of Schönlein-Henoch purpura in an adult with fever, abdominal pain, hematuria, and a rash.

Kato H, et al. Long-term consequences of Kawasaki disease. A 10- to 21-year follow-up study of 594 patients. *Circulation* 1996;94:1379–1385.
The incidence of coronary aneurysms in acute Kawasaki disease was 25%, with half the cases showing regression.

Kingston ME, Mackey D. Skin clues in the diagnosis of life-threatening infections. *Rev Infect Dis* 1986;8:1.
Examination of a Gram's-stained smear of a scraping from the base of an ulcer or of a skin biopsy specimen may establish the diagnosis. Cutaneous manifestations are illustrated in color.

Kirk JL, et al. Rocky Mountain spotted fever: a clinical review based on 48 confirmed cases, 1943–1986. *Medicine (Baltimore)* 1990;69:35.
Review. The classic triad of fever, headache, and rash was present in only 62% of patients. Two-thirds of patients noted an exposure to ticks.

Lee VTP, Chang AH, Chow AW. Detection of staphylococcal enterotoxin B among toxic shock syndrome (TSS) and non–TSS-associated *Staphylococcus aureus* isolates. *J Infect Dis* 1992;166:911.
Staphylococcal enterotoxin B was found in 62% of patients with nonmenstrual TSS who were negative for TSST-1.

Levin S, Goodman LJ. An approach to acute fever and rash (AFR) in the adult. In: Remington JS, Swartz MN, eds. *Current Clinical Topics in Infectious Diseases.* Boston, Mass: Blackwell Science; 1995:19–75.
Comprehensive review.

Litwack KD, Hoke AW, Borchardt KA. Rose spots in typhoid fever. *Arch Dermatol* 1972;105:252.
Illustrates rose spots.

Mackowiak PA, LeMaistre CF. Drug fever: a critical appraisal of conventional concepts. *Ann Intern Med* 1987;106:728.
Fever patterns were not helpful, and a rash was present in only 18% of patients.

Masters EJ, et al. Rocky Mountain spotted fever: a clinician's dilemma. *Arch Intern Med* 2003;163:769–774.
Authors emphasize diagnostic pitfalls.

Marrack P, Kappler J. The staphylococcal enterotoxins and their relatives. *Science* 1990;241:705.
Various staphylococcal toxins, TSS toxin, and streptococcal toxins activate T cells, resulting in the production of mediators such as interleukin-1 and tumor necrosis factor.

Martin DB, et al. Atypical measles in adolescents and young adults. *Ann Intern Med* 1979; 90:877.
Rash may be vesicular, petechial, and purpuric.

Mawhorter SD, et al. Cutaneous manifestations of toxoplasmosis. *Clin Infect Dis* 1992; 14:1084.
Acute toxoplasmosis may be associated with fever and a maculopapular rash.

Miller JQ, Price TR. The nervous system in Rocky Mountain spotted fever. *Neurology* 1972; 22:561.
Most frequent findings were headache and lethargy. Cerebral spinal fluid pleocytosis, usually less than 50 cells mm^3, may occur.

Parsonnet J. Nonmenstrual toxic shock syndrome: new insights into diagnosis, pathogenesis and treatment. In: Remington JS, Swartz MN, eds. *Current Clinical Topics in Infectious Diseases.* Boston, Mass: Blackwell Science; 1996:1–20.
Review. Testing for TSST-1 and its antibody may be helpful in menstrual but not non-menstrual cases of TSS.

Perez CM, et al. Adjunctive treatment of streptococcal toxic shock syndrome using intravenous immunoglobulin: case report and review. *Am J Med* 1997;102:111–113.
IV immunoglobulin was useful for streptococcal TSS.

Procop GW, et al. Immunoperoxidase and immunofluorescent staining of *Rickettsia rickettsii* in skin biopsies. A comparative study. *Arch Pathol Lab Med* 1997;121:894–899.
Immunoperoxidase and immunofluorescent staining of skin biopsy specimens were useful in diagnosing Rocky Mountain spotted fever (sensitivity of 73% and specificity of 100%).

Pruksananonda P, et al. Primary human herpesvirus 6 infection in young children. *N Engl J Med* 1992;326:1445.
An important cause of an acute febrile illness in young children.

Reingold AI, et al. Nonmenstrual toxic shock syndrome. *Ann Intern Med* 1982;96:871.
Clinical features are identical to those seen in menses-related cases, but the epidemiology differs.

Sanders CV, Lopez FA. Cutaneous manifestations of infectious diseases: approach to the patient with fever and rash. *Trans Am Clin Climatol Assoc* 2001;112:235–251.
Comprehensive review.

Sexton DJ, Corey GR. Rocky Mountain "spotless" and "almost spotless" fever: a wolf in sheep's clothing. *Clin Infect Dis* 1992;15:439.
Rash may be absent or minimal in male and black patients, making the diagnosis difficult in these populations.

Sexton DJ, Kaye KS. Tick-borne diseases. *Med Clin North Am* 2002;86:351–360.
Treatment should be given within the first 5 days of illness to avoid fatalities.

Shands KN, et al. Toxic shock syndrome in menstruating women. *N Engl J Med* 1980; 303:1436.
Classic. Associated TSS with tampon use and isolated S. aureus from vaginal cultures.

Silpapojakul K, et al. Scrub and murine typhus in children with obscure fever in the tropics. *Pediatr Infect Dis J* 1991;10:200.
Scrub typhus in children was characterized by fever, diarrhea, vomiting, and hepatosplenomegaly. Rash was rare.

Steere AC, et al. Lyme carditis: cardiac abnormalities of Lyme disease. *Ann Intern Med* 1983; 99:8.
The most common abnormality is atrioventricular block of various degrees, especially complete heart block.

Steere AC, et al. Treatment of the early manifestations of Lyme disease. *Ann Intern Med* 1983;99:22.
Penicillin is an alternative drug for treating early Lyme disease.

Steere AC, et al. The early clinical manifestations of Lyme disease. *Ann Intern Med* 1983; 99:76.
Color pictures of erythema chronicum migrans.

Steere AC, et al. The spirochetal etiology of Lyme disease. *N Engl J Med* 1983;308:733.
Isolated the spirochete from the blood, skin lesions, and cerebrospinal fluid of patients and from the ticks.

Stevens DL. The toxic shock syndromes. *Infect Dis Clin North Am* 1996;10:727–746.
Review of streptococcal and staphylococcal TSS.

Stevens DL, et al. Severe group A streptococcal infections associated with a toxic shock-like syndrome and scarlet fever toxin A. *N Engl J Med* 1989;321:1.
Patients with this life-threatening illness did not have the typical rash of scarlet fever or the erythroderma of staphylococcal TSS. Petechial and maculopapular rashes were noted.

Stevens FA. The occurrence of *Staphylococcus aureus* infection with a scarlatiniform rash. *JAMA* 1927;88:1957.
Classic.

Swartz MN. Cellulitis. *N Engl J Med* 2004;350:904–912.
Review.

Todd JK. Therapy of toxic shock syndrome. *Drugs* 1990;39:856.
Reviews management of TSS.

Todd J, et al. Toxic shock syndrome associated with phage-group-1 staphylococci. *Lancet* 1978;2:1116.
Classic.

Todd JK, et al. Corticosteroid therapy for patients with toxic shock syndrome. *JAMA* 1984;252:3399.
Corticosteroid therapy may be beneficial, but the trial was not controlled.

Toews WH, Bass JW. Skin manifestations of meningococcal infection. *Am J Dis Child* 1974;127:173.
Color pictures. Mortality was high (44%) in patients with purpuric or ecchymotic skin lesions.

Torok TJ. Parvovirus B19 and human disease. *Adv Intern Med* 1992;37:431.
Review.

Toxic shock syndrome. *Ann Intern Med* 1982;96:831.
Entire issue on TSS.

Van Nguyen O, Nguyen EA, Weiner LB. Incidence of invasive bacterial disease in children with fever and petechiae. *Pediatrics* 1984;74:77.
Twenty percent of patients with fever and petechiae had bacterial infections.

Walker DH. Rocky mountain spotted fever: a seasonal alert. *Clin Infect Dis* 1995;20:1111–1117.
A history of a tick exposure with a 3- to 12-day incubation period is key to diagnosis.

Wolfson JS, Sober AJ, Rubin RH. Dermatologic manifestations of infections in immunocompromised patients. *Medicine (Baltimore)* 1985;64:115.
Diagnosis is usually established by skin biopsy for culture and histologic examination. The gross appearance of the skin lesions is of limited value.

Woodward TE, et al. Prompt confirmation of Rocky Mountain spotted fever: identification of rickettsiae in skin tissues. *J Infect Dis* 1976;134:297.
An immunofluorescence technique identified rickettsiae in a skin biopsy specimen in 4 hours.

Working Group on Severe Streptococcal Infections. Defining the group A streptococcal toxic shock syndrome. *JAMA* 1993;269:390–391.
Cases are defined by isolation of group A streptococci from a sterile site, presence of hypotension, and presence of two or more of the following: renal impairment, coagulopathy, liver abnormalities, acute respiratory distress syndrome, tissue necrosis, and an erythematous rash.

Young NS, Brown KE. Parvovirus B19. *N Engl J Med* 2004;350:586–597.
Major diseases caused by parvovirus B19 include fifth disease, arthropathy, transient aplastic crisis, anemia, and hydrops fetalis.

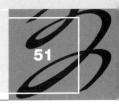
*I*nfection is the primary cause of death after renal transplantation. Nevertheless, there has been a substantial decrease in the frequency of infection, which can be attributed to improved surgical techniques, more precise immunosuppressive regimens, better matching of donor and recipient organs, improved harvesting and preservation of donor organs, and prompt diagnosis and treatment of infections. Since the introduction of cyclosporine, an 11-amino acid, cyclic polypeptide antirejection agent, the incidence of infection has decreased even further. In a randomized, prospective trial of cyclosporine versus azathioprine for immunosuppression in renal allograft recipients, the incidence of all infections in the cyclosporine-treated patients was approximately half that in the azathioprine-treated patients. The number of bacterial infections was similar in the two groups, but viral infections, particularly cytomegalovirus (CMV) infections, occurred in a significantly greater number of azathioprine-treated than cyclosporine-treated patients. There was no significant difference, however, between the two treatment groups' graft survival rates.

EARLY INFECTION

During the first month after transplantation, the chief considerations are wound-, pulmonary-, urinary tract-, and IV line-related infections caused by the usual bacterial pathogens. Perioperative antibiotics have decreased the incidence of wound infection. Prophylaxis with trimethoprim-sulfamethoxazole, daily, for the first 4 months after transplantation has decreased the incidence of urinary tract infection. Wound infections may occur without the usual signs of inflammation and fever. Ultrasound and computed tomographic (CT) scan may be helpful when the diagnosis is in doubt.

Opportunistic infections are rare during the first month after transplantation, and their occurrence suggests either an unusual nosocomial exposure or an infection that was present but unrecognized in the period before transplantation, with symptomatic disease resulting from immunosuppressive therapy, surgical manipulation, or both.

MIDDLE PERIOD INFECTION (1–4 MONTHS)

Opportunistic infections become manifest 1 to 4 months after transplantation. Infections caused by CMV, Epstein-Barr virus, varicella-zoster virus, hepatitis C and other hepatitis virus agents, *Nocardia, Listeria,* fungi, *Toxoplasma,* and *Pneumocystis carinii,* and serious bacterial infections related to the surgical procedure are common at this time.

Among these pathogens, CMV predominates. About 50% of all renal transplant recipients presenting with fever during this period have CMV disease. Infection with CMV may occur as primary disease when a seronegative recipient receives a kidney from a seropositive donor. Reactivation may occur when the donor is seropositive. The clinical presentation may be subtle and lymphadenopathy and splenomegaly are uncommon. Arthralgias and myalgias with atypical lymphocytosis are clues. CMV will induce other opportunistic infections and causes glomerulopathy. Immunoglobulin preparations with antibodies to CMV and valacyclovir have been used successfully in prevention.

Other herpes virus infections also can occur during this middle period. Herpes simplex virus may cause oral and anogenital lesions that are particularly severe. Varicella-zoster infection causes disseminated disease in nonimmune recipients and reactivation zoster in immune patients. Human herpesvirus 6, 7, and 8 are emerging pathogens in renal transplant patients. Human herpesvirus 8 has been associated with clonal gammopathy and Kaposi's sarcoma.

Epstein-Barr virus reactivation can result in extranodal proliferation of B cells causing tissue invasion into the nasopharynx and central nervous system.

Patients in this period are vulnerable to a variety of pulmonary infections that are usual with decreased T-cell immunity. Pulmonary infections are a major cause of mortality and may be difficult to distinguish from pulmonary embolus or pulmonary edema. Infections include, in addition to CMV interstitial pneumonia, *P. carinii*, *Legionella pneumophila*, *Nocardia*, tuberculosis, and *Aspergillus* spp. In endemic areas, deep-seated mycoses such as blastomycosis, histoplasmosis, and coccidioidomycosis are important pulmonary pathogens that are likely to occur with disseminated disease. *Streptococcus pneumoniae* and influenza virus will be important causes of community-acquired infection at all times.

In the late posttransplantation period, 6 months or more after the transplantation, cryptococcal meningitis occurs insidiously. Skin lesions may herald the onset of meningitis. Cryptococcal infections usually begin more than 1 year after transplantation. *Listeria* meningitis needs to be in the differential diagnosis of lymphocytic meningitis. Other infections observed in the late period are CMV infection, chorioretinitis, urinary tract infection, chronic viral hepatitis, and the usual community-acquired infections, such as pneumococcal pneumonia. Unusual organisms such as *Mycobacterium marinum* and *Protheca wickerhamii* cause nodular skin lesions. Papillomavirus warts are a late consequence of immunosuppression. Table 51-1 describes the most common infections in renal transplant patients by time period after transplantation.

Fever in a renal transplant recipient may indicate an infectious or noninfectious cause. Important noninfectious causes of fever are allograft rejection, malignancy, drug fever, and pulmonary emboli. When a renal transplant patient has a fever, the clinician should initiate an exhaustive evaluation to determine any clues to its cause. Symptoms and signs other than fever help to localize the site of infection. Clues to the presence of infection are often subtle in a renal transplant recipient. Headache, even without a stiff neck, indicates the possibility of

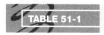 **TABLE 51-1**   **Infection in the Kidney Transplant Patient**

Period After Transplantation		
Early *Less than 1 month*	**Middle** *1–4 months*	**Late** *Longer than 6 months*
Urinary tract infection with pyelonephritis caused by gram-negative bacilli	CMV urinary tract infection	Uncomplicated urinary tract infection
Wound infection—staphylococcus and streptococci		Skin infection with *M. marinum*, Protheca, papilloma virus
Bacterial pneumonia	Pneumonia caused by CMV, *P. carinii*, tuberculosis, mycoses	*Nocardia*, *Aspergillus*, mucor pulmonary infections
		CMV retinitis cryptococcal meningitis, *L. monocytogenes* meningitis

meningitis. Travel history and place of residence are important factors if coccidioidomycosis, histoplasmosis, or parasitic disease is suspected and diagnosed. The possibility of drug fever must always be considered. The clinician should order blood, urine, and other cultures based on the clinical clues. Signs of rejection should be assessed by measuring changes in renal function. Other useful studies include urinalysis, chest radiograph, complete blood count (CBC), acute and convalescent serologies, and cultures of the urine and buffy coat for CMV. CT and ultrasound examinations are useful to evaluate the transplant site and detect any other occult intra-abdominal disease.

Infection is responsible for approximately 75% of fevers. Of these infections, viruses are the most frequent cause, responsible for more than half (55%) of all febrile episodes. Of the viral agents, CMV is by far the most frequent and can be found alone or in combination with other viruses. Most CMV disease occurs between 14 days and 4 months after transplantation, and only 17% of the febrile episodes observed more than 1 year after transplantation are associated with CMV infection. Bacterial and fungal infections are responsible for 14% and 5% of febrile episodes, respectively. The other important cause of fever is rejection, which accounts for 13% of posttransplantation fever. Infection with HIV can occur, and screening for this agent should be carried out in donors as well as recipients.

Central nervous system (CNS) infections occur in about 10% of renal transplant recipients. The CNS is second only to the lungs as a site of infection by opportunistic pathogens. Three pathogens are responsible for about 90% of the infections: *Listeria monocytogenes, Cryptococcus neoformans,* and *Aspergillus fumigatus.* Recently several cases of West Nile virus-associated encephalitis have been reported in renal transplant patients. Fever and headache are the most common symptoms of CNS infection and often are the only clues present. A minority of cases have nuchal rigidity. All renal transplant recipients with fever and headache should have a lumbar puncture analysis. CT should precede the lumbar puncture if papilledema or any focal neurologic finding is present. The use of OKT3 to reverse graft rejection after renal transplantation has been associated with an aseptic meningitis syndrome characterized by fever, headache, and an altered mental status. In this syndrome, patients have a cerebrospinal fluid pleocytosis with negative cultures.

Fever and pulmonary infiltrates in a renal transplant recipient, as in any other immunocompromised host, suggest many diagnoses, both infectious and noninfectious, and an organized approach to establish a causative diagnosis is imperative. Pulmonary infection is a major cause of mortality in renal transplant recipients. Noninfectious causes, such as pulmonary emboli and pulmonary edema, account for about 25% of the cases in one report. Clues to the cause can be obtained from assessing the course of illness and the chest roentgenographic pattern. For example, fungi and *Nocardia* produce cavitation, and the infiltrates generally develop over several weeks. Common infecting pathogens, such as *S. pneumoniae* and influenza virus, are still seen more often than opportunistic pathogens, except for CMV, and must always be considered in a patient with community-acquired pneumonia. CMV infection occurs during the 1- to 4-month interval after transplantation. In one report, mixed infections were noted in 40% of patients. If the expectorated sputum fails to yield a diagnosis, more invasive techniques are required. Treatment should be based on the specific cause.

 PROPHYLAXIS

In a survey of United States transplant centers, there was consensus on many aspects of prophylaxis against infection posttransplant. All centers screened donors and recipients for HIV, hepatitis B and hepatitis C, and CMV. Most also screened for Epstein-Barr virus and syphilis. Screening for human herpesvirus 6 and 8 was performed in some centers.

All centers provided prophylaxis against CMV with positive donors to negative recipients. Perioperative surgical prophylaxis is given to all patients. Long-term prophylaxis against pneumocystis with trimethoprim-sulfamethoxazole is used at 84% of centers. Trimethoprim-sulfamethoxazole is also used to prevent urinary tract infection.

The use of vaccines, particularly live viral vaccines, was controversial. Some centers avoided posttransplantation vaccines because of concern about inducing rejection. (SLB)

Bibliography

Arduino R, Johnson P, Miranda A. Nocardiosis in renal transplant recipients undergoing immunosuppression with cyclosporine. *Clin Infect Dis* 1993;16:505–512.
  Lung involvement predominates. Drug interaction between cyclosporine and trimethoprim-sulfamethoxazole may require use of another agent for therapy of Nocardia infection (e.g., imipenem, amikacin, minocycline, or amoxicillin-clavulanic acid).
Batiuk TD, Bodziak KA, Goldman M. Infectious disease prophylaxis in renal transplant patients: a survey of U.S. transplant centers. *Clin Transplant* 2002;16:1.
  This paper presents a consensus of the prophylactic measures used by transplant centers, including surgical prophylaxis, prophylaxis against urinary tract infections, CMV, and pneumocystis. Vaccine prophylaxis varies with centers.
Brayman KL, et al. Analysis of infectious complications occurring after solid-organ transplantation. *Arch Surg* 1992;127:38.
  Infection remains the most frequent cause of death after renal transplantation. Most life-threatening infections were noted in the first 4 months after transplantation.
Case records of the Massachusetts General Hospital (case 24-1984). *N Engl J Med* 1984;310:1584.
  Fever and pancytopenia in a renal transplant recipient from Venezuela. The diagnosis is disseminated histoplasmosis.
Dowling JN, et al. Infections caused by *Legionella micdadei* and *Legionella pneumophila* among renal transplant recipients. *J Infect Dis* 1984;149:703.
  Renal transplant recipients are at increased risk for Legionella *infection at certain transplant centers.*
Farrugia E, Schwab TR. Management and prevention of cytomegalovirus infection after renal transplantation. *Mayo Clin Proc* 1992;67:879.
  CMV disease usually occurs within 2 to 6 months after transplantation.
Finberg R, Fingeroth J. Infections in transplant recipients. In: Braunwald E, Fauci AS, Kasper DL, Hauser SL, Longo DL, Jameson JL eds. *Principles of Internal Medicine.* 15th ed. New York: McGraw Hill 2001:863.
  This chapter divides the infections that occur in renal transplant patients based on time after transplant, with early, middle, and late infections each having a different panel of likely pathogens.
Fishman JA, Rubin RH. Infection in organ-transplant recipients. *N Engl J Med* 1998;338: 1741.
  CMV is the most important pathogen affecting transplant recipients. Diagnosis is made with tests for antigenemia, polymerase chain reaction assays, or tissue biopsy.
Hadley S, Karchmer AW. Fungal infections in solid-organ transplant recipients. *Infect Dis Clin North Am* 1995;9:1045.
  Describes clinical and laboratory characteristics of fungal infection in transplant patients.
John GT, Shankar V. Mycobacterial infections in organ transplant recipients. *Semin Respir Infect* 2002;17:274.
  Prevalence of posttransplant tuberculosis was 13.7% at a center in India. Cyclosporin and tacrolimus were associated with earlier onset tuberculosis as compared with prednisolone and azathioprine.
Kontoyiannis DP, Rubin RH. Infection in the organ transplant recipient. An overview. *Infect Dis Clin North Am* 1995;9:811.
  Review. Infections result from technical problems (e.g., wound hematoma), epidemiologic exposures (e.g., Aspergillus spp.*), and net state of immunosuppression (e.g., CMV infection, drugs to prevent rejection).*
Martinez-Marcos F, et al. Prospective study of renal transplant infections in 50 consecutive patients. *Eur J Clin Microbiol Infect Dis* 1994;13:1023.
  During the first year after transplantation, urinary tract infections, especially asymptomatic bacteriuria, were most common.

Mayoral JL, et al. Diagnosis and treatment of cytomegalovirus disease in transplant patients based on gastrointestinal tract manifestations. *Arch Surg* 1991;126:202.
Clinical symptoms in patients with invasive CMV disease involving the gastrointestinal tract included abdominal pain (79%), fever (36%), diarrhea (21%), and gastrointestinal bleeding (21%).

Paterson DL, Singh N. Interactions between tacrolimus and antimicrobial agents. *Clin Infect Dis* 1997;25:1430.
Tacrolimus (FK506) is metabolized by the cytochrome P-450 3A system, and any antimicrobial drug that inhibits or induces these enzymes can alter levels of tacrolimus. Tacrolimus can cause nephrotoxicity.

Peterson PK, et al. Cytomegalovirus disease in renal allograft recipients: a prospective study of the clinical features, risk factors and impact on renal transplantation. *Medicine (Baltimore)* 1980;59:283.
Review of CMV primary and reactivation disease. Fever was present in 95% of patients.

Peterson PK, et al. Fever in renal transplant recipients: causes, prognostic significance and changing patterns at the University of Minnesota Hospital. *Am J Med* 1981;71:345.
Viral infections, primarily CMV infections, were responsible for more than 50% of the episodes.

Ravindra KV, et al. West Nile virus-associated encephalitis in recipients of renal and pancreas transplants. Case series and literature review. *Clin Infect Dis* 2004;38:1257.
Additional differential in the transplant patient with meningoencephalitis. West Nile encephalitis should be considered in endemic areas.

Regamey N, et al. Infection with human herpesvirus 8 and transplant-associated gammopathy. *Transplantation* 2004;77:1551.
Transplant recipients with herpesvirus infection had a higher incidence of clonal gammopathy than transplant patients who were human herpesvirus-8 negative.

Rubin RH, Tolkoff-Rubin NE. Antimicrobial strategies in the care of organ transplant recipients. Minireview. *Antimicrob Agents Chemother* 1993;37:619.
Review of prophylaxis. Use fluconazole for asymptomatic candiduria in diabetic renal transplant patients.

Rubin RH, et al. Infection in the renal transplant recipient. *Am J Med* 1981;70:405.
Infections are categorized according to time of onset in this classic article.

Stamm AM. Listeriosis in renal transplant recipients: report of an outbreak and review of 102 cases. *Rev Infect Dis* 1982;4:665.
The major manifestations of the disease are meningitis (50%) and primary bacteremia (30%).

Stephan RN, Munschauer CE, Kumar A. Surgical wound infection in renal transplantation: outcome data in 102 consecutive patients without perioperative systemic antibiotic coverage. *Arch Surg* 1997;132:1315–1319.
Incidence of wound infection was only 2%.

Stone RM. Case records of the Massachusetts General Hospital (case 31-1997). *N Engl J Med* 1997;337:1065–1074.
Fever and diffuse pulmonary infiltrates 5 months after renal transplantation. The diagnosis was lymphoma.

Tolkoff-Rubin NE, Rubin RH. The infectious disease problems of the diabetic renal transplant recipient. *Infect Dis Clin North Am* 1995;9:117–130.
Diabetic renal transplant recipients have the same infections as nondiabetic patients, plus infections resulting from vascular compromise (e.g., foot infections).

Tolkoff-Rubin NE, et al. A controlled study of trimethoprim-sulfamethoxazole prophylaxis of urinary tract infection in renal transplant recipients. *Rev Infect Dis* 1982;4:614.
Trimethoprim-sulfamethoxazole is effective for prophylaxis of urinary tract infection.

Toogood GJ, Roake JA, Morris PJ. The relationship between fever and acute rejection or infection following renal transplantation in the cyclosporin era. *Clin Transplant* 1994;8:373–377.
Fever in the first 2 weeks is more likely caused by rejection rather than infection.

Wagener MM, Yu VL. Bacteremia in transplant recipients: a prospective study of demographics, etiologic agents, risk factors, and outcomes. *Am J Infect Control* 1992;20:239.

The urinary tract (58%) was the most frequent source for a bacteremia in renal transplant recipients. Mortality was 11%.

Weiland D, et al. Aspergillosis in 25 renal transplant patients. *Ann Surg* 1983;622:198.
Sputum culture failed to yield the organism in 60% of patients.

Wheat LJ, et al. Histoplasmosis in renal allograft recipients. Two large urban outbreaks. *Arch Intern Med* 1983;143:703.
A diagnosis of histoplasmosis is suspected in renal transplant recipients with prolonged unexplained fever in endemic areas. Results of chest roentgenography are often negative.

Wilson JP, et al. Nocardial infections in renal transplant recipients. *Medicine (Baltimore)* 1989;68:38.
Review. Overall mortality was 25%, but 42% in patients with CNS disease.

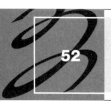

52 — FEVER FOLLOWING TRAVEL ABROAD

*W*hen patients are being evaluated, it is important to obtain a detailed history, perform a focused clinical examination, and obtain the appropriate lab tests to diagnose a travel-acquired infection. Important factors to consider would include the destination and the nature of the trip that was taken (business, leisure, and medical). It also would be helpful to know what kind of accommodations were available. Knowledge of water and insect exposures, as well as what kind of human (sexual, medical) contacts occurred can be used to help determine the degree of risk that exists for each patient. Seasonality and trip duration also are important factors. Tables 52-1 and 52-2 may provide helpful clues to determine

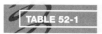

TABLE 52-1	**Risk Factors for Infection After Travel**

Exposure	Potential diseases
Undercooked food	Cholera, salmonellosis, typhoid fever, *Escherichia coli*
Milk	*Brucella*, *Salmonella*, tuberculosis
Water exposure	Leptospirosis, schistosomiasis, dracontiasis
Infected animals	Brucellosis, plague, Q fever, rabies, tularemia, monkey pox, leptospirosis
Mosquitoes	Dengue fever, malaria, encephalitis
Ticks	Rickettsial diseases, tularemia, Colorado tick fever, relapsing fever, Babesia, typhus, Lyme, Crimean hemorrhagic fever
Reduviids	American trypanosomiasis
Tsetse flies	African trypanosomiasis
Sexual contacts	Chancroid, gonorrhea, hepatitis B, herpes and HIV
Sick contacts	Meningococcal disease, tuberculosis, viral hemorrhagic fevers, severe acute respiratory syndrome (SARS)
Transfusion	Hepatitis, HIV, malaria, Chagas

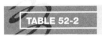

| **TABLE 52-2** | Incubation Periods |

Less than 21 days	More than 21 days
Meningococcemia	Acute HIV infection
Nontyphoidal salmonellosis	Schistosomiasis
Plague	Epstein-Barr virus
Typhoid fever	Filariasis
Typhus	Secondary syphilis
Viral hemorrhagic fevers	Amebic liver abscess
Yellow fever	Borreliosis (relapsing fever)
Campylobacter	Brucellosis
Toxigenic E. coli	Leishmaniasis
Influenza	Malaria
Rickettsial diseases	Rabies
Shigella	Tuberculosis
Measles	Viral hepatitis (A, B, C, D, E)
CMV	West African trypanosomiasis
East African trypanosomiasis	
Dengue fever	
Japanese encephalitis	
Leptospirosis	
Malaria	

an etiology. The incubation period of the illness often can help the physician formulate a differential diagnosis.

FEVER

Infection is the most common cause of fever in the returned traveler but other causes such as medications, thromboembolism, malignancy and other noninfectious causes also need to be considered. Fever patterns, although classically described, are seldom useful in the clinical setting. See Table 52-3 for specific details.

Generally, a few illnesses account for the majority of diagnoses. These would include malaria, dengue, typhoid, and viral hepatitis. Immunization history and compliance with antimalarial chemoprophylaxis are helpful clues to the etiology of fever. A tropical hospital

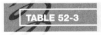

| **TABLE 52-3** | Fever Patterns |

Fever patterns	Illness	Comments
Tertian	*P. vivax*	Fever spike every other day
Quartan	*P. malariae*	Spike every third day
Saddleback	Dengue, yellow fever, and Colorado tick fever	Biphasic pattern. Febrile period between spikes
Relapsing	*Borealis* spp.	A period of days or weeks between spikes
Undulant	Brucellosis, visceral leishmaniasis	Moving like waves
Bradycardia	Typhoid and yellow fever	Relative to the temperature
Breakbone	Dengue	Severe myalgias

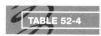

TABLE 52-4 Differential Diagnosis of Skin Lesions Associated With Travel

Maculopapular	Petechiae	Eschar	Chancre	Ulcers	Papular
Dengue	Dengue	Anthrax	Syphilis	Leishmaniasis	Syphilis
Rubella	Leptospirosis			Mycobacteria	Insect bites
EBV			African	Insect bites	Tungiasis
Rickettsia	Rickettsia	Rickettsia	trypanosomiasis	STDs	Myiasis
Meningococcemia	Meningococcemia	Scrub typhus		Sporotrichosis	Onchocerciasis
Rose spots in					
typhoid fever					
Measles					

in London found that malaria accounted for 42% of admissions. The most common illness that requires immediate treatment *is Plasmodium falciparum* malaria. This should be urgently investigated with thick and thin blood smears. The second largest group was assumed to have a nonspecific viral infection (25%). Cosmopolitan infections (urinary tract infection, community-acquired pneumonia, streptococcal sore throat, etc.) accounted for 9%. Coincidental infections (schistosomiasis, filariasis, and intestinal helminths) were found in 16%. Serology was positive for HIV infection in 3%. The most useful investigation was a malaria film, which was positive in 45% of cases in which it was performed.

RASH, SPLENOMEGALY, JAUNDICE, AND EOSINOPHILIA

The presence of a rash often will alert the physician to a specific diagnosis (Table 52-4). A biopsy with pathologic analysis and culture can be very helpful. Splenomegaly and lymphadenopathy are often present as well (Table 52-5). The most common diseases in the tropics that present with fever and eosinophilia are acute schistosomiasis (Katayama fever) and ascariasis (Table 52-6). Diseases that may be associated with jaundice are noted in Table 52-7.

MALARIA

Urgent evaluation of a potential *P. falciparum* malaria infection is required because it carries a high fatality rate of more than 20%. Attention should be given to the type of and compliance with any prescribed antimalarial medication. Perhaps out of a false sense of security, a greater prevalence of malaria is seen in residents of developing countries who have returned home to visit friends and relatives.

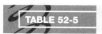

TABLE 52-5 Diseases Associated With Lympadenopathy and Splenomegaly

Lymphadenopathy Localized	Generalized	Splenomegaly Bacterial	Nonbacterial
Plague, tularemia	Brucellosis,	Enteric fever,	EBV, CMV, HIV,
African trypanosomiasis,	leptospirosis,	Brucella,	Malaria, visceral
American	melioidosis	Endocarditis,	Leishmaniasis,
trypanosomiasis,	Dengue fever, Lassa	Leptospirosis,	Trypanosomiasis,
filariasis,	fever, measles	Typhus	Schistosomiasis
toxoplasmosis	Visceral leishmaniasis		
Tuberculosis	HIV infection,		
	secondary syphilis		

TABLE 52-6 Degree of Eosinophilia

None to rare	Minimal to moderate	Moderate to significant
Protozoa (Isospora, Toxoplasma rarely) Tapeworms	Filariasis Ascariasis Clonorchiasis Enterobiasis Trichuriasis Hydatid disease Cysticercosis	Trichinosis Loaiasis Strongyloidiasis Ascariasis Hookworm Paragonimiasis Onchocerciasis Fascioliasis Schistosomiasis Paragonimiasis Fasciolopsiasis Toxocariasis Angiostrongylus Gnathostomiasis

Regardless of whether antimalarial medication was taken, patients should have thick and thin smears (at least 3 over 48 hours) ordered for malaria. Symptoms of *P. falciparum* infection are usually apparent within 2 months of returning, but those caused by other species might take longer to present (several months). Some patients, such as immigrants and visitors from endemic areas and those taking chemoprophylaxis, may have delayed onset or atypical presentation.

Almost all patients will report fever but not necessarily with classic fever pattern as noted in Table 52-3. They may also complain of malaise, headache, myalgias, and gastrointestinal symptoms. Jaundice and hepatosplenomegaly also may be seen as well. Rash and lymphadenopathy, however, are uncommon and should suggest another diagnosis. The World Health Organization (WHO) defines *severe malaria* as a parasitemic person (>5%) with one or more of the following: prostration, impaired consciousness, respiratory distress or pulmonary edema, seizures, circulatory collapse, abnormal bleeding, jaundice, hemoglobinuria, and anemia. Several complications of severe malaria can occur and include severe anemia, acute renal failure, respiratory failure, intravascular hemolysis, and cerebral malaria. Hematologic abnormalities are common, and liver function test results are often abnormal. An elevated bilirubin level in the face of a high lactate dehydrogenase level suggests hemolysis. Hypoglycemia and hyponatremia may be present as well.

The thick blood film provides enhanced sensitivity of the blood film technique and is much better than the thin film for detection of low levels of parasitemia. A recognized way of estimating the number of parasites present in 1 μL of blood is to use a standard value for the white blood cell (WBC) count (8,000 WBC/μL). Counting the number of parasites

TABLE 52-7 Causes of Jaundice

Bacterial	Nonbacterial
Leptospirosis Typhus Typhoid	Severe malaria Fascioliasis Cytomegalovirus Viral hepatitis Yellow fever

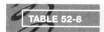

TABLE 52-8 CQ-Sensitive Strains

Organism	Treatment	Dose	Prevention	Comments
Vivax, sensitive strains	Chloroquine (CQ) plus primaquine if sensitive.	1 g P.O. (600 mg of base) then 0.5 g at 6 hr and 0.5 g daily times 2 days. Total of 1500 mg of base. *Give 30 mg of Primaquine base/day times 14 days.*	CQ 500 mg (300 mg base) P.O. q wk beginning 1–2 weeks before and continuing until 4 weeks after travel	For persons with borderline G6PD deficiency or as an alternate to the above regimen, primaquine may be given at the dose of 45 mg (base) orally one time per week for 8 weeks Primaquine must not be used during pregnancy
Ovale	CQ plus primaquine	As above	As above	G6PD as above
Malariae	CQ	As above for CQ	As above	
Falciparum, sensitive strains	CQ	As above for CQ	As above	Haiti, Central America, Parts of Middle East

present until 200 WBC have been seen and then multiplying the parasites counted by 40 will give the parasite count per microliter of blood. The sensitivity for the examination of the thick blood film procedure is about 50 parasites/μL of blood, which is equivalent to 0.001% of red blood cells (RBC) infected. The identification of the parasite to the species level is much easier and provides greater specificity.

The thin blood film is often preferred for estimation of the parasitemia. The parasitemia may be estimated by examination of a well-stained thin blood film. This is usually accomplished by noting the number of parasitized RBC (not individual parasites) seen in 10,000 RBC (equal to approximately 40 monolayer cell fields of a standard microscope using the 100× oil immersion objective; however, microscopists are advised to calculate the average number of cells per microscope field of view for their own microscopes) and expressing the number of parasitized cells seen as a percentage. The approximate numbers of parasites present in 1 μL of blood can be calculated by assuming that 1 μL of blood contains 5×10^6 RBC; therefore, a 1% parasitemia will contain 1 parasite/100 RBC or 50,000 parasites/μL of blood. Similarly, a 0.1% parasitemia will contain 5,000 parasites/μL of blood. This may be corrected to exact counts if the total RBC count per microliter is known.

Polymerase chain reaction (PCR) has been used to detect malaria as well. Its utility lies in its sensitivity, with the ability to detect five parasites or less per microliter of blood. Nested and multiplex PCR methods can give valuable information when difficult morphologic problems arise during attempts to identify parasites to the species level.

Immunochromatographic dipsticks offer the possibility of more rapid, nonmicroscopic methods for malaria diagnosis, thereby saving on training and time. The new immunochromatographic antigen capture tests are capable of detecting more than 100 parasites/μL (0.002% parasitemia) and of giving rapid results (15–20 minutes). They are commercially available in a kit with all the necessary reagents, and no extensive training or equipment is required to perform or interpret the results. The persistence of HRP-2 antigenemia beyond the clearance of peripheral parasitemia in certain cases reduces the usefulness of these assays

Treatment of CQ-Resistant Organisms

TABLE 52-9

Organism	Treatment	Dose	Comments
Vivax, CQ resistant	Quinine sulfate plus doxycycline and primaquine Mefloquine (MQ) plus primaquine	(A) 542 mg of base (650 mg of salt) P.O. t.i.d. for 3–7 days Doxycycline 100 mg P.O. b.i.d. times 7 days. Primaquine as above.	Papua New Guinea and Indonesia and other areas occasionally Atovaquone plus proguanil
		(B) MQ 684 mg base (750 mg salt) then 456 mg base (500 mg salt) P.O. given 6–12 hr after initial dose for a total of 1,250 mg salt	There are no adequate, well-controlled studies to support the use of atovaquone-proguanil to treat chloroquine-resistant *P. vivax* infections
Falciparum, resistant	(A) Quinine sulfate plus doxycycline (B) Atovaquone (250 mg) proguanil (100 mg). Known as Malarone	(A) 542 mg base (650 mg salt) P.O. t.i.d. times 7 days. (3 days for Africa) Plus 100 mg b.i.d. times 7 days for doxycycline (B) 4 tabs P.O. q day times 3 days.	Less desirable is MQ 750 mg salt P.O. as an initial dose followed by 500 mg salt 6–12 hr later
Severe Falciparum	Quinidine gluconate plus doxycycline (or clindamycin) times 7 days if necessary	Dose of quinidine is 6.25 mg base/kg loading dose IV over 2 hr, then 0.0125 mg base/kg minute continuous infusion times 24 hr	Once the parasitemia level is <1%, try oral quinine if possible

for monitoring the response to therapy. The overall sensitivity and specificity of rapid detection tests (RDTs) for the detection of *Falciparum* malaria are better than 90%. However, sensitivity falls dramatically with low-level parasitemia and at present, RDTs cannot be used alone to exclude malaria.

See Tables 52-8 through 52-10 for information regarding malaria.

 DIARRHEA

Please see Chapter 64 for information regarding traveler's diarrhea.

 LEPTOSPIROSIS

Leptospirosis is a bacterial zoonosis transmitted from animals to humans through contact with contaminated water or moist soil. People who work close to where either rats or infected livestock contact water are at a higher risk of infection. Leptospirosis is an important cause of fever in travelers returning from the tropics. Prophylaxis with 200 mg of doxycycline per week can be considered for those at highest risk.

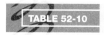

TABLE 52-10		Prevention of CQ-Resistant *Falciparum*	
Organism	Prevention	Dose	Comments
CQ-resistant Falciparum	(A) Atovaquone-proguanil (B) Doxycycline 100 mg daily (C) MQ (D) Primaquine	(A) 1 adult tablet orally, daily (B) 100 mg daily (C) 228 mg base (250 mg salt) orally, once/week 30 mg base daily	Atovaquone/proguanil primary prophylaxis should begin 1–2 days before travel to malarious areas and should be taken daily, at the same time each day, while in the malarious area, and daily for 7 days after leaving such areas Doxycycline primary prophylaxis should begin 1–2 days before travel to malarious areas. It should be continued once a day, at the same time each day, during travel in malarious areas, and daily for 4 weeks after the traveler leaves such areas MQ primary prophylaxis should begin 1–2 weeks before travel to malarious areas. It should be continued once a week, on the same day each week, during travel to malarious areas, and for 4 weeks after the traveler leaves such areas Primaquine primary prophylaxis should begin 1–2 days before travel to the malaria-risk area. It should be continued once a day, at the same time each day, while in the malaria-risk area, and daily for 7 days after leaving the malaria-risk area For MQ resistance, use either atovaquone-proguanil or doxycycline. Most likely in parts of Burma, Cambodia or Thailand

Travelers will become ill within 1 to 2 weeks after a potential exposure. The majority of patients (90%) experience a mild febrile illness, but more severe forms can affect some patients. A biphasic course of illness is characteristic. The initial or *septicemic* stage is characterized by the sudden onset of fever, retro-orbital headache, chills, myalgias, conjunctival suffusion, and skin rashes. In addition to the conjunctival injection seen in the primary stage, a uveitis can be seen in the secondary stage. Defervescence of fever occurs in 7 days in this phase and is usually followed by an interval afebrile period of 2 days. The second or *immune phase* is heralded by the appearance of IgM antibodies. The organisms usually cannot be cultured from blood or cerebrospinal fluid (CSF) during this second immune phase but can be found in the urine for months. Symptoms may recur and meningitis is noted in about 50% of cases. Severe cases are characterized by renal failure, pulmonary hemorrhage, jaundice, and myocarditis. The treatment of choice is doxycycline, 100 mg orally twice a day for 7 days.

Diagnosis can be difficult. Usually the diagnosis is made serologically but can be made by culture of the organism on special media such as Fletcher's, Stuart's, Ellinghausen-

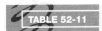

| TABLE 52-11 | Web Resources |

Site	Address
Online fever algorithm	http://www.fevertravel.ch/
Australian malaria site	http://rph.wa.gov.au/labs/haem/malaria/index.html
CDC malaria FAQ	http://www.cdc.gov/malaria/faq.htm
Navy malaria site	http://www.vnh.org/Malaria/ch4.html
CDC diarrhea	http://www.cdc.gov/travel/diarrhea.htm
ACG diarrhea primer	http://www.acg.gi.org/physicianforum/gifocus/diarrhea.html
Parasitology atlas	http://www.hamt.or.jp/KENSA/MSTAFF/PARS/
Schistosomiasis	http://www.cdc.gov/ncidod/dpd/parasites/schistosomiasis/
WHO schistosomiasis	http://www.who.int/tdr/diseases/schisto/
Japanese encephalitis	http://www.mdtravelhealth.com/infectious/japanese_encephalitis.html
Leptospirosis	http://www.cdc.gov/ncidod/dbmd/diseaseinfo/leptospirosis_g.htm
MD travel health	http://www.mdtravelhealth.com/index.html
Yellow fever vaccine	http://www.who.int/wer/2003/en/wer7840.pdf
Insect protection	http://www.mdtravelhealth.com/illness/insect_and_tick.html

McCullough-Johnson-Harris (EMJH), or Tween 80-albumin medium. Appropriate fluids to be cultured include blood and CSF during the first week of illness; urine should be cultured thereafter. Detection of leptospiral DNA by PCR is more sensitive than culture. The spirochetes can be demonstrated in tissue sections with silver stains as well.

DENGUE

Also known as *breakbone fever*, this mosquito-borne illness is typically self limited and nonfatal. After an incubation period of about 1 week, there may be the sudden onset of fever, headache, retro-orbital pain, and myalgias. A transient rash and relative bradycardia may be noted on physical examination. Marked leukopenia and thrombocytopenia are not uncommon. Typically the patient recovers in less than a week. Only minor hemorrhagic manifestations such as petechiae are present in most patients, but occasionally significant bleeding results from gastrointestinal ulcers.

Dengue hemorrhagic fever (DHF) patients are afflicted with a second phase of illness characterized by ascites, pleural effusions, and spontaneous hemorrhages, including gastrointestinal hemorrhage, ecchymoses, and epistaxis. Capillary permeability and coagulation defects lead to hemorrhagic manifestations and, in more severe cases, to hypovolemic shock. The risk factors of hemorrhage in DHF/dengue shock syndrome (DSS) are prolonged shock with a normal or low hematocrit at the time of shock. DHF and DSS appear to have an immunologic basis and occur with subsequent episodes of dengue. At present, there is no specific drug therapy for DHF beyond supportive care, as outlined previously.

For web resources regarding international travel, see Table 52-11. (JWM)

Bibliography
Advice for travelers. *Med Lett Drugs Ther* 2002;44:33–38.
Abell L, et al. Health advice for travelers. *N Engl J Med* 2000;343:1045–1046.
Cetron MS, et al. Yellow fever vaccine. Recommendations of the Advisory Committee on Immunization Practices (ACIP), 2002. *MMWR Recomm Rep* 2002;51:1–11; quiz CE1–4.
This report updates Centers for Disease Control and Prevention's (CDC's) recommendations for using yellow fever vaccine.

Cheng AC, Thielman NM. Update on traveler's diarrhea. *Curr Infect Dis Rep* 2002;4:70–77.
Fluoroquinolones effectively treat severe traveler's diarrhea, and even a single dose may be sufficient. However, with the emergence of resistance, particularly in Campylobacter infection, other agents are required; interest has focused on azithromycin and rifaximin.

D'Acremont V, et al. Practice guidelines for evaluation of fever in returning travelers and migrants. *J Travel Med* 2003;10(suppl 2):S25–S52.
Although the quality of evidence was limited by the paucity of clinical studies, these guidelines established with the support of a large and highly experienced panel should help physicians to deal with patients coming back from the tropics with fever.

Dumont L, et al. Health advice for travelers. *N Engl J Med* 2000;343:1046.

DuPont HL. Treatment of travelers' diarrhea. *J Travel Med* 2001;8(suppl 2):S31–S33.

Eichmann A. [Sexually transmissible diseases following travel in tropical countries]. *Schweiz Med Wochenschr* 1993;12324:1250–1255.
Travel to tropical countries is an important factor in the spread of sexually transmitted diseases.

Ericsson CD. Rifaximin: a new approach to the treatment of travelers' diarrhea. Conclusion. *J Travel Med* 2001;8(suppl 2):S40.

Fradin MS, Day JF. Comparative efficacy of insect repellents against mosquito bites. *N Engl J Med* 2002;347:13–18.

Freedman DO, Woodall J. Emerging infectious diseases and risk to the traveler. *Med Clin North Am* 1999;83:865–883, v.
The authors also discuss several novel pathogens, such as Ebola virus, that are clearly of insignificant or minimal risk to travelers, but are the subject of frequent questions from patients requesting pretravel advice from medical providers.

Fryauff DJ, et al. Randomised placebo-controlled trial of primaquine for prophylaxis of falciparum and vivax malaria. *Lancet* 1995;346:1190–1193.

Isaacson M. Viral hemorrhagic fever hazards for travelers in Africa. *Clin Infect Dis* 2001;33:1707–1712.
This short review covers six viral hemorrhagic fevers (VHFs) that are known to occur in Africa: yellow fever, Rift Valley fever, Crimean-Congo hemorrhagic fever, Lassa fever, Marburg virus disease, and Ebola hemorrhagic fever.

James WD. Imported skin diseases in dermatology. *J Dermatol* 2001;28:663–666.
The clinical characteristics, diagnostic tests, and therapeutic options for such imported tropical diseases will be discussed.

Jong EC. Immunizations for international travel. *Infect Dis Clin North Am* 1998;12: 249–266.

Jong EC. Risks of hepatitis A and B in the traveling public. *J Travel Med* 2001;8(suppl1): S3–S8.

Joubert JJ, et al. Schistosomiasis in Africa and international travel. *J Travel Med* 2001;8: 92–99.

Leder K, et al. Travel vaccines and elderly persons: review of vaccines available in the United States. *Clin Infect Dis* 2001;33:1553–1566.
Consideration of potential age-related differences in responses to travel vaccines is becoming increasingly important as elderly persons more frequently venture to exotic destinations.

Lo Re V 3rd, Gluckman SJ. Eosinophilic meningitis due to Angiostrongylus cantonensis in a returned traveler: case report and review of the literature. *Clin Infect Dis* 2001;33:e112–e115.
Angiostrongylus cantonensis, the rat lungworm, is the principal cause of eosinophilic meningitis worldwide. The increase in world travel and shipborne dispersal of infected rat vectors has extended this parasite to regions outside of its traditional geographic boundaries.

Magill AJ. Fever in the returned traveler. *Infect Dis Clin North Am* 1998;12:445–469.
Excellent review article.

Magill AJ. The prevention of malaria. *Prim Care* 2002;29:815–842, v–vi.

Maiwald H, et al. Long-term persistence of anti-HAV antibodies following active immunization with hepatitis A vaccine. *Vaccine* 1997;15:346–348.

Geometric mean titers *(GMTs) at protective levels higher than 20 mIU mL-L can be expected to persist for at least 15 years.*

Matteelli A, Carosi G. Sexually transmitted diseases in travelers. *Clin Infect Dis* 2001;32:1063–1067.
Prevention of sexually transmitted diseases (STDs) is a low priority among travel clinic services, despite increasing evidence that travelers have an increased risk of acquiring such infections.

Mileno MD, Bia FJ. The compromised traveler. *Infect Dis Clin North Am* 1998;12:369–412.

Monath TP. Yellow fever: an update. *Lancet Infect Dis* 2001;1:11–20.

Moody A. Rapid diagnostic tests for malaria parasites. *Clin Microbiol Rev* 2002;15:66–78.
Comparison of methods for diagnosing Plasmodium *infection in blood. Table 3 is very informative.*

O'Brien D, et al. Fever in returned travelers: review of hospital admissions for a 3-year period. *Clin Infect Dis* 2001;33:603–609.

Pollard AJ, Shlim DR. Epidemic meningococcal disease and travel. *J Travel Med* 2002;9:29–33.

Ramzan NN. Traveler's diarrhea. *Gastroenterol Clin North Am* 2001;30:665–678, viii.
This article presents a review of causes, presentation, and diagnosis of traveler's diarrhea. Treatment and prevention of this common problem is described in some detail. Finally, a practical and cost-effective approach to evaluating and treating a returning traveler is presented.

Rieder HL. Risk of travel-associated tuberculosis. *Clin Infect Dis* 2001;33:1393–1396.

Ryan ET, Calderwood SB. Cholera vaccines. *J Travel Med* 2001;8:82–91.

Sa-ngasang A, et al. Evaluation of RT-PCR as a tool for diagnosis of secondary dengue virus infection. *Jpn J Infect Dis* 2003;56:205–209.
Review of this diagnostic tool.

Samuel BU, Barry M. The pregnant traveler. *Infect Dis Clin North Am* 1998;12:325–354.
A safety profile of commonly used travel medications, antibiotics, and antiparasitic drugs is reviewed.

Steffen R. Immunization against hepatitis A and hepatitis B infections. *J Travel Med* 2001;8(suppl 1): S9–S16.

Suh KN, Kain KC, Keystone JS. Malaria. *CMAJ* 2004;170:1693–1702.
Good review article.

Taylor WR, et al. Malaria prophylaxis using azithromycin: a double-blind, placebo-controlled trial in Irian Jaya, Indonesia. *Clin Infect Dis* 1999;28:74–81.
Daily azithromycin offered excellent protection against P. vivax *malaria but modest protection against* P. falciparum *malaria.*

Virk A. Medical advice for international travelers. *Mayo Clin Proc* 2001;76:831–840.
This review primarily updates pretravel management of adults.

Wagner G, et al. Simultaneous active and passive immunization against hepatitis A studied in a population of travellers. *Vaccine* 1993;11:1027–1032.
The slight inhibition of antibody production induced by the concurrent administration of immunoglobulin does not affect the overall protection afforded by the vaccine. We conclude that simultaneous active and passive hepatitis A immunizations can be recommended.

Wilde H, et al. Rabies update for travel medicine advisors. *Clin Infect Dis* 2003;37: 96–100.

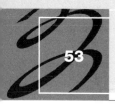

53   HYPERPYREXIA AND HYPERTHERMIA

*H*yperthermia is a temperature in excess of the normal range of 36°C (96.8°F) to 37.5°C (99.5°F). Control of thermoregulation resides within the hypothalamus, which stimulates cutaneous vasodilatation and sweating through the autonomic nervous system in response to elevation of blood temperature. Several of the conditions listed below can cause confusion when evaluating a patient with a high temperature.

 MALIGNANT HYPERTHERMIA

Malignant hyperthermia (MH) is most often diagnosed in those patients who have received halogenated inhalation agents and depolarizing muscle relaxants. MH is an autosomal-dominant abnormality of the skeletal muscle membrane with an incidence of 1:50,000 in adults. Essentially it is caused by a massive efflux of calcium from skeletal muscle sarcoplasmic reticulum, resulting in rigidity and heat production. Dantrolene sodium can be used to treat this condition because it blocks calcium release from muscle cell sarcoplasmic reticulum.

 NEUROLEPTIC MALIGNANT SYNDROME

Neuroleptic malignant syndrome (NMS) resembles MH, but in contrast, it takes about 3 days to develop and lasts longer (up to 10 days). To make a timely diagnosis of this entity, a high index of suspicion is required. This idiosyncratic disorder may occur in those patients given neuroleptic drugs, including phenothiazines, butyrophenones, thioxanthenes, lithium, and tricyclic antidepressants. The use of droperidol and metoclopramide has been reported as well. Haloperidol appears to be the most common drug implicated in this disorder. A temperature higher than 40°C, extrapyramidal symptoms such as lead pipe rigidity and autonomic instability, altered consciousness, tremor, and elevated creatine phosphokinase (CPK) should suggest the diagnosis. Dehydration, alcoholism, a history of prior brain injury, and rapid neuroleptic loading have been noted as risk factors for NMS. The condition appears to be triggered by blockade of dopaminergic receptors, resulting in spasticity of skeletal muscle, which generates excessive heat and impairs hypothalamic thermoregulation and heat dissipation.

To treat this condition, one can give dantrolene (2 to 3 mg/kg IV every 10 minutes for 3 doses), or bromocriptine at a dose of 2.5 to 10 mg three times a day. One must exclude lethal catatonia, heatstroke, serotonin syndromes, toxic encephalopathy, and central nervous system (CNS) infections to make the diagnosis of NMS. Mortality from NMS is estimated at 20% of patients who develop the condition.

 LETHAL CATATONIA

Remember that lethal catatonia emerges out of a typical excited catatonic state. Note that in lethal catatonia, rigidity is not found, in contrast to NMS. Another differentiation feature is that in lethal catatonia, the fever arises in the setting of mounting excitation, whereas in NMS it occurs in the setting of increasing rigidity.

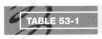

TABLE 53-1	Heat Stroke

Exertional	Classic
Younger, active patients such as athletes or recruits.	Elderly, sedentary, and chronically ill patients. They may have impaired awareness of their surroundings and of the development of heat illness.
Diaphoresis	Anhidrosis
Heat wave	Sporadic
Hypocalcemia	Normal
Rhabdomyolysis	Mild CPK elevations
Acute renal failure	Oliguria
Severe lactic acidosis	Mild
DIC	Mild
Respiratory alkalosis	Less common
Hyponatremia	Less common

 ## SEROTONIN SYNDROME

Another entity that can cause diagnostic confusion is the serotonin syndrome. Many different types of drug interactions can lead to the serotonin syndrome. It may occur with the selective serotonin reuptake inhibitors (SSRIs), monoamine oxidase inhibitors (MAOIs), tryptophan, sympathomimetics, tricyclics and other antidepressants, meperidine, dextromethorphan, and lithium. Because of the long-lasting effects of the SSRIs, the syndrome may even occur a few weeks after an SSRI has been discontinued.

This disorder is characterized by altered mental status, fever, agitation, tremor, myoclonus, hyperreflexia, ataxia, incoordination, diaphoresis, shivering, and sometimes diarrhea. Treatment is supportive and the serotonin blocker *cyproheptadine* may be of benefit in some cases.

 ## HEAT STROKE

Heat stroke includes a temperature higher than 41°C (105.8°F) and mental status changes. This form of hyperthermia is characterized by a systemic inflammatory response leading to a syndrome of multiorgan dysfunction in which encephalopathy predominates. With high temperatures, enzyme denaturation, protein coagulation, cell dysfunction, lipid liquefaction, and tissue damage occur. Patients with *exertional heat stroke* are young people who exerted themselves in a hot, humid environment. In contrast, patients with *nonexertional heat stroke* are usually elderly or sedentary. The features of the types of heat stroke are noted in Table 53-1.

It is critical that regardless of the type of heat stroke that the patient be treated immediately. Unlike patients with hypothermia in whom slow, gentle rewarming is suggested, victims of severe heatstroke must be aggressively treated with measures designed to rapidly lower the core temperature. The patient's clothing should be removed, and he or she should be rapidly cooled to 39°C (102.2°F). Ice water immersion should be stopped when the patient's core temperature reaches 39°C (102.2°F). An alternative is *evaporative cooling*, which consists of using fans and tepid water continuously applied by spray bottles or sponged onto the skin. (JWM)

Bibliography

Ali SZ, et al. Malignant hyperthermia. *Best Pract Res Clin Anaesthesiol* 2003;17:519–533. *MH is an uncommon, life-threatening, acute pharmacogenetic disorder of the skeletal muscle cell. Mortality may be as high as 70% if the syndrome is not recognized and treated. This chapter provides an overview and an update of MH.*

Ananth J, et al. Neuroleptic malignant syndrome and atypical antipsychotic drugs. *J Clin Psychiatry* 2004;65:464–570.
For NMS associated with atypical antipsychotic drugs, the mortality rate was lower than that with conventional antipsychotic drugs. However, the mortality rate may simply be a reflection of physicians' awareness and ensuing early treatment.
Barrow MW, Clark KA. Heat-related illnesses. *Am Fam Physician* 1998;58:749–756,759.
Heat-related illnesses cause 240 deaths annually. Preventive care should include drinking plenty of fluids before, during and after activities, gradually increasing the time spent working in the heat and avoiding exertion during the hottest part of the day.
Gillman PK. Comment on: serotonin syndrome due to co-administration of linezolid and venlafaxine. *J Antimicrob Chemother* 2004;54:844–845.
Hart GR, et al. Epidemic classical heat stroke: clinical characteristics and course of 28 patients. *Medicine (Baltimore)* 1982;61:189–197.
Patients with classic heat stroke are different in many ways from those with exertional injury; contrasts included differences in demographic factors, prior general health, in-hospital complications, and laboratory abnormalities (lactate, liver enzymes, pH, electrolytes).
Mieno S, et al. Neuroleptic malignant syndrome following cardiac surgery: successful treatment with dantrolene. *Eur J Cardiothorac Surg* 2003;24:458–460.
Dantrolene, which is able to impede effectively the abnormal flow of calcium from the sarcoplasmic reticulum into the muscle cytoplasm, was beneficial in reducing the clinical symptoms of NMS. We hereby present a patient with NMS following cardiac surgery and discuss its subsequent management.
Susman VL. Clinical management of neuroleptic malignant syndrome. *Psychiatr Q* 2001;72:325–336.
Pharmacologic interventions include immediate discontinuation of antipsychotics, judicious use of anticholinergics, and adjunctive benzodiazepines. The utility of specific agents in actively treating NMS is reviewed. Bromocriptine and other dopaminergic drugs and dantrolene sodium alternatively have been considered without merit or efficacious. Guidelines for using these agents are presented. Electroconvulsive therapy, also somewhat controversial, is identified as a second line of treatment. Finally, management of the post-NMS patient is also reviewed.
Thomas CR, et al. Serotonin syndrome and linezolid. *J Am Acad Child Adolesc Psychiatry* 2004;43:790.
Tomaselli G, Modestin J. Repetition of serotonin syndrome after reexposure to SSRI—a case report. *Pharmacopsychiatry* 2004;37:236–238.
Reexposure of patients with a history of serotonin syndrome to another serotoninergic drug should be avoided; if necessary, it must be carried out with the utmost caution.
Wexler RK. Evaluation and treatment of heat-related illnesses. *Am Fam Physician* 2002;65:2307–2314.
Heatstroke is a medical emergency that should be treated immediately with temperature-lowering techniques, such as immersion in an ice bath or evaporative cooling. Fluid resuscitation is important but should be closely monitored, and renal function may need to be protected with mannitol and diuretics. It is important to be vigilant for heat illnesses because they occur insidiously but progress rapidly.
Yeo TP. Heat stroke: a comprehensive review. *AACN Clin Issues* 2004;15:280–293.
The prognosis is poorest when treatment is delayed longer than 2 hours.

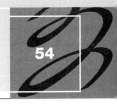

 ranulocytopenia is associated with conditions as diverse as hematologic malignancy and its treatment, adverse reactions from medications, selected infections, and hereditary conditions. Although fever can be associated with any of these, it is most feared when complicating leukemia and other hematologic malignancies. Fever in a granulocytopenic patient can be a medical emergency. It is defined as a single temperature of more than 38.3°C (101.3°F), or a sustained temperature higher than 38°C for longer than 1 hour. Elderly patients or those taking corticosteroids may not develop a fever. The definition of granulocytopenia may vary but usually is an absolute neutrophil count (ANC) of less than 500 to 1,000 cells/mL^3. Risk of infection increases substantially when ANC is less than 100 cells/mL^3 and is associated with leukemia or its chemotherapy, rather than chronic conditions such a aplastic anemia. Although at least 40% of patients with fever and neutropenia demonstrate no source of infection, they may clinically improve with antibiotics. The likelihood of response to initial antibiotics reaches 95% for those with neutropenia longer than 7 days but is only 32% in those with more than 2 weeks of fever and neutropenia. Risk of infection varies directly with both duration of granulocytopenia and rate of decline and inversely with the absolute granulocyte count. With regard to acute leukemia, infections are noted more commonly during relapse.

DIAGNOSIS

Diagnosis of infection in the granulocytopenic host is made difficult by subtleties of signs and symptoms. Frank pus is rarely encountered because polymorphonuclear leukocytes are necessary for its production. Host responses to infection may be blunted, but pain and fever are usually preserved. Thus, the afebrile individual is unlikely to be infected. Patients with pharyngitis may have pain and erythema without exudate. Skin and anorectal infections demonstrate erythema and local pain but usually lack prominent local heat, swelling, exudate, fluctuation, or regional adenopathy. Urinary tract infections often occur in the absence of irritative voiding symptoms (dysuria, frequency, urgency) and pyuria. Classic hallmarks of pneumonia (cough, sputum production, rales, and clinical consolidation) are frequently not observed. As a general rule, fever attributable to leukemia, drugs, and other noninfectious causes is usually unassociated with rigors or hypotension. Alternatively, shaking chills or a "toxic" appearance indicate probable infection, possibly bacteremia.

EVALUATION

Evaluation begins with a comprehensive history and physical examination. The history can provide evidence of localized discomfort. Sore throat associated with fever and pharyngeal ulceration caused by antineoplastic drugs may be early signs of bacteremia resulting from *Pseudomonas aeruginosa* or infection with *Herpes simplex*. Dysphagia suggests esophagitis caused by *Candida* spp., *Herpes simplex*, or other potential pathogens. Painful defecation can alert the physician to perirectal cellulitis or phlegmon, often involving *P. aeruginosa* and anaerobes. Fever, vomiting, abdominal pain, and abdominal tenderness may be symptoms of typhlitis (inflammation of the cecum) or pseudomembranous colitis from either underlying leukemia or antibiotics.

319

Physical examination should be meticulous and repeated at least on a daily basis. Special attention should be directed toward painful or erythematous skin and anorectal lesions, pharyngeal erythema, periodontal inflammation, sinus tenderness, and rales. Skin lesions of ecthyma gangrenosum (classically, necrotic centers with surrounding areolae but with many variants), indicate probable gram-negative bacteria, often *P. aeruginosa*. Such lesions provide sources for biopsy and culture, often yielding rapid bacteriologic information. Periodontal infection is manifested by local tenderness and fever accompanied by minimal signs and symptoms of inflammation. Careful attention should be paid to indwelling lines. Redness and swelling may be the only indications of infection. However, up to 50% of line-related bacteremias present without localized clinical evidence of infection.

Urine cultures, several sets of blood cultures, and chest radiographs are indicated in all patients presenting with fever and neutropenia. With pneumonia, radiographic evidence is usually present, although findings may be subtle. Presence of lung necrosis generally indicates pneumonia associated with gram-negative enteric bacilli, *Staphylococcus aureus*, *Aspergillus*, or *Mucor*. The onset of cough or pleurisy in the absence of chest radiographic findings may be indicative of invasive aspergillosis and should trigger prompt computed tomographic (CT) scanning of the lungs. Other cultures and radiographs should be obtained as clinically indicated. Routine surveillance cultures of nares, stool, and other sites are not generally recommended.

Bacteriology of infections in the granulocytopenic patient includes a wide variety of organisms and will vary to a large extent with previous use of antimicrobials and recent hospitalizations. Anaerobes are uncommonly implicated, except in anorectal infections, where they predominate and require specific therapy. Gram-negative pathogens commonly demonstrated include *Escherichia coli*, *Klebsiella* spp., *Enterobacter*, and *P. aeruginosa*. The frequent use of indwelling venous access devices has been associated with a resurgence of gram-positive infections caused by *S. aureus* (including methicillin-resistant *S. aureus*), *S. epidermidis*, streptococci, and occasionally others. Fungal infections are more commonly noted in patients maintained on prolonged broad-spectrum antimicrobials and with prolonged neutropenia. Although *Aspergillus* and *Candida* spp. have been classically implicated, recent studies demonstrate possibility for infection with diverse organisms that include *Trichosporon beigelii*, *Fusarium* species, *Geotrichum candidum*, and *Pseudallescheria boydii*. Infection with these more unusual species is often associated with sinusitis, deep organ involvement, or fungemia. Risk factors for adverse outcome include prolonged neutropenia and presence of organ involvement.

 SITE OF CARE

Selected neutropenic patients with fever may be safely managed as outpatients. This concept has been promulgated in part because of the availability of oral antipseudomonal antibiotics and the availability of an infrastructure that allows for intravenous therapy outside of the hospital. There is uniform agreement that high-risk neutropenic patients need to be treated using standard, hospital-based, parenteral, broad-spectrum antibiotics for the entire febrile episode. Many patients with fever and neutropenia do not fall in this category, but it is difficult to separate them. One classification divides patients into three high risks groups: (1) high-risk: includes severe (ANC <100 cells/mL^3) and prolonged (i.e., 14 days) neutropenia, hematologic malignancy, allogenic bone marrow/stem cell transplantation, significant medical comorbidity or poor performance status, presentation with shock, complex infection (pneumonia, meningitis); (2) intermediate risk: includes solid tumors, intensive chemotherapy, autologous hematopoietic stem cell transplantation, moderate duration of neutropenia, (i.e., 7–14 days), minimal medical comorbidities, and clinical/hemodynamic stability; and (3) low-risk: solid tumors, conventional chemotherapy, no comorbidity, short duration of neutropenia (i.e., <7 days), clinical and hemodynamic stability. Highest risk patients should be treated in-hospital with broad-spectrum parenteral therapy for the duration of febrile episode. Those with intermediate risks can be treated in the hospital with parenteral therapy followed by early discharge on a parenteral or oral regimen. Those in the low-risk category can be treated with outpatient therapy. Tables 54-1 and 54-2 summarize

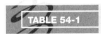

Risk group	Features	Morbidity/mortality
I	Developed in-hospital	Mortality = 13%
II	Outpatients with hypotension, altered sensoria, respiratory failure, bleeding, etc.	Serious complications in 40%; mortality: 12%
III	Outpatients without comorbidity but with uncontrolled cancer	Serious complication in 25%; mortality: 18%
IV	Stable outpatients	Serious complications in 3%; mortality: 0%

TABLE 54-1   Risk Stratification for Febrile, Neutropenic Patients

strategies for risk stratification and management of patients with fever and neutropenia. From 40 to 60% of patients fall into the category of those who can be treated outside of the hospital. Patients at low risk for adverse outcome generally do not suffer from uncontrolled cancer or concurrent associated problems requiring hospitalization. In the absence of these features, complications were noted in only 2% of patients and mortality approached 0%. Using similar parameters, patients may be safely discharged to home to complete therapy with either intravenous or oral antibiotics. All patients receiving outpatient therapy should live within a reasonable distance from the medical center where treatment is being administered. Daily follow-up by telephone is indicated, and the patients must have access to a healthcare provider.

 ANTIBIOTIC THERAPY

Outpatient treatment of the febrile neutropenic may be with either oral or parenteral antibiotics. The specific initial therapy will depend on local microflora and susceptibility patterns, allergy, organ dysfunction, and adjunctive medications. Choices generally include fluoroquinolones because of ease of oral administration and broad spectrum of coverage, including *P. aeruginosa*. They have been studied either as single agents or in conjunction with clindamycin or amoxicillin/clavulanate.

For patients to be treated in-hospital, initial therapy generally consists of broad-spectrum bactericidal agents. Controversy continues regarding the need for combination therapy versus monotherapy. Numerous studies now demonstrate efficacy of monotherapy (e.g., imipenem/cilastatin, piperacillin/tazobactam, meropenem, ceftazidime, cefepime). However, many centers continue to use combinations that include double β-lactams (e.g., ceftazidime plus piperacillin) or β-lactams plus aminoglycosides (e.g., piperacillin or ceftazidime plus gentamicin, tobramycin, or amikacin). If aminoglycosides are used, a loading dose of more than 2 mg/kg should be used to optimize initial levels. Many centers use single daily doses of 5 to 7 mg/kg of gentamicin or tobramycin as a means of maximizing peak levels while minimizing toxicity. When *P. aeruginosa* is strongly considered (based

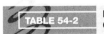

TABLE 54-2   Patients With Fever and Neutropenia: Candidates for Outpatient Therapy

Patients lack:

Hypotension (blood pressure <90 systolic)

Tachypnea (respiratory rate >30/minute)

Renal insufficiency (serum creatinine >2.5, or creatinine clearance <50 mL/minute)

Hyponatremia (serum sodium <128 mg/dL)

Altered liver function tests (serum transaminases more than four times normal)

Uncontrolled hypercalcemia

Altered sensorium

on epidemiology, ecthyma gangrenosum, etc.), two effective antipseudomonal agents are indicated. At Baystate Medical Center, no single agent is active against more than 80% of strains of *P. aeruginosa*.

Need for vancomycin in the initial regimen remains controversial. A recent investigation continues to demonstrate that its routine addition in patients with fever and neutropenia does not improve outcome. However, this issue continues to undergo reassessment as the role of serious gram-positive infection increases. Reasons for this include use of long-standing intravenous devices, appreciation of methicillin-resistant staphylococci (MRSA) as a community-acquired pathogen and increased prevalence of viridans streptococci in selected clinical circumstances. Vancomycin should be used in the initial antibiotic regimen if: (1) suspected catheter-related infection, (2) colonization with penicillin- or cephalosporin-resistant *S. pneumoniae* or MRSA, (3) positive results of blood cultures for gram-positive bacteria prior to final identification, (4) hypotension or evidence of hemodynamic instability, or (5) prior prophylaxis with fluoroquinolones or trimethoprim/ sulfamethoxazole. Additionally, initial use of a regimen including vancomycin may be indicated at hospitals that have noted fulminant gram-positive infections or if regimens that result in intense mucosal ulceration are used. Over the next several years, it is likely that studies will demonstrate enhanced efficacy of other agents that could include daptomycin or linezolid.

Generally intravenous catheters may be left in place during antibiotic treatment of fever and neutropenia. However, catheter removal is generally indicated if infection is recurrent or response to antibiotics is poor after 2 to 3 days of treatment and an alternative source of infection has not been identified. Catheters should be removed in the presence of tunnel infection, septic emboli, hypotension, or plugging. Proven line-related bacteremia generally requires removal of the catheter unless caused by coagulase-negative staphylococci. Some investigators have proposed catheter salvage by use of an antibiotic-containing heparin lock solution to supplement systemic therapy, but such practices remain controversial.

After initial treatment, 2–3 days are generally needed to assess response to treatment and cause of fever. Further management strategies are guided by these parameters. If originally used, vancomycin should be discontinued if cultures fail to substantiate need. If clinical improvement is noted and cultures define a pathogen, therapy should be optimized, but broad-spectrum therapy should be continued. If the patient's neutrophil count is higher than 500/mm^3 for two consecutive days, if there is no definite site of infection, and if cultures do not demonstrate positive results, antibiotics may be discontinued when the patient is afebrile for more than 48 hours. If the patient improves in the absence of a defined organism, therapy should be maintained for at least 1 week. Switch to oral antibiotics (e.g., fluoroquinolone, cefixime) can be undertaken if patients are stable and compliant and can be monitored as outpatients.

Failure to improve after 3 to 5 days requires meticulous reassessment of the patient and a possible change in antimicrobials. Drug fever may be considered. Ultrasonography and CT scanning of the abdomen with percutaneous sampling of collections is expeditious and reasonably well tolerated. If fever persists longer than 5 days and reassessment does not yield a cause, antifungal therapy is generally added. Up to 50% of patients will respond to this strategy, although the source of infection may not be identified. The antifungal chosen should have activity against *Candida* spp. and *Aspergillus* spp. Although amphotericin B has been the antifungal historically used, recent investigations have demonstrated roles for liposomal amphotericin B preparations, itraconazole, voriconazole, and caspofungin. These are as effective and less toxic than amphotericin B. Voriconazole and itraconazole are available intravenously and orally, so many persons can be transitioned to the oral formulation. Several forms of liposomal amphotericin B have been approved for use in the United States. All have the advantage of allowing higher dosing with enhanced safety— typically up to 5 mg/kg versus 1 mg/kg with amphotericin B. Their major role appears to be in the management of mold infections (aspergillus/mucor) and in patients who have developed significant intolerance to amphotericin B desoxycholate. Fluconazole is rarely used empirically because of its poor activity against *Aspergillus* spp. and more resistant strains of *Candida*. Improved testing for fungi is becoming available. This is badly needed as blood cultures are positive in fewer than 40% of patients with documented fungal infections.

If persons remain febrile despite the addition of an antifungal, ongoing clinical assessment is mandatory. Generally, a broad-spectrum regimen including an antifungal is continued until reversal of neutropenia. The clinician should strive toward keeping the patient stable until neutropenia corrects. Antiviral therapy with acyclovir or ganciclovir is indicated for proved or suspected infections caused by susceptible viruses, but is generally not recommended empirically.

Colony-stimulating factors (granulocyte colony-stimulating factor [GCSF] and granulocyte-macrophage colony-stimulating factor [GM-CSF]) have been used to shorten the duration of neutropenia after chemotherapy for solid tumors and hematologic malignancies. Several studies now demonstrate decreased antimicrobial needs, length of hospitalization, and shortened neutropenic periods when colony-stimulating factors are used. However, mortality related to infection has not been notably decreased. Additionally, most patients respond favorably without it, and it is expensive. Colony-stimulating factors should be considered in selected patients with severe infection, poor likelihood of rapid marrow recovery, and poor response to appropriate antimicrobials.

Normally fever resolves with the correction of neutropenia. Duration of antibiotic therapy is dependent on the process being treated. If used "empirically," and if no focus of infection was documented, antibiotics are generally discontinued when neutropenia has resolved. Focal hepatic candidiasis represents an unusual syndrome that may present with fever in the face of resolving neutropenia and often is a local manifestation of systemic disease. Abdominal pain, nausea, and diarrhea occasionally may be noted. Striking elevations of the serum alkaline phosphatase have been noted. Hepatic defects can be detected on CT or ultrasound and the diagnosis confirmed by aspiration of a lesion. Fluconazole is generally appropriate in doses of up to 400 mg daily for a median of 30 weeks. (RBB)

Bibliography

Boogaerts M, et al. Intravenous and oral itraconazole versus intravenous amphotericin B deoxycholate as empirical antifungal therapy for persistent fever in neutropenic patients with cancer who are receiving broad-spectrum antibacterial therapy. *Ann Intern Med* 2001;135:412–422.
This is another study demonstrating that satisfactory alternatives to amphotericin deoxycholate exist. These now include itraconazole, caspofungin, liposomal amphotericin B, and voriconazole. All are likely to be less toxic, equally effective, and, in the cases of voriconazole and itraconazole, allow oral administration. Best among these remains uncertain, but many institutions are shying away from amphotericin B in favor of these other products.

Cometta A, et al. Vancomycin versus placebo for treating persistent fever in patients with neutropenic cancer receiving piperacillin-tazobactam monotherapy. *Clin Infect Dis* 2003;37:382–389.
This recent investigation continues to demonstrate that routine addition of vancomycin for ongoing fever in neutropenic patients does not result in enhanced outcomes. Measures studied included time to defervescence and proven gram-positive bacteremias. However, there are clearly instances when use of vancomycin empirically is indicated, and these are summarized in the text.

Freifield A, et al. A double-blind comparison of empirical oral and intravenous antibiotic therapy for low-risk febrile patients with neutropenia during cancer chemotherapy. *N Engl J Med* 1999;341:305–311.
This prospective study in low-risk patients with fever and neutropenia demonstrated that empirical therapy with oral ciprofloxacin and amoxicillin clavulanate was safe and effective. Careful patient selection is mandatory.

Hughes WT, et al. 2002 Guidelines for the use of antimicrobial agents in neutropenic patients with cancer. *Clin Infect Dis* 2002;34:730–751.
This represents the latest effort to provide practical guidelines based on best information for the management of fever and neutropenia. A number of algorithms are given to guide the clinician through several steps of this process that include need for vancomycin, persistence of fever despite antimicrobials, and duration of treatment. An exhaustive list of excellent references is also provided.

Lin MT, Lu HC, Chen WL. Improving efficacy of antifungal therapy by polymerase chain reaction-based strategy among febrile patients with neutropenia and cancer. *Clin Infect Dis* 2001;33:1621–1627.

This is one of several articles recently published that use novel modalities for documentation of fungal infection to enhance use of antifungal agents. As more sensitive and specific tests become available that can be used "real time," need for empiric antifungal treatment should decrease.

Mermel LA, et al. Guidelines for the management of intravascular catheter-related infections. *Clin Infect Dis* 2001;32:1249–1272.

Although not strictly speaking a manuscript dealing with fever and neutropenia, use of intravascular catheters is sufficiently common in this population that an understanding of risks and management is appropriate. It should be required reading for all persons involved with catheter care and the patients requiring them.

Ramphal R, et al. Clinical experience with single agent and combination regimens in the management of infection in the febrile neutropenic patient. *Am J Med* 1996;100:83S–89S.

Cefepime is a "fourth generation" cephalosporin similar to ceftazidime but with enhanced stability against selected enteric bacilli and better gram-positive activity. Febrile neutropenic patients were randomized to receive either cefepime as monotherapy or combination antibiotic therapy. Bacterial infections were documented in 40% of patients in both groups. Outcomes as measured by fever resolution, need for alternative therapies, and survival were similar in both groups. This is another study demonstrating that for most febrile neutropenic patients monotherapy is sufficient. There are now several appropriate agents from which to choose. I would still use combination therapy for situations at high risk of infection with P. aeruginosa (i.e., ecthyma gangrenosum lesions, known positive blood cultures), but in most other instances monotherapy will suffice.

Tunkel AR, Sepkowitz KA. Infections caused by viridans streptococci in patients with neutropenia. *Clin Infect Dis* 2002;34:1524–1529.

The authors demonstrate the enhanced risk of serious infections caused by viridans streptococci. Risk factors include severe mucositis and use of antibiotic prophylaxis with either fluoroquinolones or trimethoprim-sulfamethoxazole. Other studies also demonstrate risks that include use of proton pump inhibitors and gut decontamination with oral antimicrobials. Unlike endocarditis associated with these organisms, presentation in the febrile neutropenic host may be abrupt, aggressive, and lethal. Unfortunately susceptibility to agents such as penicillin and ceftriaxone can no longer be assumed. In circumstances where these organisms are suspected, empiric treatment with vancomycin is indicated.

Walsh TJ, et al. Liposomal amphotericin B for empirical therapy in patients with persistent fever and neutropenia. *N Engl J Med* 1999;340:764–771.

This prospective study demonstrated that liposomal amphotericin B was as effective as conventional amphotericin B for empirical antifungal therapy in patients with fever and neutropenia, and was associated with fewer breakthrough fungal infections, less-infusion–related toxicity, and less nephrotoxicity However, liposomal products may still cause severe initial toxicities and should be used with caution during initial doses.

Walsh TJ, et al. Voriconazole compared with liposomal amphotericin B for empirical therapy in patients with neutropenia and persistent fever. *N Engl J Med* 2002;346:225–234.

This study showed that voriconazole is a suitable alternative to amphotericin B preparations for empirical antifungal therapy in patients with neutropenia and persistent fever. It has advantages that include availability of an oral preparation and decreased toxicities. When used in ambulatory patients, advice regarding potential visual toxicities should be given.

Walsh TJ, et al. Caspofungin versus liposomal amphotericin B for empirical antifungal therapy in patients with persistent fever and neutropenia. *N Engl J Med* 2004;351: 1391–1402.

This prospective trial shows that in patients with persistent fever and neutropenia, empirical therapy with caspofungin is as effective as, and generally better tolerated than, liposomal amphotericin B. Caspofungin, however, lacks activity against Cryptococcus spp. and cannot be recommended in situations in which this pathogen is considered.

FEVER OF UNKNOWN ORIGIN

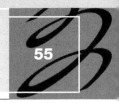

In 1961, Petersdorf and Beeson defined the clinical syndrome of fever of unknown origin (FUO) as continuous fever of at least 3 weeks' duration, with temperatures of 101°F or more, that remains unexplained despite 1 week of complete investigation. Using this definition, the authors studied 100 patients at a university teaching hospital. This study, which divided the causes of FUO into infections, malignancy, and rheumatic diseases and described drug fevers, factitious fevers, and cranial arteritis as additional diagnoses, demonstrated that patients may often have atypical manifestations of common diseases. The authors recommended no one battery of tests and discouraged therapeutic trials unless treatment was directed at a particular disease. Biopsy specimens were frequently required for specific diagnosis.

Petersdorf and colleagues looked again at FUO between the years 1970 and 1980. This second study, of 105 patients was somewhat different from the initial one of 20 years earlier:

1. Neoplastic disease became the most common cause of FUO. Most neoplastic cases were secondary to Hodgkin's or non-Hodgkin's lymphoma. In these cases, peripheral lymphadenopathy was absent, and disease was confined to retroperitoneal nodes or the liver. Patients were usually elderly. Not all recent studies support the high incidence of malignancy. Knockaert et al., in a study from Belgium, found tumor to be a less important cause of FUO in a 1980–1989 prospective series.
2. Bacterial endocarditis, which caused 5 of 100 cases of FUO in the first study, did not occur in any patient during the 1970–1980 study. Better culture methods, echocardiography, and appreciation of the causes of culture-negative endocarditis may explain this change. Tuberculosis also became less common. Biliary tract infection continued to be an important cause of FUO, even in an era of better imaging techniques.
3. Rheumatic fever was a cause of FUO in only one patient in the second study, compared with six patients in the first. However, rheumatic fever has reemerged in some parts of the United States in the past several years; young clinicians who are unfamiliar with the disease might overlook it as a cause of fever.
4. Systemic lupus erythematosus is no longer a cause of FUO owing to better serologic methods.
5. Cytomegalovirus caused FUO in four patients in the second study and in none in the first. Patients presented with a mononucleosis-like syndrome, had self-limited disease, and had often undergone transfusion or coronary artery bypass surgery.

Continued technologic improvements make some types of FUO less common. Progress in transesophageal echocardiography has made endocarditis increasingly less common as a cause of FUO. Improved methods of computed tomography (CT) and magnetic resonance imaging (MRI) make it possible for most intra-abdominal abscesses to be diagnosed in less than 3 weeks. Better serologic tests have made most collagen vascular diseases less likely to become FUOs.

The distribution of causes of FUO continues to change with the availability of newer diagnostic methods. FUO as defined by the initial criteria of Petersdorf is a disease that is becoming less common. The distribution of diagnoses can be seen in Table 55-1.

There are relatively few important new causes of FUO. Cunha describes histiocytic necrotizing adenitis (Kikuchi's disease) and hypergammagobulinemia IgD syndrome, but these diseases are rare.

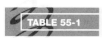

| TABLE 55-1 | Most Common Diagnoses in Fever of Unknown Origin |

1. Infectious diseases—estimated to cause 20 to 40% of FUO. Tuberculosis will still be the most important etiologic agent. Some cases of malaria continue to be reported as FUO. Unusual and atypical infections remain common in HIV-positive patients. Endocarditis will be much less common with transesophageal echocardiography, better serology for *Bartonella, Chlamydia,* and *Coxiella burnetii,* and molecular bacterial methods. Intra-abdominal abscess less common cause of FUO, with ease and relative inexpensiveness of abdominal ultrasound. Viral causes still common, such as cytomegalovirus and Epstein-Barr, although paired serology will often be diagnostic.
2. Neoplasms—estimated to cause 5 to 31% of FUO. Lymphoma is likely to remain an important cause. More widespread use of CT scans, MRI, and ultrasound make diagnosis of malignancy more rapid and less likely to result in FUO.
3. Collagen vascular disease—estimated to cause 10 to 30% of FUO, particularly the diagnosis of temporal arteritis and polymyalgia rheumatica in older patients. Systemic lupus erythematosus, rheumatoid arthritis are more easily diagnosed by serology.
4. Miscellaneous—estimated to be 15 to 25%. This group is likely increasing as percentage of total FUO. Includes diseases for which history is crucial, such as factitious fever and drug fever. Recurrent pulmonary emboli, particularly in community hospitals, may be an important diagnosis.

The workup of a patient with FUO is now usually performed on an outpatient basis. Although procedures such as bone marrow biopsy, transesophageal echocardiography, liver biopsy, and CT or MRI are now easily performed in an outpatient setting, the overall evaluation must be organized in a logical order and completed in a timely manner. Factors such as the overall toxicity of the patient, vital signs during febrile episodes, and rate of weight loss may help determine whether the workup requires a period of hospitalization. In general, basic aspects of the evaluation, such as history and physical examination, complete blood count (CBC), erythrocyte sedimentation rate, blood cultures, liver function tests, and urinalysis, should be completed before hospitalization. Although cost effectiveness remains important, it is tempting to consider the usually assessable CT of the thorax and abdominal ultrasound in an ill-appearing patient with fever and no definite etiology after careful history and physical exam.

The rising incidence of tuberculosis in the United States will likely be reflected in more cases of this disease presenting as FUO. The enhancing or boosting phenomenon in serial tuberculin testing will help exclude false-negative tests. Older patients in particular may have a positive purified protein derivative (PPD) test result when given a second test 1 week after a negative result on the first test. When tuberculosis presents as an FUO, it will usually be associated with miliary disease. Disseminated pulmonary lesions may be so small that they are not appreciated on chest radiographs. This is particularly likely to occur in older individuals.

Extrapulmonary tuberculosis may also present as FUO, although better imaging techniques should help in the diagnosis. Sterile pyuria in a patient with an FUO should suggest renal tuberculosis. In some cases, the urinary sediment may be unremarkable but the urine culture is positive. Tuberculosis of mesenteric lymph nodes may present without abdominal pain but can be diagnosed by abdominal CT scan. Tuberculosis of the endometrium and fallopian tubes usually causes fever and menstrual irregularities. Tuberculous pericarditis should be suggested by changing cardiac silhouette on chest radiographs, with confirmation of pericardial effusion on echocardiogram.

The literature on the FUO syndrome has recognized that the problem varies with the patient population studied. Durack and Street have redefined FUO to include (1) classic FUO, (2) nosocomial FUO, (3) neutropenic FUO, and (4) HIV-associated FUO. FUO that develops in a hospitalized patient, although not well studied, requires a different approach than does classic FUO. The history and physical examination, particularly in the ICU

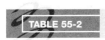

| TABLE 55-2 | Causes of Fever of Unknown Origin in the Elderly |

Giant cell arteritis	Tuberculosis
Intra-abdominal abscess	Pulmonary emboli
Lymphoma	Drug fever

setting, may be less reliable, making clinical diagnosis more difficult. Diseases causing FUO may include pulmonary embolism, transfusion-related hepatitis or cytomegalovirus infection, drug fever, IV line infection, intubation-related sinusitis, or *Clostridium difficile* colitis. FUO in neutropenic patients requires a modification in definition. These fevers of unknown cause occur abruptly and tend not to be prolonged, as patients usually respond to treatment or succumb to infection. Unlike the treatment of classic FUO, empiric treatment of neutropenic FUO must be begun quickly. Most cases of FUO in neutropenic patients are bacterial infections without an obvious source. Disseminated candidemia and aspergillosis are also common. Careful, repeated physical examination, including examination of the anorectal area, is important. FUO is extremely common in AIDS patients, although it has not been studied well as an entity. Fever may be caused by HIV infection itself. *Mycobacterium avium-intracellulare* infection, tuberculosis, and cytomegalovirus infection are among the common causes of FUO in AIDS patients, often taking weeks to declare themselves as clinical entities. *Salmonella* infection, fungal infection, and lymphoma are also well described.

Several studies have assessed FUO in the elderly patient population (Table 55-2). Giant-cell arteritis was responsible in 16% of elderly patients with classically defined FUO in one study. This syndrome may include headaches, transient visual loss, and polymyalgia rheumatica symptoms. Respiratory tract symptoms of cough, sore throat, and hoarseness have been described more recently. The temporal artery may be tender, nodular, and pulseless. Often in the FUO patient, these symptoms are not prominent and may be absent altogether. The erythrocyte sedimentation rate is almost always very high in giant-cell arteritis; however, an elevated erythrocyte sedimentation rate is common in many cases of FUO. Temporal biopsy is the diagnostic intervention of choice when the disease is suspected. Results of empiric therapy with steroids may be dramatic and is indicated when vision is threatened. However, a definitive diagnosis is necessary to justify long-term steroid therapy.

Biliary tract and intra-abdominal infection are also common causes of FUO in the older patient. Hepatic abscess, cholecystitis, and empyema of the gallbladder may present with fever alone, particularly in the debilitated patient.

Weinstein has described the clinically benign FUO syndrome. These patients may have persistent fever that is clinically unimportant. Temperature elevation may be minimal or reach 102°F to 104°F. Despite persistent fever, patients generally appear well nourished. Malaise and aching joints are common for patients with low-grade fever. Diurnal variations, ovulation, use of tobacco and chewing gum, and exercise can cause these low-grade fevers. In patients who appear well but have a high-grade fever, drugs, occupational exposures, and metabolic disorders may be causative.

Another subcategory of FUO has been defined by Knockaert. Some patients have recurrent or episodic fevers that may last months or years. Subacute cholangitis, chronic prostatitis, adults Still's disease, and familial Mediterranean fever are common diagnoses in these patients.

Mackowiak has reviewed the characteristics of drug-induced fever, an increasingly common problem. Fifty-one episodes of drug fever and 97 cases from the literature were analyzed. Hectic fever patterns and shaking chills were common. Rashes were seen in only 18% of patients and eosinophilia in 22%. The time between initiation of the drug and development of fever averaged 8 days. Patients tended to tolerate drug fever well, and exaggerated or dangerous reactions did not develop when the patients were rechallenged. Antimicrobials appear to be becoming a more common cause of drug fever in several studies.

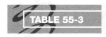

TABLE 55-3	Initial Work-Up in Fever of Unknown Origin

1. Complete blood count and microscopic exam
2. Urinalysis
3. Liver function studies
4. Chest radiograph
5. Blood and urine culture
6. Purified protein derivative
7. Abdominal ultrasound or CT of chest
8. Blood and urine culture

When FUO is studied in a community hospital, the etiologies may be somewhat different than in a referral hospital. Pulmonary emboli and alcoholic hepatitis may cause prolonged fever in this setting, whereas illnesses such as familial Mediterranean fever will be rare. One recent study found AIDS and Lyme disease to be causes of FUO in a community hospital.

Recent literature on the FUO syndrome has focused on the role of imaging in diagnosis. Schmidt et al., using granulocyte scintigraphy with indium-111, studied 32 patients who had at least 3 weeks of unexplained fever. Focal infections were identified in five patients—four with abdominal infection and one with dental abscess. Intestinal activity was observed in one patient found to have Whipple's disease. McNeil et al. prospectively compared CT, ultrasound, and gallium imaging in patients thought to have a focal source of sepsis. The diagnoses of the patient population studied were uncertain after standard diagnostic evaluation. All three modalities had a similar ability to detect sepsis, but sensitivity was increased by the use of any two. Rowland and Del Bene studied the impact of CT in the workup of FUO. They found that CT reduced the incidence of biopsy of normal tissue, with CT of the abdomen often correctly directing the investigation to laparotomy. Kjaer recently studied the use of both positron emission tomography and indium-111 granulocyte scintigraphy in patients with FUO. Scintigraphy was superior in identifying localized inflammatory or neoplastic areas.

Several authors have proposed algorithms and standard workup for FUO. The workup shown in Table 55-3 is usually recommended as an initial assessment. However, history, physical examination, and clinical judgment will continue to dictate a patient-oriented approach to the diagnosis of this syndrome. (SLB)

Bibliography

Amin K, Kauffman CA. Fever of unknown origin. *Postgrad Med* 2003;114:69.
  Reviews causes and approach to FUO, including recommendations for standard workup. Emphasizes increasing importance of drug fever.
Brusch JL, Weinstein L. Fever of unknown origin. *Med Clin North Am* 1988;72:1247.
  Basic review of FUO that includes many clinical insights and contains an interesting section on miscellaneous causes.
Chang JC, Gross HM. Utility of naproxen in the differential diagnosis of fever of undetermined origin in patients with cancer. *Am J Med* 1984;76:597.
  Of 15 patients with neoplastic fever, 14 responded to naproxen. None of five cases of infectious fever resolved.
Chan-Tack KM, Bartlett J. Fever of unknown origin. [eMedicine Web site]. Available at: www.emedicine.com/med/topic785.htm. Accessed July 5, 2004.
  Up-to-date review of causes of FUO and list of routine and specialized diagnostic tests.
Cunha BA. Fever of unknown origin. *Infect Dis Clin North Am* 1996;10:111.
  Updates the causes of FUO and describes the ambulatory workup appropriate for most patients. Categorizes diseases by laboratory abnormality, history, and physical examination clues.
Dinarello CA, Wolff SM. Molecular basis of fever in humans. *Am J Med* 1982;72:799.
  Insights into the pathogenesis of fever are useful in the understanding of FUO.

Drenth JPH, et al. Hyperimmunoglobulinemia D and periodic fever syndrome. *Medicine* 1994;73:133.
This syndrome presents with prolonged fevers, arthritis of large joints, and rash. Serum levels of IgD are greater than 100 U/mL.

Ghose MK, Shensa S, Lerner PI. Arteritis of the aged (giant-cell arteritis) and fever of unexplained origin. *Am J Med* 1976;60:429.
Giant-cell arteritis may present with prolonged fever but without headache, visual disturbance, or arthralgias.

Gleckman R, Crowley M, Esposito A. Fever of unknown origin: a view from the community hospital. *Am J Med Sci* 1977;274:21.
In a community hospital, pulmonary emboli and alcoholic hepatitis were common causes of prolonged fever.

Kauffman CA, Jones PG. Diagnosing fever of unknown origin in older patients. *Geriatrics* 1984;39:46.
Excellent review of FUO in elderly patients. Giant-cell arteritis, biliary tract infection, and drug fever are particularly important in this group.

Kjaer A, et al. Fever of unknown origin: prospective comparison of diagnostic value of 18F-FDG PET and 111 In-granulocyte scintigraphy. *Eur J Nucl Med Imaging* 2004;31: 622.
Scintigraphy had better positive and negative predictive value in the diagnosis of FUO as compared to positron emission tomography.

Knockaert DC, Vaneste LJ, Bobbaers HJ. Recurrent or episodic fever of unknown origin. Review of 45 cases and review of the literature. *Medicine (Baltimore)* 1993;72:184.
Long-standing recurrent fevers have a smaller differential diagnosis. Bacterial infections include chronic biliary tract or prostatic infection. Still's disease, familial Mediterranean fever, Crohn's disease, and lymphoma are examples of this type of FUO.

Larson EB, Featherstone HJ, Petersdorf RG. Fever of undetermined origin: diagnosis and follow-up of 105 cases, 1970–1980. *Medicine (Baltimore)* 1982;61:269.
Follow-up study by Petersdorf group (see also Petersdorf RG, Beeson PM, 1961). Neoplastic disease was the most common cause of FUO.

Mackowiak PA. Southwestern Internal Medicine Conference. Drug fever: mechanisms, maxims and misconceptions. *Am J Med Sci* 1987;294:275.
Excellent detailed review of the clinical picture of drug fevers. Some findings go against standard teachings on drug fever.

Mourad O, Palda V, Desky AS. A comprehensive-evidence based approach to fever of unknown origin. *Arch Intern Med* 2003;163:545.
Systematic review to develop evidence-based recommendations for the workup of FUO. Concludes that diagnosis is assisted by CT scan of abdomen, nuclear scanning, and liver biopsy. Empiric bone marrow culture not supported by literature review. Most patients with FUO (50–100%) recover spontaneously.

Murray HW, et al. Urinary temperature: a clue to early diagnosis of factitious fever. *N Engl J Med* 1977;296:23.
Urinary temperature can be used to diagnose factitious fever.

Musher DM. Fever of unknown origin: diagnostic principles. *Hosp Pract* 1982;17:89.
Excellent description of the traditional case-by-case approach to the diagnosis of FUO.

Musher DM, et al. Fever patterns: their lack of clinical significance. *Arch Intern Med* 1979;139:1225.
Fever patterns were not helpful in assessing the etiology of fever on an infectious disease consultation service.

Petersdorf RG. Fever of unknown origin. *Arch Intern Med* 1992;152:21.
Petersdorf's most recent reflections on FUO (see also Petersdorf RG, Beeson PM, 1961; Larson EB, Featherstone HJ, Petersdorf RG, 1982.) Patients with a diagnosis of FUO should rarely die.

Petersdorf RG, Beeson PM. Fever of unexplained origin: report of 100 cases. *Medicine (Baltimore)* 1961;40:1.
Initial, classic paper that defined FUO, its etiologies, and diagnostic approach.

Pizzo PA, Lovejoy FH, Smith DH. Prolonged fever in children: review of 100 cases. *Pediatrics* 1975;5:468.

Children are more likely to have viral and collagen inflammatory causes of FUO than adults.

Quinn MJ, et al. Computed tomography of the abdomen in evaluation of patients with fever of unknown origin. *Radiology* 1980;136:407.
Results of 29% of 78 CT scans were positive in FUO patients.

Rowland MD, Del Bene VE. Use of body computed tomography to evaluate fever of unknown origin. *J Infect Dis* 1987;156:408.
Documents role of CT in the workup of FUO.

Vanderschueren S, et al. Lack of value of the naproxen test in the differential diagnosis of prolonged febrile illness. *Am J Med* 2003;115:572.
Contradicts earlier studies that suggested that the naproxen test could distinguish fever caused by malignancy from fever caused by infection.

Young EJ, Fainstain V, Musher DM. Drug-induced fever: cases seen in the evaluation of unexplained fever in a general hospital population. *Rev Infect Dis* 1982;4:69.
Antimicrobial agents were responsible for most cases of drug fever.

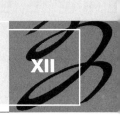

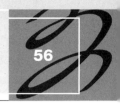

A furuncle is a deep inflammatory nodule that occurs around a hair follicle. Furuncles arise around these follicles because of friction, perspiration, and occlusion of the follicle. Such furuncles can occur in otherwise healthy patients. However, factors such as obesity, diabetes mellitus, immunologic deficiencies, neutrophil disorders, glucocorticoids, can all predispose to furuncles and result in recurrent furunculosis.

The furuncle, which might start as a tender nodule, eventually develops to become a fluctuant pustule. The lesion is either drained or rupture occurs, resulting in the discharge of pus and necrotic material. Drainage or rupture decreases the pain and associated tenderness.

Although many organisms can cause skin infections, *Staphylococcus aureus* is the most likely etiologic agent by far to cause these lesions. Folliculitis, a more superficial skin infection, can lead to furunculosis. Folliculitis may be caused by *Pseudomonas aeruginosa*, other kinds of gram-negative rods, dermatophytes, and viruses. Table 56-1 lists organisms than can cause folliculitis.

Furunculosis can result in extensive cellulitis or bacteremia because of the deep nature of the skin infection. When occurring on the face, infection of the emissary veins to the cavernous sinus can produce life-threatening infection of the central nervous system.

Recurrent furunculosis may occur frequently over many years and therefore requires careful evaluation and management. The history is important in evaluating potential causes of recurrence. The following factors predispose to recurrence:

1. Industrial exposure to chemicals or oils
2. Poor hygiene
3. Ingrown hairs
4. Hyperhidrosis
5. Tight belts or clothing
6. Pyogenic infections in children or families
7. Contact sports
8. Nasal carriage of *Staphylococcus aureus*
9. Defects in neutrophil function
10. Immune globulin deficiency
11. Treatment with glucocorticoids or cytotoxic agents

Hyperimmunoglobulin E syndrome is a primary immunodeficiency disease that presents with high titers of IgE, eczema, and chronic staphylococcal infection, including furuncles. There is an associated impairment of neutrophil chemotaxis and impaired lymphocyte proliferation. IgG subclass deficiency may also predispose to furuncles.

MANAGEMENT OF RECURRENT FURUNCULOSIS

One important measure is to reduce the number of colonizing staphylococci on the skin. Good skin care, including washing frequently with soap and water or with a 4% chlorhexidine solution, is recommended. Strong irritants such as deodorants and perfumes or colognes should be avoided. Sheets and towels may harbor staphylococci that may be reintroduced to the skin. These items may need to be washed daily to prevent spread and recurrence.

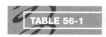

TABLE 56-1	Causes of Folliculitis
Staphylococcus aureus	From skin colonization
P. aeruginosa	From hot tubs
Gram-negative folliculitis	From acne treatment, after antibiotics
Fungal folliculitis	Tinea capitis and tinea barbae
Viral folliculitis	Herpes simplex and molluscum contagiosum
Irritant folliculitis	From mineral oil, tar products

If the work environment is suspected as the cause of the cycle of infection, breaking the routine by reassignment if possible or vacation may be the solution for some patients. Vacation to a cool and dry climate might be particularly effective.

Measures to eliminate colonization or carriage of staphylococci also are part of preventing recurrence. Intranasal application of 2% mupirocin ointment can eliminate carriage in most patients for several months. A 5-day course, every month, for a year or more may be necessary to prevent recurrent furunculosis in some patients. Oral rifampin with or without a penicillinase-resistant penicillin (such as oxacillin) also has been used. The two antibiotics together may be synergistic for methicillin-sensitive or methicillin-resistant staphylococci.

Treating the acute infection aggressively may help to prevent recurrences. A furuncle with surrounding cellulitis should always be treated with systemic antibiotics. Again, penicillinase-resistant penicillins usually have been considered the antibiotic of choice. However, in recent years more methicillin-resistant community-acquired infections have occurred so that vancomycin will be used more frequently as initial therapy. When lesions are painful and fluctuant, drainage is required. Antibiotic therapy is continued until inflammation is resolved.

Several studies have suggested that the use of vitamin C can prevent recurrent furuncles. The vitamin C effect has been shown to be on neutrophil chemotaxis, phagocytosis, and superoxide generation. Vitamin C was successful in the treatment of a group of 23 patients with recurrent furunculosis and negative nasal cultures. Twelve of the patients had initial abnormal neutrophil function that improved with vitamin C. In one study, a subgroup of patients with recurrent furunculosis had low iron levels and their condition improved with iron therapy. (SLB)

Bibliography

Demircay Z, et al. Phagocytosis and oxidative burst by neutrophils in patients with recurrent furunculosis. *Br J Dermatol* 1998;138:1036.
In patients with hypoferremia, neutrophil oxidative burst was abnormal and might predispose to neutrophil dysfunction, contributing to furunculosis.
Hsu CT, et al. The hyperimmunoglobulin E syndrome. *J Microbiol Immunol Infect* 2004;37: 121.
This syndrome may present with recurrent furunculosis, high IgE levels, and defective neutrophil chemotaxis.
Iyer S, Jones DH. Community-acquired methicillin-resistant Staphylococcus aureus skin infections: a retrospective analysis of clinical presentation and treatment of a local outbreak. *J Acad Dermatol* 2004;50:854.
Increasing reports of community-acquired methicillin-resistant staphylococcus infection. Incision and drainage plus use of vancomycin or linezolid was curative.
Levy R, et al. Vitamin C for the treatment of recurrent furunculosis in patients with impaired neutrophil function. *J Infect Dis* 1996;173:1502.
Study of 23 patients showed improvement of neutrophil function and treatment success.
Levy R, Schaeffler F. Successful treatment of a patient with recurrent furunculosis by vitamin C: improvement of clinical course and impaired neutrophil function. *Int J Dermatol* 1993;32:832.
Describes patient who responded to vitamin C, including documented improvement in neutrophil function.

Mahe E, et al. Furunculosis and IgG subclass deficiency. *Dermatology* 2004;208:84.
IgG subclass deficiency has been implicated as an underlying problem in recurrent furunculosis.

Raz R, et al. A 1-year trial of nasal mupirocin in the prevention of recurrent staphylococcal nasal colonization and skin infections. *Arch Intern Med* 1996;156:1109.
Mupirocin reduced the incidence of nasal colonization and chronic skin infection in chronic carriers.

Stulberg DL, Penrod MA, Blatny RA. Common bacterial skin infections. *Am Fam Physician* 2002;66:119.
Description of spectrum of staphylococcal soft-tissue infections, including furunculosis.

Wheat LJ, et al. Long-term studies on the effect of rifampin on nasal carriage of coagulase-positive staphylococci. *Rev Infect Dis* 1983;5:S459.
Staphylococci was eradicated from 50 to 70% of patients when rifampin was used with oxacillin in nasal carriers.

Nosocomial Infections 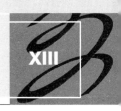 XIII

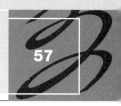

$\mathcal{I}$n the numerous discussions of the problem of postoperative fever, certain causes of fever, such as atelectasis or wound or urinary tract infection, are associated with a variety of surgical procedures. Others, such as mediastinitis or a prosthetic graft infection after the insertion of a heart valve, are specific for the particular type of operation performed. Occasionally, the fever represents an infectious disease problem unrelated to the surgical procedure, such as acute cholecystitis after a hernia repair. Any major surgical procedure can produce a fever for a few days after the operation. This is usually a low-grade, self-limited fever, and no cause is determined. However, a localized or systemic infectious disease is always a consideration, especially with a high, persistent, or recurrent fever.

In evaluating a patient with postoperative fever, it is helpful to note the temporal relationship of the fever to the operation. Causes of fever during the procedure or within the first 24 hours include malignant hyperthermia, transfusion reactions, atelectasis, aspiration pneumonia, wound infection, drug reactions, or endocrine disorders, such as acute adrenal insufficiency, thyroid storm, or pheochromocytoma. Malignant hyperthermia is a rare but life-threatening cause in which high fever occurs immediately after the introduction of anesthesia. It is triggered by halogenated inhalational anesthetics, such as enflurane, isoflurane, and the muscle relaxant succinylcholine. The disorder is dominantly inherited, and a family history of fatal reactions associated with anesthesia may be the only clue. High fever and muscle rigidity occur, resulting from elevated cytoplasmic calcium levels triggered by various anesthetic agents. The disorder is diagnosed by a muscle biopsy and an in vitro muscle contracture test. In the future, genetic testing will play a role in diagnosis. Therapy consists of supportive measures and dantrolene.

Another disorder that can cause fever is the neuroleptic malignant syndrome. Fever also occurs commonly with blood transfusions. Although these reactions are usually self limited, they may represent red cell or granulocyte incompatibility or contamination of the blood with microorganisms. Atelectasis, although this is controversial, may be the most frequent cause identified for fever during the first 24 hours and responds to vigorous chest physiotherapy. The aspiration of a foreign body, such as a denture, should be excluded. Although wound infections are usually detected after several days, those caused by group A streptococci or *Clostridium* organisms may occur during the first 24 hours.

Fever may begin after the initial 24 to 48 postoperative hours. The possibilities are numerous, but five causes are most frequent: infection in an IV site, wound, or urinary tract; deep venous thrombosis; or a pulmonary source. Two uncommon but potentially lethal infections should be considered when a patient has high fever in the initial 24 to 48 hours after surgery: toxic shock syndrome associated with *Staphylococcus aureus* or a group A streptococcal wound infection or bowel perforation. After an abdominal operation, an unnoticed injury to the bowel or an anastomotic leak may cause high fever and shock. In patients with toxic shock syndrome, the signs of a wound infection may be minimal, and the clinical picture is characterized by fever, diarrhea, erythroderma, and shock.

"Third-day surgical fever" has been used to describe fever occurring on the third postoperative day as a result of an infection at the IV site. Such fevers are not limited to the third day and may result from contaminated IV fluid or infection at the catheter site. Inflammation may be absent from the IV site, making the diagnosis more difficult. Therapy consists of removing the catheter, culturing its tip, and obtaining several blood cultures.

Most wound infections are seen from 4 to 10 days after an operation. Increased warmth, redness, pain, and tenderness, along with purulent drainage, may be detected.

A Gram's stain and culture of the discharge should identify the etiologic agent. Adequate drainage and antimicrobials are usually required. A urinary tract infection should be suspected in any patient who has an indwelling catheter or has undergone urinary tract instrumentation. Although urinary tract infection occurs infrequently, the source of the fever may be in the prostate; thus, rectal examination should not be neglected. Fever developing 5 to 7 days or longer after an operation should always raise the possibility of deep venous thrombosis. An asymptomatic presentation, except for fever, can occur. The lungs are the other common site of infection. Atelectasis, aspiration, bacterial pneumonia, and pulmonary embolism are the most likely possibilities. Atelectasis with or without pleural effusion may be a clue to an intra-abdominal abscess beneath the diaphragm. Another cause of postoperative fever is antimicrobial-associated colitis caused by *Clostridium difficile*. The onset is usually 4 to 9 days after operation. Diarrhea, abdominal pain and tenderness, and fever often are present. Some patients have little or no diarrhea and have fever and abdominal pain. Fecal leukocytes are present in the stool in half the patients, and the diagnosis is confirmed by identifying *C. difficile* toxin in the stool.

Fever with an onset at least 24 hours after an operation suggests other causes, such as complications associated with anesthesia, hepatitis, infection with cytomegalovirus (CMV) or Epstein-Barr virus, malaria transmitted through the blood, sterile or infected hematomas, drugs, and infections unrelated to the operation (e.g., acute cholecystitis). Chemical and bacterial meningitis are other reported febrile complications that may occur with spinal anesthesia or after neurosurgical procedures. Transmission of CMV is not restricted to patients after open heart surgery, and CMV infection can develop after any blood transfusion. Fever developing 2 to 4 weeks after an operation and accompanied by atypical lymphocytes is a clue to mononucleosis. Drugs are an important noninfectious cause of persistent postoperative fever, especially in patients on antimicrobials, phenytoin, allopurinol, or medications for sleep. However, drug fever may be caused by any drug, and the associated rash and eosinophilia may be absent. Finally, always consider the possibility of an infection unrelated to an operation, such as acute cholecystitis caused by biliary stones, acalculous cholecystitis, pancreatitis, or hospital-acquired influenza.

In addition to the complications that can occur with various surgical procedures, the cause of the fever may be closely related to the particular kind of operation performed. An intra-abdominal, subphrenic hepatic abscess or pancreatitis may develop after abdominal surgery. A pelvic operation may be complicated by septic pelvic thrombophlebitis, pelvic abscess, or cellulitis. After cardiovascular surgery, sternal osteomyelitis, endocarditis, mediastinitis, or the postcardiotomy syndrome are diagnostic considerations. Similarly, in neurosurgical, orthopedic, and other surgical specialty operations, the causes of fever may be unique to the procedure. Only after analysis of the patient's complaints, the physical and laboratory findings, and the fever onset and its relationship to surgery in general or the particular operation can the cause of the fever become apparent. (NMG)

Bibliography

Adelson-Mitty J, Fink MP, Lisbon A. The value of lumbar puncture in the evaluation of critically ill, non-immunosuppressed surgical patients: a retrospective analysis of 70 cases. *Intensive Care Med* 1997;23:749–752.
In surgical patients who are not immunosuppressed and have no history of recent head trauma or neurosurgery, a lumbar puncture has a low yield.

Altemeier WA, McDonough JJ, Fuller WD. Third-day surgical fever. *Arch Surg* 1971;103:158.
Septic thrombophlebitis related to IV infusion catheters is emphasized.

Badillo AT, Sarani B, Evans SRT. Optimizing the use of blood cultures in the febrile postoperative patient. *J Am Coll Surg* 2002;194:477–487.
Fever is a poor marker of postoperative bacteremia, with rates of positivity of 0 to 3%. Yield is higher in an intensive care unit or immunocompromised patient.

Bartlett JG, Gorbach SL, Finegold SM. The bacteriology of aspiration pneumonia. *Am J Med* 1974;56:202.
The importance of anaerobes in aspiration pneumonia is stressed. A mixture of anaerobes and aerobes was common in hospital-acquired infections.

Bell DM, et al. Unreliability of fever and leukocytosis in the diagnosis of infection after cardiac valve surgery. *J Thorac Cardiovasc Surg* 1978;75:87.
These two tests were not useful in distinguishing infected from uninfected patients after cardiac valve surgery.

Bennett SN, et al. Postoperative infections traced to contamination of an intravenous anesthetic, propofol. *N Engl J Med* 1995;333:147–154.
Postoperative fever and a bloodstream infection were caused by contamination of a multidose vial of an anesthetic agent, propofol.

Borger MA, et al. Deep sternal wound infection: risk factors and outcomes. *Ann Thorac Surg* 1998;65:1050–1056.
Male sex and diabetes were risk factors for deep sternal wound infections.

Bornstain C, et al. Sedation, sucralfate, and antibiotic use are potential means for protection against early-onset ventilator-associated pneumonia. *Clin Inf Dis* 2004;38:1401–1408.
An increased risk of pneumonia was seen in patients given sucralfate and having an unplanned extubation.

Clancy CJ, Nguyen MH, Morris AJ. Candidal mediastinitis: an emerging clinical entity. *Clin Infect Dis* 1997;25:608–613.
A rare cause of mediastinitis. An intraoperative sternal culture for Candida *should not be readily dismissed as a contaminant.*

Craven DE, Steger KA, Barber TW. Preventing nosocomial pneumonia: state of the art and perspectives for the 1990s. *Am J Med* 1991;91:44S.
A review of pathogenesis and prophylaxis.

Cruse PJE, Foord R. A 5-year prospective study of 23,649 surgical wounds. *Arch Surg* 1973;107:206.
A comprehensive study of wound infections.

de la Toore SH, Mandel L, Goff BA. Evaluation of postoperative fever: usefulness and cost-effectiveness of routine workup. *Am J Obstet Gynecol* 2003;188:1642–1647.
Pneumonia was the most frequent cause.

Drew WL, Miner RC. Transfusion-related cytomegalovirus infection following noncardiac surgery. *JAMA* 1982;247:2389.
Consider this diagnosis in a postoperative patient with fever in the presence or absence of atypical lymphocytes 3 weeks after a blood transfusion.

Durand ML, et al. Acute bacterial meningitis in adults. *N Engl J Med* 1993;328:21.
Recent neurosurgery (45%) or the presence of a neurosurgical device (21%) such as a shunt were the major predisposing factors in patients with nosocomial meningitis.

Eason E, Aldis A, Seymour RJ. Pelvic fluid collections by sonography and febrile morbidity after abdominal hysterectomy. *Obstet Gynecol* 1997;90:58–62.
The presence of pelvic fluid as determined by endovaginal ultrasound was not helpful in determining the cause of fever after abdominal hysterectomy.

Engoren M. Lack of association between atelectasis and fever. *Chest* 1995;107:81–84.
Fever should not be attributed to atelectasis in patients who have undergone cardiac surgery.

Fischer SA, et al. Infectious complications in left ventricular assist device recipients. *Clin Infect Dis* 1997;24:18–23.
The mean onset of infection of a left ventricular assist device was 23 days after implantation. Cure of infection did not always require removal of the device.

Fitzgerald RH, et al. Deep-wound sepsis following total hip arthroplasty. *J Bone Joint Surg Am* 1977;59:847.
An extensive review of hip infections that may present during the immediate postoperative period or after several years. A spontaneously draining hematoma with hip pain and an elevated sedimentation rate are clues to an early hip infection.

Forgacs P, Geyer CA, Friedberg SR. Characterization of chemical meningitis after neurological surgery. *Clin Infect Dis* 2001;32:179–185.
Chemical meningitis occurs as a common complication after neurosurgery. Patients with chemical meningitis lack purulent drainage and cerebrospinal fluid rhinorrhea or otorrhea.

Garibaldi RA, et al. Evidence for the non-infectious etiology of early postoperative fever. *Infect Control* 1985;6:273.

Most of the causes of fever during the first 48 hours after surgery were not infectious in origin.

Gaynes R, et al. Mediastinitis following coronary artery bypass surgery: a 3-year review. *J Infect Dis* 1991;163:117.

Risk factors for infection included prolonged duration of surgery (>210 minutes), low preoperative levels of serum albumin (<3.0 g/dL), and a resident with a positive nasal culture for methicillin-resistant S. aureus.

Gur E, et al. Clinical-radiological evaluation of poststernotomy wound infection. *Plast Reconstr Surg* 1998;101:348–355.

Computed tomography is useful in the detection and staging of poststernotomy infections.

Hall SC. Pediatric emergencies. *Anesthesiol Clin North Am* 2001;19:367–382.

Diagnosis is usually made by muscle biopsy measuring contraction in the presence of halothane and caffeine.

Henle W, et al. Antibody responses to the Epstein-Barr virus and cytomegaloviruses after open heart and other surgery. *N Engl J Med* 1970;282:1068.

The postperfusion syndrome may result from the transfusion of blood with CMV or, less often, Epstein-Barr virus.

Holt HM, et al. Infections following epidural catheterization. *J Hosp Infect* 1995;30:253–260.

Infection, both local at the catheter exit site or generalized (e.g., meningitis), can complicate epidural catheterization. Most frequent causative organisms included coagulase-negative staphylococci (41%), S. aureus (35%), and gram-negative bacilli.

Hopkins PM. Malignant hyperthermia: advances in clinical management and diagnosis. *Br J Anaesth* 2000;85:118–128.

Review.

Hubmayr RD, et al. Statement of the 4th International Consensus Conference in critical care on ICU-acquired pneumonia-Chicago, Illinois, May 2002. *Intensive Care Med* 2002;28:1521–1536.

Early-onset pneumonia occurs during the first 5 days of intubation.

Ishikawa S, et al. Management of postoperative fever in cardiovascular surgery. *J Cardiovasc Surg* 1998;39:95–97.

Only 28% of patients with postoperative fever had a bacteriologic cause.

Johnson LB. The importance of early diagnosis of acute acalculous cholecystitis. *Surg Gynecol Obstet* 1987;164:197.

Fever is often the initial finding, and normal liver function test results should not exclude the diagnosis. An ultrasound study showing a thickening of the gallbladder (≥ 3 mm) was helpful in the diagnosis.

Johnson S, et al. Prospective, controlled study of vinyl glove use to interrupt *Clostridium difficile* nosocomial transmission. *Am J Med* 1990;88:137.

Hand carriage of C. difficile is an important factor in the transmission of this disease.

Lee Y-H, Kerstein MD. Osteomyelitis and septic arthritis: a complication of subclavian venous catheterization. *N Engl J Med* 1971;285:1179.

Osteomyelitis and septic arthritis are potential risks after subclavian vein catheterization.

Lim E, et al. Pyrexia after cardiac surgery: natural history and association with infection. *J Thorac Cardiovasc Surg* 2003;126:1013–1017.

Fever is frequent after cardiac surgery and usually resolves by day 5. Leukocytosis is of limited value in diagnosing infection in the first 5 days.

Loeber B, Swenson RM. Bacteriology of aspiration pneumonia. *Ann Intern Med* 1974;81:329.

The bacteriology of community-acquired and hospital-acquired aspiration pneumonia differs and reflects pharyngeal colonization.

Mellors JW, et al. A simple index to estimate the likelihood of bacterial infection in patients developing fever after abdominal surgery. *Am Surg* 1988;54:558.

After abdominal surgery, only 16% of patients with postoperative fever had a bacterial infection.

Negishi C. Fever during anaesthesia. *Best Pract Res Clin Anaesthesiol* 2003;17:499–517.

Fever in the postoperative period is usually the result of noninfectious causes.

O'Grady NP, et al. Practice guidelines for evaluating new fever in critically ill adult patients. *Clin Infect Dis* 1998;26:1042–1059.
Review. Fever in the initial 48 hours after surgery is usually noninfectious.
Ottinger LW. Acute cholecystitis as a postoperative complication. *Ann Surg* 1976;184:162.
Acute cholecystitis may be a cause of fever after an operation for unrelated disease. An atypical presentation is emphasized, with a mortality of 47%.
Perlino CA. Postoperative fever. *Med Clin North Am* 2001;85:1141–1149.
Review.
Perry JW, et al. Wound infections following spinal fusion with posterior segmental spinal instrumentation. *Clin Infect Dis* 1997;24:558–561.
Most wound infections were caused by gram-negative aerobic bacilli. Removal of the hardware (rods or wires) was not required for cure.
Rello J, Diaz E. Pneumonia in the intensive care unit. *Crit Care Med* 2003;31:2544–2551.
Review.
Robson MC, Krizek TJ, Heggers JP. Biology of surgical infections. *Curr Probl Surg* 1973;10: 1–62.
Classic. A monograph on surgical wound infections.
Sarubbi FA, Vasquez JE. Spinal epidural abscess associated with the use of temporary epidural catheters: report of two cases and review. *Clin Infect Dis* 1997;25:1155–1158.
Fever and localized back pain may be caused by an abscess associated with an epidural catheter.
Schlenker JD, Hubay CA. The pathogenesis of postoperative atelectasis. *Arch Surg* 1973;107:846.
This is an early, noninfectious cause of postoperative fever.
Schoenbaum SC, Gardner P, Shillito J. Infections in cerebrospinal fluid shunts: epidemiology, clinical manifestations, and therapy. *J Infect Dis* 1975;131:543.
Shunt replacement and antimicrobials are usually required for cure.
Shapira OM, et al. Unexplained fever after aortic valve replacement with cryopreserved allografts. *Ann Thorac Surg* 1995;60:S151–S155.
Unexplained fever was noted in 26% of patients undergoing allograft aortic valve replacement after the third postoperative day. It lasted 24 to 48 hours and resolved without antibiotics.
Siegel SE, et al. Transmission of toxoplasmosis by leukocyte transfusion. *Blood* 1971;37: 388.
Toxoplasma was transmitted to four patients with leukemia by granulocyte transfusions.
Soto-Hernandez JL, et al. Secondary adrenal insufficiency manifested as an acute febrile illness. *South Med J* 1989;82:384.
In this case report, fever 5 weeks after surgery was caused by adrenal insufficiency.
Talmore M, Li P, Barie PS. Acute paranasal sinusitis in critically ill patients: guidelines for prevention, diagnosis, and treatment. *Clin Infect Dis* 1997;25:1441–1446.
Computed tomography of the paranasal sinus is the best test for diagnosis. Sinusitis develops in about 25% of nasally endotracheally intubated patients.
Wolfe JE, Bone RC, Ruth WE. Effects of corticosteroids in the treatment of patients with gastric aspiration. *Am J Med* 1977;63:719.
No beneficial effect was noted in a controlled study. Gram-negative pneumonia occurred more frequently in the steroid-treated patients, which suggests a harmful effect.
Wynne JW, Modell JH. Respiratory aspiration of stomach contents. *Ann Intern Med* 1977;87:466.
Reviews the pathophysiology and therapy of gastric aspiration.

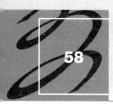

URINARY CATHETER-RELATED INFECTIONS

*T*he urinary catheter is an extremely useful device but a nosocomial infection hazard. More than 4 decades ago, in an editorial entitled "Case against the Catheter," the importance of the urinary catheter was noted and its dangers emphasized. Today, the urinary tract is still the most common site of nosocomial infection, accounting for approximately 40% of infections.

The two most effective measures to prevent nosocomial urinary tract infections—decreasing the duration of catheterization and use of a closed, sterile drainage system—were described 3 decades ago. Few advances have occurred since then, except for the use of medicated urinary catheters. Approximately 85% of cases of urinary tract infections are catheter-associated, and another 5% follow other types of urologic instrumentation, such as cystoscopy. Prevalence studies show that about 10% of patients in acute care hospitals have a urinary catheter; in an intensive care unit (ICU), the rate of urinary catheter use is even higher.

Nosocomial urinary tract infections vary from asymptomatic conditions that resolve spontaneously on catheter removal to infections associated with complications that include pyelonephritis, bacteremia, perinephric abscess, renal stones, renal failure, and death. Bloodstream invasion occurs at a rate of nearly 3% among cases of nosocomial bacteriuria. The rate of bacteremia in patients with a *Serratia* urinary tract infection was four times that of patients with nosocomial urinary tract infections caused by other organisms. Bacteremia developed in men with nosocomial urinary tract infections twice as often as in women. In fact, the urinary tract is the most common portal of entry for bacteria in patients with gram-negative bacteremia. The mortality rate of bacteremia from a catheter-associated urinary tract infection is estimated to be 10 to 30%. In one study, the mortality was three times higher among patients with nosocomial bacteriuria than in uninfected controls, although bacteremias were not documented in the group with the increased mortality rate. In a subsequent study, a significant reduction was noted in the frequency of infections and death rate after introduction of a catheter bag drainage system that did not disconnect at the junction of the catheter and collection tube. Other investigators in a case-control study found no relationship between nosocomial urinary tract infections and death. Catheter-related urinary tract infections also increase health care costs.

RISK FACTORS

A number of factors are linked to an increased rate of catheter-associated nosocomial bacteriuria, including female sex, age older than 50, and the presence of a rapidly progressive, fatal underlying illness. Using an aseptic technique during catheter insertion and maintaining a closed, sterile drainage system are key factors in determining the incidence of bacteriuria. The average rate of acquisition of bacteriuria is 5 to 10% for each day of catheterization; thus, after 10 days, about 50% of patients have bacteriuria. Breaks in the closed drainage system and improper care of the drainage bag occurred in 30% of catheterized patients. Other investigators found that in patients whose urinary catheters had sealed catheter-drainage tube junctions that could not be disconnected, the rate of infection was nearly three times lower than in patients assigned to catheters with unsealed junctions.

Systemic antimicrobials can decrease the rate of bacteriuria but are effective only for the initial 4 days of catheterization. When infection does occur in patients receiving systemic antimicrobials, however, the organisms isolated are generally more resistant. Having more than one patient with a urinary catheter in a room is another risk factor. This is especially a problem if one patient already has bacteriuria, because the hands of medical personnel have been shown to spread organisms from one drainage bag to another.

 ## PATHOGENESIS

Organisms appear to enter the urinary tract by one of three routes: (1) from the urethra into the bladder by way of the catheter, (2) at the urethral meatus around the catheter, or (3) by an intraluminal route from the drainage bag or the junction between the catheter and collecting tube during a disconnection. The majority of infections result when bacteria ascend from the periurethral area by means of a thin layer of fluid on the outside of the catheter at the catheter-meatal junction or by the intraluminal route during disconnection of the junction between the catheter and the collection tube. Studies have emphasized the importance of the meatal route in the pathogenesis of bacteriuria; 70% of catheterized patients acquire bacteriuria with the same organism isolated from the urethral meatus before the development of bacteriuria. In another study assessing the importance of prior urethral and rectal colonization in the pathogenesis of catheter-associated bacteriuria, prior urethral colonization was observed in 67% of women and 29% of men in whom bacteriuria developed. Antecedent rectal colonization was noted in 78% of women and 29% of men. In catheterized women, the majority of episodes of bacteriuria develop through the periurethral route, and the source is usually the rectal flora. In contrast, in male patients, most infections develop through the intraluminal route; the source of bacteria is not the rectum, but rather cross-infection. This study suggests that different prevention strategies may be needed for male and female patients.

 ## ETIOLOGY

Escherichia coli is the most common cause of nosocomial bacteriuria, accounting for about one-third of infections. Other common pathogenic agents are *Proteus* spp. (15%), *Klebsiella* spp. (10%), *Pseudomonas* spp. (10%), *Enterobacter* spp. (5%), enterococci (10–15%), and *Candida* (5%). Other organisms, such as *Serratia* and *Providencia,* account for the remaining 7 to 12%. In general, the organisms responsible for nosocomial bacteriuria are more resistant to antimicrobials than are the strains that cause community-acquired infections. The patient's own gastrointestinal flora is the source of many gram-negative bacilli that cause catheter-associated infections. Outbreaks of nosocomial urinary tract infections have been linked to contaminated rectal thermometers, cystoscopes, irrigation solutions, and disinfectants. Medical personnel who do not wash their hands after caring for each patient can transmit gram-negative bacilli from one urinary drainage bag to another.

 ## DIAGNOSIS

The diagnosis of a nosocomial urinary tract infection in a catheterized patient is based on a urine culture showing significant bacteriuria. Formerly, counts of more than 10^5 colony-forming units (CFU) per milliliter were required to establish a diagnosis; however, according to a study by Maki and associates, counts as low as 10^2 CFU/mL are probably significant and should not be ignored. Low-level counts of bacteria or *Candida* in the urine usually increase within 3 days to concentrations above 10^5 CFU/mL. Pyuria usually occurs with infections caused by gram-negative bacilli but less often because of gram-positive cocci or yeasts. When a urinary tract infection is responsible for fever, pyuria (more than five white cells per high-power field) should be present. One or more organisms per oil-immersion field in a Gram's-stained drop of unspun urine may provide a clue to the identity of the pathogen and help guide the initial selection of antimicrobial therapy. Polymicrobial bacteriuria occurs in about 75% of patients with long-term indwelling urethral catheters, with a mean of more than two organisms per specimen. The duration of bacteriuric episodes varies with each species. Gram-positive organisms such as coagulase-negative staphylococci persist for about 1 week, whereas *Providencia stuartii* may be present for 10 weeks or longer. Routine bacteriologic monitoring of urine from asymptomatic catheterized patients, however, is not a cost-effective approach to decrease or predict the frequency of symptomatic, catheter-related urinary tract infections.

The clinical features of nosocomial bacteriuria in a catheterized patient vary; the patient often has no symptoms or may have chills, fever, flank pain, oliguria, disseminated intravascular coagulation, or shock. Lower urinary tract symptoms such as frequency and dysuria are absent. In older catheterized patients, manipulation and change of the urinary catheter are frequent predisposing factors of urosepsis. In this group of patients, gastrointestinal complaints may predominate and direct attention away from the urinary tract.

 TREATMENT

All patients with a symptomatic, catheter-related urinary tract infection should be treated with a drug to which the causative organism is susceptible. If possible, the catheter should be removed if not needed or changed. The optimal duration of therapy is unknown, and the patient should be treated at least until the symptoms resolve if the catheter remains in place. For patients with a secondary bacteremia, which indicates a renal or prostatic source, drugs should be used that provide adequate levels in both urine and serum. Patients who have candiduria without candidemia may respond to catheter removal alone, amphotericin B bladder irrigation, or fluconazole. If clinical evidence of systemic candidiasis is lacking and there is no indication that pyelonephritis is present, then amphotericin B bladder irrigation may be tried if the catheter cannot be removed. Amphotericin B bladder irrigation consists of infusion of 5 to 10 mg of amphotericin B in 250 mL of sterile water into the bladder once daily; the catheter is cross-clamped for 1 hour. The appropriate duration of therapy is unknown, but 2 to 7 days is usually adequate. Most *Candida* organisms are susceptible to less than 1 μg of amphotericin B per milliliter, and the concentrations achieved with the suggested mixture are 20 to 40 μ/mL. In patients without renal insufficiency, fluconazole can be given at a dosage of 200 mg orally followed by 100 mg once daily for 4 days. Fluconazole is preferred for therapy of candiduria if therapy is used for a symptomatic patient.

Generally, patients with catheter-associated bacteriuria who are asymptomatic do not require therapy because of the risk of selecting for resistant organisms. One exception may be patients with asymptomatic bacteriuria and a prosthetic graft or heart valve; such patients are at risk for seeding of the foreign body. The most effective measure is to remove the catheter and, if the urine culture remains positive, to then treat the patient. In patients without prosthetic devices, the management of catheter-acquired bacteriuria after catheter removal is controversial. In one report, patients often became symptomatic after the catheter was removed. A single dose of oral trimethoprim-sulfamethoxazole (TMP-SMX) after catheter removal was usually effective in preventing symptomatic disease, particularly in patients younger than age 65. Antimicrobial impregnated catheters using silver-coated catheters, minocycline and rifampin-coated catheters, and nitrofurazone decrease the frequency of urinary tract infections for short-term catheterization (2–3 weeks).

Recommendations by the Centers for Disease Control and Prevention to prevent catheter-related bacteriuria are listed in Table 58-1. Use of a closed, sterile drainage system and hand washing before and after a urinary catheter or drainage bag is handled are two measures to prevent nosocomial bacteriuria. The use of meatal disinfectants, such as a povidone-iodine solution or silver sulfadiazine cream, antimicrobial-impregnated catheters, silver oxide-coated catheters, antibacterial urethral lubricants, and antibacterial bladder irrigation has failed to decrease the incidence of bacteriuria. The addition of disinfectants such as hydrogen peroxide to the drainage bag is not effective in reducing the incidence of catheter-related bacteriuria.

The value of prophylactic systemic antimicrobials in preventing or delaying bacteriuria remains unclear. The possible benefits must be balanced against cost, adverse effects, and selecting for resistant flora. In one study, there was no benefit from the use of TMP-SMX to reduce the incidence of urinary tract infections in patients with long-term indwelling catheters. Resistant organisms such as *Pseudomonas aeruginosa* and *P. stuartii* were

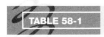

TABLE 58-1 Summary of Recommendations for Prevention of Catheter-Associated Urinary Tract Infections

Strongly recommended for adoption
Educate personnel in correct techniques of catheter insertion and care.
Catheterize only when necessary.
Emphasize hand washing.
Use aseptic technique and sterile equipment to insert catheter.
Secure catheter properly.
Maintain closed sterile drainage.
Obtain urine samples aseptically.
Maintain unobstructed urine flow.

Moderately recommended for adoption
Periodically reeducate personnel in catheter care.
Use smallest-bore catheter that is suitable.
Avoid irrigation unless necessary to prevent or relieve obstruction.
Refrain from daily meatal care with either povidone-iodine solution or soap and water.
Do not change catheters at arbitrarily fixed intervals.

Weakly recommended for adoption
Consider alternative techniques of urinary drainage before using an indwelling urethral catheter.
Replace the collecting system when sterile closed drainage has been breached.
Spatially separate infected and uninfected patients with indwelling catheters.
Avoid routine bacteriologic monitoring.

(Adapted from Centers for Disease Control Working Group. Guidelines for prevention of catheter-associated urinary tract infections. In: *Guidelines for the Prevention and Control of Nosocomial Infections.* Atlanta: U.S. Department of Health and Human Services, Public Health Service, 1981.)

identified more often in the antimicrobial-treated group than in the control group. For selected patients, condom catheters can be used to prevent nosocomial bacteriuria. Condoms, however, can produce gangrene and serve as reservoirs for resistant bacteria. The technique of intermittent catheterization appears effective, but controlled studies evaluating this approach are necessary. Hospital-acquired urinary tract infections cause considerable patient suffering and economic loss, and new approaches to dealing with this common problem are needed. (RBB)

Bibliography
Beeson PB. Case against the catheter. *Am J Med* 1958;24:1.
Classic.
Breitenbucher RB. Bacterial changes in the urine samples of patients with long-term indwelling catheters. *Arch Intern Med* 1984;144:1585.
Neither monthly cultures nor prophylactic TMP-SMX were of value.
Burke JP, Larsen RA, Stevens LE. Nosocomial bacteriuria: estimating the potential for prevention by closed sterile urinary drainage. *Infect Control* 1986;7:96.
Bacteriuria, particularly in female patients, was associated with improper suspension of the drainage bag.
Burke JP, et al. Prevention of catheter-associated urinary tract infections: efficacy of daily meatal care regimens. *Am J Med* 1981;70:655.
Daily meatal care was of no benefit in preventing bacteriuria.
Classen DC, et al. Daily meatal care for prevention of catheter-associated bacteriuria: results using frequent applications of polyantibiotic cream. *Infect Control Hosp Epidemiol* 1991;12:157.
Use of an antimicrobial cream containing polymyxin B, neomycin, and gramicidin applied to the urethral meatus three times daily did not reduce the rate of bacteriuria.
Cornia PB, et al. Computer-based order entry decreases duration of indwelling urinary catheterization in hospitalized patients. *Am J Med* 2003;114:404–407.

Early removal of a urinary catheter decreases the frequency of urinary tract infections.
Filice GA, et al. Nosocomial febrile illnesses in patients on an internal medicine service. *Arch Intern Med* 1989;149:319.
Pneumonia and urinary tract infection were the two most common causes for nosocomial fever in patients on the medical service.
Fisher JF, Newman CL, Sobel J. Yeast in the urine: solutions for a budding problem. *Clin Infect Dis* 1995;20:183–189.
Patients with candiduria should be evaluated for possible candidemia or a deep-seated infection.
Garibaldi RA, et al. Factors predisposing to bacteriuria during indwelling urethral catheterization. *N Engl J Med* 1974;291:215.
Risk factors are outlined. Antimicrobials were effective during the initial 4 days of catheterization.
Garibaldi RA, et al. Meatal colonization and catheter-associated bacteriuria. *N Engl J Med* 1980;303:316.
Bacteria can often be isolated in the periurethral space before the development of bacteriuria.
Gleckman R, et al. Catheter-related urosepsis in the elderly: a prospective study of community-derived infections. *J Am Geriatr Soc* 1982;30:255.
Usually a polymicrobial infection. A traumatic catheter event often precedes the acute symptomatic episode.
Haley RW, et al. The nationwide nosocomial infection rate. *Am J Epidemiol* 1985;121:159.
Nosocomial urinary tract infections accounted for 42% of all infections.
Harding GKM, et al. How long should catheter-acquired urinary tract infection in women be treated? A randomized, controlled study. *Ann Intern Med* 1991;114:713.
After catheter removal, asymptomatic bacteriuria frequently becomes symptomatic. Single-dose therapy with oral TMP-SMX was effective after short-term catheter use.
Hirsh DD, Fainstein V, Musher DM. Do condom catheter collecting systems cause urinary tract infections? *JAMA* 1979;242:340.
Cooperative patients with condom catheters had lower rates of urinary tract infections than patients with indwelling catheters.
Jacobs LG, et al. Oral fluconazole compared with bladder irrigation with amphotericin B for treatment of fungal urinary tract infections in elderly patients. *Clin Infect Dis* 1996;22:30–35.
Both amphotericin B bladder irrigation and oral fluconazole were effective treatments for patients with candiduria.
Johnson ET. The condom catheter: urinary tract infection and other complications. *South Med J* 1983;76:579.
Long-term use of a condom catheter drainage system was associated with urinary tract infections and penile complications.
Karchmer TB, et al. A randomized crossover study of silver-coated urinary catheters in hospitalized patients. *Arch Intern Med* 2000;160:3294–3298.
Silver alloy, hydrogel-coated catheters decreased the frequency of catheter-related urinary tract infections compared with a noncoated catheter.
Krieger JN, Kaiser DL, Wenzel RP. Urinary tract etiology of bloodstream infections in hospitalized patients. *J Infect Dis* 1983;148:57.
Bacteremia developed in almost 39% of patients with nosocomial bacteriuria.
Kunin CM, Finkelberg Z. Evaluation of an intraurethral lubricating catheter in prevention of catheter-induced urinary tract infections. *J Urol* 1971;106:928.
Classic. Ineffective approach to preventing urinary tract infections.
Kunin CM, McCormack RC. Prevention of catheter-induced urinary tract infections by sterile closed drainage. *N Engl J Med* 1966;274:1155.
Classic.
Leu HS, Huang CT. Clearance of funguria with short-course antifungal regimens: a prospective, randomized, controlled study. *Clin Infect Dis* 1995;20:1152–1157.
Spontaneous clearance rate in the control group was 40%. Systemic regimens with amphotericin B or oral fluconazole were more effective than local irrigation with amphotericin B.

Maki DG, Tambyah PA. Engineering out the risk of infection with urinary catheters. *Emerg Infect Dis* 2001;7:1–6.
  Medicated urinary catheters may reduce the frequency of urinary tract infections for short-term catheterization not exceeding 2 to 3 weeks.
Maki DG, et al. Nosocomial urinary tract infection with *Serratia marcescens:* an epidemiologic study. *J Infect Dis* 1973;128:579.
  An infected, catheterized patient should not share a room with another catheterized patient.
Pappas PG, et al. Guidelines for treatment of candidiasis. *Clin Infect Dis* 2004;30:161–189.
  Review.
Platt R, et al. Mortality associated with nosocomial urinary tract infection. *N Engl J Med* 1982;307:637.
  Nosocomial bacteriuria was associated with a threefold increase in mortality.
Platt R, et al. Reduction of mortality associated with nosocomial urinary tract infections. *Lancet* 1983;1:893.
  Fewer infections and deaths were noted in patients whose bladder catheters had preconnected, sealed junctions.
Platt R, et al. Prevention of catheter-associated urinary tract infection: a cost-benefit analysis. *Infect Control Hosp Epidemiol* 1989;10:60.
  Analysis supporting the use of sealed-junction catheters.
Saint S, Chenoweth CE. Biofilms and catheter-associated urinary tract infections. *Infect Dis Clin North Am* 2003;17:411–432.
  Review. Before treatment, the urinary catheter should be replaced if still needed.
Saint S. Clinical and economic consequences of nosocomial catheter-related bacteriuria. *Am J Infect Control* 2000;28:68–75.
  A symptomatic catheter-related urinary tract infection costs about $676 and a catheter-related bacteriuria about $2,836.
Sanford JP. The enigma of candiduria: evolution of bladder irrigation with amphotericin B for management—from anecdote to dogma and a lesson from Machiavelli. *Clin Infect Dis* 1993;16:145.
  Guidelines for treating candiduria.
Sobel JD, et al. Candiduria: a randomized, double-blind study of treatment with fluconazole and placebo. *Clin Infect Dis* 2000;30:19–24.
  No treatment for asymptomatic candiduria. Treat symptomatic patients 7 to 14 days. After stopping therapy, the recurrence rate is high.
Stamm WE. Catheter-associated urinary tract infections: epidemiology, pathogenesis, and prevention. *Am J Med* 1991;91(suppl 3B):65S.
  Comprehensive review.
Stark RP, Maki DG. Bacteriuria in the catheterized patient. *N Engl J Med* 1984;311:560.
  Quantitative cultures showing fewer than 10^5 CFU/mL are significant.
Tambyah PA, Maki DG. Catheter-associated urinary tract infection is rarely symptomatic: a prospective study of 1,497 catheterized patients. *Arch Intern Med* 2000;160:678–682.
  Catheter-related urinary tract infections are usually asymptomatic.
Tambyah PA, Knasinski V, Maki DG. The direct costs of nosocomial catheter-associated urinary tract infection in the era of managed care. *Infect Control Hosp Epidemiol* 2002;23:27–31.
  Catheter-related urinary tract infections are costly.
Tambyah PA, Maki DG. The relationship between pyuria and infection in patients with indwelling urinary catheters. *Arch Intern Med* 2000;160:673–677.
  In a patient with a catheter related urinary tract infection, pyuria is present if the etiology is gram-negative bacilli but often absent if the cause is gram-positive cocci or yeast.
Trautner BW, Darouiche RO. Catheter-associated infections: pathogenesis affects prevention. *Arch Intern Med* 2004;164:842–850.
  Review. Few advances have occurred in the prevention of catheter-related urinary tract infections.
Warren JW. Catheter-associated bacteriuria in long-term care facilities. *Infect Control Hosp Epidemiol* 1994;15:557–562.

Review. Closed catheter drainage is the only effective method to prevent bacteriuria.
Warren JW. Catheter-associated urinary tract infections. *Infect Dis Clin North Am* 1997;11:609–622.
Review.
Warren JW, et al. Antibiotic irrigation and catheter-associated urinary tract infections. *N Engl J Med* 1978;299:570.
Antimicrobial irrigation is not effective in preventing bacteriuria.

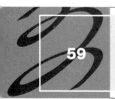

59 HEALTHCARE-ASSOCIATED PNEUMONIA

$\mathcal{H}$ospital-acquired (nosocomial) infections occur in more than 5% of patients hospitalized for at least 48 to 72 hours. The rate is highest for critically ill patients in intensive care units (ICUs). In most studies, pneumonia is the second or third most common type identified, accounting for 13 to 18% of all cases. It occurs at rates of four to seven cases per 1,000 hospitalizations. Mortality from nosocomial pneumonia is higher than 30%, and pneumonia is the most common fatal nosocomial infection. Best estimates are that approximately 140,000 deaths occur annually.

Ventilator-associated pneumonia (VAP) represents an important subset of nosocomial pneumonia. Almost 20% of all nosocomial pneumonia occurs in the 1% of patients who are ventilated. Incidence of VAP generally has been noted at 15 to more than 50% and is tenfold to twentyfold higher than in nonventilated individuals. Duration of ventilation is an important variable. Mortality from VAP is 20 to more than 70%.

Up to 25% of ICU patients become colonized with resident gram-negative bacilli within 24 hours. This increases to almost 50% by 5 days. Nosocomial pneumonia is more common (23% vs. 3%) in patients who have become colonized. Sources of bacteria are often the patient's own upper respiratory flora. Patients with endotracheal tubes are at risk because these devices bypass respiratory tract host defense mechanisms and allow bacteria to be deposited directly into the lower respiratory tract. Additionally, secretions may pool in the subglottic area above the endotracheal cuff and slowly "leak" into the lower respiratory tract. The other major source of bacteria for nosocomial pneumonia is colonization of the stomach with subsequent microaspiration. Rarely, nosocomial pneumonia is caused by penetrating trauma or hematogenous spread.

BACTERIOLOGY

Bacteriology of nosocomial pneumonia is complex. The likelihood of specific pathogens is dependent on factors that include (1) duration of hospitalization/ICU stay, (2) prior antimicrobial therapy, (3) underlying comorbidities, and (4) specifics of an individual institution. Core pathogens include common Enterobacteriaceae (e.g.,*Escherichia coli* and *Klebsiella pneumoniae*), *Staphylococcus aureus*, *Streptococcus pneumoniae*, and *Haemophilus influenzae*. Persons on recent antibiotics or with prolonged stay (i.e., >7 days) in an ICU are predisposed to resistant organisms such as *Pseudomonas aeruginosa*, *Acinetobacter* spp., and methicillin-resistant *S. aureus* (MRSA). Witnessed aspiration predisposes to infection with anaerobes. Except in this context, importance of anaerobic infection is controversial. Selected hospitals have also been associated with *Legionella* spp. infections. Nosocomial pneumonias associated with viruses, such as respiratory syncytial virus and influenza virus, have been less thoroughly investigated, in part because of difficulties with cultures.

Organisms infrequently associated with nosocomial pneumonia include *Candida* spp., *Enterococcus* spp., and coagulase (−) staphylococci.

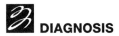 DIAGNOSIS

The clinical diagnosis of nosocomial pneumonia is imprecise, and there is currently no "gold standard" other than positive cultures directly from lung tissue. The Clinical Pulmonary Infection Score (CPIS) has been developed to help assist with diagnosis. Table 59-1 depicts criteria and points. As used, a score of less than 6 indicates a low likelihood of pneumonia and may allow a shortened antibiotic course (see below). This score also may be used to follow-up on response to treatment, although it has not been validated for this use.

As noted below, quantitative cultures from bronchoalveolar lavage (BAL) and flexible fiberoptic bronchoscopy (FFB) are considered accurate, but they have limitations. Pneumonia should be suspected in patients with progressive pulmonary infiltrates or a new infiltrate consistent with this diagnosis, plus adjunctive evidence of infection that could include purulent secretions, fever, and leukocytosis, coupled with ultimate bacteriologic confirmation. Alternatively, a negative chest radiograph excludes this diagnosis. However, in the presence of endotracheal tubes or tracheostomy, purulent secretions may be indicative of local irritation rather than true infection, and for similar reasons polymorphonuclear leukocytes (PMNs) may be present when endotracheal material is Gram's-stained. Cultures of lower respiratory secretions obtained through endotracheal tubes or tracheostomies (blind bronchial sampling) may reveal potential pathogens that may reflect colonization or tracheobronchitis only. The severely ill individual may develop fever and leukocytosis for many reasons other than lower respiratory tract infection. Alternatively, the patient with pneumonia may fail to mount a fever or elevation of white blood cell (WBC) count for reasons that include old age, renal failure, or effects of medication. Well-defined infections may be unaccompanied by fever in up to 30% of cases. Similarly, radiographs of the chest may prove unreliable. Among

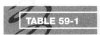 **Clinical Pulmonary Infection Score**

TABLE 59-1

Feature	Value	# Points
Temperature (C)	>36.5, <38.4	0
	>38.5, <38.9	1
	<36.5, >39.0	2
WBC count	>4000, <11,000	0
	<4000, >11,000 or	1
	>500 bands	1
Pulmonary secretions	None	0
	Nonpurulent	1
	Purulent	2
Oxygenation (PaO$_2$/FiO$_2$)	>240 or ARDS	0
	<240, no ARDS	2
Radiographic infiltrate	None	0
	Diffuse or patchy	1
	Localized	2
Radiographic progression	None	0
	Progression (No CHF, ARDS)	2
Bacteriology	None cultured	0
	Pathogens cultured or	1
	Pathogens on smear	1

(Adapted from DeRosa FG, Craven DE. Ventilator-associated pneumonia: current management strategies. *Infect Med* 2003;20:248–259 *CHF*, Congestive heart failure.)

the numerous other causes for pulmonary infiltrates are adult respiratory distress syndrome (ARDS), congestive heart failure, and malignancy. Autopsies performed on patients with ARDS suspected of having nosocomial pneumonia have failed to corroborate clinical and radiographic findings in up to 30% of cases.

Need for bacteriologic diagnosis of nosocomial pneumonia is controversial but increasingly preferred. Cultures from sterile sites such as blood or pleural effusion are rarely positive. Expectorated secretions may be contaminated. Recommendations range from empiric antibiotic therapy through invasive procedures that include flexible fiberoptic bronchoscopy with protected brush (FFPB) and quantitative bacteriology or bronchoalveolar lavage (BAL). Endpoints that differentiate true pathogens from contaminants are more than 10^3 (FFB) and more than 10^4 (BAL). Potential advantages of invasive diagnosis of nosocomial pneumonia include (1) a sense of security with the diagnosis; (2) the ability to discontinue antibiotics in a timely fashion (based on organism identified); and (3) the capacity *not* to use antibiotics if pneumonia is not proven. These advantages may be lost if new antibiotics for pneumonia are initiated prior to etiologic documentation.

Two investigations using quantitative bacteriology from specimens obtained by endotracheal aspiration demonstrate a 70% correlation with gold standards. Cutoffs of 10^5 and 10^6 were used. Other investigations of ventilator-associated pneumonia compared FFPB, BAL, and quantitative endotracheal aspirates, with mortality as the endpoint. There was no mortality advantage to use of data from FFPB or BAL when compared with that available from quantitative endotracheal aspirates. Limitations of invasive techniques include (1) sampling error, (2) no conclusive evidence documenting enhanced survivorship, and (3) costs/risks. It is the opinion of the author that endotracheal aspirate with quantitation may be the most cost-effective method of diagnosing nosocomial pneumonia in ventilated patients and should be obtained prior to antibiotic changes or initiation of antibiotics.

 MANAGEMENT

Respiratory support, treatment of ancillary conditions, and antimicrobial therapy are the cornerstones of management. Antibiotics should be administered in full therapeutic doses, generally intravenously, with dosing and choice consistent with end-organ function and other host factors. Recent recommendations from the American Thoracic Society suggest antibiotics based on risks for "severe" pneumonia (those requiring ICU care, rapid radiologic progression, acute renal failure, or respiratory failure), underlying host conditions, and time of onset. Early pneumonia is that which occurs within the first 5 days of hospitalization, often associated with trauma. Underlying conditions include risk of aspiration, structural lung disease, and risks for legionellosis. Table 59-2 provides antibiotic recommendations based on "core" pathogens. Table 59-3 expands antibiotic recommendations in the presence of mitigating factors.

The most important consideration in the management of nosocomial pneumonia is to use the correct agent from the outset. Inappropriate initial antibiotic therapy is correlated

TABLE 59-2	Patients with Mild/Moderate Nosocomial Pneumonia, No Unusual Risk Factors, Onset Anytime or Patients with Severe Nosocomial Pneumonia and Early Onset

Likely (core) organisms	Appropriate antibiotics
Enteric gram-negative bacilli (*E. coli*, *Klebsiella* spp., *Enterobacter* spp., *Serratia*, *Proteus* spp.) *S. pneumoniae*	Either second-generation cephalosporin, or non-*Pseudomonas* third-generation cephalosporin, or β-lactam/β-lactamase combination
H. influenzae Methicillin-sensitive *S. aureus*	If allergic to β-lactam: fluoroquinolone or clindamycin plus aztreonam

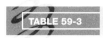

| **TABLE 59-3** | **Patients with Mild/Moderate Nosocomial Pneumonia; with Risk Factors** |

Organism based on risk factor	Core antibiotics plus:
Anaerobes (recent abdominal surgery, witnessed aspiration)	Clindamycin or β-lactam/β-lactamase inhibitor
S. aureus (coma, head trauma, diabetes mellitus, renal failure)	$+/-$ vancomycin (until MRSA ruled out)
Legionella (high-dose corticosteroids)	Erythromycin $+/-$ rifampin(or quinolone alone)
P. aeruginosa (prolonged ICU stay, corticosteroids, prior antibiotics, structural lung disease)	Aminoglycoside or ciprofloxacin plus one of the following: Imipenem/cilastatin Aztreonam β-lactam/β-lactamase inhibitor

with enhanced mortality, even if "correct" agent(s) are later used. In many instances a single effective antibiotic suffices. Two agents may be indicated for pneumonia caused by *P. aeruginosa*, and when no single agent will cover likely pathogens (e.g., considerations of MRSA or legionellosis). Multiple antibiotics also may be indicated for empiric therapy if resistance patterns within an ICU dictate this (e.g., no single antibiotic covers more than 70% of isolates of *P. aeruginosa*). Third-generation cephalosporins, imipenem-cilastatin, piperacillin/tazobactam, and parenteral quinolones are effective against susceptible gram-negative pathogens. Aminoglycosides remain valuable agents for many enteric gram-negative bacilli and *P. aeruginosa*. Dosing regimens using single daily doses of 5 to 7 mg/kg are generally more efficacious and may be safer than those using more classic thrice-daily regimes. For considerations of *P. aeruginosa,* two effective agents are advised by the author, although not conclusively proven to be beneficial when compared to a single effective agent. For the consideration of *Legionella pneumophila*, either a macrolide or quinolone should be in the antibiotic regime. Gram-positive pneumonias can be treated with a single appropriate antimicrobial. Those caused by MRSA may be more favorably managed with linezolid than vancomycin.

Acinetobacter baumannii has recently emerged as a nosocomial pulmonary pathogen. Mortality rates approach more than 50% (overall) with almost 40% attributable. Although some are sensitive to carbapenems, others required colistin for treatment. The two agents appear comparable, and colistin, when appropriately dosed for renal function, has been found to be well tolerated.

The optimal length of therapy for nosocomial pneumonia is unknown. Patients with initial CPIS scores of less than 6 that remain below that level at day 3 may be effectively managed with 3 days of antibiotics. To date, only ciprofloxacin has been studied in this manner. Recent data indicates that nosocomial pneumonia caused by most pathogens can now be managed by eight days of effective therapy. However, infections due to *Acinetobacter* spp. and other nonfermenters may prove an exception and be better managed with 10–14 days of treatment. Thus the need for etiologic diagnosis. Patients with suppurative complications will require longer courses, generally more than 3 weeks. Those with pneumonia caused by *L. pneumophila* generally are treated for up to 21 days. A number of agents, including fluoroquinolones, trimethoprim/sulfamethoxazole, and linezolid, have excellent oral bioavailability, and for the person capable of oral intake there is no need for intravenous agents.

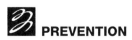

PREVENTION

Respiratory support paraphernalia that bypasses normal respiratory defenses should be used judiciously, and noninvasive pulmonary support is preferred when appropriate. Postoperative patients should have cough and deep-breathing exercises, and positioning patients so as to decrease vomiting is sensible. Somnolent patients should be turned regularly. Patients in ICUs should be positioned to maintain the head at 30 to 45°, although this may prove difficult. Endotracheal or tracheostomy tubes should be suctioned as necessary. Routine treatment of colonizing bacteria in the absence of clinical or radiographic lower respiratory infection is not indicated. Such therapy enhances the emergence of resistant organisms and the potential for clinical infection. Adherence to infection control procedures, including hand washing and use of personal protective equipment as necessary, is mandatory. Availability of alcohol-based portable products may improve hand hygiene, especially in busy ICUs with poor availability of sinks.

Gastric colonization with potentially pathogenic bacteria is known to be associated with rising gastric pH, as may occur with H_2 antagonists (and even sucralfate) used for stress ulcer prophylaxis. Although some data demonstrate benefits of sucralfate (compared to H_2 antagonists) at preventing nosocomial pneumonia, this potential benefit needs to be weighed against the decreased efficacy of this agent in preventing gastrointestinal bleeding. Other attempts at decreasing oral colonization are ongoing, with preliminary results encouraging.

Occasional outbreaks of nosocomial pneumonia caused by specific pathogens may occur in hospital areas. Prophylactic administration of aerosolized polymyxin B has been shown to be effective in decreasing both transmission and infection with *P. aeruginosa* during respiratory outbreaks with this pathogen. All at-risk persons entering the ICU should receive the aerosol for several weeks after the last isolate. However, prolonged prophylaxis results in higher mortality rates due to pneumonia caused by pathogens resistant to polymyxin (e.g., *Flavobacterium meningosepticum*). Thus, the routine use of this aerosol as a preventive measure is not encouraged.

Preventing nosocomial pneumonia, especially ventilator-associated pneumonia (VAP), is difficult and generally unrewarding. Attention to small details is important. Adherence to infection control policies and procedures, to help prevent individual cases and to abort transmission among patients, is encouraged. (RBB)

Bibliography

Bartlett JG, et al. Bacteriology of hospital-acquired pneumonia. *Arch Intern Med* 1986; 146:868–871.
  This is one of the few reports on the etiology of nosocomial pneumonia that used transtracheal aspiration and anaerobic bacteriology. A Veterans Administration population was studied that was unassociated with endotracheal intubation and ventilation. A diverse group of organisms was identified that included many anaerobes, common bacteria (S. pneumoniae and H. influenzae), and enteric gram-negative bacilli. Almost 50% of patients had at least two organisms identified.
Chastre J, Fagon J-Y. Ventilator-associated pneumonia. *Am J Respir Crit Care Med* 2002; 165:867–903.
  This article represents the best single source for information about VAP. The authors review available literature concerning epidemiology, diagnosis, management, and prevention. They have contributed much of the literature concerning invasive diagnostic techniques, and it is their bias (openly mentioned in the review) that invasive bacteriologic diagnosis should be obtained in most patients in whom the diagnosis is entertained.
Chastre J, et al. Comparison of 8 vs 15 days of antibiotic therapy for ventilator-associated pneumonia in adults. *JAMA* 2003;290:2588–2598.
  The authors conducted a prospective, randomized, double-blinded trial in numerous French critical care units to assess adequacy of shorted therapy for VAP. Major outcomes were 28-day mortality, recurrence of infection, and antibiotic-free days. The choice of antibiotic was left up to the prescribing physician, but guidelines for use were provided. Treatment for 8 days was not associated with excess mortality, but did result in more antibiotic-free days (as expected). However, patients with nonfermenting organisms that included P. aeruginosa and Acinetobacter spp. had more infection recurrence when they received the shorter therapy. Such information is noteworthy and makes bacteriologic diagnosis important if considering shorter courses of antibiotics. Alternatively, they can probably be used if nonfermenters are unlikely to be encountered (e.g., early VAP in the absence of prior antibiotic therapy).
DeRosa FG, Craven DE. Ventilator-associated pneumonia: current management strategies. *Infect Med* 2003;20:248–259.

An excellent overview of this disease with good explanations of the pneumonia clinical infection score, bacteriology based on risk factors, and excellent management tables.

Driks MR, et al. Nosocomial pneumonia in intubated patients given sucralfate as compared with antacids or histamine type-2 blockers. *N Engl J Med* 1987;317:1376–1382.

An excellent study comparing two methods commonly used for prevention of stress ulceration in ICU patients. It demonstrates that sucralfate, not primarily associated with elevating gastric pH, was less likely to result in gastric colonization with enteric gram-negative bacilli and was associated with a lower incidence of nosocomial pneumonia. However, sucralfate now appears to be less effective in preventing gastrointestinal bleeding. It probably has benefit in patients not at high risk for bleeding.

Fowler RA, et al. Variability in antibiotic prescribing patterns and outcomes in patients with clinically suspected ventilator-associated pneumonia. *Chest* 2003;123: 835–844.

An observational prospective investigation was performed to assess adequacy of initial antibiotic therapy and outcomes in VAP. Overall mortality in 156 patients with VAP was 34%, and more than 90% of individuals received appropriate antibiotics based on available bacteriology obtained primarily by blind endotracheal aspirates. About 30% of patients were bacteremic. Of note, almost 60% of patients had recently received antibiotics, specifics not given. Methicillin-sensitive S. aureus and P. aeruginosa were the most commonly encountered pathogens. The lowest in-hospital mortality was seen when initial treatment included piperacillin/tazobactam and, possibly, aminoglycosides. Outcomes were poorer with β-lactams or fluoroquinolones. Monotherapy or dual treatment did not matter, nor whether treatment was "appropriate" or "inappropriate." The latter result was likely influenced by the small numbers who received inappropriate treatments. Initial antibiotic treatment should be appropriate to organisms likely to be confronted and may vary among hospitals and regions. There should be no advantage to dual therapy regimens unless they enhance coverage.

Garnacho-Montero J, et al. Treatment of multidrug-resistant *Acinetobacter baumannii* ventilator-associated pneumonia (VAP) with intravenous colistin: a comparison with imipenem-susceptible VAP. *Clin Infect Dis* 2003;203:1111–1118.

An outbreak of VAP associated with A. baumannii was identified. Two-thirds of isolates were exclusively sensitive to colistin; the others remained sensitive to imipenem/cilastatin. Overall mortality was higher than 50% in both groups. Treatment with colistin resulted in (bad) outcomes similar to those seen with imipenem/cilastatin. In the patients assessed for neurotoxicity from colistin, none was noted. Acinetobacter VAP is a bad disease; however, therapy with colistin can be used with apparent safety when indicated.

Hofken G, Niederman MS. Nosocomial pneumonia. The importance of a de-escalating strategy for antibiotic treatment of pneumonia in the ICU. *Chest* 2002;122:2183–2196.

The authors review nosocomial pneumonia in the ICU and point out that inappropriate initial treatment portends bad outcomes, and that this is one factor that can be potentially controlled. "Hit early, hit hard" appears to be the best strategy for initial management of this disease. The most common reason for inappropriate initial treatment was identification of resistant gram-negative pathogens. Once further information becomes available, antibiotics can be tailored. Such a strategy requires knowledge of ICU-specific pathogens and resistance patterns and should take into account duration of ICU stay and prior antibiotic usage. In a perfect world, bacteriologic confirmation prior to antibiotic changes should be available.

Sanchez-Nieto JM, et al. Impact of invasive and noninvasive quantitative culture sampling on outcome of ventilator-associated pneumonia. *Am J Respir Crit Care Med* 1998;157:371–376.

The authors conducted an open, prospective, randomized study in 51 ventilated patients to determine if they could identify benefits of invasive diagnostic procedures in the management of ventilator-associated pneumonia. In one group, decision making was made on the basis of either FFPB or BAL (both with quantitative bacteriology), whereas in the second group it was made on the basis of endotracheal aspirates with quantitative bacteriology. There was no difference in mortality with the use of the invasive procedures, although there were more changes in antibiotic treatment. The authors conclude that they could not identify benefits of the more invasive procedures in this pilot study.

Singh N, et al. Short-course empiric antibiotic therapy for patients with pulmonary infiltrates in the intensive care unit. *Am J Respir Crit Care Med* 2000;162:505–511.

The authors conducted a prospective study using the CPIS to determine the need for antibiotic therapy beyond 3 days. Patients with CPIS lower than 6 (i.e., low likelihood for nosocomial pneumonia) were randomized to either standard antibiotic therapy or ciprofloxacin for 3 days. Ciprofloxacin was discontinued at 3 days if the CPIS remained less than 6. The patients who received 3 days of ciprofloxacin did as well as those on prolonged treatment and had lower antibiotic costs and fewer secondary infections. The authors conclude that a subset of patients with low likelihood of pneumonia can be successfully treated with a short course of antibiotics. The CPIS needs further validation as a discriminatory tool, but it appears to be a good one.

Wunderink RG, et al. Linezolid vs vancomycin. Analysis of two double-blind studies of patients with methicillin-resistant *Staphylococcus aureus* nosocomial pneumonia. *Chest* 2003;124:1789–1797.

The authors conducted a retrospective analysis of two prospective double-blind studies of these agents for nosocomial pneumonia, and then also performed a subset analysis of patients with MRSA. It has been criticized for the methodology. However, conclusions that linezolid was associated with significantly better outcomes that included mortality and clinical cure are substantiated by the pulmonary pharmacokinetics of these agents. Vancomycin penetrates pulmonary tissue poorly at prescribed dosing. Anecdotally, many clinicians would favor linezolid for this condition, but cost becomes problematic. Prospective data are awaited.

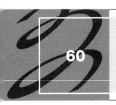

60 MANAGEMENT OF THE EMPLOYEE WITH A NEEDLESTICK INJURY

*A*ccidental needle punctures are a frequent hospital problem and a threat to the health of medical personnel. The reported rate is approximately 19 sharp injuries per 100 employees annually. Many needlestick injuries are not reported; in one study, 90% went unreported. Needlestick injuries account for nearly one-third of all work-related accidents in the hospital and are second only to musculoskeletal injuries as a cause of work-related illness. Of the reported needlesticks, about 90% occur among nursing personnel, housekeepers, and laboratory technicians. Registered nurses experience at least half of all needlestick injuries. The nursing activities during which most of the needlesticks occur are recapping needles, drawing blood, and administering an injection or infusion. Among housekeeping personnel, needlesticks usually result from handling trash containing improperly disposed needles. Laboratory workers report that most of the needle punctures happen while they are drawing blood and recapping needles. IV systems without needles have decreased the rate of sharp injuries. However, needlesticks still occur because compliance with these devices may be only 50%.

 ## EVALUATION OF EXPOSURE

When a needlestick occurs, the record of the patient who is the source should be reviewed with respect to status of hepatitis B virus (HBV), hepatitis C virus (HCV), and HIV. If the status is not known, the source person should be informed of the needlestick injury and serologic studies should be performed to evaluate for these bloodborne viral infections. Testing of needles themselves, regardless of whether the source is known, is not recommended.

In the patient who is HIV positive, additional information from the chart, such as CD4 count, viral load, and viral resistance testing may also be important.

MANAGEMENT OF EXPOSURE TO HBV

The Centers for Disease Control and Prevention (CDC), in 2001, updated guidelines for the management of and postexposure prophylaxis (PEP) for HBV, HVC, and HIV disease.

HBV infection is a risk to healthcare personnel because of needlesticks and other sources of blood exposure. Needlestick injury is among the most efficient methods of HBV transmission. Risk of infection is related to amount of blood exposure and the hepatitis B e antigen (HbeAG) status of the source. In studies of healthcare workers who sustained needlestick injuries with HBV-contaminated blood that was also HBeAG positive, risk of developing hepatitis was 22 to 31%. If HBeAG of the source is negative, the risk of transmission is much less—1 to 6%.

The centerpiece of prevention of hepatitis B in healthcare personnel is the hepatitis B vaccination. All personnel at risk of needlestick injuries should have already received the hepatitis B vaccine. The vaccine is extremely safe and effective. The CDC has not found associations with Guillain-Barré syndrome, multiple sclerosis or other autoimmune diseases. It is a three-dose series given by intramuscular injection in the deltoid. Those who do not respond to the series may be given a second series and have a 30 to 50% chance of responding.

When a needlestick occurs, the vaccination status and vaccine response status of the exposed person is reviewed. Recommendations for prophylaxis are based on this vaccine status and the HBsAg status of the exposure source. Table 60-1 summarizes these recommendations.

If a healthcare worker receives a needlestick from an HBsAg-positive source and the worker has not received the hepatitis B vaccine then the recommendation is for both vaccination with the hepatitis B series and one dose of hepatitis B immune globulin (HBIG). If the employee was a vaccine nonresponder, then the same recommendation stands. If the employee was a nonresponder to two regimens of the vaccine, then two doses of HBIG are recommended. If the employee has had a documented response to previous vaccination, then no prophylaxis is necessary for the needlestick. If the source is HBsAg negative, then again no prophylaxis is necessary. If the HBsAg source is not known, then a decision must be made based on the risk of the source; if the risk is high, then treatment would follow the same recommendations as if the source were HBsAg positive.

MANAGEMENT OF EXPOSURE TO HIV

The management of a needlestick exposure to an HIV-positive source has become more complex as more antiretroviral options become available and viral resistance becomes an increasing problem. Table 60-2 summarizes recommendations for management of needlestick injury from an HIV-positive source.

The decision to use a two-drug antiviral regimen versus a three-drug regimen depends on two factors:

1. The severity of exposure described by the CDC as less severe or more severe. *Less severe* suggests a solid needle and superficial injury. *More severe* describes a stick with a large bore needle, deep puncture, visible blood on the device, or needle used in a patient's artery or vein.
2. HIV-positive classification of the source. Class 1 describes an HIV-positive patient who is asymptomatic or has a low viral load. Class 2 is a patient with AIDS or symptomatic disease, seroconversion, or a high viral load.

The type of HIV exposure should be evaluated within hours. If the source person is seronegative, no further action is necessary. If antiretroviral therapy is to be started, it should be done as soon as possible.

Most exposures will require the two-drug regimen usually using two nucleoside analogues. Zidovudine and didanosine, lamivudine and stavudine, or stavudine and didanosine

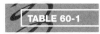

TABLE 60-1	Recommended Postexposure Prophylaxis for Exposure to HBV		
Vaccination and antibody response status of exposed workers*	Treatment		
	Source HBsAg† positive	Source HBsAg† negative	Source unknown or not available for testing
Unvaccinated	HBIG§ × 1 and initiate HB vaccine series¶	Initiate HB vaccine series	Initiate HB vaccine series
Previously vaccinated Known responder** Known nonresponder††	No treatment	No treatment	No treatment
Antibody response unknown	HBIG§§ × 1 and initiate revaccination or HBIG × 2	No treatment	If known high risk source, treat as if source were HBsAg positive
Antibody response unknown	Test exposed person for anti-HBs¶ 1. If adequate,** no treatment is necessary 2. If inadequate,¶ administer HBIG × 1 and vaccine booster	No treatment	Test exposed person for anti-HBs 1. If adequate,¶ no treatment is necessary 2. If inadequate,¶ administer vaccine booster and recheck titer in 1–2 months

*Persons who have previously been infected with HBV are immune to reinfection and do not require postexposure prophylaxis.
†Hepatitis B surface antigen.
§Hepatitis B immune globulin; dose is 0.06 mL/kg intramuscularly.
¶Hepatitis B vaccine.
** A responder is a person with adequate levels of serum antibody to HBsAg (i.e., anti-HBs ≥10 mIU/mL).
†† A nonresponder is a person with inadequate response to vaccination (i.e., serum anti-HBs <10 mIU/mL).
§§ The option of giving one dose of HBIG and reinitiating the vaccine series is preferred for nonresponders who have not completed a second 3-dose vaccine series. For persons who previously completed a second vaccine series but failed to respond, two doses of HBIG are preferred.
(Updated U.S. Public Health Service Guidelines for the Management of Occupational Exposures to HBV, HCV, and HIV and Recommendations for Postexposure Prophylaxis. *MMWR Morb Mortal Wkly Rep* 2001;50:1–42.)

all have been used. Expert consultation is advised when a three-drug regimen is chosen and when the source's virus is known and shows resistance.

 POSTEXPOSURE HIV TESTING

The individual with a needlestick exposure should receive follow-up counseling and postexposure testing. If given antiviral agents, he or she will require medical evaluation for potential side effects (hyperglycemia, anemia, crystalluria, depending on regimen used). HIV antibody testing should be performed at 6 weeks, 12 weeks, and 6 months. Testing with electroimmunoassay is recommended; direct viral assays have a higher false-positive rate and are discouraged. Individuals should be warned to use precautions to prevent secondary transmission during the follow-up period.¶

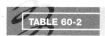

TABLE 60-2 Recommended HIV Postexposure Prophylaxis for Percutaneous Injuries

| Exposure type | Infection status of source | | | | |
	HIV-Positive Class 1*	HIV-Positive Class 2*	Source of unknown HIV-status†	Unknown source††	HIV-Negative
Less severe¶	Recommend basic 2-drug PEP	Recommend expanded 3-drug PEP	Generally, no PEP warranted; however, consider basic 2-drug PEP** for source with HIV risk factors††	Generally, no PEP warranted; however, consider basic 2-drug PEP** in settings where exposure to HIV-infected persons is likely	No PEP warranted
More severe¶¶	Recommend expanded 3-drug PEP	Recommend expanded 3-drug PEP	Generally, no PEP warranted; however, consider basic 2-drug PEP** for source with HIV risk factors††	Generally, no PEP warranted; however, consider basic 2-drug PEP** in settings where exposure to HIV-infected persons is likely	No PEP warranted

*HIV-Positive, Class 1—asymptomatic HIV infection or known low viral load (e.g., <1,500 RNA copies/mL). HIV-Positive, Class 2—symptomatic HIV infection, AIDS, acute seroconversion, or known high viral load. If drug resistance is a concern, obtain expert consultation. Initiation of postexposure prophylaxis (PEP) should not be delayed pending expert consultation, and because expert consultation alone cannot substitute for face-to-face counseling, resources should be available to provide immediate evaluation and follow-up care for all exposures.
†Source of unknown HIV status (e.g., deceased source person with no samples available for HIV testing).
††Unknown source (e.g., a needle from a sharps disposal container).
¶Less severe (e.g., solid needle and superficial injury).
**The designation "consider PEP" indicates that PEP is optional and should be based on an individualized decision between the exposed person and the treating clinician.
††If PEP is offered and taken and the source is later determined to be HIV-negative, PEP should be discontinued.
¶¶More severe (e.g., large-bore hollow needle, deep puncture, visible blood on device, or needle used in patient's artery or vein).

MANAGEMENT OF EXPOSURE TO HCV

HCV generally is not effectively transmitted through occupational exposure to blood. The incidence of conversion after needlestick from an HCV-positive source is only 1.8%. There appears to be little convincing data that the use of immune globulin prevents seroconversion. Interferon also has not been proved effective as postexposure prophylaxis and is not approved for this purpose by the Food and Drug Administration. Intervention with interferon when HCV DNA first becomes detectable may be beneficial. However, this too is controversial, as 25% of infected patients resolve spontaneously and a beneficial effect of treating acute infection is still not proved.

The postexposure management of HCV includes:

1. Perform baseline testing for anti-HCV and ALT activity.
2. Perform follow-up testing at 4 to 6 months
3. Confirm anti-HCV tests with a recombinant immunoblot assay.

The exposed employee does not need to take precautions to prevent secondary transmission but should refrain from donating blood or other body fluids through the evaluation period. When seroconversion is documented, the individual should be referred to a specialist for follow-up evaluation. (SLB)

Bibliography

Bell DM, Gerberding JL. Human immunodeficiency virus (HIV) postexposure management of health care workers. *Am J Med* 1997;102:1–126.
>*The entire issue is devoted to HIV postexposure management. The Public Health Service suggests that an exposed healthcare provider be followed for 6 months (e.g., 6 weeks, 12 weeks, and 6 months) to detect HIV seroconversion.*

Cardo DM, et al. A case-control study of HIV seroconversion in health care workers after percutaneous exposure. *N Engl J Med* 1997;337:1485–1490.
>*Factors associated with an increased risk for HIV transmission include deep injury, injury with a device that is visibly contaminated with blood, procedures that involve inserting a needle into the source patient's artery or vein, and a terminally ill source patient.*

Centers for Disease Control and Prevention. Updated U.S. Public Health Service Guidelines for the Management of Occupational Exposures to HBV, HCV, and HIV and Recommendations for Postexposure Prophylaxis. *MMWR Morb Mortal Wkly Rep* 2001;50:1–42.

Centers for Disease Control and Prevention. Evaluation of safety devices for preventing percutaneous injuries among health care workers during phlebotomy procedures, Minneapolis-St. Paul, New York City, and San Francisco, 1993–1995. *MMWR Morb Mortal Wkly Rep* 1997;46:21–25.
>*Injuries associated with phlebotomy account for 39% of cases of HIV seroconversion. Use of safety devices can decrease the sharp injuries related to phlebotomy.*

Centers for Disease Control and Prevention. Evaluation of blunt suture needles in preventing percutaneous injuries among health care workers during gynecologic surgical procedures, New York City, March 1993–June 1994. *MMWR Morb Mortal Wkly Rep* 1997;46:25–29.
>*Blunt rather than curved suture needles were associated with fewer sharp injuries.*

Centers for Disease Control and Prevention. Recommendations for follow-up of health care workers after occupational exposure to hepatitis C virus. *MMWR Morb Mortal Wkly Rep* 1997;46:603–606.
>*Guidelines for the management of an HCV exposure, now updated.*

Dienstag JL, et al. Hepatitis B vaccine in health care personnel: safety, immunogenicity, and indicators of efficacy. *Ann Intern Med* 1984;101:34.
>*Ninety-seven percent of vaccine recipients responded to three doses of vaccine.*

Gerberding JL, et al. Risk of exposure of surgical personnel to patients' blood during surgery at San Francisco General Hospital. *N Engl J Med* 1990;322:1788.
>*Parenteral exposures occurred in 1.7% of operations. Risk was greatest with procedures lasting more than 3 hours, blood loss exceeding 300 mL, and major vascular and intra-abdominal gynecologic surgery.*

Hoofnagle JH, et al. Passive-active immunity from hepatitis B immune globulin. *Ann Intern Med* 1979;91:813.
>*Efficacy of HBIG documented.*

Ippolito G, et al. The risk of occupational human immunodeficiency virus infection in health care workers. *Arch Intern Med* 1993;153:1451.
>*The rate of seroconversion was 0.25% after percutaneous exposure and 0.09% after mucous membrane contamination. The rate of seroconversion after HIV contamination of nonintact skin is even lower than with a mucous membrane exposure.*

Lawrence LW, et al. The effectiveness of a needleless intravenous connection system: an assessment by injury rate and user satisfaction. *Infect Control Hosp Epidemiol* 1997; 18:175–182.
Use of a needleless IV connection system was associated with about a 50% reduction in needlesticks.

L'Ecuyer PB, et al. Randomized prospective study of the impact of three needleless intravenous systems on needlestick injury rates. *Infect Control Hosp Epidemiol* 1996;17:803–808.
Needlestick injuries can occur despite the availability of needleless devices.

Mangione CM, Gerberding JL, Cummings SR. Occupational exposure to HIV: frequency and rates of underreporting of percutaneous and mucocutaneous exposures by medical house staff. *Am J Med* 1991;90:85.
Only 30% of sharp injuries were reported by the house staff.

Manian FA, Meyer L, Jenne J. Puncture injuries due to needles removed from intravenous lines: should the source patient routinely be tested for blood-borne infections? *Infect Control Hosp Epidemiol* 1993;14:325.
Testing of source blood is unnecessary in injuries caused by needles from peripheral IV lines and distal ports of central lines unless blood is seen.

McCormick RD, et al. Epidemiology of hospital sharps injuries: a 14-year prospective study in the pre-AIDS and AIDS eras. *Am J Med* 1991;91(suppl 3B):301S–307S.
Injuries occurred during disposal of used procedure trays (20%), administration of parenteral drugs (16%), surgery (16%), blood drawing (13%), and recapping of used needles (10%).

Patel N, Tignor GH. Device-specific sharps injury and usage rates: an analysis by hospital department. *Am J Infect Control* 1997;25:77–84.
Reported injury rates per 100,000 devices. Injury rates were 11.1/100,000 for butterfly needles and 8.5/100,000 for IV catheters.

Petrosillo N, et al. The risks of occupational exposure and infection by human immunodeficiency virus, hepatitis B virus, and hepatitis C virus in the dialysis setting. *Am J Infect Control* 1995;23:278–285.
In this dialysis unit, a seroprevalence survey revealed HIV antibody (0.1%), HBsA (5.1%), and HCV antibody (39.4%).

Puro V, Petrosillo N, Ippolito G. Risk of hepatitis C seroconversion after occupational exposures in health care workers. *Am J Infect Control* 1995;23:273–277.
Risk for HCV seroconversion after a hollow-bore needlestick was 1.2% and 0 after mucous membrane contamination.

Resnic FS, Noerdlinger MA. Occupational exposure among medical students and house staff at a New York City Medical Center. *Arch Intern Med* 1995;155:75–80.
Half the surgical house officers, 27% of students, and 20% of medical house staff noted an exposure (sharp injury, mucous membrane, or broken skin) to a patient's blood within the past 6 months.

Seef LB, et al. Long-term mortality and morbidity of transfusion-associated non-A, non-B and type C hepatitis: a National Heart, Lung, and Blood Institute collaborative study. *Hepatology* 2001;33:455.
In patients with acute HCV infection, 15 to 25% resolve their infection spontaneously.

Tack PC, et al. Genotypic analysis of HIV-1 isolates to identify antiretroviral resistance mutations from source patients involved in health care worker occupational exposures. *JAMA* 1999;281:1085.
Describes emergence of drug-resistant HIV as source of healthcare worker exposures.

Tokars JI, et al. Surveillance of HIV infection and zidovudine use among health care workers after occupational exposure to HIV-infected blood. *Ann Intern Med* 1993;118:913.
Rate of seroconversion after percutaneous exposure to HIV-infected blood was 0.36%. Failures of zidovudine prophylaxis have occurred.

Wang SA, et al. Experience of healthcare workers taking postexposure prophylaxis after occupational HIV exposures. *Infect Control Hosp Epidemiol* 2000;21:780.
Describes safety of PEP regimens, specifically in employees with accidental exposures.

Zoonoses 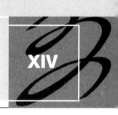 XIV

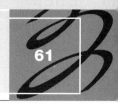

HUMAN INFECTIONS AFTER ANIMAL BITES **61**

$\mathcal{E}$ach year millions of people in the United States are bitten by animals. Approximately 2 to 5% of all typical dog bite wounds seen in emergency departments become infected. Most animal bites are from dogs; cat bites are second most common. However, the risk of infection from a cat bite is much higher than from a dog bite. Cat bites have a high incidence of infection (approximately 50%), but dog bites may cause severe injury to tissues. Dogs have wider canines, unlike cats which have thinner ones. Approximately 15% of dog bites are to the head and neck, 20% to the leg or foot and 15% to the upper extremity. Cat bites are typically characterized by puncture wounds.

Bite wounds in joint spaces may be complicated by septic arthritis. Deep wounds may be complicated by bone infections, such as osteomyelitis.

 INITIAL ASSESSMENT

It is important to determine the risk of rabies from each potential exposure. A careful history and physical should be performed as soon as possible. The physician should explore for damage to tissues caused by crushing or tearing and search for damaged tendons, blood vessels, joints, and bones. Attention to the details of a biting incident can be critical to management (Table 61-1). Foreign bodies, such as tooth fragments, may be demonstrated on radiographs. Any available discharge should be cultured and baseline complete blood count (CBC) and chemistry obtained. Culture specimens for both aerobic and anaerobic bacteria should be obtained from animal bite wounds. In wounds that are contaminated by soil or vegetative debris, cultures for mycobacteria and fungi should be done. The use of Gram's stain as an indicator of the presence of pathogens in the wound can be of assistance. Blood cultures may be useful in more critically ill patients, especially those missing a spleen (*Capnocytophaga canimorsus*).

 GENERAL MANAGEMENT

Whether bite wounds that are clinically uninfected and are seen within 24 hours should be surgically closed remains controversial. Surgical consultation is advised. Rabies prevention should be instituted after dog bites, if indicated, and a tetanus toxoid booster should be administered if the patient has been adequately immunized previously and has received the last dose within the past 10 years. Tetanus immune globulin (human) is required if tetanus immunization has not taken place or is inadequate.

Antibiotic Therapy

Antibiotic prophylaxis is considered reasonable if the risk of infection is 5 to 10%. Dog bite wounds carry reported infection rates from 1.6 to 30%. As noted earlier, cat bites carry a greater risk of infection. The clinical features of the wound and type of injury are important factors to consider when choosing to give antibiotic prophylaxis. The location (hand, wrist,

TABLE 61-1   Initial Assessment of Bite Victims

History	Physical	Assess rabies risk	Wound care	Reasons to admit
Important details in the history include the type of animal that attacked the patient, behavior of the animal, and time of day the bite occurred. Document the address or location of the attack and the time of the attack. Ascertain ownership of the animal, current location of the animal, and rabies vaccination status. Document prehospital care (e.g., wound cleansing). Document the patient's allergies, current medications, medical history, immunization status, and the time of the last meal.	Ensure that no compromise of circulation, motor skills, or sensation exists. Nerve function Tendon function Blood supply (pulses) Bone penetration Cat bites may appear innocuous but may penetrate deeper than expected from initial inspection. Animal bites might leave teeth fragments and require radiographs. Be sure to photograph the wounds, if possible	Provoked attacks Antagonizing an animal Hurting an animal Unprovoked attacks Approaching the young of an animal Approaching an animal that is eating Entering the property of a territorial animal	Irrigation Debridement Elevation	Fever > 100.5°F Sepsis Compromised host Acute septic arthritis or bone injury Tendon/nerve injury

foot, scalp, face, joint) of a wound is important, as is the type (puncture, laceration, crush injury, edema) of wound present. The species of the animal will help determine the flora that might be present in the wound (see Tables 61-2 and 61-3).

Some patients appear to be at a higher risk of infection or will have more complications after a bite. These types of patients would include, but not be limited to, diabetics, cirrhotics, asplenics, transplants, those taking immunosuppressives, and those at the extremes of age. Duration of therapy is listed in Table 61-4. Generally amoxicillin-clavulanate is the drug of choice for prophylaxis as it covers the most common pathogens. Alternatives for penicillin-allergic patients are listed in Table 61-5. Empiric therapy for established infection would typically include a parental form of the drugs listed in Table 61-5, but definitive treatment should be based on culture results.

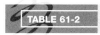

TABLE 61-2 Microbiology of Common Animal Bites

Species	Organism	Prevention of infection	Other information
Cat bite	*Pasteurella multocida, Staphylococcus aureus,* streptococci	Amoxicillin-clavulanic acid, 875 mg bid or 500 mg tid for 3–5 days	A high percentage of cat bites become infected without prophylaxis First-generation cephalosporins not as active as penicillin against *P. multocida,* which is present in oral flora of 50–70% of cats
Dog bite	Viridans streptococci, oral anaerobes, *S. aureus, P. multocida, Capnocytophaga canimorsus* (formerly DF-2)	Amoxicillin-clavulanic acid, 875 mg bid or 500 mg tid for 3–5 days	Infection less common than with cat or human bites; need for routine prophylaxis for all bites uncertain; persons without spleens at risk of overwhelming *Capnocytophaga* sepsis, should receive prophylaxis following any dog bite

TABLE 61-3 Less Common Animal Bites

Species	Microbiology
Monkey bites	B virus (also known as *Herpesvirus simiae* or Cercopithecine herpes virus 1)
Bird pecking and bites	*Streptococcus bovis, Clostridium tertium,* and *Aspergillus niger. Bacteroides* species *Pseudomonas aeruginosa.*
Ferrets	*Staphylococcus aureus*
Horse bites	*S. aureus, Streptococcus* spp., *Neisseria* spp., *Escherichia coli, Actinobacillus lignieresii, Pasteurella* species, *Bacteroides ureolyticus, B. fragilis,* other anaerobic gram-negative bacilli, *Prevotella melaninogenica,* and *P. heparinolytica*
Pig bites	*Staphylococcus* spp., *Streptococcus* spp. (including *S. sanguis, S. suis,* and *S. milleri*), diphtheroids, *Pasteurella multocida,* other *Pasteurella* spp., *Haemophilus influenzae, Actinobacillus suis, Flavobacterium* IIb–like organisms, *Bacteroides fragilis,* and other anaerobic gram-negative bacilli
Sheep bites	*Actinobacillus* spp.
Rat	*Streptobacillus moniliformis, Spirillum minus*
Freshwater injury	Snake and leech bites have also resulted in *Aeromonas* infections
Saltwater injury	Vibrio species

TABLE 61-4 Duration of Antibiotics	
Type of wound	**Duration of treatment**
If seen < 8 hr after injury*	Prophylaxis for 3–5 days
Cellulitis	7–14 days
Bone/Joint	Treat for 3–8 weeks

*Considerations for antibiotic prophylaxis should include:
   Wounds seen less than 8 hours after infliction that are moderate or severe, with crush injury or
     edema
   Those that might involve bones or joints
   Cat bites may penetrate deeper than expected
   Punctures, especially those that occur near a joint
   Hand wounds
   Wounds in those with comorbid conditions such as immunosuppression

Rabies Assessment

Rabies is a viral infection transmitted through the saliva of infected mammals. The virus spreads to the central nervous system, causing an encephalomyelitis that progresses to coma and death. On average, one to two cases of human rabies and 5,000 to 10,000 cases of animal rabies are reported in the United States each year. The World Health Organization (http://www.rabnet.who.int) keeps a list of countries supposedly free of rabies.

Rabies virus is transmitted in the saliva of mammals, almost always by a bite. Rabies in humans has an incubation period of 1 to 3 months, but occasionally periods may be as short as a week or may last as long as several years. In about 75% of cases, the incubation period is between 20 and 90 days. If the bite was caused by an animal that is likely to have rabies in that particular geographic location, that animal should be confined or euthanized.

If the animal tests positive or if it is unavailable for testing, the patient should receive rabies postexposure prophylaxis (PEP; Table 61-6). Regardless of the length of the interval between true rabies exposure and presentation of the healthy patient, PEP should be initiated as soon as possible after the bite. A healthy domestic dog, cat, or ferret that bites a person should be confined and observed for 10 days. Any illness in the animal should be evaluated by a veterinarian and reported immediately to the local health department and attending physician. If signs suggestive of rabies develop, human prophylaxis is begun without delay. If the suspected animal is determined to be a stray dog, cat, or ferret, rather than being confined as above, it may be euthanized, the head removed and the package shipped, under refrigeration, for examination by a qualified diagnostic laboratory to make an assessment.

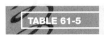

TABLE 61-5 Prophylactic Choice of Antibiotic*	
Not allergic to penicillins	**Allergic**
Amoxicillin-clavulanate 875/125 mg P.O. b.i.d.	Clindamycin plus either ciprofloxacin or TMP-SMX
Covers gram-positive, *Pasteurella*, some gram-negative rods and anaerobes	Combination therapy will cover the above pathogens. Give Bactrim to children if possible. Doxycycline has activity against *Pasteurella* as well. Give for 3–5 days

*Consider giving the first dose intravenously if possible.
TMP-SMX, trimethoprim-sulfamethoxazole.

TABLE 61-6 **PEP Recommendations for Rabies**

Geography	Animals	Bite *	Nonbite†
Group 1: Rabies enzootic or suspected in species involved in the exposure	Bat, raccoon, skunk, fox, coyote; mongoose in Puerto Rico; stray dogs and cats along border with Mexico	Offer PEP	Offer PEP
Group 2: Rabies not enzootic in species involved in the exposure but reported in other animals in region (e.g. most of continental USA)	Most wild carnivores (wolf, cougar, bobcat, bear, etc.)	Offer PEP	Offer PEP or consult with public health authorities
	Domestic dogs, cats, and ferrets	Observe or consult. Can observe for 10 days	Observe or consult
	Wild rodents and lagomorphs, except groundhogs	Consult or do not treat	No PEP offered
	Livestock	Consult or do not treat	No PEP offered
Group 3: Rabies not enzootic in species involved in the exposure and only sporadic reports in region (e.g., Pacific Northwest)	Dogs, cats, other domestic animals and many wild terrestrial animals	Consult or do not treat	Consult or do not treat
Group 4: Rabies not reported in region (e.g., Hawaii, Guam, Samoa, Virgin Islands, etc.)	Any terrestrial mammal	No PEP offered	No PEP offered

*Any penetration of the skin by teeth constitutes a bite exposure. All bites, regardless of location, represent a potential risk of rabies transmission. Bites by some animals, such as bats, can inflict minor injury and thus remain undetected.
†Nonbite exposures from terrestrial animals rarely cause rabies. However, occasional reports of transmission by nonbite exposure suggest that such exposures constitute sufficient reason to consider postexposure prophylaxis. The nonbite exposures of highest risk appear to be among persons exposed to large amounts of aerosolized rabies virus and surgical recipients of corneas transplanted from patients who died of rabies. The contamination of open wounds, abrasions, mucous membranes, or theoretically, scratches, with saliva or other potentially infectious material (such as neural tissue) from a rabid animal also constitutes a nonbite exposure. Other contact by itself, such as petting a rabid animal and contact with blood, urine, or feces (e.g., guano) of a rabid animal, does not constitute an exposure and is not an indication for prophylaxis. Because the rabies virus is inactivated by desiccation and ultraviolet irradiation, in general, if the material containing the virus is dry, the virus can be considered noninfectious. (Adapted from http://www.cdc.gov/epo/mmwr/preview/mmwrhtml/00056176.htm.)

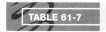

TABLE 61-7 **PEP Administration for Rabies***

Intramuscular vaccine	Rabies immune globulin (RIG)
The standard regimen is one dose of tissue culture vaccine (1 mL or 0.5 mL, depending on the product) intramuscularly into the deltoid on days 0, 3, 7, 14, and 28.	A single dose of 20 IU/kg of human RIG or 40 IU/kg of equine RIG is given at the same time as the first dose of vaccine. As much as possible is infiltrated into and around the wound, but care is needed when injecting into fingers or other tight tissue compartments. Any remaining vaccine is injected intramuscularly away from the vaccine site

*Postexposure treatment of previously vaccinated patients.
RIG treatment is unnecessary. Treatment is always urgent, but provided that the patient has previously had a complete pre-exposure or postexposure course of tissue culture vaccine or if a neutralizing antibody level has been over 0.5 I U/mL at some time, only two doses of intramuscular vaccine are needed on days 0 and 3.

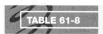

TABLE 61-8 **Information for Patients**

First aid for bites	Preventing bites
Don't put the bitten area in your mouth! You will just be adding the bacteria in your mouth to that already in the wound. If the wound is superficial, wash the area thoroughly. Use soap and water or an antiseptic such as hydrogen peroxide or alcohol. Apply an antibiotic ointment and cover with a nonstick bandage. Watch the area carefully to see if there are signs of damaged nerves or tendons. Some bruising may develop, but the wound should heal within a week to 10 days. If it does not, or if you see signs of infection or damage to nerves and tendons, seek medical help. If there is bleeding, apply direct pressure with a clean, dry cloth. Elevate the area. Do not clean a wound that is actively bleeding. Cover the wound with a clean sterile dressing and always seek medical help. If the wound is to the face or head and neck area, seek medical help immediately. Contact your physician to see whether additional treatment is needed. Report the incident to your public health department. They may ask your assistance in locating the animal so that it can be confined and observed for symptoms of rabies.	Do not try to separate fighting animals. Avoid animals that appear sick or act strangely. Keep pets on a leash when out in public. Never leave a young child alone with a pet. Do not allow children to tease an animal by waving sticks, throwing stones, or pulling a tail. Be sure pets are vaccinated. Teach children not to pet strange animals, even pets on a leash, without asking permission of the owner first.

(Adapted from http://www.orthoinfo.org/fact/thr_report.cfm?Thread_ID=390&topcategory=Hand.)

Two types of rabies immunizing products are available in the United States (Table 61-7).

1. Rabies vaccines induce an active immune response that includes the production of neutralizing antibodies. This antibody response requires approximately 7 to 10 days to develop and usually persists for 2 years or longer.

2. Rabies immune globulin (RIG) provides a rapid, passive immunity that persists for only a short time (half-life of approximately 21 days).

In all postexposure prophylaxis regimens, except for persons previously immunized, both products should be used concurrently (Table 61-7). The deltoid area is an acceptable site of vaccination in adults and older children; the outer aspect of the thigh may be used in younger children. Vaccine should never be administered in the gluteal area. People who have been vaccinated previously are those with a history of pre-exposure vaccination with human diploid cell rabies vaccine (HDCV), purified chick embryo cell (PCEC) or rabies vaccine activated (RVA), prior postexposure prophylaxis with HDCV, PCEC, or RVA or previous vaccination with any other type of rabies vaccine and documented history of antibody response to the prior vaccination.

Table 61-8 provides information for patients regarding animal bites. (JWM)

Bibliography

Brook I. Microbiology and management of human and animal bite wound infections. *Prim Care* 2003;30:25–39, v.
> *This article describes the microbiology, diagnosis, and management of human and animal bite wound infections. Superb review article.*

Cummings P. Antibiotics to prevent infection in patients with dog bite wounds: a meta-analysis of randomized trials. *Ann Emerg Med* 1994;23:535–540.
> *The full costs and benefits of antibiotics in this situation are not known. It may be reasonable to limit prophylactic antibiotics to patients with wounds that are at high risk for infection.*

De Roodt AR, et al. [Poisoning by spiders of Loxosceles genus]. *Medicina (B Aires)* 2002;62: 83–94.
> *Despite the great number of spiders in the world, only a small group of them is capable of producing death in humans. These data provide biological and biochemical tools to understand the course of poisoning and to have better criteria for the treatment and prevention of these accidents and their complications.*

Dieter RA Jr, et al. Bear mauling: a descriptive review. *Int J Circumpolar Health* 2001;60: 696–704.
> *The chance of a human encountering a bear increases as the remote bear territory diminishes. Bear incidents are widely publicized, though few serious incidents occur.*

Durrheim DN, Leggat PA. Risk to tourists posed by wild mammals in South Africa. *J Travel Med* 1999;6:172–179.
> *Local advice on personal safety in wildlife reserves and the credentials of trail guides should be obtained from lodge or reserve management, tourism authorities, or the travel industry before travel to game reserves.*

Elston DM. What's eating you? Centipedes (Chilopoda). *Cutis* 1999;64:83.

Elston DM. What's eating you? Echidnophaga gallinacea (the sticktight flea). *Cutis* 2001;68:250.

Elston DM, Stockwell S. What's eating you? Bedbugs. *Cutis* 2000;65:262–264.

Elston DM, Stockwell S. What's eating you? Centruroides exilicauda. *Cutis* 2002;69: 16, 20.

Forks TP. Brown recluse spider bites. *J Am Board Fam Pract* 2000;13:415–423.
> *Most brown recluse spider bites are asymptomatic. All bites should be thoroughly cleansed and tetanus status updated as needed. Patients who develop systemic symptoms require hospitalization. Surgical excision of skin lesions is indicated only for lesions that have stabilized and are no longer enlarging. Steroids are indicated in bites that are associated with severe skin lesions, loxoscelism, and in small children. Dapsone should be used only in adult patients who experience necrotic arachnidism and who have been screened*

for glucose-6-phosphate dehydrogenase deficiency. Topical nitroglycerin can be of value in decreasing the enlargement of necrotic skin ulcers.

Gibbons RV. Cryptogenic rabies, bats, and the question of aerosol transmission. *Ann Emerg Med* 2002;39:528–536.

The known pathogenesis of rabies and available data suggest that all or nearly all cases of human rabies attributable to bats were transmitted by bat bites that were minimized or unrecognized by the patients.

Glaser C, et al. Pet-, animal-, and vector-borne infections. *Pediatr Rev* 2000;21:219–232.

Goldstein EJ Current concepts on animal bites: bacteriology and therapy. *Curr Clin Top Infect Dis* 1999;19: 99–111.

Greenstein P. Tick paralysis. *Med Clin North Am* 2002;86:441–446.

Tick paralysis is a preventable cause of morbidity and death that, when diagnosed promptly, requires a simple low-cost intervention. The key to success is to consider tick paralysis in the differential diagnosis of ascending weakness, particularly in children, in geographic areas where this disease predominates.

Heard K, et al. Antivenom therapy in the Americas. *Drugs* 1999;58:5–15.

Envenomations are an important cause of injury in the Americas. Supportive care alone may result in an acceptable outcome; however, antivenom offers a specific therapy that can significantly reduce the injury and symptoms of the envenomation.

Hirschhorn RB, Hodge RR Identification of risk factors in rat bite incidents involving humans. *Pediatrics* 1999;104:e35.

Risk factors for potential rat bite victims still exist and can be identified for additional planning of intervention and prevention strategies.

Juckett G, Hancox JG. Venomous snakebites in the United States: management review and update. *Am Fam Physician* 2002;65:1367–1374.

Venomous snakebites, although uncommon, are a potentially deadly emergency in the United States.

Kemp SF, et al. Expanding habitat of the imported fire ant (Solenopsis invicta): a public health concern. *J Allergy Clin Immunol* 2000;105:683–691.

This article reviews the medically important entomology, clinical aspects of stings, and the current approaches to chemical control of fire ants. We also propose directions for future research and treatment.

Medeiros I, Saconato H. Antibiotic prophylaxis for mammalian bites. *Cochrane Database Syst Rev* 2001;2:CD001738.

There is evidence from one trial that prophylactic antibiotics reduce the risk of infection after human bites, but confirmatory research is required. There is no evidence that the use of prophylactic antibiotics is effective for cat or dog bites. There is evidence that the use of antibiotic prophylactic after bites of the hand reduces infection, but confirmatory research is required.

Messenger SL, et al. Emerging epidemiology of bat-associated cryptic cases of rabies in humans in the United States. *Clin Infect Dis* 2002;35:738–747.

In the United States during the past half-century, the number of humans to die of rabies dramatically decreased to an average of 1 to 2 per year. Although the number of deaths is low, most deaths occur because individuals are unaware that they had been exposed to and infected with rabies virus and, therefore, do not seek effective postexposure treatment. Molecular epidemiologic studies have linked most of these cryptic rabies exposures to rabies virus variants associated with insectivorous bats. In particular, virus variants associated with two relatively reclusive species, the silver-haired bat (Lasionycteris noctivagans)and the eastern pipistrelle (Pipistrellus subflavus), are the unexpected culprits of most cryptic cases of rabies in humans.

Noah DL, et al. Epidemiology of human rabies in the United States, 1980 to 1996. *Ann Intern Med* 1998;128:922–930.

In the United States, human rabies is rare but probably underdiagnosed. Rabies should be included in the differential diagnosis of any case of acute, rapidly progressing encephalitis, even if the patient does not recall being bitten by an animal. In addition to situations involving an animal bite, a scratch from an animal, or contact of mucous membranes with infectious saliva, postexposure prophylaxis should be considered if the history indicates that a bat was physically present, even if the person is unable to reliably report contact that could have resulted in a bite. Such a situation may arise when a bat bite causes an insignificant wound or the circumstances do not allow recognition of contact, such as when a bat is found in the room of a sleeping person or near a previously unattended child.

Parola P, Raoult D. Ticks and tickborne bacterial diseases in humans: an emerging infectious threat. *Clin Infect Dis* 2001;32:897–928.

Ticks are currently considered to be second only to mosquitoes as vectors of human infectious diseases in the world. Methods are described for the detection and isolation of bacteria from ticks and advice is given on how tick bites may be prevented and how clinicians should deal with patients who have been bitten by ticks.

Presutti RJ. Prevention and treatment of dog bites. *Am Fam Physician* 2001;63:1567–1572.

The dog bite injury should be documented with photographs and diagrams when appropriate. Family physicians should educate parents and children on ways to prevent dog bites.

Rhoades R. Stinging ants. *Curr Opin Allergy Clin Immunol* 2001;1:343–348.

Ants belong to the order Hymenoptera, along with bees, wasps, yellow jackets, etc., and are the most successful animal genera in this world. This article reviews the history and recent developments regarding stinging ants around the world.

Smith PF, et al. Treating mammalian bite wounds. Antibiotic prophylaxis for mammalian bites. *J Clin Pharm Ther* 2000;25:85–99.

Review article.

Woolgar JD, et al. Shark attack: review of 86 consecutive cases. *J Trauma* 2001;50:887–891.

Victims of shark attack usually sustain only minor injuries. In more serious cases, particularly if associated with a major vascular injury, hemorrhage control and early resuscitation are of utmost importance during the initial management if these patients are to survive.

Newly Appreciated Infections

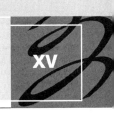

XV

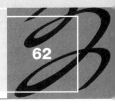

62

$\mathcal{S}$ince 1999, when infection secondary to West Nile virus was first reported in New York, this virus should be added to the differential diagnosis of patients presenting with a febrile illness with a rash, aseptic meningitis, encephalitis, or a polio-like illness. The virus was first described in a woman with a febrile illness in 1937 in the West Nile district of Uganda. The disease continued to occur in Africa, Israel, Romania, and Russia. In the United States, West Nile virus infection was reported for the first time in 1999 in New York City. Since that time, the virus has spread dramatically across the United States with about 10,000 cases reported in the year 2003 and one-third of those infections being reported from Colorado. In 2004, there were more than 2,000 cases across the United States, with California and Arizona leading the nation. Most states reported human cases in the year 2004.

West Nile virus is an arbovirus (arthropod-borne agent) and a member of the flavivirus genus which also includes yellow fever virus, dengue virus, St. Louis encephalitis virus, Japanese encephalitis virus and tickborne encephalitis virus (Powassan virus). West Nile is a single strain RNA virus.

EPIDEMIOLOGY

West Nile virus is transmitted by the bite of an infected mosquito (primarily *Culex pipiens* or *Culex tarsales*) in the United States. The mosquito acquires the virus from feeding on an infected bird, the amplifying host. Humans and other vertebrates such as horses, dogs, and cats are incidental hosts. Mosquitoes cannot transmit the infection by biting an infected human or other vertebrate. Nearly all human cases are due to a mosquito bite. Rarely, transmission occurs through a transplanted organ, transfused blood, transplacentally, from breast milk, or by a needlestick. Some wild birds develop prolonged high levels of viremia but may be asymptomatic. Other birds such as crows, ravens, and jays may die of the infection. The incubation period ranges from 3 to 14 days but may be longer in the compromised host. Dogs and cats can be infected in the same way as humans. Horses with West Nile virus encephalitis have a 40% mortality rate. A vaccine to prevent West Nile virus is available for horses.

PATHOGENESIS

The pathogenesis of severe infection with West Nile virus is unknown, but older people and compromised hosts have a higher morbidity and mortality rate. The virus can cause destruction of spinal anterior horn cells and infiltrates in the posterior thalamus, basal ganglia, and brainstem. Since 1996, the West Nile virus has become more virulent, resulting in more severe disease.

CLINICAL MANIFESTATIONS

Approximately 80% of persons infected with West Nile virus are asymptomatic, resulting in antibody production and probably lifelong immunity. Some patients have a febrile illness with headache, myalgias, rash, nausea, and vomiting. The illness resembles dengue fever.

377

The rash is maculopapular in appearance and is not pruritic. The rash mimics that seen in patients with enteroviral infection, which occurs during the same season. Neuroinvasive disease is characterized by encephalitis, meningoencephalitis, or acute flaccid paralysis resembling polio. Movement disorders, such as a tremor or myoclonus, may be prominent. Ataxia may occur with symptoms resembling Parkinson's disease. Among survivors, long-term cognitive and neurologic impairment may occur. Rarely, myocarditis, pancreatitis, or hepatitis may occur. Ocular manifestations include bilateral vitreitis and chorioretinitis. Typically, symptomatic West Nile virus infection does not usually cause a self-limited viral illness.

 DIAGNOSIS

West Nile virus infection should be considered in the differential diagnosis of febrile patients in the late summer and fall in the northern and western states and year-round in the more southern states. The peripheral white cell count is normal or increased. In patients with meningitis, the cerebrospinal fluid shows an increased cell count of 300 to 1,500 cells/mm^3 with a lymphocyte predominance, elevated protein, and normal glucose. The diagnosis is usually established by serologic testing. The serum will show elevated IgM and IgG antibodies to West Nile virus, and the spinal fluid will demonstrate an elevated West Nile virus IgM antibody. Antibody production can be delayed as long as 30 days in compromised hosts. The diagnosis can be confirmed with viral neutralization studies in special laboratories. Nuclear acid amplification tests (polymerase chain reaction [PCR]) lack the sensitivity for diagnosis using serum or cerebrospinal fluid (CSF). Serum IgM antibody may be detected for 1 year after the diagnosis, and the IgG antibody probably remains elevated for life. Other flaviviruses may produce antibodies that cross-react with West Nile virus, resulting in false-positive test results. Blood used for donation is screened for West Nile virus since 2003. Blood donors with low levels of viremia may not be detected.

 TREATMENT

There is no specific therapy to treat West Nile virus infection. It is critical to establish diagnosis and provide supportive care. Data available are anecdotal and include the use of interferon, specific intravenous immune globulin derived from Israeli donors with high-titer IgG, ribavirin, and antisense therapy. Steroids do not appear to be beneficial, but again, controlled trials are lacking.

A vaccine for humans is being studied. Because specific therapy is lacking, prevention by avoiding mosquito bites is critical. Peak mosquito biting times span from dusk to dawn. Apply insect repellant containing N, N-diethyl-meta-toluamide (DEET). DEET can be used in pregnancy and for children older than age 2 months. A concentration of 23.8% DEET provides about 5 hours of protection. Concentrations of DEET higher than 25% are unnecessary. Some products with 2% soybean oil may provide protection. Other protective measures include using protective clothing, mosquito proofing your home, and draining standing water where mosquitoes can breed. Remember the 4 Ds: DEET, Dress, Dusk to Dawn, and Drain).

 PROGNOSIS

Morbidity and mortality are higher in older and immunosuppressed patients with a fatality rate of 15 to 20 % in patients with central nervous system (CNS) disease. Persistent neurologic defects are common. In a study of outcomes for New York, more than 5% of patients have persistent symptoms at 1 year after infection. This can be a devastating illness for some patients with neuroinvasive disease. (NMG)

Bibliography

Anninger WV, et al. West Nile virus-associated optic neuritis and chorioretinitis. *Am J Ophthalmol* 2003;136:1183–1185.
A review of eye findings.

Emig M, Apple DJ. Severe West Nile virus disease in healthy adults. *Clin Infect Dis* 2004;38: 289–292.
Review.

Gea-Banacloche J, et al. West Nile virus: pathogenesis and therapeutic options. *Ann Intern Med* 2004;140:545–553.
Review.

Guarner J, et al. Clinicopathologic study and laboratory diagnosis of 23 cases with West Nile virus encephalomyelitis. *Hum Pathol* 2004;35:983–990.
Review.

Iwamoto M, et al and the West Nile Virus in Transplant Recipients Investigation Team. Transmission of West Nile virus from an organ donor to four transplant recipients. *N Engl J Med* 2003;348:2196–2203.
Review.

Kleinschmidt-DeMasters BK, et al. Naturally acquired West Nile virus encephalomyelitis in transplant recipients: clinical, laboratory, diagnostic, and neuropathological features. *Arch Neurol* 2004; 61:1210–1220.
Review.

Nash D, et al. The outbreak of West Nile virus infection in the New York City area in 1999. *N Engl J Med* 2001;344:1807–1814.
Initial description of outbreak in New York in 1999.

Petersen LR, Marfin AA. West Nile virus: a primer for the clinician. *Ann Intern Med* 2002;137:173–179.
Review.

Pealer LN, et al, and the West Nile Virus Transmission Investigation Team. Transmission of West Nile virus through blood transfusion in the United States in 2002. *N Engl J Med* 2003;349:1236–1245.
An unusual form of transmission that should be prevented by screening blood donors for West Nile virus.

Ravindra KV, et al. West Nile virus-associated encephalitis in recipients of renal and pancreas transplants: case series and literature review. *Clin Infect Dis* 2004;38:1257–1260.
Consider West Nile virus infection in transplant recipients presenting with unexplained fever or neurologic symptoms in the West Nile virus season.

Sejvar JJ, et al. Neurologic manifestations and outcome of West Nile virus infection. *JAMA* 2003;290:511–515.
Although many infections are asymptomatic, neurologic manifestations may be irreversible.

Smithburn KC, et al. A neurotropic virus isolated from the blood of a native of Uganda. *Am J Trop Med* 1940;20:471–492.
Initial report from Uganda.

Solomon T. Flavivirus encephalitis. *N Engl J Med* 2004;351:370–378.
Review. Groups at greater risk for severe disease include older, immunosuppressed, and chronically ill individuals.

Tyler KL. West Nile virus infection in the United States. *Arch Neurol* 2004;61:1190–1195.
Review.

Watson JT, et al. Clinical characteristics and functional outcomes of West Nile fever. *Ann Intern Med* 2004;141:360–365.
Patients with West Nile fever often had persistent fatigue, fever, and headache.

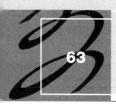

63 BIOTERRORISM

$\mathcal{T}$he Centers for Disease Control and Prevention (CDC) and a panel of other experts previously formed a strategic work group to outline steps to strengthen the U.S. public health infrastructure and healthcare capacity to protect against bioterrorism. They helped to identify a list of "critical biological agents" that, if released, would have the greatest impact. Those of greatest concern were designated *category A* and were chosen because of their ease of dissemination or ability for person-to-person transmission, high mortality rate, potential major impact on public health, ability to incite panic and social disruption, and the requirement for additional major public health preparedness measures. Other potential agents of concern were assigned to *categories B or C* by using the above criteria to rate each pathogen's impact on the medical and public health systems. We will focus on two of the potential threats in greater detail and summarize several others in tabular form and reference material (Tables 63-1 and 63-2).

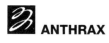 **ANTHRAX**

Anthrax is not contagious; the illness cannot be transmitted from person to person. *Bacillus anthracis* spores can live in the soil for many years, and humans can become infected with anthrax by handling products from infected animals or by inhaling anthrax spores from contaminated animal products. Anthrax also can be spread by eating undercooked meat from infected animals. Anthrax occurs in three major clinical types in humans: inhalational, cutaneous, and gastrointestinal. Endospores are resistant to drying, heat, ultraviolet light, gamma radiation, and some disinfectants.

In a biologic attack, aerosol exposure would be the most likely scenario. It has been demonstrated that significant dispersion of spores can occur by opening a contaminated envelope. In this form, the spores behave like a gas and can disperse over wide areas with the potential to infect high numbers of people. In inhalational anthrax, 1 to 5 μm spores are deposited in the terminal airways or alveoli. The spores are then phagocytized by alveolar macrophages and transported to regional (mediastinal) lymph nodes. Spores may stay in the mediastinal lymph nodes for extended periods and can germinate for up to 60 days or longer. Tissue damage is caused by two toxins: edema toxin and lethal toxin. These two toxins are composed of three components called edema factor, lethal factor, and protective antigen, which are produced by vegetative cells, which also produce an antiphagocytic capsule. Together, edema toxin and lethal toxin cause edema, hemorrhage, necrosis, and shock.

Unlike patients with inhalational anthrax, adults with influenza or other viral respiratory illnesses do not usually have shortness of breath and vomiting but often have sore throat or rhinorrhea. Initial symptoms of inhalation anthrax may resemble a common cold. Patients may complain of a sore throat, mild fever, muscle aches, and malaise. The incubation period for inhalational disease is 1 to 6 days. After several days, the symptoms may progress to severe breathing problems and shock, and ultimately to death.

Presumptive identification to identify to species level (*B. anthracis*) requires tests for motility, lysis by gamma phage, capsule production and visualization, hemolysis, wet mount, and malachite green staining for spores. Confirmatory identification of *B. anthracis* carried out by CDC may include phage lysis, capsular staining, and direct fluorescent antibody (DFA) testing on capsule antigen and cell wall polysaccharide. *B. anthracis* is detectable

TABLE 63-1   Bioweapons Characteristics

Agent/organism	Incubation period	Symptoms	Laboratory diagnosis	Person to person	Vaccine	Treatment	Isolation
Anthrax	1–6 days	Lung/skin/CNS	Stain, culture, PCR (LRN)*	No	Yes	Ciprofloxacin, doxycycline initially	Standard
Smallpox	12 days	Skin/systemic	Culture, PCR (LRN)	Yes	Yes	Supportive	Airborne, contact
Plague	3 days	Lung, not skin	Stain, culture, PCR (LRN)	Yes	Research area	Streptomycin, Gentamicin, Doxycycline	Droplet plus eye protection
Tularemia	4 days	Lung, glands	Culture, DFA (LRN)	No	Research area	Streptomycin, Gentamicin, Doxycycline, Ciprofloxacin	Standard
Botulism	1–5 days	Afebrile paralysis	Toxin (LRN)	No	IND toxoid	Supportive, antitoxin	Standard
Viral HFs	4–21days	Systemic	Culture, ELISA, PCR (LRN)	Yes	Yellow fever	Ribavirin?	Airborne, contact
Ricin	18–24 hr	Respiratory, GI	ELISA assay	No	IND toxoid	Supportive	Decontaminate
T2 mycotoxins (Oily liquid)	2–4 hr	Systemic, respiratory	Gas chromatography-mass spectrometry	No	No	Supportive care	Decontaminate

LRN, Lab Response Network; DFA, Direct Flourescent Antibody; IND, Investigational New Drug; HF, Hemorrhagic Fevers.

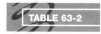

TABLE 63-2	Bioterrorism Web Sites
Blue Book	http://www.usamriid.army.mil/education/bluebook.htm
JAMA	http://jama.ama-assn.org/cgi/collection/bioterrorism
Infectious Diseases Society of America	http://www.idsociety.org/Template.cfm?Section=Bioterrorism
CDC FAQ	http://www.bt.cdc.gov/DocumentsApp/faq.asp
CDC smallpox	http://www.cdc.gov/nip/ed/smallpox-trg/clinician-should-know/default.htm
American Society for Microbiology	http://www.asm.org/Policy/index.asp?bid=6342
Emerging Infectious Diseases Journal	http://www.cdc.gov/ncidod/eid/index.htm
Johns Hopkins University Center	http://www.hopkins-id.edu/
FDA	http://www.fda.gov/oc/opacom/hottopics/bioterrorism.html
ACP	http://www.acponline.org/bioterro/
APIC	http://www.apic.org/Content/NavigationMenu/PracticeGuidance/Topics/Bioterrorism/Bioterrorism.htm
SHEA	http://www.shea-online.org/bioterrorism/organizations.cfv

by Gram's stain of the blood, blood culture on routine media, and by enzyme-linked immunosorbent assay (ELISA), but often not until later in the course of the illness. Approximately 50% of cases are accompanied by hemorrhagic meningitis, and therefore organisms also may be identified in cerebrospinal fluid (CSF). Blood cultures and *B. anthracis*-specific polymerase chain reaction (PCR) of sterile fluids (e.g., blood and pleural fluid) are important in the diagnosis of inhalational anthrax. Serologic testing also has been valuable. An ELISA to detect immunoglobulin IgG response to *B. anthracis* protective antigen (PA) is highly sensitive (detects 98.6% of true positives) but is only approximately 80% specific. To improve specificity, a PA-competitive inhibition ELISA is used as a second, confirmatory step. Preliminary studies indicate that specific IgG anti-PA antibody can be detected as early as 10 days, but peak IgG may not be seen until 40 days after onset of symptoms. Immunohistochemical examination of pleural fluid or trans-bronchial biopsy specimens, using antibodies to *B. anthracis* cell wall and capsule, also has an important role in the diagnosis of inhalational anthrax, especially in patients who have received prior antibiotics. Immunohistochemical examination can detect intact bacilli or *B. anthracis* antigens. PCR, serologic tests, and immunohistochemical tests are currently available at CDC or at certain laboratories in the Laboratory Response Network (LRN).

Standard precautions are recommended for patient care because person-to-person spread does not occur. After any invasive procedure or autopsy, instruments and the local area should be disinfected with a sporicidal agent.

Treatment and Prophylaxis

The CDC has advised that ciprofloxacin or doxycycline should be used for initial intravenous therapy until antimicrobial susceptibility results are known. Because of the mortality associated with inhalational anthrax, they recommend that two or more antimicrobial agents predicted to be effective be used. Other agents to be considered for use in conjunction with ciprofloxacin or doxycycline include rifampin, vancomycin, imipenem, chloramphenicol, penicillin and ampicillin, clindamycin, and clarithromycin; but other than for penicillin,

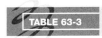

TABLE 63-3	Anthrax Web Sites
Basics	http://www.bt.cdc.gov/agent/anthrax/basics/factsheets.asp
Diagnosis	http://www.bt.cdc.gov/agent/anthrax/diagnosis/index.asp
Vaccine	http://www.bt.cdc.gov/agent/anthrax/vaccination/index.asp
Exposure management	http://www.bt.cdc.gov/agent/anthrax/exposure/index.asp
Images	http://www.bt.cdc.gov/agent/anthrax/anthrax-images/index.asp
Lab testing	http://www.bt.cdc.gov/agent/anthrax/lab-testing/index.asp
Treatment	http://www.bt.cdc.gov/agent/anthrax/treatment/index.asp
Infection control	http://www.bt.cdc.gov/agent/anthrax/infection-control/index.asp
Infectious Diseases Society of America	http://www.idsociety.org/Template.cfm?Section=Bioterrorism
Medscape	http://www.medscape.com/pages/editorial/resourcecenters/public/bioterr/rc-bioterr.ov
JAMA	http://jama.ama-assn.org/cgi/collection/bioterrorism
Management	http://www.bt.cdc.gov/documentsapp/anthrax/12212001/PreventiveTreatment/SummaryTreatmentOptions.PDF
References	http://www.bt.cdc.gov/agent/anthrax/reference/index.asp

limited or no data exist regarding the use of these agents in the treatment of inhalational *B. anthracis* infection. Treatment duration is 60 days. Also note that in the case of cutaneous anthrax associated with bioterrorism, a full 60-day course of antibiotics is recommended instead of the usual 10- to 14-day course recommended in naturally occurring cutaneous anthrax. Do not use extended-spectrum cephalosporins or trimethoprim/sulfamethoxazole because anthrax may be resistant to these drugs.

The CDC initially recommended prophylaxis with ciprofloxacin (500 mg P.O. b.i.d.) or doxycycline (100 mg P.O. b.i.d.). If confirmed that anthrax has been used as a biologic weapon, antibiotics should be continued for at least 60 days in all exposed individuals, and patients should be closely followed after antibiotics are stopped. Newer options are being considered. These include extending antibiotics for some individuals for 100 days and adding anthrax vaccination as well (Table 63-3).

 SMALLPOX

Smallpox was felt to be eradicated in 1980, 3 years after the last naturally occurring case was reported from Somalia, but recent terrorist activity has caused renewed interest in this pathogen. Traditionally, the World Health Organization (WHO) has classified smallpox into five clinical forms: ordinary, flat-type, hemorrhagic, modified, and sine eruptione. Classic, "ordinary" smallpox accounted for 90% of cases in the WHO study and had an average case-fatality rate of 30%. Both direct contact and inhalation can spread the disease. Typically, the incubation period is 7 to 17 days (mean, 10–12 days) after exposure. Symptoms of the prodromal phase are nonspecific and include the acute onset of high fever, malaise, headache, backache, and prostration.

An enanthem involving the oropharyngeal mucosa precedes the characteristic rash by a day. The characteristic rash occurs 3 days after the prodromal phase, appearing first on the face and forearms. It progresses slowly in the classic form, going from macules to papules to vesicles and pustules and finally to scabs, with each stage lasting about 1 to 2 days. Unlike chickenpox, lesions are in the same stage of development on any given part of the body. A patient's pustules remain for 5 to 8 days, after which umbilication and crusting occur. Many patients will experience an extensive desquamation that clinically resembles burns. Other complications include bronchitis and pneumonitis; panophthalmitis and blindness from viral keratitis or secondary infection of the eye; arthritis (developing in up to 2% of children); and encephalitis (less than 1% of cases). Death caused by smallpox results from toxemia associated with circulating immune complexes and variola antigens.

The disease most commonly confused with smallpox is chickenpox. With chickenpox, scabs, vesicles, and pustules may be seen simultaneously on adjacent areas of skin. Moreover, the rash in chickenpox is more dense over the trunk (the reverse of smallpox), and chickenpox lesions are almost never found on the palms or soles, unlike smallpox. The CDC has developed a protocol in poster format for evaluating patients with an acute vesicular or pustular rash illness and for determining the risk of smallpox. The protocol, including color pictures of smallpox lesions, is available on the Internet at the following address: www.bt.cdc.gov/agent/smallpox/index.asp.

The characteristic brick-shaped virions may be seen in preparations of vesiculopustular fluid or homogenates of scab material by electron microscopy. PCR methods are now available at CDC for identification. The local or state health department should be contacted to facilitate specimen collection for smallpox testing (www.statepublichealth.org).

Treatment of smallpox is supportive at this time. Cidofovir has shown some in vitro and in vivo (animal studies) activity against orthopoxviruses.

Vaccination

Vaccination administered within 3 to 4 days postexposure can prevent disease or severe illness caused by variola virus. Smallpox (vaccinia) vaccine and vaccinia human immunoglobulin (VIG), which is licensed to treat certain postvaccinial-vaccination adverse effects, are both available through the CDC.

Patients who appear to be at increased risk for complications include persons with eczema or other significant exfoliative conditions; patients with leukemia, lymphoma, or generalized malignancy who are receiving therapy with alkylating agents, antimetabolites, radiation, or large doses of corticosteroids; patients with HIV infection; persons with hereditary immune disorders; and pregnant women. Perhaps the risk can be reduced by giving vaccinia immune globulin simultaneously with vaccination.

Complications of Vaccination

1. Progressive vaccinia (vaccinia gangrenosa) can occur in persons with deficiencies of the cell-mediated immune system.

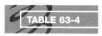

TABLE 63-4	Smallpox Web Sites
Overview	http://www.bt.cdc.gov/agent/smallpox/clinicians.asp
Diagnosis	http://www.bt.cdc.gov/agent/smallpox/diagnosis/
Lab testing	http://www.bt.cdc.gov/agent/smallpox/lab-testing/
Infection Control	http://www.bt.cdc.gov/agent/smallpox/infection-control/
Exposure	http://www.bt.cdc.gov/agent/smallpox/exposure/
Vaccination	http://www.bt.cdc.gov/agent/smallpox/vaccination/
Images	http://www.bt.cdc.gov/agent/smallpox/smallpox-images/
Infectious Diseases Society of America	http://www.idsociety.org/Template.cfm?Section=Bioterrorism
Medscape	http://www.medscape.com/pages/editorial/resourcecenters/public/bioterr/rc-bioterr.ov
Cardiac events with vaccination	http://www.cdc.gov/ncidod/eid/vol10no5/03-0967_04-0235.htm
JAMA	http://jama.ama-assn.org/cgi/content/short/281/22/2127
References	http://www.bt.cdc.gov/agent/smallpox/reference/

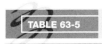

TABLE 63-5	Useful Pathogen Web Sites
Anthrax	http://www.idsociety.org/Template.cfm?Section=Bioterrorism& CONTENTID=5035&TEMPLATE=/ContentManagement/ContentDisplay.cfm
Smallpox	http://www.idsociety.org/Template.cfm?Section=Smallpox1&Template=/ TaggedPage/TaggedPageDisplay.cfm&TPLID=46&ContentID=6647
Plague	http://www.idsociety.org/Template.cfm?Section=Plague1&CONTENTID= 8210& TEMPLATE=/ContentManagement/ContentDisplay.cfm
Tularemia	http://www.idsociety.org/Template.cfm?Section=Tularemia1&CONTENTID= 8211& TEMPLATE=/ContentManagement/ContentDisplay.cfm
Botulism	http://www.idsociety.org/Template.cfm?Section=Botulism1&CONTENTID= 8212& TEMPLATE=/ContentManagement/ContentDisplay.cfm
VHF	http://www.acponline.org/bioterro/hemo_fevers.htm
Ricin	http://www.bt.cdc.gov/agent/ricin/index.asp
Mycotoxin	http://www.acponline.org/bioterro/biotoxin.htm
Radiation	http://www.afrri.usuhs.mil/www/outreach/pdf/pcktcard.pdf

Differential
  diagnosis by
  Symptom
	http://www.idsociety.org/Template.cfm?Section=Bioterrorism&CONTENTID=
	6612& TEMPLATE=/ContentManagement/ContentDisplay.cfm

2. Eczema vaccinatum may occur in persons who suffer from eczema (either from primary vaccination or contact with a person who has a nonscabbed vaccination site that contains live vaccinia virus).
3. Generalized vaccinia comprises a generalized skin rash, sometimes covering the whole body, which may occur 6 to 9 days after vaccination.
   Generalized vaccinia is not associated with the presence of immunodeficiency, and therefore has a good prognosis. The rash is generally self limited and requires minor or no therapy except in patients whose condition might be toxic or who have serious underlying immunosuppressive illnesses.
4. Post-vaccination encephalitis is an unpredictable complication that only occurs in primary vaccinees.

VIG is administered intramuscularly at a dose of 0.6 mL/kg in divided doses over a 24- to 36-hour period. A second dose may be given 2 to 3 days later if improvement does not occur. It is possibly effective for treatment of eczema vaccinatum and certain cases of progressive vaccinia; it might be useful also in the treatment of ocular vaccinia resulting from inadvertent implantation. VIG is contraindicated for the treatment of vaccinial keratitis and provides no benefit at all in the treatment of postvaccinial encephalitis.

Smallpox infected patients should be admitted to the hospital and confined to negative pressure rooms with high-efficiency particulate air (HEPA) filtration. Standard, contact, and airborne precautions, including use of gloves, gowns, and masks, should be strictly observed. Unvaccinated medical personnel should wear fit-tested N95 respirators. Once successful vaccination is confirmed, care providers are no longer required to wear an N95 mask (Table 63-4).

Please see Table 63-5 for information on the other potential agents of bioterrorism. (JWM)

Bibliography

Centers for Disease Control and Prevention. Use of onsite technologies for rapidly assessing environmental Bacillus anthracis contamination on surfaces in buildings. *JAMA* 2002;287:183.
Bioterrorism watch. Smallpox or chickenpox? How to make the diagnosis. *ED Manag* 2002;14(suppl):3–4.
Bartlett J, et al. Smallpox vaccination in 2003: key information for clinicians. *Clin Infect Dis* 2003;36:883–902.

Breman JG, Henderson DA. Diagnosis and management of smallpox. *N Engl J Med* 2002; 346:1300–1308.

Cobbs CG, Chansolme DH. Plague. *Dermatol Clin* 2004;22:303–312, vi.
When there is a strong suspicion of plague, treatment should be instituted immediately, as delaying therapy will result in increased morbidity and mortality.

Coffield JA. Botulinum neurotoxin: the neuromuscular junction revisited. *Crit Rev Neurobiol* 2003;15:175–196.
This narrative reviews our current understanding of the actions of botulinum neurotoxin at the neuromuscular junction, presents recent findings from our own work in neuromuscular tissues, and encourages future studies regarding botulinum neurotoxin at its target site.

Cronquist SD. Tularemia: the disease and the weapon. *Dermatol Clin* 2004;22:313–320, vi–vii.
An awareness of potential clinical presentations of tularemia will facilitate timely intervention, appropriate diagnostic testing, and decreased morbidity in the event of a biologic attack with Francisella tularensis.

Cuneo BM. Inhalational anthrax. *Respir Care Clin North Am* 2004;10:75–82.

Darling RG, et al. Threats in bioterrorism. I: CDC category A agents. *Emerg Med Clin North Am* 2002;20:273–309.

Dixon TC, et al. Anthrax. *N Engl J Med* 1999;341:815–826.

Doan LG. Ricin: mechanism of toxicity, clinical manifestations, and vaccine development. A review. *J Toxicol Clin Toxicol* 2004;42:201–208.
This paper reviews the mechanism of toxicity, major clinical manifestations, treatment, current methods of detection, and vaccine development.

Drazen JM. Smallpox and bioterrorism. *N Engl J Med* 2002;346:1262–1263.

Dull PM, et al. Bacillus anthracis aerosolization associated with a contaminated mail sorting machine. *Emerg Infect Dis* 2002;8:1044–1047.

Greenfield RA, Bronze MS. Current therapy and the development of therapeutic options for the treatment of diseases due to bacterial agents of potential biowarfare and bioterrorism. *Curr Opin Investig Drugs* 2004;5:135–140.
Novel vaccine strategies for plague, tularemia, and botulism are also reviewed.

Hassani M, et al. Vaccines for the prevention of diseases caused by potential bioweapons. *Clin Immunol* 2004;111:1–15.

Henghold WB 2nd. Other biologic toxin bioweapons: ricin, staphylococcal enterotoxin B, and trichothecene mycotoxins. *Dermatol Clin* 2004;22:257–262, v.

Inglesby TV, et al. Anthrax as a biological weapon, 2002: updated recommendations for management. *JAMA* 2002;287:2236–2252.

Jones ME, et al. Antibiotic susceptibility of isolates of Bacillus anthracis, a bacterial pathogen with the potential to be used in biowarfare. *Clin Microbiol Infect* 2003;9:984–986.
All isolates tested were susceptible to ciprofloxacin and doxycycline. Penicillin and amoxicillin, with or without clavulanate, showed in vitro activity against all B. anthracis isolates. Ceftriaxone demonstrated lower level in vitro activity compared with penicillin-related compounds against B. anthracis. *In vitro data from this study are in keeping with available guidelines.*

Lane JM. Smallpox and smallpox vaccination. N Engl J Med 2002;347:691–692; author reply 691–692.

Lazarus, A. A. and C. F. Decker (2004). Plague. *Respir Care Clin N Am* 10(1):83–98.

Lo Re V 3rd, Fishman NO. Recognition and management of anthrax. *N Engl J Med* 2002;346:943–945; discussion 943–945.

Papaparaskevas J, et al. Ruling out Bacillus anthracis. *Emerg Infect Dis* 2004;10:732–735.
Optimization of methods for ruling out B. anthracis leads to increased yields, faster turnaround times, and a lighter workload. We used 72 environmental non–B. anthracis bacilli to validate methods for ruling out B. anthracis. Most effective were the use of horse blood agar, motility testing after isolates had a 2-hour incubation in trypticase soy broth, and screening isolates with a B. anthracis-selective agar.

Parrish JS, Bradshaw DA. Toxic inhalational injury: gas, vapor and vesicant exposure. *Respir Care Clin North Am* 2004;10:43–58.

Rantakokko-Jalava K, Viljanen MK. Application of Bacillus anthracis PCR to simulated clinical samples. *Clin Microbiol Infect* 2003;9:1051–1056.

Evaluated PCR for the detection of B. anthracis *DNA from simulated clinical specimens relevant for the microbiological diagnosis of anthrax or exposure to* B. anthracis *spores.*

Salvaggio MR, Baddley J.W. Other viral bioweapons: Ebola and Marburg hemorrhagic fever. *Dermatol Clin* 2004;22:291–302, vi.

Shafazand S. When bioterrorism strikes: diagnosis and management of inhalational anthrax. *Semin Respir Infect* 2003;18:134–145.

Review article.

Snyder KM. Smallpox and smallpox vaccination. *N Engl J Med* 2003;348:1920–1925; author reply 1920–1925.

Swartz MN. Recognition and management of anthrax—an update. *N Engl J Med* 2001;345: 1621–1626.

Varma-Basil M, et al. Molecular beacons for multiplex detection of four bacterial bioterrorism agents. *Clin Chem* 2004;50:1060–1062.

Wortmann G. Pulmonary manifestations of other agents: brucella, Q fever, tularemia and smallpox. *Respir Care Clin North Am* 2004;10:99–109.

Zapor M, Fishbain JT. Aerosolized biologic toxins as agents of warfare and terrorism. *Respir Care Clin North Am* 2004;10:111–122.

Prophylaxis of Infection in Travelers

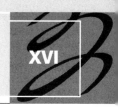

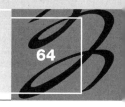

XVI

*I*f possible, the initial consultation about travel abroad should occur at least six weeks to 2 months before the patient's departure date to allow adequate time to give the appropriate immunizations and for assessment of any serious reactions. Patients may have special needs that require additional pretravel interventions or cause modifications to their itineraries. For example travel, particularly to developing countries, can carry significant risks for exposure to opportunistic pathogens for HIV-infected travelers, especially those who are severely immunosuppressed. Also counseling about preventing sexually transmitted diseases may be helpful, given that many travelers may acquire a sexually transmitted disease (STD) abroad.

The pretravel history should include information about the places the patient plans to visit, the season of the year, and the duration of the trip. Ideally one should review the patient's vaccination status at this time. Routine immunizations that need to be evaluated would include the pneumococcal vaccine, measles, mumps and rubella, polio, tetanus, varicella, and influenza. Recommendations for adult vaccinations may be found on the Centers for Disease Control and Prevention (CDC) Web site listed in Table 64-1.

Issues regarding safe consumption of water need to be addressed at the pretravel visit. Only boiled water, hot beverages (such as coffee or tea), canned or bottled carbonated beverages, beer, and wine can be considered safe. A common error committed by travelers is to add ice to their soft drinks. Ice may be made from unsafe water and should be avoided if possible. As an alternative to boiling, chemical disinfection can be achieved with either iodine or chlorine.

As a general rule, if you can peel fruit yourself, it is safe. Foods that are more worrisome include salads, uncooked vegetables and fruit, unpasteurized milk and milk products, raw meat, and shellfish. The traveler is at risk to acquire salmonellosis, toxoplasmosis, trichinosis, or cysticercosis from inadequately cooked meat; salmonellosis, shigellosis, leptospirosis, amebiasis, giardiasis, dracunculiasis, or hepatitis A from contaminated ice cubes or drinking water; brucellosis, salmonellosis, campylobacteriosis, or tuberculosis from unpasteurized milk or milk products, including cheese and ice cream; and salmonellosis, hepatitis A, fish roundworm infection, Gnathostomiasis, or infection with liver or lung flukes from raw or undercooked fish or shellfish.

Some fish are not guaranteed to be safe even when cooked because of the presence of toxins in their flesh. Some species of fish and shellfish can contain poisonous biotoxins, even when well cooked. The most common type of biotoxin in fish is ciguatoxin. The barracuda and puffer fish are usually toxic, and should be avoided. Tropical reef fish, red snapper, amber jack, grouper, and sea bass can occasionally be toxic as well.

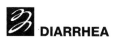

DIARRHEA

Please see chapters 16 and 23 for information on this subject.

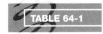

TABLE 64-1	Useful Web Sites
Adult vaccination	http://www.cdc.gov/mmwr/preview/mmwrhtml/mm5140a5.htm
DEET	http://www.deet.com
Travel vaccines	http://www.cdc.gov/travel/vaccinat.htm
Mosquito protection	http://www.cdc.gov/travel/bugs.htm
Destination information	http://www.cdc.gov/travel/destinat.htm
Specific information for travel-related infections	http://www.cdc.gov/travel/destinat.htm
Safe food and water	http://www.cdc.gov/travel/foodwater.htm
Travel clinics	http://www.cdc.gov/travel/travel_clinics.htm
International Society of Travel Medicine	http://www.istm.org/
The American Society of Tropical Medicine and Hygiene	http://www.astmh.org/
U.S. State Department	http://travel.state.gov/
WHO	http://www.who.int/en/
CDC malaria site	http://www.cdc.gov/travel/yb/index.htm
Special travel needs	http://www.cdc.gov/travel/spec_needs.htm
Alternate CDC malaria site	http://www.cdc.gov/malaria/
Malaria pocket guide	http://www.vnh.org/Malaria/Malaria.html
Diarrhea site	http://www.travelhealthline.com/z_diarrhea.html

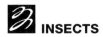

INSECTS

Many travel-related illnesses, such as malaria, are transmitted by insect vectors. Precautions against infection include the use of insect repellents, mosquito netting, and screened windows. Insect repellents should be applied only to exposed skin and should be washed off as soon as possible after exposure. They should contain DEET (30–35% diethylmethylbenzamide). The DEET concentration alone may not predict toxicity, but a standard maximum concentration of 10% for children and 30% for adults usually provides hours of safe protection without significant toxicity. Light, long-sleeved clothing and long pants should be worn where appropriate and pants should be tucked into socks. Permethrin-coated clothing and bed nets provide additional protection against insects. DEET is far less toxic than many people believe. Adverse effects, though documented, are infrequent and are generally associated with gross overuse of the product. The risk of DEET-related adverse effects pales in comparison with the risk of acquiring vector-borne infection in places where such diseases are endemic. More information about DEET can be found in Table 64-1.

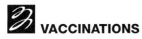 VACCINATIONS

General information about vaccination requirements for adults can be found on the CDC Web site listed in Table 64-1. Specific requirements for certain countries can be found there as well. Pretravel counseling is a good time to do routine health maintenance, including vaccination status for some patients.

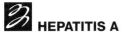 HEPATITIS A

Hepatitis A can be prevented by vaccination. The risk of hepatitis A in nonimmune travelers to developing countries has been estimated at 1 per 1,000 travelers per week for most tourists, but as high as 1 per 200 per week for backpackers. As a result, the CDC recommends hepatitis A vaccine be given for all international travelers except those going to low-risk countries such as Canada, Australia, New Zealand, Japan, or most of western Europe. HAVRIX is formulated with 2-phenoxyethanol as a preservative, unlike VAQTA which is formulated without a preservative. These two vaccines are available in pediatric (ages 2–18) and adult (older than age18) formulations, administered intramuscularly in a two-dose schedule. Also a combination hepatitis A and hepatitis B vaccine (TWINRIX, GlaxoSmithKline) is available as well and it contains 720 ELU of HAV antigen and 20 μg of recombinant hepatitis B surface antigen. Unlike the previous vaccines, the combination vaccine is given as a three-dose schedule.

Immune globulin (IG) is effective, providing 85 to 90% protection, but provides only short-term (i.e., months) protection. In general, even a single dose of the vaccine induces higher levels of antibodies than achieved with use of IG, but lower than levels induced by natural infection. However levels of neutralizing antibodies are lower immediately after active immunization than after administration of IG. Antibody production is somewhat slower and antibody levels are lower when IG and vaccine are given simultaneously, but still reach protective levels in healthy adults.

Testing for antibodies to hepatitis A after vaccination to assess for adequacy of response is not recommended. Commercially available tests for hepatitis A antibodies were developed to assess immunity to natural infection, so the vaccine does not cause a long-lasting false-positive result or diagnostic dilemmas. Protection from the vaccine is expected to be long lasting. Exposure to wild virus after receiving the vaccine will most likely lead to a booster effect. Mathematical models have predicted that protective levels of antibodies will persist for 24 to 47 years, with an average annual decrease of 25% in anti-HAV. Nevertheless, long-term follow-up studies are required to assess duration of protection.

 RABIES

Rabies is a disease of both domestic and wild mammals, particularly dogs and related species, raccoons, mongooses, skunks, and bats. Although often thought of as being a domestic illness, rabies prevention should be part of pretravel counseling. In Asia, Africa, Russia, Latin America, and other countries, dogs are the vector of rabies. Travelers should be aware that appropriate postexposure prophylaxis (PEP) treatment might unfortunately not be available in most of the third world. Also, neurologic complications associated with Semple (sheep brain-derived) vaccine may be as high as 1 case per 200 recipients.

Postexposure management includes immediate wound washing, followed by the use of human or equine rabies immunoglobulin (HRIG or ERIG) and a World Health Organization (WHO)-approved vaccination series. The postexposure regimen recommended in the United States and by WHO is rabies immune globulin (RIG) on day 0 and human diploid cell rabies vaccine (HDCV) on each of days 0, 3, 7, 14, and 28; 1 mL of vaccine is administered intramuscularly in the deltoid area only. To be optimally effective, RIG must be injected into and around wounds to neutralize virus before it enters peripheral nerves, where, once established, it is in an immune-protected environment.

Vaccines require up to 10 days to induce detectable neutralizing antibodies in most patients. Preexposure vaccination may be used for those who may come in contact with the virus or rabid animals. Because chloroquine may cause interference with the immune response, WHO recommends that preexposure treatment should be administered intramuscularly when a patient is receiving malaria prophylaxis concurrently. Those who have received prior preexposure or postexposure treatment with a cell culture vaccine, or who have proven viral neutralizing antibody (VNA) to rabies after other vaccines, should receive an intramuscular injection on each of days 0 and 3, without RIG. Information about rabies can be found at this and other Web sites (www.who.int/emc/diseases/zoo/rabies.html).

 ## JAPANESE B ENCEPHALITIS

The risk of Japanese B encephalitis (JE) virus infection appears to be very low for most travelers despite the fact that almost 50,000 cases are reported annually. JE is a mosquito-transmitted viral infection that is endemic in rural parts of Asia. The risk is felt to be highest in China, Korea, the Indian subcontinent, and Southeast Asia, especially in areas where pig farming is common. Occasionally cases have been reported in Japan, Hong Kong, southeastern Russia, Singapore, Malaysia, the Philippines, Taiwan, and parts of Oceania. Most infections are asymptomatic, but among people who develop a clinical illness, the case-fatality rate can be as high as 30%. Neuropsychiatric sequelae are reported in 50% of survivors. A higher case-fatality rate is usually reported in older persons. Both domestic pigs and wild birds serve as the reservoirs of this infection, with *Culex* mosquitoes being the principal vectors. This species of mosquito feeds outdoors beginning at dusk and during evening hours until dawn. Larvae are typically found in flooded rice fields, marshes, and small stable collections of water around cultivated fields. In temperate zones, the vectors are present in greatest numbers from June through September and are inactive during winter months.

Individuals visiting endemic areas for stays of longer than 30 days are candidates for vaccination. Short-term travelers who engage in outdoor activities with exposure to mosquito bites and long-term travelers going to endemic areas for more than 1 month should follow personal insect precautions, including the use of bed nets and insect repellents when outdoors. The vaccine should be administered at least 2 weeks before departure to allow time for monitoring of possible adverse reactions. Mild-to-moderate adverse reactions occur in about 20% of those vaccinated and consist of fever, headache, myalgia, and malaise. The risk of a possible allergic reaction to the JE vaccine has estimated to vary between 50 and 100 cases per 10,000 of those vaccinated. More serious reactions, such as urticaria and angioedema, occur at a rate of about one case per 250 persons receiving the vaccine, and usually occur within minutes after a vaccine dose, but may take up to 1 week after. A history of urticaria seems to be associated with an increased risk of a serious allergic reaction to JEV. If there is insufficient time to give the standard three-dose series, one may administer two doses of JEV 1 week apart to provide short-term protective immunity in up to 80% of vaccine recipients and may be considered for individuals with high-risk itineraries. The JEV primary immunization series consists of three doses, given by subcutaneous injection, with 1 week between the first two doses, and 1 to 2 weeks between the second and third doses. A booster dose is recommended after 3 years for continuing risk of exposure.

 ## YELLOW FEVER

Yellow fever occurs in tropical regions of Africa and South America, but it has never emerged in Asia, and vaccination for travel is currently not indicated for travel there. Yellow fever is a zoonotic infection, maintained in nature by wild nonhuman primates and diurnally active mosquitoes. In a study of 103 patients, the average stay in hospital for surviving patients was 14 days and the average duration of acute illness was 17 days. Serologic diagnosis is accomplished principally by measurement of IgM antibodies by enzyme-linked immunosorbent assay (ELISA). A certificate of vaccination is required under the International Health Regulations for entry into yellow fever-endemic countries or travel from endemic countries to *Aegypti*-infested countries at risk of introduction. Information on vaccination requirements can be obtained from travel clinics and on the CDC Web site (www.cdc.gov/travel/reference.htm).

Yellow fever 17D is a highly effective, well-tolerated live, attenuated vaccine produced from embryonated eggs. As a result, egg-allergic patients should not be immunized or should be skin tested and desensitized. Protective levels of neutralizing antibody are found in 90% of vaccinees within 10 days and in 99% within 30 days. Most likely, vaccination provides lifelong protection after a single dose, but revaccination after 10 years is required under International Health Regulations for a valid travel certificate. The vaccine may be simultaneously administered with measles, polio, DPT, hepatitis B, hepatitis A, oral cholera, and oral or parenteral typhoid. The vaccine is very well tolerated; in practice few patients complain of side effects. Adverse events may be more likely in older persons.

Yellow fever vaccine is contraindicated during pregnancy, but pregnant women who inadvertently get vaccinated should be reassured that there is no risk to themselves and no or low risk to the fetus. However they should be followed up to determine the outcome of pregnancy. On theoretical grounds the vaccine is also contraindicated in patients with immunodeficiency resulting from cancers, HIV/AIDS, or treatment with immunosuppressive agents, as prolonged viremia may increase the risk of encephalitis. In the United States it is recommended that people with a risk of exposure to yellow fever who have symptomless HIV infection without immune suppression (CD41 cell counts $>200/\mu L$) should be immunized because there is no evidence that adverse events are more frequent in HIV-infected people, although immune responses to yellow fever vaccine may be impaired.

TYPHOID FEVER

Typhoid is the second most common vaccine-preventable disease affecting travelers. Estimates of risk for contracting typhoid for short-stay travelers have ranged from 1 in 30,000 to 10 in 30,000 for trips to North Africa, India, and Senegal. Two vaccines are recommended in the United States, both of which give only about 70% protection. The newer vaccines became available during the 1990s and, although they do not result in improved vaccine efficacy, they do offer better ease of administration and fewer adverse reactions.

A parenteral capsular polysaccharide vaccine (Typhim Vi) given in a single dose will give protection for 2 years. An oral, live attenuated vaccine (Vivotif Berna) is administered in capsules, with one capsule taken every other day for 4 days; a booster series is required every 5 years for those still at risk. It is not licensed for children younger than age 6 in the United States, and administration of this vaccine may be limited by the ability of small children to ingest capsules. The oral vaccine results in fever or headache in up to 5% of recipients. In general, either the oral vaccine or the Vi capsular polysaccharide vaccine is the vaccine of choice for all individuals except for children between the ages of 6 months and 2 years, for whom the whole-cell vaccine is the only option available. The oral typhoid vaccine is a live virus preparation and cannot be given to those travelers with HIV infection.

Growth of the live Ty21a strain is inhibited by some antimicrobial agents and by the antimalarial agent *mefloquine,* so the series should be completed before beginning antimalarials, or doses of each should be separated by at least 24 hours. Fortunately chloroquine does not inhibit the growth of Ty21a. Vaccine may be administered at the same time as immune globulin. The safety of vaccines against typhoid during pregnancy has not been established.

ANTIMALARIAL CHEMOPROPHYLAXIS

Travelers should be aware that the peak biting time of mosquitoes is between dusk and dawn. Travelers should be advised to wear light-colored, long-sleeved clothing and socks and pants to minimize exposure. Also DEET may be used in combination with barrier protection, and

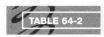

Drug	Dose	Other
Mefloquine	The adult dosage is 250 mg salt (1 tablet) once a week. Take the first dose of mefloquine 1 week before arrival in the malaria-risk area, once a week, on the same day of the week, in the malaria-risk area, and once a week for 4 weeks after leaving the malaria-risk area. Mefloquine should be taken on a full stomach, for example, after dinner.	See Table 64-3 for adverse reactions to Larium.
Doxycycline	The adult dosage is 100 mg once a day. Take the first dose of doxycycline 1 or 2 days before arrival in the malaria-risk area, once a day, at the same time each day, in the malaria-risk area, and once a day for 4 weeks after leaving the malaria-risk area.	Potential for photosensitivity. Avoid in pregnancy. Potential drug interactions.
Malarone	The adult dosage is 1 adult tablet (250 mg atovaquone/100 mg proguanil) once a day. Take the first dose of Malarone 1 to 2 days before travel in the malaria-risk area. Take Malarone once a day in the malaria-risk area. Take Malarone once a day for 7 days after leaving the malaria-risk area. Take the dose at the same time each day with food or milk.	Malarone is a combination of two drugs (atovaquone and proguanil) and is an effective alternative for travelers who cannot or choose not to take doxycycline or mefloquine.
Chloroquine	The adult dosage is 500 mg (salt) chloroquine phosphate once a week. Take the first dose of chloroquine 1 week before arrival in the malaria-risk area, once a week on the same day of the week in the malaria-risk area, and once a week for 4 weeks after leaving the malaria-risk area. Chloroquine should be taken on a full stomach, for example, after dinner, to minimize nausea.	Potential for ocular toxicity, drug interactions, marrow suppression, skin eruptions, and resistance.

(Adapted from http://www.cdc.gov/travel/malariadrugs2.htm.)

mosquito netting should be used if possible. In general, *Anophelines* prefer to bite the lower extremities, often the ankles.

Apart from those remaining areas with chloroquine-sensitive strains, mefloquine is usually the drug of choice for prevention. See Table 64-2 for information about the dosing of antimalarial drugs.

Mefloquine has a very long half-life, and is recommended for prophylaxis and therapy in chloroquine-resistant areas. Resistance to mefloquine appears to depend on export by the pfmdr1 transporter protein. Pfmdr1 amplification is associated with mefloquine resistance. Resistance to mefloquine is seen in much of Southeast Asia, although it appears to be effective in Africa. Mefloquine also has been used as solo treatment in much of Southeast Asia, although high levels of resistance have been noted. Mefloquine is still effective in most African countries and can be used in areas of chloroquine resistance. Mefloquine and halofantrine show a high degree of in vitro cross-resistance, and although evidence of

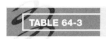

TABLE 64-3	Side Effects of Mefloquine

Adverse reactions

The most frequently reported adverse events are nausea, vomiting, loose stools or diarrhea, abdominal pain, dizziness or vertigo, loss of balance, and neuropsychiatric events, such as headache, somnolence, and sleep disorders (insomnia, abnormal dreams). These are usually mild and may decrease despite continued use.

Halofantrine must not be given simultaneously with or subsequent to Lariam, because significant, potentially fatal prolongation of the QTc interval of the electrocardiogram may result.

Concomitant administration of Lariam and quinine or quinidine may produce cardiographic abnormalities. Administration of Lariam with quinine or chloroquine may increase the risk of convulsions.

Mefloquine may cause psychiatric symptoms in a number of patients, ranging from anxiety, paranoia, and depression to hallucinations and psychotic behavior. On occasions, these symptoms have been reported to continue long after mefloquine has been stopped. Rare cases of suicidal ideation and suicide have been reported, although no relationship to drug administration has been confirmed. To minimize the chances of these adverse events, mefloquine should not be taken for prophylaxis in patients with active depression or with a recent history of depression, generalized anxiety disorder, psychosis, or schizophrenia or other major psychiatric disorders. Lariam should be used with caution in patients with a previous history of depression.

Lariam may increase the risk of convulsions in patients with epilepsy. Caution should be exercised with regard to activities requiring alertness and fine motor coordination, because dizziness, a loss of balance, or other disorders of the central or peripheral nervous system have been reported during and following the use of Lariam.

Periodic liver function tests and ophthalmic examinations are recommended during prolonged administration.

Lariam should be used during pregnancy only if the potential benefit justifies the potential risk to the fetus or nursing infant. Women of childbearing potential should be warned against becoming pregnant while taking Lariam.

Mefloquine is excreted in human milk. Because of the potential for serious adverse reactions in nursing infants, a decision should be made whether to stop taking Lariam, taking into consideration the importance of the drug to the mother.

(Adapted from http://www.lariam.com/about_lariam.asp#safety_info and http://www.fda.gov/cder/foi/label/2003/19591s19lbl_Lariam.pdf.)

in vivo cross-resistance is limited, it indicates that increasing levels of resistance to mefloquine may limit the effective chemotherapy lifetime of both mefloquine and halofantrine. Mefloquine has been the subject of much controversy regarding its side effects but six randomized, double-blind trials and seven prospective comparative studies failed to find significant differences in the rates of adverse events or drug discontinuation between subjects taking mefloquine and those taking other antimalarial drugs (see Tables 64-2 and 64-3).

If mefloquine cannot be tolerated, an alternative is daily doxycycline. Doxycycline is the preferred agent for persons unable to take mefloquine and for those traveling to areas where there is mefloquine resistance, that is, the western provinces of Cambodia and the border regions between Thailand and Cambodia and between Thailand and Myanmar (Burma). Regional information regarding antimalarial resistance can be found on the Internet (www.cdc.gov/travel/regionalmalaria/index.htm).

An alternative for travelers who are unable to take mefloquine or doxycycline is the combination of weekly chloroquine plus daily proguanil (the product is not available in the United States). However, chloroquine plus proguanil is significantly less effective than doxycycline or mefloquine in areas where these agents have been studied.

Primaquine is aimed at the preerythrocytic stage and thus may be a potential causal-prophylactic treatment that can abolish the need for long postexposure therapy. A potential advantage of primaquine, because of its activity against the liver stages of parasites, is that prophylaxis may be discontinued 1 week after the recipient has left the endemic area. Primaquine is not yet approved for this indication. For prophylaxis against *Plasmodium falciparum* malaria, primaquine has an efficacy and toxicity competitive with those of standard agents. Potential side effects include oxidant-induced hemolytic anemia and methemoglobinemia; its use is contraindicated in pregnant women and in persons with glucose-6-phosphate dehydrogenase deficiency. It appears that the addition of chloroquine did not increase the prophylactic efficacy of primaquine.

In combination with proguanil, the ability of atovaquone to inhibit parasitic mitochondrial electron transport is markedly enhanced. Evidence suggests that this drug combination has activity against a liver stage of the malaria parasite, allowing travelers to discontinue it 1 week after leaving a malarious area. Atovaquone/proguanil is highly effective against drug-resistant strains of *P. falciparum,* and cross-resistance has not been observed between atovaquone and other antimalarial agents. Halofantrine, artemisinin derivatives, and azithromycin should not be considered as first-line agents for prevention of malaria.

The use of doxycycline or primaquine is contraindicated during pregnancy, but chloroquine is safe in all trimesters. Mefloquine may be considered for use during pregnancy when exposure to chloroquine-resistant *P. falciparum* is anticipated. Also the combination of chloroquine plus proguanil is considered to be safe.

Please see Table 64-1 for information about useful Web sites. (JWM)

Bibliography

Compendium of Animal Rabies Prevention and Control, 2001. National Association of State Public Health Veterinarians, Inc. *MMWR Recomm Rep* 2001;50:1–9.
  The purpose of this compendium is to provide rabies information to veterinarians, public health officials, and others concerned with rabies prevention and control. Vaccination procedure recommendations are contained in Part I; all animal rabies vaccines licensed by the United States Department of Agriculture (USDA) and marketed in the United States are listed in Part II; Part III details the principles of rabies control.
Advice for travelers. *Med Lett Drugs Ther* 2002;44:33–8.
Abell L, et al. Health advice for travelers. *N Engl J Med* 2000;343:1045–1046.
Altekruse SF, et al. Factors in the emergence of food borne diseases. *Vet Clin North Am Food Anim Pract* 1998;14:1–15.
  This article examines these factors and briefly addresses prevention and control of foodborne diseases.
Caeiro JP, et al. Oral rehydration therapy plus loperamide versus loperamide alone in the treatment of traveler's diarrhea. *Clin Infect Dis* 1999;28:1286–1289.
  Administration of loperamide plus oral rehydration therapy (ORT) for the management of traveler's diarrhea, in cases in which subjects were encouraged to drink ad libitum, offered no benefit over administration of loperamide alone.
Camus D, et al. [Clinical studies using the combination atovaquone-proguanil as malaria prophylaxis in non-immune adult and child travelers]. *Med Trop (Mars)* 2002;62: 225–228.
  The combination of atovaquone/proguanil (Malarone) could provide an answer as it is not only effective on multiresistant strains of P. falciparum,*but also simplifies the conditions of administration and shows good tolerance in adults and children.*
Cetron MS, et al. Yellow fever vaccine. Recommendations of the Advisory Committee on Immunization Practices (ACIP), 2002. *MMWR Recomm Rep* 2002;51:1–11; quiz 1–4.
Dick L. Travel medicine: helping patients prepare for trips abroad. *Am Fam Physician* 1998;58:383–398; 401–402.
  Excellent review article. One-third of persons who travel abroad experience a travel-related illness, usually diarrhea or an upper respiratory infection. Medical advice for

patients planning trips abroad must be individualized and based on the most current expert recommendations.

Dumont L, et al. Health advice for travelers. *N Engl J Med* 2000;343:1046.

Eichmann A. [Sexually transmissible diseases following travel in tropical countries]. *Schweiz Med Wochenschr* 1993;123:1250–1255.
Travel to tropical countries is an important factor in the spread of sexually transmitted diseases. In spite of intensive anti-AIDS campaigns, some 30% of Swiss tourists have casual sexual contacts abroad.

Ericsson CD, et al. Treatment of traveler's diarrhea with sulfamethoxazole and trimethoprim and loperamide. *JAMA* 1990;263:257–261.
The combination of sulfamethoxazole-trimethoprim plus loperamide can be highly recommended for the treatment of most patients with traveler's diarrhea.

Fradin MS, Day JF. Comparative efficacy of insect repellents against mosquito bites. *N Engl J Med* 2002;347:13–18.
Currently available non-DEET repellents do not provide protection for durations similar to those of DEET-based repellents and cannot be relied on to provide prolonged protection in environments where mosquito-borne diseases are a substantial threat.

Freedman DO, Woodall J. Emerging infectious diseases and risk to the traveler. *Med Clin North Am* 1999; 83:865–883, v.
This article examines the relationship between travel and emerging infections. The authors also discuss several novel pathogens, such as Ebola virus, that are clearly of insignificant or minimal risk to travelers, but are the subject of frequent questions from patients requesting pretravel advice from medical providers.

Fryauff DJ, et al. Randomised placebo-controlled trial of primaquine for prophylaxis of falciparum and vivax malaria. *Lancet* 1995;346:1190–1193.
Malaria prophylaxis with primaquine was evaluated in Irian Jaya during 1 year in Javanese men who were not deficient in glucose-6-phosphate dehydrogenase (G-6-PD). One hundred twenty-six volunteers were randomized to receive 0.5 mg/kg primaquine base or placebo daily (double-blinded), or 300 mg chloroquine base weekly (open). When used daily for 1 year by men with normal G-6-PD activity, primaquine was well tolerated and effective for prevention of malaria.

Glandt M, et al. Enteroaggregative Escherichia coli as a cause of traveler's diarrhea: clinical response to ciprofloxacin. *Clin Infect Dis* 1999;29:335–338.
This study provides additional evidence that enteroaggregative Escherichia coli (EAEC) *should be considered as a cause of antibiotic-responsive traveler's diarrhea.*

Heppner DG Jr., et al. Primaquine prophylaxis against malaria. *Ann Intern Med* 1999;130:536; author reply 536–537.

Hogh B, et al. Atovaquone-proguanil versus chloroquine-proguanil for malaria prophylaxis in non-immune travellers: a randomised, double-blind study. Malarone International Study Team. *Lancet* 2000;356:1888–1894.
Chloroquine plus proguanil is widely used for malaria chemoprophylaxis despite low effectiveness in areas where multidrug-resistant malaria occurs. Studies have shown that atovaquone and proguanil hydrochloride is safe and effective for prevention of falciparum malaria in lifelong residents of malaria-endemic countries, but little is known about nonimmune travelers. METHODS: "In a double-blind equivalence trial, 1,083 participants traveling to a malaria-endemic area were randomly assigned to two treatment groups: atovaquone-proguanil plus placebos for chloroquine and proguanil; or chloroquine, proguanil, and placebo for atovaquone-proguanil. Overall the two preparations were similarly tolerated. However, significantly fewer adverse gastrointestinal events were observed in the atovaquone-proguanil group than in the chloroquine-proguanil group."

Jong EC. Immunizations for international travel. *Infect Dis Clin North Am* 1998;12: 249–266.
Immunization recommendations for international travelers is a complex subject that takes into consideration the geographic destination, planned activities during travel, health conditions at destination, length of trip, and underlying health status of the traveler.

Jong EC. Travel immunizations. *Med Clin North Am* 1999;83:903–922, vi.
An updated approach to selecting and prioritizing immunizations for the international traveler is presented. This article addresses vaccines against yellow fever, typhoid fever, cholera, meningococcal meningitis, rabies, tetanus, diphtheria, measles, mumps, rubella, polio, varicella, and influenza. Vaccine preparations, dosing regimens, efficacy, adverse effects, indications, and contraindications are discussed in the context of pretravel preparation.

Kain KC, et al. Imported malaria: prospective analysis of problems in diagnosis and management. *Clin Infect Dis* 1998;27:142–149.
Imported malaria is an increasing problem in many countries. The diagnosis of malaria was initially missed in 59% of cases. Community-based microscopic diagnosis provided incorrect species identification in 64% of cases. After presentation, the average delay before treatment was 7.6 days for falciparum malaria and 5.1 days for vivax malaria. Overall, 7.5% of P. falciparum-infected patients developed severe malaria, and in 11% of all cases, therapy failed. Patients who come to a center that has no expertise in tropical medicine receive suboptimal treatment. Improvements in recognition, diagnosis, and treatment of malaria are essential to prevent morbidity and death among travelers.

Laursen SB, Jacobsen E. [Air travel and deep venous thrombosis]. *Ugeskr Laeger* 1998;160:4079–4080.
A case of deep venous thrombosis (DVT) in a woman with polio sequelae is reported. Guidelines for air travelers to prevent the economy class syndrome are presented.

Lavelle O, Berland Y. [Travel and renal insufficiency]. *Med Trop (Mars)* 1997;57:449–451.
Traveling can be dangerous for subjects with kidney insufficiency. Pretravel evaluation is necessary to determine metabolic, nutritional, and immune status. Subjects with kidney insufficiency and transplanted kidneys should be informed of the dangers and appropriate action in case of trouble.

Lemon SM, et al. Immunoprecipitation and virus neutralization assays demonstrate qualitative differences between protective antibody responses to inactivated hepatitis A vaccine and passive immunization with immune globulin. *J Infect Dis* 1997;176:9–19.
These results are best explained by differences in the affinity of antibodies for virus following active versus passive immunization.

Magill AJ. The prevention of malaria. *Prim Care* 2002;29:815–842, v–vi.
In this article, the author focuses on practical uses of currently available prevention tools.

Maiwald H, et al. Long-term persistence of anti-HAV antibodies following active immunization with hepatitis A vaccine. *Vaccine* 1997; 15:346–348.
Seventy-one anti-hepatitis A virus (HAV)-negative volunteers were immunized against hepatitis A. The annual decrease of anti-HAV titers was 25%. Based on these data, the antibody persistence was calculated over time. Geometric mean titers (GMTs) at protective levels higher than 20 mIU mL-1 can be expected to persist for at least 15 years.

McKeage K, Scott L. Atovaquone/proguanil: a review of its use for the prophylaxis of Plasmodium falciparum malaria. *Drugs* 2003;63:597–623.
In combination with proguanil, the ability of atovaquone to inhibit parasitic mitochondrial electron transport is significantly enhanced. Both atovaquone and proguanil are effective against hepatic stages of P. falciparum, which means that treatment need only continue for 7 days after leaving a malaria-endemic region. Atovaquone/proguanil is generally well tolerated and was associated with fewer gastrointestinal adverse events than chloroquine plus proguanil and fewer neuropsychiatric adverse events than mefloquine. Thus, atovaquone/proguanil provides effective prophylaxis of P. falciparum malaria and, compared with other commonly used antimalarial agents, has an improved tolerability profile. Overall, it offers a more convenient dosage regimen, particularly in the posttravel period.

Mileno MD, Bia FJ. The compromised traveler. *Infect Dis Clin North Am* 1998;12:369–412.
Compromised travelers represent a diverse and challenging group of individuals. These patients are also at greater risk for acquisition of tuberculosis, severe

community-acquired pneumonia, urinary tract infections, and pyomyositis. Older travelers present both the infectious disease and travel medicine specialist with issues such as malignancy-related infections, myocardial infarction, and other forms of cardiopulmonary compromise, which the authors address in this article.

Miltgen, J., G. N'Guyen, et al. [Travel and patients with allergies]. Med Trop (Mars) 1997;57:469–472.

By changing their surroundings and lifestyle, travelers with allergic conditions exposed themselves to new risks. Travelers with allergic conditions should carry alert identification cards and medications for routine as well as emergency treatment including self-injectable adrenaline.

Monath TP. Yellow fever: an update. Lancet Infect Dis 2001; 1:11–20.

Yellow fever, the original viral hemorrhagic fever, was one of the most feared lethal diseases before the development of an effective vaccine. Today the disease still affects as many as 200,000 persons annually in tropical regions of Africa and South America and poses a significant hazard to unvaccinated travelers to these areas. New applications of yellow fever 17D virus as a vector for foreign genes hold considerable promise as a means of developing new vaccines against other viruses, and possibly against cancers.

Mulhall BP. Sexually transmissible diseases and travel. Br Med Bull 1993;49:394–411.

STDs continue to be the most common notifiable infectious conditions worldwide. Their unacceptably high incidence is underlined by the recent emergence of a (presently) incurable and lethal STD, HIV infection, which merits its description as a pandemic, and with which other STDs interact in an epidemiologic synergy.

Ohrt C, et al. Mefloquine compared with doxycycline for the prophylaxis of malaria in Indonesian soldiers. A randomized, double-blind, placebo-controlled trial. Ann Intern Med 1997;126:963–972.

Mefloquine and doxycycline are the two drugs recommended for prophylaxis of malaria for visitors to areas where P. falciparum *is resistant to chloroquine. Mefloquine and doxycycline were both highly efficacious and well tolerated as prophylaxis of malaria in Indonesian soldiers.*

Ostroff SM, Kozarsky P. Emerging infectious diseases and travel medicine. Infect Dis Clin North Am 1998;12:231–241.

International movement of individuals, populations, and products is one of the major factors associated with the emergence and reemergence of infectious diseases as the pace of global travel and commerce increases rapidly. Because of the unique role of travel in emerging infections, efforts are underway to address this factor by agencies such as the CDC, WHO, the International Society of Travel Medicine, and the travel industry.

Overbosch D, et al. Atovaquone-proguanil versus mefloquine for malaria prophylaxis in nonimmune travelers: results from a randomized, double-blind study. Clin Infect Dis 2001;33:1015–1021.

Concerns about the tolerability of mefloquine highlight the need for new drugs to prevent malaria. Atovaquone-proguanil was better tolerated than was mefloquine, and it was similarly effective for malaria prophylaxis in nonimmune travelers.

Petruccelli BP, et al. Treatment of traveler's diarrhea with ciprofloxacin and loperamide. J Infect Dis 1992;165:557–560.

Although not delivering a remarkable therapeutic advantage, loperamide appears to be safe for treatment of non-enterotoxic Escherichia coli(ETEC) causes of traveler's diarrhea. Two of 54 patients with Campylobacter *enteritis had a clinical relapse after treatment that was associated with development of ciprofloxacin resistance.*

Pollack RJ, et al. Repelling mosquitoes. N Engl J Med 2002;347:2–3.

Ramzan NN. Traveler's diarrhea. Gastroenterol Clin North Am 2001;30:665–78, viii.

This article presents a review of causes, presentation, and diagnosis of traveler's diarrhea. Treatment and prevention of this common problem is described in some detail. Finally, a practical and cost-effective approach to evaluating and treating a returning traveler is presented.

Robert E, et al. Exposure to yellow fever vaccine in early pregnancy. Vaccine 1999;17:283–285.

Although the sample is too small to rule out a moderate increased risk of adverse reproductive effect of yellow fever vaccine, it gives no argument for such an effect and should help to reassure pregnant women who might be inadvertently vaccinated.

Ryan ET, Kain KC. Health advice and immunizations for travelers. *N Engl J Med* 2000;342:1716–1725.

Samuel BU, Barry M. The pregnant traveler. *Infect Dis Clin North Am* 1998;12:325–354.
The care of the pregnant traveler is both challenging and rewarding. A safety profile of commonly used travel medications, antibiotics, and antiparasitic drugs is reviewed.

Schwartz E, Regev-Yochay G. Primaquine as prophylaxis for malaria for nonimmune travelers: a comparison with mefloquine and doxycycline. *Clin Infect Dis* 1999;29:1502–1506.
Malaria prophylaxis for travelers is a controversial issue. Primaquine was shown to be a safe and effective prophylactic drug against both P. falciparum *malaria and* P. vivax *malaria in travelers.*

Shanks GD, et al. Effectiveness of doxycycline combined with primaquine for malaria prophylaxis. *Med J Aust* 1995;162:306–307, 309–310.
To assess the causal prophylactic activity (activity against the preerythrocytic liver stage) of a daily regimen of doxycycline combined with low-dose primaquine against malaria in Australian Defence Force personnel deployed to Papua New Guinea (PNG). Although doxycycline generally provides good protection against malaria infection, it cannot be relied on for causal prophylaxis, even when combined with low-dose primaquine. Because the malaria infections occurred only after return to Australia, doxycycline appears to be effective in suppressing malaria while the drug is being taken. Intense, repeated exposure to malaria may require an extended period of chemoprophylaxis on return from an endemic area.

Shanks GD, et al. Efficacy and safety of atovaquone/proguanil as suppressive prophylaxis for Plasmodium falciparum malaria. *Clin Infect Dis* 1998; 27:494–499.
Both atovaquone/proguanil prophylactic regimens were as well tolerated as placebo. Thus, atovaquone/proguanil appears to be highly efficacious and safe as prophylaxis for P. falciparum *malaria.*

Shouval D, et al. Single and booster dose responses to an inactivated hepatitis A virus vaccine: comparison with immune serum globulin prophylaxis. *Vaccine* 1993;11(suppl 1): S9–S14.

Soto J, et al. Primaquine prophylaxis against malaria in nonimmune Colombian soldiers: efficacy and toxicity. A randomized, double-blind, placebo-controlled trial. *Ann Intern Med* 1998;129:241–244.
For prophylaxis against P. falciparum *malaria, primaquine has an efficacy and toxicity competitive with those of standard agents. A potential advantage of primaquine is that prophylaxis may be discontinued 1 week after the recipient has left the endemic area.*

Soto J, et al. Double-blind, randomized, placebo-controlled assessment of chloroquine/primaquine prophylaxis for malaria in nonimmune Colombian soldiers. *Clin Infect Dis* 1999;29:199–201.
To improve upon the efficacy of primaquine prophylaxis for malaria (94%, Plasmodium falciparum *malaria; 85%,* Plasmodium vivax *malaria), we administered chloroquine (300 mg weekly) in combination with primaquine (30 mg daily) to nonimmune Colombian soldiers during 16 weeks of patrol in a region of endemicity and for a further 1 week in base camp. Comparison of these data with data from a previous study indicates that the addition of chloroquine did not increase the prophylactic efficacy of primaquine.*

Taylor DN, et al. Treatment of travelers' diarrhea: ciprofloxacin plus loperamide compared with ciprofloxacin alone. A placebo-controlled, randomized trial. *Ann Intern Med* 1991;114:731–734.
To compare the safety and efficacy of loperamide used in combination with ciprofloxacin or ciprofloxacin alone for the treatment of travelers' diarrhea. In a region where enterotoxigenic E. coli *was the predominant cause of travelers' diarrhea, loperamide combined with ciprofloxacin was not better than treatment with ciprofloxacin alone. Loperamide appeared to have some benefit in the first 24 hours of treatment in patients infected with enterotoxigenic* E. coli. *Both regimens were safe.*

Taylor WR, et al. Malaria prophylaxis using azithromycin: a double-blind, placebo-controlled trial in Irian Jaya, Indonesia. *Clin Infect Dis* 1999;28:74–81.
New drugs are needed for preventing drug-resistant P. falciparum *malaria. Daily azithromycin offered excellent protection against* P. vivax *malaria but modest protection against* P. falciparum *malaria.*

Virk A. Medical advice for international travelers. *Mayo Clin Proc* 2001;76:831–840.
Each year, approximately 30 to 40 million Americans travel outside the United States. This review primarily updates pretravel management of adults.

Wagner G, et al. Simultaneous active and passive immunization against hepatitis A studied in a population of travellers. *Vaccine* 1993;11:1027–1032.
Three hundred travelers, seronegative for hepatitis A, were enrolled into this study to evaluate a new inactivated hepatitis A vaccine. The slight inhibition of antibody production, induced by the concurrent administration of IG, does not affect the overall protection afforded by the vaccine. We conclude that simultaneous active and passive hepatitis A immunizations can be recommended.

Wiedermann G, et al. Estimated persistence of anti-HAV antibodies after single dose and booster hepatitis A vaccination (0-6 schedule). *Acta Trop* 1998;69:121–125.
Even when taking the minimum observed titers in the older age group into account, the duration of protection will be more than 10 years. Considering at the same time its good tolerability and compliance, the single-dose hepatitis A vaccination appears highly recommendable in travel medicine.

Wilde H, et al. Rabies update for travel medicine advisors. *Clin Infect Dis* 2003;37:96–100.
Rabies is a neglected disease in many developing countries. It is preventable, and the tools to prevent it are known. There is urgent need for more funding, for study of innovative dog population-control measures, and for sustainable canine immunization. Travelers who leave the safe environments of tourist hotels and buses in regions of Asia, Russia, Africa, and Latin America where canine rabies is endemic may be at risk of life-threatening exposure to rabies.

Wilson ME. Travel-related vaccines. *Infect Dis Clin North Am* 2001;15:231–251.
Studies on special and travel vaccines in older individuals are needed urgently to define how these vaccines should be used in older populations and whether alternative means for protection are needed.

Tuberculosis   XVII

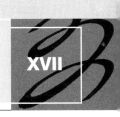

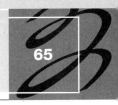
$\mathcal{T}$he clinician frequently must determine whether a patient has tuberculosis. Part of the evaluation involves tuberculin skin testing. One preparation of tuberculin is available for use in the United States: purified protein derivative (PPD).

The intradermal PPD skin test is administered using the Mantoux procedure. One concentration of PPD antigen is available: intermediate strength (5 TU). Tuberculin protein is absorbed by plastic, and the detergent polysorbate 80 is added to the diluent to prevent this reaction. After 48 to 72 hours, the extent of induration, not erythema, is determined by palpation and measured in millimeters. In the past, an area of induration of 10 mm or more was considered evidence of past or present infection with *Mycobacterium tuberculosis*. Reactions measuring 5 to 9 mm in a normal host usually represent prior infection with atypical mycobacteria that cross-react with PPD-S (*M. tuberculosis* preparation; PPD-standard).

In 1990, the American Thoracic Society and the Centers for Disease Control revised the criteria defining a positive tuberculin skin test result in an effort to decrease the number of false-negatives in high-risk persons, such as those with HIV infection, and decrease the number of false-positives in low-risk groups. Three criteria were adopted for tuberculin reactivity based on risk factors for disease and the probability of having a true infection with *M. tuberculosis*:

1. A skin test reaction of 5 mm or more of induration is considered positive in persons likely to be infected with *M. tuberculosis*, such as persons with HIV disease, close contacts of infected patients, and those with chest roentgenographic findings consistent with old, healed tuberculosis.
2. A reaction of 10 mm or more of induration is considered positive in foreign-born persons from Asia, Africa, and Latin America; IV drug users; medically underserved, low-income groups; residents of long-term care facilities; and other immunosuppressed hosts, such as persons with silicosis, gastrectomy, chronic renal failure, diabetes mellitus, or underlying hematologic or other malignancies, or who are receiving high-dose corticosteroids or other cytotoxic therapy. Additionally, a reaction in employees of an institution where a person with tuberculosis would pose a risk to a large number of susceptible persons should be considered positive at 10 mm of induration. Also considered a high-risk group are children less than 4 years of age.
3. A reaction of more than 15 mm of induration is positive in persons with no other risk factors (Table 65-1).

About 80% of normal hosts with active tuberculosis have a positive reaction to a 5-TU PPD test. The result of a 5-TU PPD skin test will be negative in 20% of seriously ill patients with active tuberculosis when first seen. In the evaluation of patients with suspected tuberculosis for delayed hypersensitivity, a number of factors can be considered that can explain false-negative tuberculin reactions (Table 65-2). Testing for anergy using a variety of antigens is no longer recommended.

A negative reaction to an intermediate-strength PPD skin test in patients who are not anergic does not exclude tuberculosis. It was found in one study that one-third of patients with active tuberculosis had a negative 5-TU PPD skin test result. Another test using whole blood called the QuantiFERON-TB test (QFT) is available for diagnosing latent tuberculosis. The test uses antigens from *M. tuberculosis* and *M. avium* complex and measures the release of interferon-gamma after a 16- to 24-hour incubation period. This test is not useful for diagnosing active tuberculosis or *M. avium* complex disease. This test may be useful to screen

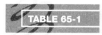

TABLE 65-1 Interpretation of Purified Protein Derivative (PPD) Tuberculin Skin Test Results

1. An induration of ≥5 mm is classified as positive in
    persons who have HIV infection
    persons who have had recent close contact with persons who have active TB
      (e.g., household contact)
    persons who have fibrotic areas on chest radiographs (consistent with healed TB)
2. An induration of ≥10 mm is classified as positive in all persons who do not meet any of the
    criteria above but who have other risk factors for TB, including
    High-risk groups–
      injecting drug users
      persons who have other medical conditions (e.g., silicosis, gastrectomy or jejunoileal
        bypass, body weight ≥10% below ideal; chronic renal failure, diabetes mellitus,
        high-dose corticosteroid or other immunosuppressive therapy, malignancies)
      children <4 years of age
    High-prevalence groups–
      persons born in countries in Asia, Africa, the Caribbean, and Latin America that have a
        high prevalence of TB
      persons from medically underserved, low-income populations
      residents of long-term care facilities (e.g., correctional institutions and nursing homes)
3. An induration of ≥15 mm is classified as positive in persons who do not meet any of the
    above criteria (e.g., health care workers) unless other risk factors are present.

(Modified from *MMWR Morb Mortal Wkly Rep* 2000;49:1–54.)

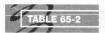

TABLE 65-2 Reasons for False-Negative Tuberculin Reactions

Technical errors
Measurement of skin induration
Faulty antigen or administration (rare)
Impaired cellular immunity
Nonspecific
Hypoalbuminemia (<2 g/dL)
Old age (>70 y)
Leukocytosis >15,000/mm^3
Anemia
Fever
Azotemia
Drugs and other therapy
Immunosuppressive drugs (corticosteroids)
Irradiation
Live viral vaccines
Specific diseases
Viral infections and vaccines (e.g., rubella, infections mononucleosis, mumps, influenza, HIV)
Overwhelming infection (e.g., tuberculosis, deep mycoses)
Sarcoidosis
Neoplasma (e.g., Hodgkin's disease, leukemia)
Too early for skin test conversion
Requires 3–6 weeks

persons at high risk for latent tuberculosis, such as recent immigrants and intravenous drug users. A tuberculin skin test can be useful in confirming a positive QFT result. The role of this new test in the diagnosis of latent tuberculosis remains to be determined.

Another problem is to distinguish between a positive tuberculin reaction in a person who has received a bacille Calmette-Guérin (BCG) vaccination and one caused by an injection of *M. tuberculosis*. Tuberculin skin reactions caused by BCG vaccination wane with time, and large reactions are likely to indicate an infection with *M. tuberculosis*. In an adult who was given BCG vaccine as an infant, a tuberculin reaction of more than 10 mm of induration is unlikely to be caused by the BCG vaccine. It is more difficult to interpret the size of a tuberculin skin test reaction in an adult who received BCG vaccine after infancy.

Repeated tuberculin skin testing can also increase the reaction size from 5 to 9 mm to more than 10 mm. This boosting reaction can occur with skin tests performed from 1 to several weeks apart. In elderly subjects, the size of the tuberculin reaction decreases with age because of a waning of cell-mediated immunity to the tuberculin antigen. When older subjects are tested twice in a 3-week interval, a positive reaction may be detected on the second skin test as a result of immunologic recall. This must not be interpreted as a recent skin test conversion but as a false-negative skin test result on the initial tuberculin test. Progressive increase in the size of the tuberculin skin test reaction has been noted when a third and a fourth boosting test is used. Although the American Thoracic Society and Centers for Disease Control and Prevention suggest that an increase of more than 10 mm of induration likely represents the occurrence of infection, in one study in older individuals, large increases were noted that did not indicate true conversions. Better tests are needed to identify persons at an increased risk for development of active disease. Rarely, an atypical mycobacterial infection will cause a reaction to the PPD-S skin test antigen that is larger than 10 mm.

A positive tuberculin skin test result in patients with suspected active tuberculosis, together with negative results on acid-fast smears, provides indirect evidence for the diagnosis pending cultures. A negative result on a properly performed tuberculin skin test is evidence against the diagnosis in a normal host. (NMG)

Bibliography

American Thoracic Society and Centers for Disease Control. Diagnostic standards and classification of tuberculosis in adults and children. *Am J Respir Crit Care Med* 2000;161: 1376–1395.
  Guidelines for use and interpretation of the tuberculin skin test.
American Thoracic Society and Centers for Disease Control. Targeted tuberculin testing and treatment of latent tuberculosis infection. *MMWR* 2000;49:1–54.
  Recommends targeted tuberculin skin testing only for those at high risk.
Buoros D, et al. Palpation vs. pen method for the measurement of skin tuberculin reaction (Mantoux test). *Chest* 1991;99:416.
  Use either the palpation or pen method to measure tuberculin skin test reactivity.
Centers for Disease Control and Prevention. Guidelines for using the QuantiFERON-TB test for diagnosing latent *Mycobacterium tuberculosis* infection. *MMWR* 2003;52:15–18.
  A blood test to diagnose latent tuberculosis.
Centers for Disease Control. Anergy skin testing and preventive therapy for HIV-infected persons: revised recommendations. *MMWR Morb Mortal Wkly Rep* 1997;46:1–10.
  Guidelines for anergy testing. Anergy testing is no longer recommended as a routine component of screening for tuberculosis among HIV-infected persons.
Centers for Disease Control. Tuberculin skin test survey in a pediatric population with high BCG vaccination coverage Botswana, 1996. *MMWR Morb Mortal Wkly Rep* 1997;46:846–851.
  A tuberculin skin test of 10 mm or more of induration is likely to be a consequence of tuberculous infection and not previous BCG vaccination.
Comstock GW, Woolpert SF. Tuberculin conversions: true or false. *Am Rev Respir Dis* 1978;118:215.
  Describes the use of two tuberculin tests given at least 1 week apart to detect true but not necessarily recent conversions resulting from the booster phenomenon.

Doto IL, Furcolow ML, MacInnis FE. Size of tuberculin reaction. *Arch Environ Health* 1971;23:392.
   The probability that reactivation tuberculosis will develop increases with the size of the skin test reactions.

Edwards PQ. Tuberculin negative? *N Engl J Med* 1972;286:373.
   The causes of false-negative test results include anergic states, faulty antigenic material, improper administration, and errors in reading the reaction.

Gershon AS, et al. Health care workers and the initiation of treatment for latent tuberculosis infections. *Clin Infect Dis* 2004;39:667–672.
   Healthcare workers are less likely than non-healthcare workers to receive treatment for latent tuberculosis.

Harrison BDW, Tugwell P, Fawcett IW. Tuberculin reaction in adult Nigerians with sputum-positive pulmonary tuberculosis. *Lancet* 1975;1:421.
   Lack of reaction to tuberculin skin test correlates with low serum albumin levels (< 2 g/dL).

Holden M, Dubin MR, Diamond PH. Frequency of negative intermediate-strength tuberculin sensitivity in patients with active tuberculosis. *N Engl J Med* 1971;285:1506.
   With 5 TU of polysorbate 80-stabilized PPD skin test antigen, 20% of results were negative.

Howard TP, Solomon DA. Reading the tuberculin skin test: who, when, and how? *Arch Intern Med* 1988;148:2457.
   Patients' readings of their own skin tests are inaccurate.

Huebner RE. The tuberculin skin test. *Clin Infect Dis* 1993;17:968.
   A review of administration, reading, and interpretation of tuberculin skin tests.

Johnson MP, et al. Tuberculin skin test reactivity among adults infected with human immunodeficiency virus. *J Infect Dis* 1992;166:194.
   Among HIV-positive persons, use a cut point of 5 mm or more of induration to increase the test sensitivity.

Levin S. The fungal skin test as a diagnostic hindrance. *J Infect Dis* 1970;122:343.
   Fungal skin tests (blastomycin, histoplasmin, and coccidioidin) should not be part of a workup for either fever of unknown origin or fungal infection.

Menzies R, Vissandjee B. Effect of bacille Calmette-Guérin vaccination on tuberculin reactivity. *Am Rev Respir Dis* 1992;145:621.
   In adults who have received BCG vaccine as infants, the tuberculin reactivity is usually less than 10 mm of induration.

Present PA, Comstock GW. Tuberculin sensitivity in pregnancy. *Am Rev Respir Dis* 1975;112:413.
   Pregnancy has no effect on the tuberculin test.

Reichman LB, O'Day R. The influence of a history of a previous test on the prevalence and size of reactions to tuberculin. *Am Rev Respir Dis* 1977;115:737.
   On retesting, a history of a positive tuberculin skin test result was confirmed in only 42% of patients. Severe reactions to the repeated test ("slough") were not a problem.

Rhoades ER, Bryant RE. The effect of injection technique upon the size of the tuberculin reaction. *Am Rev Respir Dis* 1973;107:1089.
   The route of administration (intradermal or subcutaneous) has little effect on reaction size.

Robertson JM, et al. Delayed tuberculin reactivity in persons of Indochinese origin: implications for preventive therapy. *Ann Intern Med* 1996;124:779–784.
   Some patients (26%) had a negative tuberculin skin test result at 48 to 72 hours that became positive at 6 days. This delayed response can be detected with the booster technique.

Rooney JJ, et al. Further observations on tuberculin reactions in active tuberculosis. *Am J Med* 1976;60:517.
   Of patients who were seriously ill, 20% had a negative intermediate PPD skin test result. The majority (94%) reacted after the protein depletion was corrected.

Sepkowitz KA, et al. Benefit of two-step PPD testing of new employees at a New York City hospital. *Am J Infect Control* 1997;25:283–286.
   Without use of the two-step testing technique, 10% of new employees would have been classified falsely as new tuberculin converters.

Singh D, Sutton C, Woodcock A. Tuberculin test measurement: variability due to the time of reading. *Chest* 2002;122:1299–1301.
Tuberculin skin tests should be read at 72 hours, not 48 hours.

Sokal JE. Measurement of delayed skin-test responses. *N Engl J Med* 1975;293:501.
A discussion of how to identify a positive reaction.

Squier CL, et al. The anergy panel: an ineffective tool to validate tuberculin skin testing. *Am J Infect Control* 2004;32:243–245.
Anergy testing is not useful.

Stead WW, To T. The significance of the tuberculin skin test in elderly persons. *Ann Intern Med* 1987;107:837.
An increase of at least 12 mm in the size of a tuberculin skin test reaction is evidence of a new M. tuberculosis *infection.*

ISONIAZID TREATMENT OF LATENT TUBERCULOSIS INFECTION-INDICATIONS AND MANAGEMENT

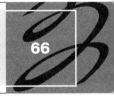

66

*J*soniazid (INH) has been used to treat latent tuberculous infection to prevent reactivation disease. The terms "preventive therapy" and "chemoprophylaxis" have been used for decades. However, they are confusing, and it is recommended that the terminology "treatment of latent tuberculosis" be used. Although the therapy of active pulmonary tuberculosis has improved considerably with highly effective short-course regimens, little progress has been made in the treatment of latent tuberculosis.

Daily therapy with INH for 12 months has been the standard regimen for several decades. Currently, using INH daily for a 9-month course of therapy is preferred. An acceptable alternative is to use isoniazid daily for 6 months or rifampin daily for 4 months. A 2-month course of daily rifampin and pyrazinamide is effective but because of death from hepatotoxicity, the American Thoracic Society and Centers for Disease Control and Prevention no longer recommend this treatment for latent tuberculosis. One controversial issue concerns the old recommendations of the American Thoracic Society and the Centers for Disease Control and Prevention that all tuberculin skin test reactors younger than age 35 with no other risk factors should receive INH. Currently, persons with latent tuberculosis who are at high risk for developing active tuberculosis should be treated irrespective of age. Table 66-1 lists some of the underlying conditions associated with developing active tuberculosis if not treated for latent tuberculosis.

An extensive controlled study involving almost 28,000 patients with positive Mantoux skin test reactions and fibrotic lesions detected by chest roentgenography was published in 1982 and provided important data on INH preventive therapy. In this study, patients were treated with either INH or placebo for 12, 24, or 52 weeks and were then followed up for 5 years. Using data from this study to conduct a cost-effectiveness analysis of the three treatment durations, Snider et al. (1986) concluded that a 24-week regimen was the most cost-effective duration. A 12-week course of INH was felt to be inadequate, and the danger of a 24-week regimen was that patients might shorten their therapy even further. Other reports based on the application of decision-analysis techniques to the management of low-risk tuberculin reactors have failed to resolve the controversy.

A positive induration after testing with intermediate-strength (5 tuberculin units) purified protein derivative (PPD-S) stabilized with polysorbate 80 indicates recent or remote infection, usually with *Mycobacterium tuberculosis* (see Chapter 65). In the absence of evidence of active disease, a positive delayed-hypersensitivity reaction to tuberculosis means that the primary infection has been arrested by the host; thus, the tuberculin-positive person

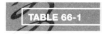

TABLE 66-1	Persons at High Risk for Developing Active Tuberculosis

Recent tuberculosis infection within the past year.
Injection drug user
Silicosis
HIV seropositivity
Radiographic finding consistent with prior tuberculosis
Underweight by > 5%
Diabetes mellitus
Chronic renal failure/hemodialysis
Gastrectomy
Jejunoileal bypass
Solid organ transplantation
Carcinoma of head or neck

has viable tubercle bacilli that, although contained by acquired cellular immunity, may multiply in subsequent years with alterations in host-resistance factors. In fact, 92% of all new cases of active pulmonary tuberculosis represent reactivation disease in a small proportion (7%) of the tuberculin-positive population. The old term *INH chemoprophylaxis* does not, in fact, indicate prophylaxis but rather actual treatment of a subclinical infection to prevent the development of active tuberculosis. Single-drug therapy is effective because the number of organisms is small; thus, there is little chance of selecting out resistant mycobacteria.

 EFFICACY

INH was commercially released in 1952, and since then numerous controlled studies have shown that a 9- to 12-month course of INH therapy is effective in preventing reactivation of disease in tuberculin reactors. The risk for active disease in a placebo group was found to be as many as 61 times that in patients treated with INH. Eighty percent of the active cases in a placebo group occurred within the first year after diagnosis, but the onset of active disease in the placebo group might be delayed as long as 8 years. The protective effect of INH is more impressive for children than for adults. Compliance is the key to the effectiveness of INH, and success rates approach 100% when the drug is given under direct supervision. One year of treatment is effective for at least 19 years and probably for the life of the patient. In summary, there is no controversy that INH treatment is effective for symptomless tuberculin reactors, tuberculin-positive household contacts, and persons with positive skin test reactions and inactive fibrotic lesions revealed by chest roentgenography. See Table 66-1.

 ISONIAZID HEPATITIS

The major disadvantage of INH is the risk for drug-induced hepatitis. The risk for hepatitis is age related and is increased with daily alcohol consumption. This complication is extremely rare in a person younger than age 20 but occurs in 2.1 to 4.3% of persons older than age 50. Although the exact pathogenic mechanism of INH-associated hepatitis remains unknown, certain features are clear. Women may be at an increased risk for development of fatal INH hepatitis. Elevations in liver enzymes with or without symptoms develop in about 10 to 20% of those taking INH. In a small percentage (1%) of patients, jaundice and fatal hepatitis develop. The onset of the liver function abnormalities varies widely, from 1 week to 11 months after the start of treatment. Half the reactions occur within 2 months, mostly during the second month. Fatal hepatitis is more common in patients taking INH for at least 8 weeks than in those on therapy for a shorter period, and it often occurs in patients who continue therapy even after symptoms of hepatitis develop.

Clinical monitoring of symptoms of liver disease—anorexia, malaise, nausea, and vomiting—are indicated for all patients receiving treatment. Biochemical monitoring is required in patients whose baseline liver function tests are abnormal and for other persons at risk for hepatic disease. It is recommended that if a patient's transaminase level is three times the upper limit of normal and he or she is symptomatic, and five times the upper limit of normal and the patient is asymptomatic, that isoniazid be stopped. Only 7% of the patients in one large study had their INH treatments stopped because of symptoms or asymptomatic elevations of transaminase levels. Clinically, biochemically, and histologically, the liver injury is indistinguishable from viral hepatitis. Contrary to what was observed in earlier studies, the incidence is not increased in rapid acetylators. In fact, slow acetylators older than age 35 appear to be at an increased risk. The mechanism of the hepatitis appears to be conversion of INH to one or more toxic metabolites. The fatality rate is about 10% for icteric cases, and the illness is usually preceded by gastrointestinal symptoms. The majority of patients who have died of INH hepatitis continued to receive the drug despite clinical evidence of hepatitis.

 ## DECISION TO USE ISONIAZID

The decision to treat a tuberculin reactor with INH is not an easy one to make and should be individualized. Active tuberculosis must be excluded, because usually four drugs are required. The clinician must weigh the risk for development of active tuberculosis and the consequences of infection in each patient. Children younger than age 5 and adolescents tend to have more serious disease than older persons. Patients of low body weight also are at increased risk for tuberculous disease. Finally, the younger a tuberculin reactor is, the greater the number of years there are in which reactivation disease may occur. In a patient who has coexisting illnesses or is taking drugs with which adverse interactions are possible, deferring INH therapy should always be considered. INH should not be deferred in pregnancy.

 ## INDICATIONS

Table 66-2 lists the indications for INH therapy in patients at high risk. All household contacts who are tuberculin positive should receive INH unless active disease is documented, in which case two drugs are given. Children who are household contacts and are tuberculin negative should be given INH for 3 months; a skin test is then repeated. If the test result remains negative and there is no further risk for exposure, INH can be discontinued. For tuberculin-negative adult household contacts, therapy with INH is optional, depending on the infectiousness of the source. Skin testing should be repeated after 3 months. Newly infected persons (documented to have a negative PPD skin test result within the past 2 years) should receive INH.

It is important to distinguish persons who are new, true tuberculin-positive reactors from those who are new positive reactors as a result of the booster phenomenon. The booster effect, which refers to an increase in the size of the tuberculin skin reaction as a consequence of serial tuberculin testing, can be demonstrated as early as 1 to 3 weeks after an initial tuberculin test. This diminished skin reactivity occurs more often in the elderly, and the repeated skin test can erroneously be interpreted as a new positive skin test reaction (conversion). Rather, the initial negative skin test reaction represents a false-negative result, and the result of the repeated test with an increase in size is positive but does not necessarily indicate a recent conversion.

The efficacy of INH is well documented in patients with a positive tuberculin skin test reaction and a fibrotic pulmonary lesion revealed by chest roentgenography. No studies support the efficacy of INH and the risk for disease in tuberculin reactors in special clinical situations, and the recommendations are based on uncontrolled studies of tuberculosis in the various groups outlined (Table 66-3). Patients to be placed on either long-term prednisone or other cytotoxic drugs should undergo skin testing before starting the drugs to establish their tuberculin status before the immunosuppressive therapy.

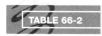

TABLE 66-2	Indications for Treatment of Latent Tuberculosis Infection

Tuberculin-positive with HIV infection
Tuberculin-negative with HIV infection in high-risk group (e.g., drug users)
Tuberculin-positive household contacts
Tuberculin-negative household contacts——children
New tuberculin reactor
Tuberculin-positive* with parenchymal scarring revealed on chest roentgenogram
   (excluding isolated calcifications)
Tuberculin reactors with special circumstances:
   Underlying neoplasm such as Hodgkin's disease
   Prednisone (>15 mg/day) or its equivalent or other immunosuppressive drugs for a
     prolonged time
   Silicosis
   Solid organ transplants
   Poorly controlled diabetes mellitus
   Long-term hemodialysis
   Postgastrectomy
   Intestinal bypass surgery for obesity
   End-stage renal disease
Tuberculin reactors from Latin America, Asia, or Africa or from low-income groups.
Tuberculin-positive residents of long-term care facilities (e.g., correctional institutions, nursing
   homes)
Tuberculi-positive staff of facilities in which many people could be exposed

*Patient has never received a full course of antituberculous therapy.

Recommendations on the use of INH for immunosuppressed patients differ widely. Some authors advocate INH; others recommend deferring therapy because of the risk for hepatitis, such as that observed in renal transplant recipients. The duration of therapy for immunosuppressed patients is also unclear; some experts favor 1 year of therapy and others recommend treatment for the duration of the immunosuppressed state. I favor using INH carefully for 9 months for the tuberculin-positive immunosuppressed patient.

INH, the drug of choice for latent treatment, is given in a dose of 300 mg daily for adults and 10 mg/kg of body weight (up to 300 mg) in children. It is usually recommended for 6 to 9 months. No more than a 1-month supply of INH should be given at any one time. In the recent trial of INH and placebo in Europe, patients randomly received 12, 24, or 52 weeks of treatment. There was a 93% reduction in tuberculosis for those with good compliance in the 52-week group. A 12-week treatment was too brief and eliminated fewer than one-third of cases; 24 weeks of treatment eliminated 69% of the cases. INH for 1 year was particularly effective in patients with fibrotic lesions larger than 2 cm^2. There were more cases of hepatitis (than in controls) in patients being treated for 1 year, but the test population had a median age of 50 years. Nearly half the cases of hepatitis were observed during the initial 3 months of therapy. This study also demonstrated the importance of compliance for successful therapy. Rifampin (10 mg/kg of body weight, up to 600 mg) is recommended for 4 months for contacts who have presumably been infected by a source shedding INH-resistant bacilli. Twice-weekly INH treatment in a high dose (15 mg/kg of body weight) for 6 to 9 months may be tried if compliance is a problem.

The optimal preventive regimen for persons exposed to a source patient infected with multidrug-resistant *M. tuberculosis* is unknown. Susceptibility test results of the source-infecting strain may be helpful to guide therapy. If the infecting strain is less than 100% resistant to INH or rifampin, these drugs can be used. Potential alternative regimens include a combination of pyrazinamide plus ethambutol, or pyrazinamide plus either ofloxacin or

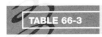

TABLE 66-3	Indications for Isoniazid Therapy

Tuberculin-positive with HIV infection
Tuberculin-negative with HIV infection in high-risk group (e.g., drug users)
Tuberculin-positive household contacts
Tuberculin-negative household contacts—children
New tuberculin reactor*
Tuberculin-positive** with parenchymal scarring revealed on chest x-ray films (excluding isolated calcifications)
Tuberculin reactors with special circumstances:
   Underlying neoplasm such as Hodgkin's disease
   Prednisone (>15 mg/d) or its equivalent or other immunosuppressive drugs for a prolonged time
   Silicosis
   Poorly controlled diabetes mellitus
   Long-term hemodialysis
   Postgastrectomy
   Intestinal bypass surgery for obesity
   End-stage renal disease
Tuberculin reactors under age 35 years from Latin America, Asia, or Africa or from low-income groups
Tuberculin-positive residents of long-term care facilities (e.g., correctional institutions, nursing homes)
Tuberculin-positive staff of facilities in which many people could be exposed
Tuberculin-positive under age 35 years with no other risk factors (?)

---

*Increase ≥10 mm within a 2-year period for those under age 35 years; increase ≥15 mm for those age 35 years or older.
**Patient has never received a full course of antituberculous therapy.

ciprofloxacin. Clinical data are lacking on preventive therapy regimens that do not include INH, as this is the only drug approved for treatment of latent tuberculosis. Shortening the duration of therapy with other drug combinations, as well as developing other regimens for prevention, should be a goal of future investigations. (NMG)

Bibliography

American Thoracic Society/CDC. Update: adverse event data and revised American Thoracic Society/CDC recommendations against the use of rifampin and pyrazinamide for treatment of latent tuberculosis infection—United States, 2003. *MMWR* 2003;52:735–739.
   Rifampin and pyrazinamide for 2 months cannot be recommended for treatment of latent tuberculosis because of severe hepatotoxicity.
American Thoracic Society, CDC, Infectious Diseases Society of America. Treatment of tuberculosis. *Am J Respir Crit Care Med* 2003;167:603–662.
   Guidelines for treatment.
American Thoracic Society, CDC. Targeted tuberculin testing and treatment of latent tuberculosis infection. *Am J Respir Crit Care Med* 2000;161:221–247.
   Review of indications and treatment of latent tuberculosis.
American Thoracic Society, CDC. Diagnostic standards and classification of tuberculosis in adults and children. *Am J Respir Crit Care Med* 2000;161:1376–1395.
   Guidelines for testing.
Asch S, et al. Relationship of isoniazid resistance to human immunodeficiency virus infection in patients with tuberculosis. *Am J Respir Crit Care Med* 1996;153:1708–1710.
   INH-resistant tuberculosis was not more frequent in HIV-infected patients.
Black M, et al. Isoniazid-associated hepatitis in 114 patients. *Gastroenterology* 1975;69:289.

A review of the cases of 114 patients with INH hepatitis, who had a 12% fatality rate. The clinical picture is indistinguishable from that of viral hepatitis.

Byrd RB, Nelson R, Elliott RC. Toxic effects of isoniazid in tuberculosis chemoprophylaxis. *JAMA* 1979;241:1239.
Ten percent of patients were unable to complete therapy with INH.

Centers for Disease Control. Management of persons exposed to multidrug-resistant tuberculosis. *MMWR Morb Mortal Wkly Rep* 1992;41:61.
An approach to a tuberculin-positive contact suspected of having acquired infection with multidrug-resistant M. tuberculosis. Preventive therapy consists of pyrazinamide plus ethambutol, or pyrazinamide plus a fluoroquinolone.

Centers for Disease Control. Prevention and treatment of tuberculosis among patients infected with human immunodeficiency virus: principles of therapy and revised recommendations. *MMWR* 1998;47:1–58.
Describes use of a 2-month regimen of rifampin or rifabutin combined with pyrazinamide to prevent tuberculosis in patients with HIV infection.

Centers for Disease Control. Transmission of *Mycobacterium tuberculosis* associated with failed completion of treatment for latent tuberculosis infection—Chickasaw County, Mississippi, June 1999–March 2002. *MMWR* 2003;52:222–224.
Patients who fail to receive treatment for latent tuberculosis may develop active tuberculosis and transmit disease.

Comstock GW, Baum C, Snider DE. Isoniazid prophylaxis among Alaskan Eskimos: a final report of the bethel isoniazid studies. *Am Rev Respir Dis* 1979;119:827.
Documents INH effectiveness in preventing tuberculosis.

Comstock GW, Ferebee SH, Hammes LM. A controlled trial of community-wide isoniazid prophylaxis in Alaska. *Am Rev Respir Dis* 1967;95:935.
Documents INH effectiveness in preventing tuberculosis.

Curry FJ. Prophylactic effect of isoniazid in young tuberculin reactors. *N Engl J Med* 1967;277:562.
Documents INH effectiveness in preventing tuberculosis.

Ferebee SH. Controlled chemoprophylaxis trials in tuberculosis. A general review. *Adv Tuber Res* 1970;17:28.
Review of INH efficacy.

Glassroth J, et al. Why tuberculosis is not prevented. *Am Rev Respir Dis* 1990;141:1236.
This report cites three reasons why tuberculosis is not prevented: (1) patients are not in the healthcare system until active tuberculosis occurs, (2) patients do not receive a tuberculin skin test or INH, or (3) patients fail to react to the skin test.

Halsey NA, et al. Randomised trial of isoniazid versus rifampicin and pyrazinamide for prevention of tuberculosis in HIV-1 infection. *Lancet* 1998;351:786–792.
Twice-weekly isoniazid for 6 months or rifampin and pyrazinamide for 2 months were equally effective for chemoprophylaxis.

Hawken MP, et al. Isoniazid preventive therapy for tuberculosis in HIV-1-infected adults: results of a randomized controlled trial. *AIDS* 1997;11:875–882.
INH is not indicated for all HIV-infected persons.

Hong Kong Chest Service, Tuberculosis Research Centre, Madras, British Medical Research Council. A double-blind, placebo-controlled clinical trial of three anti-tuberculosis chemoprophylaxis regimens in patients with silicosis in Hong Kong. *Am Rev Respir Dis* 1992;145:36.
At 5 years, the rate of active tuberculosis was halved in patients with silicosis receiving chemoprophylaxis with rifampin for 3 months, INH and rifampin for 3 months, or INH for 6 months, compared with those given placebo.

Hsu KHK. Thirty years after isoniazid. *JAMA* 1984;251:1283.
No control group. Effectiveness of INH prophylaxis was best demonstrated in children infected before age 4.

Huang YS, et al. Polymorphism of the N-acetyltransferase 2 gene as a susceptibility risk factor for antituberculosis drug-indicated hepatitis. *Hepatology* 2002;35:883–889.
Slow acetylatose are at an increase risk for hepatotoxicity than rapid acetylatose.

International Union Against Tuberculosis Committee on Prophylaxis. Efficacy of various durations of isoniazid preventive therapy for tuberculosis: 5 years of follow-up in the IUAT trial. *Bull World Health Organ* 1982;60:555.
A 24-week regimen of INH was effective.

Israel HL, Gottlieb JE, Maddrey WC. Perspective: preventive isoniazid therapy and the liver. *Chest* 1992;101:1298.
INH hepatic toxicity is reviewed, and three cases of fatal INH hepatitis are reported.

Jasmer RM, Nahid P, Hopewell PC. Latent tuberculosis infection. *N Engl J Med* 2002;347:1860–1866.
Review.

Livengood JR, et al. Isoniazid-resistant tuberculosis: a community outbreak and report of a rifampin prophylaxis failure. *JAMA* 1985;253:2847.
Three options are available for the management of contacts of persons with known INH-resistant tuberculosis: (1) INH, (2) rifampin alone or in combination with INH, or (3) no antituberculous therapy and close observation of the patient for development of active disease. A possible case of rifampin prophylaxis failure is presented.

Moreno S, et al. Isoniazid preventive therapy in human immunodeficiency virus-infected persons. *Arch Intern Med* 1997;157:1729–1734.
INH prophylaxis in HIV-positive patients decreased the incidence of active tuberculosis and improved overall survival.

Moulding TS, Redeker AG, Kanal GC. Twenty isoniazid-associated deaths in one state. *Am Rev Respir Dis* 1989;140:700.
INH was used for prevention in 19 cases.

Nazar-Stewart V, Nolan CM. Results of a directly observed intermittent isoniazid preventive therapy program in a shelter for homeless men. *Am Rev Respir Dis* 1992;146:57.
In a supervised program, INH could be given safely to the homeless in a dosage of 900 mg twice weekly.

Passannante M, Gallagher CT, Reichman LB. Preventive therapy for multidrug-resistant tuberculosis, MDRTB: a Delphi survey. *Chest* 1994;106:431–434.
No evidence that multidrug-resistant tuberculosis is more invasive than susceptible strains. Optimal therapy is unknown in this setting.

Priest DH, et al. Use of intermittent rifampin and pyrazinamide therapy for latent tuberculosis infection in a targeted tuberculin testing program. *Clin Infect Dis* 2004;39:1764–1771.
Despite monitoring, avoid using rifampin and pyrazinamide for latent tuberculosis because of hepatotoxicity.

Singh N, Wagener MM, Gayowski T. Safety and efficacy of isoniazid chemoprophylaxis administered during liver transplant candidacy for the prevention of posttransplant tuberculosis. *Transplantation* 2002;74:892–895.
A 12-month course of isoniazid was well tolerated.

Smieja MJ, et al. Isoniazid for preventing tuberculosis in non-HIV infected persons. *Cochrane Database Syst Rev* 2004:4.
Review. A 6- or 12-month course had a similar efficacy in preventing active tuberculosis.

Snider DE Jr. Pyridoxine supplementation during isoniazid therapy. *Tubercle* 1980;61:191.
Useful in older individuals, alcoholics, and pregnant women to prevent peripheral neuropathy.

Snider DE Jr, Caras GJ. Isoniazid-associated hepatitis deaths: a review of available information. *Am Rev Respir Dis* 1992;145:494.
Deaths reviewed. Women may be at an increased risk for fatal INH-related hepatitis.

Snider DE Jr, Caras GJ, Koplan JP. Preventive therapy with isoniazid: cost effectiveness of different durations of therapy. *JAMA* 1986;255:1579.
According to a cost effectiveness analysis, a 6-month course of INH had an advantage over a 1-year regimen.

Stead WW. Management of health care workers after inadvertent exposure to tuberculosis: a guide for the use of preventive therapy. *Ann Intern Med* 1995;122:906–912.
In a heavily exposed healthcare worker, start INH even if the tuberculin skin test reaction is negative. If the skin test reaction is still negative at 3 months, discontinue INH.

Stead WW, et al. Benefit-risk considerations in preventive treatment for tuberculosis in elderly persons. *Ann Intern Med* 1987;107:843.
Among older persons, INH hepatic toxicity developed in 4.4%.
Steiger Z, et al. Pulmonary tuberculosis after gastric resection. *Am J Surg* 1976;131:668.
Tuberculosis is likely to be reactivated after a gastrectomy in patients with chest roentgenographic evidence of inactive tuberculosis who have not been previously treated.
Whalen CC, et al. A trial of three regimens to prevent tuberculosis in Ugandan adults infected with the human immunodeficiency virus. *N Engl J Med* 1997;337:801–808.
A 6-month course of INH in PPD-positive, HIV-infected adults was effective in reducing the risk for active tuberculosis. Also effective in reducing the risk for tuberculosis were INH and rifampin for 3 months and INH, rifampin, and pyrazinamide for 3 months.

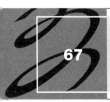

67   TREATMENT OF TUBERCULOSIS

The modern era of tuberculosis (TB) treatment began in 1944, when streptomycin was first administered to a critically ill patient with dramatic effect. Shortly thereafter streptomycin monotherapy was found to promote clinical relapse with the emergence of drug-resistant organisms. In the 1950s and 1960s, however, prolonged courses of combination antituberculosis chemotherapy successfully prevented drug resistance, ushering in an era in which public health policy makers in this country began to plan for TB control and even elimination. To illustrate this, the TB case rate declined more than tenfold since midcentury, from 53 cases per 100,000 in 1953 to 5.2 cases per 100,000 in 2002. Nevertheless, the clinician who treats a patient today with active TB has a challenging responsibility.

The goals of active TB treatment are to kill *Mycobacterium tuberculosis* organisms rapidly, to prevent the emergence of drug resistance, and to eliminate persistent bacilli to prevent relapse. Therapy benefits both the patient and the community by preventing the spread of disease. The most effective management plan adheres to several essential principles of care. First, the decision to treat assumes acceptance of the collaboration and relative responsibilities of the treating provider and the local health department in identifying all persons suspected of having TB, evaluating them, and ensuring that an effective treatment plan is not just initiated but completed as well. Second, success is best ensured with a patient-centered plan based on the patient's clinical condition and tailored with the patient as an active participant, together with a team of physician and nurse, outreach worker, and case manager or social worker. Third, direct observation of therapy (DOT), in which the patient is observed swallowing the medications, is the preferred strategy for all patients and a priority for patients with positive sputum smears, previous treatment failure or relapse, drug resistance, HIV infection, substance abuse, psychiatric illness, memory impairment, previous nonadherence to therapy, and all children and adolescents.

The American Thoracic Society and the Centers for Disease Control and Prevention have offered guidelines for the management of TB since 1971. The most recent guidelines, released in 2003, were cosponsored also by the Infectious Diseases Society of America. The guidelines emphasize that the responsibility for successful treatment of TB is placed primarily on the provider or program initiating therapy. They also address the choice of treatment regimen based on evidence from clinical trials, the increasing importance of drug-susceptibility testing of the cultured organism, and reevaluation of the sputum smear and culture after the first 2 months of therapy—the so-called initial phase—to guide the subsequent course of therapy—the so-called continuation phase.

 INITIAL MANAGEMENT

The decision to initiate treatment should be based on epidemiologic information, such as history of exposure or risk factors for infection, the patient's clinical condition, including pathology, radiographic findings, results of acid-fast bacilli (AFB)-staining of sputum smears and other specimens, and mycobacterial cultures. If the suspicion of disease is high or the patient is seriously ill, treatment should be initiated before the results of sputum culture are obtained. If the diagnosis is confirmed by isolation of *M. tuberculosis* or by a positive nucleic acid amplification test, treatment should be continued to complete a standard course of therapy.

Patients with suspected TB should have sputum and other clinical specimens collected for AFB smear, culture, and drug-susceptibility testing. Baseline testing in patients begun on therapy should include measurement of serum amino transferases, bilirubin, alkaline phosphatase, and creatinine, a platelet count, an HIV screening antibody test and, if ethambutol (EMB) is to be used, testing of visual acuity and red-green color discrimination.

 RECOMMENDED TREATMENT REGIMENS

Culture-Positive Drug-Susceptible Active TB

The recommended regimens for patients with drug-susceptible organisms are based on evidence from clinical trials (Table 67-1). Each of the four regimens for patients with culture-positive pulmonary TB include an initial 2-month phase using three or four drugs, then obtaining sputum cultures to identify patients at increased risk of relapse, then choosing one of several options for a 4- or 7-month continuation phase of two drugs. The 4-month continuation phase should be used for the majority of patients. The 7-month continuation phase is recommended only for: patients with cavitary pulmonary TB caused by drug-susceptible organisms and whose sputum culture at the time of completion of the initial phase is positive; patients whose initial phase did not include pyrazinamide (PZA); and patients being treated with once-weekly isoniazid (INH) and whose sputum culture at the time of completion of the initial phase is positive. A three-drug regimen of INH, rifampin (RIF), and PZA can be used if the likelihood of INH resistance is less than 4% in a community, and if there are no risk factors for multiple-drug resistant TB (MDR-TB). The same regimens can be used in patients who are HIV positive; however, the length of therapy must be extended to at least 9 months, or 6 months beyond sputum culture conversion.

Culture-Negative Active TB

If initial AFB smears and cultures are negative, a diagnosis other than TB should be considered. If no other diagnosis is found and the purified protein derivative (PPD)-tuberculin skin test is positive, empirical combination chemotherapy should be started using one of the recommended initial-phase regimens (Table 67-1). If there is a clinical or radiographic response after 2 months of therapy, a diagnosis of culture-negative TB can be made. Treatment should be continued with a 2-month continuation phase of INH and RIF. A 4-month total course of therapy is effective for culture-negative active TB.

Culture-Negative Latent TB Infection

If initial AFB smears are negative and the suspicion for active TB is low, treatment can be deferred until the results of mycobacterial cultures and repeat chest radiograph at 2 months are available. If the culture is negative and follow-up clinical information suggests the patient does not have active TB, patients with positive PPD-tuberculin skin tests should be treated for latent TB infection.

TABLE 67-1 Drug Regimens for Culture-Positive Pulmonary Tuberculosis Caused by Drug-Susceptible Organisms

Initial phase			Continuation phase			Range of total doses (minimum duration)	Rating (evidence)*	
Regimen	Drugs	Interval and doses† (minimum duration)	Regimen	Drugs	Interval and doses‡‡ (minimum duration)		HIV−	HIV+
1	INH RIF PZA EMB	Seven days per week for 56 doses (8 wk) or 5 days/wk for 40 doses (8 wk)§	1a	INH/RIF	Seven days per week for 126 doses (18 wk) or 5 days/wk for 90 doses (18 wk)	182–130 (26 wk)	A (I)	A (II)
			1b¶	INH/RIF	Twice weekly for 36 doses (18 wk)	92–76 (26 wk)	A (I)	A (II)
			1c#	INH/RPT	Once weekly for 18 doses (18 wk)	74–58 (26 wk)	B (I)	E (I)
2	INH RIF PZA EMB	Seven days per week for 14 doses (2 wk), then twice weekly for 12 doses (6 wk) or 5 days/wk for 10 doses (2 wk),§ then twice weekly for 12 doses (6 wk)	2a¶	INH/RIF	Twice weekly for 36 doses (18 wk)	62–58 (26 wk)	A (II)	B (II)
			2b#	INH/RPT	Once weekly for 18 doses (18 wk)	44–40 (26 wk)	B (I)	E (I)
3	INH RIF PZA EMB	Three times weekly for 24 doses (8 wk)	3a	INH/RIF	Three times weekly for 54 doses (18 wk)	78 (26 wk)	B (I)	B (I)
4	INH RIF EMB	Seven days per week for 56 doses (8 wk) or 5 days/wk for 40 doses (8 wk)§	4a	INH/RIF	Seven days per week for 217 doses (31 wk) or 5 days/wk for 155 doses (31 wk)§	273–195 (39 wk)	C (I)	C (II)
			4b	INH/RIF	Twice weekly for 62 doses (31 wk)	118–102 (39 wk)	C (I)	C (II)

RPT, Rifapentine.

Rating: A = preferred; B = acceptable alternative; C = offer when A and B cannot be given; E = should never be given. Evidence: I = randomized clinical trial; II = data from clinical trials that were not randomized or were conducted in other populations.

† When DOT is used, drugs may be given 5 days/week and the necessary number of doses adjusted accordingly. Although there are no studies that compare five with seven daily doses, extensive experience indicated this would be effective practice.

‡ Patients with cavitation on initial chest radiograph and positive cultures at completion of 2 months of therapy should receive a 7-month (31 week; either 217 doses [daily] or 62 doses [twice weekly]) continuation phase.

§ Five-day-a-week administration is always given by DOT.

¶ Not recommended for HIV-infected patients with CD4 cell counts less than 100 cells/μL.

Options 1c and 2b should be used only in HIV-negative patients who have negative sputum smears at the time of completion of 2 months of therapy and who do not have cavitation on initial chest radiograph. For patients started on this regimen and found to have a positive culture from the 2-month specimen, treatment should be extended an extra 3 months.

(Source: Official Joint Statement of the American Thoracic Society, Centers for Disease Control and Prevention and the Infectious Diseases Society of America [see references].)

FIRST-LINE ANTITUBERCULOSIS DRUGS

Six first-line antimicrobial drugs are used in the recommended regimens for active TB (Table 67-2). Among them INH, rifampin (RIF), EMB, and PZA form the core of TB therapy for patients with drug-susceptible organisms. Rifabutin is useful for treating TB in patients concurrently taking drugs that have unacceptable interactions with other rifamycins, such as antiretroviral protease inhibitors. Rifapentine is a recently FDA-approved rifamycin taken once weekly for use in the continuation phase, but should be used only in HIV-negative patients who have negative sputum smears at the time of completion of the initial phase and who do not have cavitation on initial chest radiograph.

Isoniazid

INH is a first-line agent for the treatment of all forms of TB caused by drug-susceptible organisms. It has profound early bactericidal activity against rapidly dividing cells. INH is safe for use in pregnancy. Central nervous system (CNS) penetration is excellent. Asymptomatic elevation of aminotransferases up to five times the upper limit of normal occurs in 10 to 20% of persons receiving INH alone for treatment of latent TB infection. The enzyme levels usually return to normal even with continued administration. Clinical hepatitis is a serious complication of INH administration, with an incidence of approximately 0.6% in patients given INH alone (nearly 2% in persons ages 50–64), 1.6% when INH is given with other agents not including RIF, and 2.7% when combined with RIF. Incidence may be enhanced by underlying liver disease, heavy alcohol consumption, and perhaps also the peri-partum period, particularly among Hispanic women. Continued administration can lead to death. All persons taking INH should have a baseline measurement of hepatic function and should be informed of symptoms of hepatitis; use of INH should be discontinued if such symptoms arise. Peripheral neuropathy occurs in fewer than 0.2%, and the risk is increased in persons with other diseases associated with neuropathy such as nutritional deficiency, diabetes, HIV infection, renal failure, alcoholism, pregnancy, and breastfeeding women. Prevention in patients with these conditions consists of pyridoxine 25 mg/day. Clinically significant drug interactions exist between INH and disulfiram or phenytoin; such interactions can result in psychosis or phenytoin toxicity.

Rifampin

RIF is a first-line agent for the treatment of all forms of TB caused by drug-susceptible organisms and is an essential component of all short-course regimens. It is bactericidal against organisms that are dividing rapidly and against semidormant organisms. RIF imparts an orange color to bodily fluids (sputum, urine, sweat, tears), and soft contact lenses and clothing may become stained. Pruritus may occur in up to 6% of patients but is generally self-limited; true hypersensitivity is uncommon. When RIF is used intermittently in doses above 600 mg per day, a flulike syndrome and thrombocytopenia may occur (incidence 0.4–0.7% of patients on twice-weekly RIF). Transient asymptomatic hyperbilirubinemia may occur in 0.6% of patients. Severe clinical hepatitis typically with a cholestatic pattern is rare when RIF is used alone and approximately 2.7% when used with INH. No routine monitoring tests are recommended. RIF can induce hepatic enzymes that increase the metabolism of common drugs (e.g., oral contraceptives, warfarin, methadone), often to ineffective levels. There are important bidirectional interactions between rifamycins and antiretroviral agents, and dosage adjustments are often necessary. RIF is safe for use in pregnancy. Cerebrospinal fluid (CSF) concentrations are 10 to 20% of serum levels, but this is sufficient for clinical effectiveness.

Rifabutin

Rifabutin is a substitute for RIF and is used for patients who are receiving any medication having unacceptable interactions with RIF or who have intolerance with RIF. It commonly is used in patients receiving antiretroviral therapy with protease inhibitors or nonnucleoside reverse transcriptase inhibitors, and in these circumstances, the dose may need to be adjusted.

TABLE 67-2 First-Line Drugs Used for the Treatment of Tuberculosis

Drug, route	Age group	Dose (maximum dose)			Comments
		Daily	Twice weekly	Three times weekly	
Isoniazid Oral, IM, IV	Children	10–15 mg/kg (300 mg)	20–30 mg/kg (900 mg)	—	Adverse effects: hepatitis, peripheral neuropathy, CNS effects; monitoring of liver function tests necessary only for patients with liver disease or symptoms of abnormal liver function
	Adults	5 mg/kg (300 mg)	15 mg/kg (900 mg)	15 mg/kg (900 mg)	
Rifampin Oral, IV	Children	10–20 mg/kg (600 mg)	10–20 mg/kg (600 mg)	—	Adverse effects: hepatitis, thrombocytopenia, fever, orange discoloration of bodily fluids, many drug interactions
	Adults	10 mg/kg (600 mg)	10 mg/kg (600 mg)	10 mg/kg (600 mg)	
Rifabutin Oral	Children	Unknown	Unknown	Unknown	Not FDA approved for treatment of tuberculosis; indicated for patients receiving antiretroviral or other drugs that interact with rifampin or who do not tolerate rifampin
	Adults	5 mg/kg (300 mg)	5 mg/kg (300 mg)	5 mg/kg (300 mg)	
Rifapentine Oral	Children	Not approved	Not approved	Not approved	Once-weekly dose during continuation phase: 10 mg/kg (600 mg maximum dose); use only in patients who meet criteria
	Adults	—	—	—	

Drug/Route	Population				Adverse effects
Pyrazinamide Oral	Children Adults	15–30 mg/kg (2 g) Weight 40–55 kg: 1.0 g Weight 56–75 kg: 1.5 g Weight 76–90 kg: 2.0 g	50 mg/kg (2 g) Weight 40–55 kg: 2.0 g Weight 56–75 kg: 3.0 g Weight 76–90 kg: 4.0 g	– Weight 40–55 kg: 1.5 g Weight 56–75 kg: 2.5 g Weight 76–90 kg: 3.0 g	Adverse effects: asymptomatic hyperuricemia, acute gout rare, routine monitoring of uric acid levels not necessary but can be used to measure compliance; hepatotoxicity rate 1% or less, monitor liver function tests when used in patients with preexisting liver disease; teratogenicity data uncertain, may be safe in pregnancy
Ethambutol Oral	Children Adults	15–20 mg/kg (1 g) Weight 40–55 kg: 0.8 g Weight 56–75 kg: 1.2 g Weight 76–90 kg: 1.6 g	50 mg/kg (2.5 g) Weight 40–55 kg: 2.0 g Weight 56–75 kg: 2.8 g Weight 76–90 kg: 4.0 g	– Weight 40–55 kg: 1.2 g Weight 56–75 kg: 2.0 g Weight 76–90 kg: 2.4 g	Adverse effect: optic toxicity manifested as decreased acuity or decreased red-green discrimination; monitor visual acuity and color vision at baseline and monthly, use with caution in children too young to assess visual acuity

IM, Intramuscular; IV, Intravenous; FDA, Food and Drug Administration.

In severely immunocompromised HIV-infected patients, it has been found to be associated with neutropenia (incidence 2%) or gastrointestinal symptoms (incidence 3%). Asymptomatic elevation of liver enzymes occurs at a frequency similar to that of RIF. Flulike syndrome is rare and orange discoloration of bodily fluids is universal.

Rifapentine

Rifapentine is used once weekly with INH in the continuation phase of treatment. It is reserved for patients without HIV infection, with noncavitary pulmonary TB caused by drug-susceptible organisms, who have negative sputum smears at the completion of the 2-month initial phase of treatment. The adverse effects are similar to those associated with RIF.

Pyrazinamide

PZA is a first-line agent for the treatment of all forms of TB caused by drug-susceptible organisms. It exerts its greatest activity against dormant or semidormant organisms within macrophages or the acidic environment of caseous foci. Mild anorexia and nausea are common side effects. Hepatotoxicity is rare (although it was 1% in one study) when administered at the currently recommended dose (25 mg/kg per day) but very common at the higher doses prescribed in past decades. Polyarthralgias occur in up to 40% of patients taking daily PZA; the pain responds to nonsteroidal anti-inflammatory drugs. Asymptomatic hyperuricemia is an expected effect and is without adverse consequence. Acute gout is rare, and a history of gout is a contraindication. There is little information about safety in pregnancy, but the benefits of PZA may outweigh the possible risks.

Ethambutol

EMB is a first-line agent for the treatment of all forms of TB caused by drug-susceptible organisms. It is included in initial regimens primarily to prevent emergence of RIF resistance when primary resistance to INH may be present. It can cause retrobulbar neuritis, manifested as decreased visual acuity or decreased red-green color discrimination. The effect is dose-related, with a minimal risk at a dose of 15 mg/kg per day; higher doses can be given safely twice or three times weekly. EMB is generally not recommended for routine use in children whose visual acuity cannot be monitored. EMB does not have efficacy in tuberculous meningitis. Patients should have baseline visual acuity and color discrimination testing; at monthly visits patients should be questioned regarding possible visual disturbances. Monthly testing is recommended for patients taking more than 15 to 25 mg/kg per day, for patients taking EMB longer than 2 months, and for any patient with renal insufficiency.

 MANAGEMENT DURING THERAPY

During treatment for pulmonary TB, sputum should be collected and tested for AFB smear and culture at monthly intervals until two consecutive specimens are negative on culture. Patients should be evaluated each month for treatment adherence and adverse medication effects. Routine measurements of hepatic and renal function and platelet count are not necessary during treatment unless patients have baseline abnormalities or risk factors for hepatotoxicity.

After 2 months of four-drug therapy, approximately 80% of patients with pulmonary TB caused by drug-susceptible organisms will have negative sputum cultures. The most common reason for positive cultures at this time is nonadherence to the regimen, which can be prevented by DOT. Other causes include extensive cavitary disease, drug resistance, malabsorption of drugs, and many bacilli on initial sputum smear. Treatment failure (positive cultures after 4 months of treatment) or relapse (recurrence after completion of treatment and cure) occurs at increased rates in patients who have cavitation on the initial chest radiograph combined with positive sputum cultures after the 2-month initial phase of treatment.

Completion of treatment is determined by the total number of doses taken, not on the duration of the treatment regimen. In the event of interruption of the regimen, the goal is to deliver the specified number of doses within a recommended maximum time. For example, for a 6-month daily regimen, the 182 doses should be administered within 9 months of beginning treatment.

Drug-induced hepatitis is the most serious common adverse effect of therapy, defined as a serum AST level more than three times the upper limit of normal in the presence of symptoms or five times the upper limit of normal in the absence of symptoms. INH, RIF, PZA and all other causes of hepatic injury should be stopped immediately, and testing for viral causes should be performed. Two or more antituberculosis drugs without hepatotoxicity may be used until the cause of the hepatitis is known. Once the AST level decreases to less than twice the upper limit of normal and symptoms have improved, first-line medications should be restarted in sequential fashion.

The prognosis for patients with active TB treated with a recommended regimen is excellent; the case-fatality rate worldwide for patients with smear-positive pulmonary TB is 3.8%. Among patients in the United States with HIV infection and silicosis, the TB case-fatality rate was 10%. Factors associated with a higher case-fatality rate are drug resistance, lack of DOT, and inadequate treatment regimen. In a recent analysis of patients treated with an adequate regimen, a high case-fatality rate was found to be associated with older age and underlying diabetes mellitus and renal failure.

 SPECIAL SITUATIONS

HIV Infection

Recent studies of newly diagnosed patients with TB have observed that up to 30% are simultaneously infected with HIV. Additionally, patients with HIV are more likely to reactivate latent infection, to have extrapulmonary disease, and to progress more rapidly to active TB. The rate of development of active disease in patients with latent TB and HIV dual infection is approximately 8% per year, compared with 10% in a lifetime for individuals with latent TB infection without HIV infection.

Recommendations for active TB treatment in HIV-infected patients are the same as for HIV-uninfected patients, with a few exceptions. The once-weekly rifapentine-containing regimen is contraindicated. RIF resistance occurs frequently in patients with advanced HIV disease who are treated with twice-weekly RIF or rifabutin regimens, and therefore daily or three times-weekly regimens are recommended. DOT is especially important in these regimens and for any HIV-infected patient on TB treatment.

The management of HIV-associated active TB is complex and requires expertise. Early consultation at a specialty center is recommended. Two sets of complex drug regimens with bidirectional interactions requires experienced decision making. Of particular concern is use of the rifamycins combined with antiretroviral protease inhibitors or nonnucleoside reverse transcriptase inhibitors. Furthermore, the likelihood of extrapulmonary disease increases with more advanced HIV infection. Fortunately, in the absence of MDR-TB, response to antituberculous therapy is similar to that seen in non–HIV-infected individuals. The likelihood of adverse reactions to antituberculous medications is probably higher in HIV-infected patients, so these patients should be closely monitored. Paradoxical reactions that mimic worsening of TB are more common in HIV-infected patients and may complicate therapy.

Extrapulmonary TB

The 6-month regimens that include INH and RIF are thought to be effective for extrapulmonary TB, with the exception of meningeal TB, for which a 9- to 12-month regimen is recommended. Prolonged courses are also recommended for infection in any organ slow to resolve clinically. Adjunctive therapy with corticosteroids is recommended for TB pericarditis and TB meningitis.

TABLE 67-3 Second-Line Drugs Used for the Treatment of Tuberculosis

Drug, route	Daily dose (maximum)	Adverse effects	Comments
Capreomycin IM, IV	Children: 15–30 mg/kg (1 g). Adults: 15mg/kg (1 g), 10 mg/kg (750 mg) in persons older than age 59	Nephrotoxic: reduced creatinine clearance, hypokalemia, hypomagnesemia. Ototoxic: vestibular deafness, tinnitus	Administration as a single dose 5–7 days/wk, can be reduced to 2–3 times per week after the first 2–4 months or after culture conversion; does not penetrate the CSF. Use with caution in renal insufficiency
Cycloserine Oral	Children: 10–15 mg/kg (1 g). Adults: 10–15 mg/kg (1 g) in two doses	Central nervous system effects: headache, restlessness, psychosis, seizures (pyridoxine 100–200 mg/day may prevent neurotoxic side effects)	Reduce dosage in renal insufficiency. Monitor neuropsychiatric symptoms monthly. Consider measurements of serum concentration until appropriate dose is established
Ethionamide Oral	Children: 15–20 mg/kg (1 g). Adults: 15–20 mg/kg (1 g)	Gastrointestinal (common): metallic taste, nausea, vomiting, anorexia, hepatotoxicity (incidence 2%). Neurotoxicity: peripheral neuritis, optic neuritis, depression, psychosis. Endocrine: gynecomastia, hypothyroidism, worsens diabetes control	Administration usually as 500–750 mg/day in a single dose or two divided doses. Reduce dosage in renal insufficiency. In patients with liver disease, use with caution, monitor liver function tests
Streptomycin IV, IM	Children: 20–40 mg/kg (1 g). Adults: 15mg/kg (1 g), 10 mg/kg (750 mg) in persons older than age 59	Ototoxicity: vestibular and hearing disturbances (higher incidence with age, loop diuretics). Neurotoxicity: circumoral paresthesias. Nephrotoxicity: renal insufficiency (incidence 2%). Teratogenic: congenital deafness	Administration as a single dose 5–7 days/wk, can be reduced to two–three times per week after the first 2–4 months or after culture conversion. Baseline testing: audiogram, vestibular, serum creatinine; monthly renal function monitoring

Drug	Dose	Adverse effects	Comments
p-Aminosalicylic acid Oral	Children: 200–300 mg/kg in two–four divided doses (10 g) Adults: 8–12 g in two or three doses	Gastrointestinal: intolerance (incidence 11%), steatorrhea Hypothyroidism, common; increased prothrombin time Hepatitis (incidence 0.3–0.5%)	Marginal efficacy in meningitis
Amikacin and kanamycin IV, IM	Children: 15–30 mg/kg (1 g) Adults: 15 mg/kg (1 g), 10 mg/kg (750 mg) in persons older than age 59	Nephrotoxicity: renal insufficiency (incidence 3% in patients without risk factors, 9% in patients with risk factors: baseline elevated creatinine, higher dose, other nephrotoxic drugs) Ototoxicity: deafness, less vestibular dysfunction than with streptomycin	Administration as a single dose 5–7 days/wk, can be reduced to two–three times per week after the first 2–4 months or after culture conversion
Levofloxacin, Moxifloxacin, Gatifloxacin Oral, IV	Levofloxacin: children: not approved; adults: 500–1,000 mg Moxifloxacin and Gatifloxacin: children: not approved; adults: 400 mg	Children: long-term use not approved because of concern about effects on bone and cartilage growth Gastrointestinal: nausea, bloating; neurological: dizziness, insomnia; cutaneous: rash, pruritus	Though not approved for use in children and adolescents, consider use in children with tuberculosis caused by organisms resistant to both INH and RIF Antacids decrease absorption of fluoroquinolones Avoid in pregnancy (teratogenic)

IM, Intramuscular; IV, Intravenous.

Infants, Children, and Adolescents

Infants and children younger than age 4 have high rates of disseminated TB, and therefore treatment should be started as soon as the diagnosis of TB is suspected. The regimens recommended for adults are also the regimens of choice for infants, children, and adolescents, with the exception that EMB is not routinely used in children. Acquired drug resistance is less likely in children because of the lower bacillary burden. Most studies of TB treatment in children have used a 6-month regimen of 2 months of INH, RIF plus PZA followed by 4 months of INH and RIF. The success rate is greater than 95% and the adverse reaction rate is less than 2%.

Pregnancy

The risk of active TB to the fetus is great, and therefore treatment should be initiated whenever the probability of disease is moderate to high. The initial treatment regimen should consist of INH, RIF, and EMB. If PZA is not used in the initial phase, the minimum duration of treatment is 9 months. The safety of PZA in pregnancy is uncertain. The World Health Organization and the International Union against Tuberculosis and Lung Disease state that PZA can probably be used safely in pregnancy.

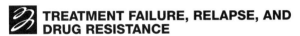# TREATMENT FAILURE, RELAPSE, AND DRUG RESISTANCE

Treatment failure, defined as recurrently positive cultures after 4 months of treatment, is most frequently caused by nonadherence to the regimen, but also by drug resistance, malabsorption of drugs, laboratory error, extensive cavities at the initiation of treatment, and biological variation of the response to therapy. Early consultation at a specialty center is recommended. If the patient is not seriously ill and the failure is thought to be caused by drug resistance, drug susceptibility testing should be performed. An empirical retreatment regimen can be begun or therapy can be delayed until the results of drug susceptibility testing guide the choice of regimen.

Never add a single drug to a failing regimen. Doing so is the equivalent of monotherapy and rapidly results in resistance to the new drug. At least two or preferably three new drugs to which susceptibility is likely should be added to lessen further new drug resistance. Empirical regimens might include second-line antituberculosis agents such as a fluoroquinolone, an injectable agent such as streptomycin, amikacin, kanamycin, or capreomycin, and an additional oral agent, such as *p*-aminosalicylic acid (PAS), cycloserine, or ethionamide (Table 67-3). The regimen can be adjusted when the results of drug-susceptibility testing are reported. Disease caused by organisms resistant to both INH and RIF are at higher risk of treatment failure and further drug resistance.

Relapse, defined as recurrence after completion of treatment and cure, should prompt culture confirmation and drug-susceptibility testing. Most relapses occur within 6 to 12 months after completion of therapy. In patients with drug-susceptible organisms originally treated with a DOT regimen containing RIF, most relapses are caused by susceptible organisms. For such patients, a standard four-drug regimen is an appropriate choice for empirical retreatment. (Patients with critical illness should also be treated with at least three additional drugs.) In patients originally treated with self-administered regimens or regimens that did not include a rifamycin, acquired drug resistance is likely. For such patients, empirical retreatment is advised with an expanded regimen of INH, RIF, PZA and two or three additional drugs, administered using DOT methods (Table 67-3). Length of therapy is not defined but should probably be 18 to 24 months if MDR-TB is identified.

Multidrug resistance (MDR) increases the risk of TB-associated death. Case-fatality rates approached 90% in early reports, although recent studies of patients treated with three drugs for which the organism is susceptible demonstrate treatment failure in 8% and case-fatality in 4%. These studies demonstrate that early identification of at-risk patients and use of effective combination therapies can result in earlier bacteriologic conversion and prolonged survival. Factors that have been shown to impact on survival with MDR-TB include: initiation of treatment within 4 weeks of diagnosis, treatment with at least two effective agents for at least 2 consecutive weeks, and disease limited to the lungs. Appropriate treatment for at least 2 consecutive weeks is probably the most important of these. Drug resistance often extends beyond INH and RIF. Consideration for MDR-TB is made on epidemiologic grounds, because most cases have occurred in closed populations within hospitals or prisons and in localized geographic areas, including Florida and New York. Healthcare workers exposed to actively infected individuals have also become ill. Recent national data suggest that 7 to 8% of *M. tuberculosis* isolates are now INH-resistant, whereas 1 to 2% of strains are multidrug resistant. Forty-three states plus the District of Columbia reported strains of MDR-TB between 1993 and 1997. Other data from New York, an area with increased numbers of patients with AIDS, demonstrate that approximately 33% of isolates of *M. tuberculosis* are resistant to one drug and 19% are multiply resistant. Knowledge of applicable resistance patterns is mandatory in order to effect treatment. (RBB)

Bibliography

Centers for Disease Control and Prevention. Treatment of Tuberculosis, American Thoracic Society, CDC, and Infectious Diseases Society of America. *MMWR* 2003;52: 1–77.

A consensus statement released by the CDC and two professional societies. This is the most recent in a series of such statements since 1971. The content includes a detailed presentation of antituberculosis drugs, drug regimens, principles of treatment, practical management advice, drug interactions, treatment in special situations, management of relapse, treatment failure and drug resistance, treatment of TB in low-income countries, and a research agenda for TB treatment. The evidence for and the strength of the recommendations are rated on the basis of a system developed by the United States Public Health Service and the Infectious Diseases Society of America. An excellent source of information for most clinicians.

Dean GL, et al. Treatment of tuberculosis in HIV-infected persons in the era of highly active antiretroviral therapy. *AIDS* 2002;16:75–83.

The authors evaluated the benefits and risks of starting highly active antiretroviral therapy (HAART) during the treatment of TB in HIV-infected patients in 12 centers in England. Initiating HAART resulted in significant reductions in HIV viral load, HIV-associated disease and mortality. Ten percent of patients with CD4 counts higher than 100 cells/μL developed an AIDS-defining illness (ADI), but 20% of patients with CD4 counts less than 100 cells/μL developed an ADI. Adverse events of HAART occurred in 54% of patients. The authors recommend starting HAART early in patients with advanced HIV disease and deferring HAART until the continuation phase of TB treatment for stable patients with CD4 counts higher than 100 cells/μL.

Fielder JF, et al. A high tuberculosis case-fatality rate in a setting of effective tuberculosis control: implications for acceptable treatment success rates. *Int J Tuberc Ling Dis* 2002;6:1114–1117.

The TB case-fatality rate in persons on treatment is 3.8% worldwide. Among adequately treated patients in Baltimore with an especially high case-fatality rate, independent risk factors for death were found to be older age, underlying diabetes mellitus, or underlying renal failure.

Saloman N, et al. Predictors and outcome of multidrug-resistant tuberculosis. *Clin Infect Dis* 1995; 21:1245–1252.

The investigators identified 88 HIV-infected patients, 18 of whom had MDR-TB. Use of at least two in vitro effective agents resulted in enhanced 1-year survivorship and more rapid sputum conversion. Presence of MDR-TB did not predict poor outcome. This study reemphasizes the need for earlier and better identification of patients, use of multiple drug regimens, and expanded susceptibility testing of patients at risk for MDR-TB.

Tahaoğlu K, et al. The treatment of multidrug-resistant tuberculosis in Turkey. *N Engl J Med* 2001;345:170–174.

The authors report the results of treatment of 158 patients with MDR-TB. The patients had previously received a mean of 5.7 antituberculosis drugs and were infected with organisms that were resistant to a mean of 4.4 drugs. Patients were treated for 18 to

24 months with at least three drugs thought to be active. Surgical resection was performed in 36 patients. Cultures became negative in 95% of patients after a mean of 1.9 months. The overall success rate of treatment was 77%, with cures in 49% and probable cures in 27%. Treatment failed in 8% and the death rate was 4%. The authors conclude that MDR-TB can be cured with the use of appropriate, intensive treatment regimens.

Tuberculosis Trials Consortium. Rifapentine and isoniazid once a week versus rifampin and isoniazid twice a week for treatment of drug-susceptible pulmonary tuberculosis in HIV-negative patients: a randomised clinical trial. *Lancet* 2002;360:528–534.

The authors conducted a trial of the continuation phase of TB treatment in 1,004 patients who had completed the first 2 months of a 6-month treatment regimen. Failure or relapse occurred in 9.2% of those on the once weekly regimen and 5.6% in those on the twice weekly regimen (relative risk 1.64, 95% confidence interval [CI] 1.04–2.58). Characteristics independently associated with failure were sputum culture positive at 2 months, cavitation on chest radiograph, being underweight, bilateral pulmonary involvement, and being a non-Hispanic white person. Among subjects without cavitation, rates of failure or relapse were 2.9% in the once-weekly group and 2.5% in the twice-weekly group. Rates of adverse events and death were similar in the two treatment groups.

Selected Laboratory Procedures XVIII

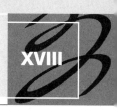

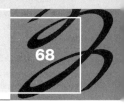
henever the microbiology laboratory reports that a blood culture is positive for a gram-negative bacillus, it must be assumed that the patient is bacteremic and a life-threatening infection is present. The report of a gram-negative rod on smear is important to the clinician who will then reassess the evaluation and antibiotic selection made when blood cultures were first taken. This chapter describes some of the clinical scenarios associated with a gram-negative rod in the bloodstream. Specific identification of the gram-negative bacillus will also sometimes be helpful in identifying a primary infection. Current automated continuous-monitoring blood culture systems will help shorten the waiting time for notification and identification, decrease hospital stay, and improve patient care.

ETIOLOGIC AGENTS

Several studies have classified gram-negative bacteremia according to most common etiologic agent and most frequent source of infection. Kreger and associates, for example, reviewed 612 episodes of gram-negative bacteremia during a 10-year period. Table 68-1 shows the distribution of etiologic agents. *Escherichia coli* was the most common gram-negative rod causing bacteremia, being responsible for 31% of cases. Table 68-2 shows the sources of gram-negative bacteremia. Urinary tract infection is by far the most common source, with infection of the gastrointestinal and biliary tract second. The respiratory tract (i.e., bacteremic pneumonia) was the source in only 9% of cases, and skin and soft tissue in 6.5%.

A recent survey of bloodstream infection resulting from gram-negative bacilli around the world showed a similar distribution of organisms, with *E. coli* responsible for 41% of all gram-negative bacteremia, *Klebsiella* spp. 17.9%, and *Pseudomonas* 10.6%.

The gram-negative organism most likely to cause bacteremia varies with several factors. If the bacteremia is acquired in the community, *E. coli* is the most common organism. Organisms such as *Pseudomonas aeruginosa* and *Serratia marcescens* are most likely to occur in the hospital. The longer the length of stay, the more likely it is that relatively antimicrobial-resistant organisms will be found. The population studied will also affect the distribution of etiologic agents in gram-negative bacteremia. *P. aeruginosa* is more likely to occur in the neutropenic patient, whereas *E. coli* is by far the most common agent in the healthy young patient. Each hospital has its own profile of etiologic agents. Some organisms, such as *Acinetobacter* spp., may be common in one hospital and unusual in another. The site of infection may also predict the etiologic agent. For example, *Proteus mirabilis* or *Providencia* spp. isolated from blood cultures suggest urinary tract infection. In bacteremic pneumonia, *Klebsiella pneumoniae* and *P. aeruginosa* are much more common than *Proteus* spp., *Providencia*, or even *E. coli*. *Bacteroides* bacteremia suggests anaerobic infection of the colon or female genital tract, a liver abscess, or postoperative wound infection.

The pattern of gram-negative bacteremia has been changing with the introduction of new antimicrobials. For example, *Stenotrophomonas maltophilia* (formerly *P. maltophilia*) infection has been increasing because of the aminoglycoside resistance of this organism. Isolates can be cultured from the hospital environment, and common-source outbreaks can occur. *Burkholderia cepacia* also has caused an increasing incidence of bacteremia and outbreaks associated with hospital devices, such as a blood gas analyzer. An increasing number of *Pseudomonas* spp. have been implicated in bacteremia. Newer trends in antibiotic resistance to gram-negative bacilli include ciprofloxacin-resistant *E. coli*, with 6% of all

433

TABLE 68-1 | **Etiologic Agents in Gram-Negative Bacteremia**

Agent	Frequency (%)
Escherichia coli	31
Klebsiella-Enterobacter-Serratia	22
Pseudomonas species	10
Proteus and *Providencia*	8
Bacteroides	7
Other	6
Polymicrobial	16

species in the United States and ceftazidime-resistant *Klebsiella* now accounting for 5% of all species.

Enterobacter bacteremia has been caused by contaminated blood products and contaminated intravenous fluids. A recent outbreak occurred in a neonatal unit secondary to contaminated dextrose-saline infusions.

Acinetobacter spp. are causing more cases of nosocomial bacteremia, in part because of their relative resistance to third-generation cephalosporins. Bacteremia is frequently associated with an IV catheter or is secondary to pneumonia. In one recent study, patients with *A. baumannii* bacteremia had more hemodynamic instability and longer hospital stays than those with other bloodstream infections. The organism, on Gram's stain, frequently appears as a gram-negative coccus or diplococcus rather than as a rod.

A gram-negative bacillus on smear may represent bacteremia from a nonenteric gram-negative rod. For example, a group of slow-growing gram-negative bacilli, including *Haemophilus aphrophilus*, *Actinobacillus actinomycetemcomitans*, *Cardiobacterium hominis*, *Eikenella corrodens*, and *Kingella* species (HACEK group), can cause a picture of subacute bacterial endocarditis. These organisms are often difficult to grow, requiring prolonged incubation and subculturing to chocolate agar. *H. influenzae* can cause bacteremia secondary to pneumonia, otitis media, meningitis, or epiglottitis. These small, gram-negative coccobacilli usually can be distinguished from the larger enteric gram-negative rods on smear.

Dysgonic fermenter-2, now called *Capnocytophaga canimorsus*, is a slow-growing gram-negative bacillus that causes a zoonotic infection acquired through dog bites. It can cause fulminating bacteremia in splenectomized and alcoholic patients.

Salmonella bacteremia has become an increasing problem in patients with AIDS. Recurrent episodes of fever and chills and positive blood cultures are common. *Campylobacter* may also cause disease with bacteremia. *Shigella* spp., rarely a cause of bacteremia, have been more commonly reported, particularly in AIDS patients.

Flavobacterium spp., particularly *Flavobacterium meningosepticum*, are nonmotile, catalase-positive, gram-negative bacilli that have become ubiquitous in some hospital environments. Hospital outbreaks of bacteremia can occur. The organism has an unusual

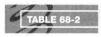

TABLE 68-2 | **Primary Sources of Gram-Negative Bacteremia**

Source	Frequency (%)
Urinary tract	34.0
Gastrointestinal tract	14.0
Respiratory tract	9.0
Skin	6.5
Biliary tract	2.0
Reproductive tract	3.0
Unknown	30.0

sensitivity pattern, generally being sensitive to trimethoprim-sulfamethoxazole and vancomycin, but it is resistant to aminoglycosides.

New genera and species of Enterobacteriaceae continue to emerge. In 1972, there were 11 genera and 26 species; in 1995, there were 28 genera and 115 species. Newer genera, which may cause episodes of urinary tract infection, wound infection, or bacteremia, include *Hafnia, Edwardsiella, Ewingella, Kluyvera,* and *Cedecea.* Many of these newer genera are particularly antibiotic resistant.

 CLINICAL APPROACH

An internal medicine or infectious disease consultant often will be asked to assess a patient when the laboratory calls with the positive blood culture report. A history and physical examination should be directed at the most likely sources of infection (a urinary tract infection; gastrointestinal infection; pneumonia; skin, soft-tissue, or catheter infection). Urine Gram's stain and culture should be obtained. Chest roentgenography and sputum Gram's stain are necessary if pneumonia is suspected. A complete physical examination will include a pelvic examination in a woman in whom no other definite source of infection can be defined. IV lines should be removed, and the patency of indwelling Foley catheters or nephrostomy tubes should be checked. Abdominal tenderness in the setting of gram-negative bacteremia will usually require a surgical consult and appropriate imaging examination.

Most patients reported to have gram-negative rods in a blood culture will require therapy with an antimicrobial that has a broad spectrum of gram-negative activity. In the case of a patient who appears well at the time of the report, blood cultures can be repeated while the patient is being closely observed. However, few blood cultures positive for gram-negative bacilli represent contamination. The great majority of such cases require rapid antimicrobial therapy. When infection caused by *H. influenzae,* endocarditis-causing organisms of the HACEK group, dysgonic fermenter-2, or anaerobes is suspected, a different approach to antimicrobial therapy will be required than in infection with the more common enteric gram-negative bacilli. (SLB)

Bibliography

Beekman SE, et al. Effects of rapid detection of bloodstream infection on length of hospitalization and hospital charges. *J Clin Microbiol* 2003;41:3119.
Current automated continuous-monitoring blood culture systems have decreased the time from obtaining blood cultures to time of call about positive Gram's stain. This results in better patient care and shorter hospitalizations.

Blot S, Vandewoude K, Colardyn F. Nosocomial bacteremia involving *Acinetobacter baumannii* in critically ill patients: a matched cohort study. *Intensive Care Med* 2003; 29:471.
A. baumannii bacteremia patients had more hemodynamic instability, longer stays, and more ventilator dependence than matched control patients with other types of bacteremia.

Diekma DJ, et al. Survey of bloodstream infections due to gram-negative bacilli: frequency of occurrence and antimicrobial susceptibility of isolates collected in the United States, Canada, and Latin America for the SENTRY antimicrobial surveillance program. *Clin Infect Dis* 1999;29:595.
Distribution of gram-negative bacilli causing bacteremia has changed little over the past 30 years. E. coli is the most common isolate, Klebsiella spp. second, and Pseudomonas third.

Diekma DJ, et. al. Antimicrobial resistance trends and outbreak frequency in United States hospitals. *Clin Infect Dis* 2004;38:78.
Ceftazidime-resistant Klebsiella has become 5% of all Klebsiella isolates, ciprofloxacin-resistant E. coli, 6% of all isolates.

DuPont HL, Spink WW. Infections due to gram-negative organisms: an analysis of 860 patients with bacteremia at the University of Minnesota Medical Center, 1958–1966. *Medicine (Baltimore)* 1969;48:307.
An analysis of the portal of entry in 655 adults with gram-negative bacteremia.

Edmondson EB, Sanford JP. The *Klebsiella-Enterobacter (Aerobacter)-Serratia* group: a clinical and bacteriological evaluation. *Medicine (Baltimore)* 1967;46:323.
The lung is an important primary source for Klebsiella *bacteremia.*

Freney J, et al. Postoperative infant septicemia caused by *Pseudomonas luteola* (CDC Group Ve-1) and *Pseudomonas orzihabitans* (CDC Group Ve-2). *J Clin Microbiol* 1988;26:1241.
Several unusual Pseudomonas *species have caused bacteremia—in this case, in an infant after open heart surgery.*

Glew RH, Moellering RC Jr, Kunz LJ. Infections with *Acinetobacter calcoaceticus* (*Herellea vaginicola*): clinical and laboratory studies. *Medicine (Baltimore)* 1977;56:79.
The sources of bacteremia include intravascular cannulas and respiratory infections.

Hicklin H, Verghese A, Alvarez S. Dysgonic fermenter-2 septicemia. *Rev Infect Dis* 1987;9:884.
Dysgonic fermenter-2 causes bacteremia after dog bites, particularly in splenectomized and alcoholic patients.

Kang CI, et al. Pseudomonas aeruginosa bacteremia: risk factor for mortality and influence of delayed receipt of effective antimicrobial therapy on clinical outcome. *Clin Infect Dis* 2003;37:745.
More recent data again showing that delay in proper antibiotic therapy results in higher mortality rate. It is important to predict likelihood of Pseudomonas *when therapy for bacteremia is being considered.*

Kang CI, et al. Risk factors for ciprofloxacin resistance in bloodstream infections due to extended spectrum beta lactamase producing *E. coli* and *K. pneumoniae. Microb Drug Resist* 2004;10:71.
Ciprofloxacin resistance among E. coli *and* Klebsiella *spp. are best predicted by previous antibiotic therapy with quinolones and use of indwelling Foley catheters.*

Kang CI, et al. Bloodstream infections caused by Enterobacter species: predictors of 30-day mortality rate and impact of broad spectrum cephalosporin resistance on outcome. *Clin Infect Dis* 2004;39:12.
Broad-spectrum cephalosporin resistance adversely affected 30-day mortality rate in patients with Enterobacter *bacteremia.*

Kreger BE, et al. Gram-negative bacteremia. III. Reassessment of etiology, epidemiology and ecology in 612 patients. *Am J Med* 1980;68:332.
Definitive study on the clinical picture of gram-negative bacteremia, including etiologic agents and sources of infection.

McCue JD. Improved mortality in gram-negative bacillary bacteremia. *Arch Intern Med* 1985;145:1212.
Compares etiologic agents in community-acquired versus hospital-acquired gram-negative bacteremia.

McGowan JE Jr. Changing etiology of nosocomial bacteremia and fungemia and other hospital-acquired infections. *Rev Infect Dis* 1985;7(suppl 3):357.
Describes changing trends between 1935 and 1983, which is of historical interest in following gram-negative rod susceptibility to antibiotics.

Miller PJ, Wenzel RP. Etiologic organisms as independent predictors of death and morbidity associated with bloodstream infection. *J Infect Dis* 1987;156:471.
Compares mortality rates and incidence of shock associated with various etiologic agents in gram-negative bacteremia. Mortality is more related to patient underlying disease than organism.

Morduchowicz G, et al. *Shigella* bacteremia in adults: a report of five cases and review of the literature. *Arch Intern Med* 1987;147:2034.
Report of five cases of Shigella *bacteremia. Patients were malnourished but did not have AIDS.*

Munson EL, et al. Detection and treatment of bloodstream infection: laboratory reporting and antimicrobial management. *J Clin Microbiol* 2003;41:495.
Most therapy interventions occur at the time of phlebotomy for initial blood cultures and when Gram's stain results are called. Broad-spectrum agents, of necessity, are increasingly being used.

Smego RA Jr. Endemic nosocomial *Acinetobacter calcoaceticus* bacteremia. *Arch Intern Med* 1985;145:2174.

> A. calcoaceticus *causes nosocomial bacteremia. The lungs and IV catheters are the most common primary sources.*

BLOOD CULTURE GROWING A GRAM-POSITIVE ROD

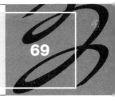

A report from the laboratory that a blood culture contains a gram-positive rod suggests that the organism is a diphtheroid or *Corynebacterium* spp., *Clostridium* spp., *Propionibacterium acnes*, *Listeria monocytogenes*, or *Bacillus* spp. Other possibilities, although they are much less common, include *Rhodococcus equi*, *Erysipelothrix rhusiopathiae*, *Gardnerella vaginale*, or *Lactobacillus* spp. Some *Corynebacterium* spp., *P. acnes*, and *Bacillus* spp. are part of the indigenous flora of the skin, and their isolation in a blood culture may represent nothing more than contamination. Other organisms, such as *Listeria*, *Clostridium*, or *Bacillus anthracis* may produce life-threatening disease, and their recovery from a blood culture may indicate the need for prompt therapy. A clinician who is assessing the importance of a blood culture positive for a gram-positive rod should consider the following factors:

1. *Does the patient have a single positive blood culture or multiple sets of positive blood cultures obtained during several days?* The finding of a single positive culture for a *Corynebacterium* spp., *P. acnes*, or *Bacillus* spp., except for *B. anthracis* or *B. cereus*, may represent nothing more than contamination. If the patient is febrile or has an implanted device, blood cultures should be repeated because, in selected clinical settings, these organisms can produce disease such as infective endocarditis. The patient with endocarditis will have multiple positive blood cultures because the bacteremia is generally continuous. In contrast, a single blood culture positive for an organism such as *Listeria* or, rarely, *Rhodococcus* or *Erysipelothrix* always indicates disease rather than contamination. Repeated blood cultures are indicated to determine if the patient has an illness associated with a sustained bacteremia. A single blood culture positive for a *Clostridium* sp. may be unimportant and secondary to a transient bacteremia, or it may reflect a life-threatening illness. Repeated blood cultures are indicated only if the patient is "ill." Often, a blood culture positive for *Clostridium* becomes evident after the patient has been sent home from the hospital. In this situation, antimicrobial therapy is usually unnecessary.

2. *Is the patient a normal or a compromised host?* Although any of the gram-positive rods can infect a normal host, *Listeria* has a predilection to produce infection in patients with impaired cellular immunity. Pregnant women and neonates also are susceptible to *Listeria*. *Rhodococcus* also is an intracellular pathogen that has a predilection for infecting the compromised host. *C. jeikeium* usually causes infection in neutropenic patients with central venous catheters.

3. *Does the patient have an implanted device, such as a cardiac valve prosthesis, arterial graft, ventriculoatrial shunt, or skeletal prosthesis?* Although *Staphylococcus epidermidis* is a major pathogen in patients with implanted devices, rarely *Corynebacterium* spp., *P. acnes*, or a *Bacillus* sp. can cause an infection in this setting. The finding of multiple positive blood cultures for one of these organisms during several days suggests an infection of a prosthetic device, regardless of how innocuous the organism is considered. If a

patient has a single positive blood culture for a gram-positive rod and has an implanted device, obtain two to three sets of blood cultures within 24 hours. In a patient who is not receiving antimicrobials, this approach should detect the vast majority of cases of bacteremia. If the patient has an IV line and is febrile, the line should be changed and the tip cultured.

Corynebacterium spp. and *P. acnes* are the dominant organisms on the skin of adults. They are often called diphtheroids because they resemble, but do not include, *C. diphtheriae*. Diphtheroids are aerobic gram-positive rods, do not form spores, and are not acid-fast. *P. acnes* organisms resemble diphtheroids and are anaerobic. The documentation of endocarditis caused by a diphtheroid may be difficult because the blood cultures may require prolonged incubation before demonstrating positivity, and *Corynebacterium* or *Propionibacterium* organisms frequently contaminate blood cultures. *Propionibacterium* is usually susceptible to penicillin, a cephalosporin, and the macrolides. Although it is an anaerobe, the organism is resistant to the imidazoles, such as metronidazole. Bacteremia caused by *Corynebacterium* spp. may be treated with a combination of penicillin with an aminoglycoside. If the patient is allergic to penicillin, vancomycin can be used.

Listeria is a β-hemolytic, aerobic, gram-positive rod that may be mistaken for a diphtheroid. In the laboratory, the organism has a characteristic tumbling motility. Both epidemic and sporadic disease occurs. Foodborne outbreaks were recognized in the 1980s, with coleslaw, milk, and cheese responsible for several outbreaks. *Listeria* has been isolated from uncooked beef, poultry, processed meats, and raw vegetables. It has been recommended that compromised hosts, pregnant women, and older individuals avoid soft cheeses, such as Mexican-style or feta cheese. In addition, beef, pork, and poultry should be thoroughly cooked and raw vegetables well washed. Disease occurs mainly in pregnant women, neonates, and immunocompromised persons. Bacteremia and meningitis are the most common manifestations in nonpregnant persons. Focal infections, such as endophthalmitis or a liver abscess are rare. In patients with meningitis, the cerebrospinal fluid glucose level is normal in more than 60% of patients, and the Gram's stain shows organisms in fewer than 40% of cases. In patients with bacteremia, gastrointestinal symptoms such as nausea, vomiting, and diarrhea may be prominent.

Ampicillin plus an aminoglycoside, such as gentamicin, is the therapy of choice in a patient without a history of penicillin allergy. If the patient is allergic to penicillin, then trimethoprim-sulfamethoxazole (TMP-SMX) or vancomycin can be selected. Cephalosporins should be avoided. Although controlled studies are lacking, patients with meningitis should be treated for 3 weeks to prevent relapse, and those with endocarditis should be treated for 4 weeks. The management of patients with infected synthetic grafts should consist of surgical resection in combination with 6 weeks of antimicrobial therapy.

Most *Bacillus* spp. isolated in the laboratory, except for *B. anthracis*, are contaminants. The organism is an aerobic, gram-positive rod that forms spores. *B. cereus* and *B. subtilis* have been associated with posttraumatic endophthalmitis. Bacteremia generally occurs in the compromised patient with a central venous line. The IV catheter should be removed, and vancomycin plus an aminoglycoside should be administered. The organism is often resistant to penicillin and other β-lactam drugs, including the new cephalosporins. Clindamycin is an alternative drug in patients unable to tolerate vancomycin.

R. equi is a recently recognized human pathogen that can cause cavitary pulmonary disease and bacteremia in the compromised host. Although the optimal therapy is unknown, the organism is susceptible to vancomycin, erythromycin, clindamycin, or TMP-SMX. Most authors favor selecting two agents, with possible surgical drainage for an abscess. Prolonged therapy is usually required.

Clostridium spp. are anaerobic rods that are usually gram-positive. In clinical specimens, the organisms may appear to stain as gram-negative bacilli. Spore formation occurs but may not be present in clinical specimens. Clostridia are an interesting group of organisms, in that a positive blood culture has been associated with life-threatening disease or an "insignificant transient bacteremia." *C. perfringens* accounts for about 60% of blood culture isolates. An intra-abdominal focus should be searched for in an ill patient with clostridial bacteremia. Some patients will have colon cancer. *C. septicum* bacteremia is unusual; when present, it is often associated with an occult colon malignancy (about 40%). *C. septicum* bacteremia also occurs in patients with leukemia or in diabetic patients with infected foot ulcers. *C. perfringens* and *C. septicum* usually respond to penicillin or clindamycin. Approximately 25% of strains of *C. perfringens* are resistant to metronidazole. Rarely, a patient will have a blood culture positive for *C. tertium*. Infection with *C. tertium* usually has a gastrointestinal source and often will respond without surgery to vancomycin or TMP-SMX. Interestingly, *C. tertium* is often resistant to clindamycin, penicillin, and metronidazole. (NMG)

Bibliography

Bodey GP, et al. Clostridial bacteremia in cancer patients: a 12-year experience. *Cancer* 1991;67:1928.
Review. Fatality rate was 42%.

Brook I, Frazier EH. Infections caused by *Propionibacterium* species. *Rev Infect Dis* 1991; 13:819.
Usually causes bacteremia in the presence of a foreign body. The organism is commonly susceptible to penicillin and resistant to metronidazole.

Claeys G, et al. Endocarditis of native aortic and mitral valves due to *Corynebacterium accolens*: report of a case and application of phenotypic and genotypic techniques for identification. *J Clin Microbiol* 1996;34:1290–1292.
A rare cause of endocarditis, which responded to penicillin.

Dalton CB, et al. An outbreak of gastroenteritis and fever due to *Listeria monocytogenes* in milk. *N Engl J Med* 1997;336:100–105.
Gastroenteritis caused by contaminated milk.

Funke G, et al. Clinical microbiology of coryneform bacteria. *Clin Microbiol Rev* 1997;10: 125–159.
Comprehensive review of the various coryneform bacteria.

Gaur AH, et al. *Bacillus cereus* bacteremia and meningitis in immunocompromised children. *Clin Infect Dis* 2001;32:1456–1462.
A recognized cause of food poisoning in normal hosts, B. cereus can cause bacteremia and meningitis in the immunocompromised patient.

Gorbach SL, Thadepalli H. Isolation of *Clostridium* in human infections: evaluation of 114 cases. *J Infect Dis* 1975;131(suppl):S81.
Clostridial bacteremia may be clinically unimportant.

Hof H, Nichterlein T, Kretschmar M. Management of listeriosis. *Clin Microbiol Rev* 1997;10:345–357.
Ampicillin plus gentamicin remains the therapy of choice because the combination is bactericidal. TMP-SMX is an alternative in the penicillin-allergic patient.

Hong T, Heibler N, Tang Y. *Bacillus hackensackii* sp. nov., a novel carbon dioxide sensitive bacterium isolated from blood culture. *Diagn Microbiol Infect Dis* 2003;45;143–147.
A gram-positive rod inhibited by 5% carbon dioxide.

Husni RN, et al. *Lactobacillus* bacteremia and endocarditis: review of 45 cases. *Clin Infect Dis* 1997;25:1048–1055.
Lactobacilli occur as part of the normal gastrointestinal and genitourinary flora. Bacteremia is often (60%) polymicrobial in patients with underlying illnesses.

Jacobs A, et al. Extracolonic manifestations of *Clostridium difficile* infections: presentation of 2 cases and review of the literature. *Medicine (Baltimore)* 2001;80:88–101.
An infrequent cause of bacteremia and extraintestinal infection usually in patients with malignancy or chronic renal disease.

Johnson WD, Kaye D. Serious infections caused by diphtheroids. *Ann N Y Acad Sci* 1970;174:568.
Classic review. The majority of patients had endocarditis.

Kaplan K, Weinstein L. Diphtheroid infections of man. *Ann Intern Med* 1969;70:919.
Classic review. Penicillin is usually effective.

Kedlaya I, Ing MB, Wong SS. *Rhodococcus equi* infections in immunocompetent hosts: case report and review. *Clin Infect Dis* 2001;32:E39–47.
A rare cause of pneumonia in immunocompetent hosts. Most infections occur in compromised patients.

Kudsk KA. Occult gastrointestinal malignancies producing metastatic *Clostridium septicum* infections in diabetic patients. *Surgery* 1992;112:765.
In a patient with a soft-tissue infection caused by C. septicum *in the absence of trauma, search for a gastrointestinal malignancy.*

Lorber B. Listeriosis. *Clin Infect Dis* 1997;24:1–11.
Review.

Mayer TA, et al. Clinical presentation of inhalational anthrax following bioterrorism exposure. *JAMA* 2001;286:2549–2553.
Consider anthrax in a patient with a gram-positive rod in the blood and a widened mediastinum on chest radiograph. See also Dixon TC, et al. Anthrax. N Engl J Med 1999;341:815–826.

Morris A, Guild I. Endocarditis due to *Corynebacterium pseudodiphtheriticum:* five case reports, review, and antibiotic susceptibilities of nine strains. *Rev Infect Dis* 1991;13:887.
Penicillin plus an aminoglycoside should be effective.

Mylonakis E, Hohmann EL, Calderwood S. Central nervous system infection with *Listeria monocytogenes:* 33 years' experience at a general hospital and review of 776 episodes from the literature. *Medicine* 1998;77:313–316.
Review.

Ognibene FP, et al. *Erysipelothrix rhusiopathiae* bacteremia presenting as septic shock. *Am J Med* 1985;78:861.
A rare cause of bacteremia in fishermen and meat handlers.

Perez MGV, Vassilev T, Kemmerly SA. *Rhodococcus equi* infection in transplant recipients: a case of mistaken identity and review of the literature. *Transpl Infect Dis* 2002;4:52–56.
Consider as a cause of pulmonary infiltrates or lung abscess in solid organ transplant recipients.

Pinner RW, et al. Role of foods in sporadic listeriosis: II. Microbiologic and epidemiologic investigation. *JAMA* 1992;267:2046.
Listeria was isolated from food in the refrigerators in 64% of infected patients. Ready-to-eat foods often grew serotype 4b, a disease-producing strain.

Rechner PM, et al. Clinical features of clostridial bacteremia: a review from a rural area. *Clin Infect Dis* 2001;33:349–353.
67% of patients were elderly and half had a gastrointestinal source.

Salminen MK, et al. *Lactobacillus* bacteremia, clinical significance, and patient outcome, with special focus on probiotic *L. rhamnosus* GG. *Clin Infect Dis* 2004;38:62–69.
The drug of choice for treatment is unknown, but imipenem and aminoglycosides may be effective. Usually occurs in patients with immunosuppression. Mortality was 26%.

Saxelin M, et al. Lactobacilli and bacteremia in southern Finland, 1989–1992. *Clin Infect Dis* 1996;22:564–566.
Lactobacilli are found in dairy products and colonize the gastrointestinal tract. Despite their widespread occurrence, bacteremia is rare.

Schuchat A, et al. Role of foods in sporadic listeriosis: I. Case-control study of dietary risk factors. *JAMA* 1992;267:2041.
Patients were likely to have eaten soft cheese, sliced meats, cheese from a store delicatessen, or poultry products.

Sliman R, Rehm S, Shlaes DM. Serious infections caused by *Bacillus* sp. *Medicine (Baltimore)* 1987;66:218.
Underlying conditions included IV drug use, intravascular catheters, and malignancy.

Speirs G, Warren RE, Rampling A. *Clostridium tertium* septicemia in patients with neutropenia. *J Infect Dis* 1988;158:1336.
An uncommon cause of bacteremia in patients with a hematologic malignancy and granulocytopenia.

Spitzer PG, Hammer SM, Karchmer AW. Treatment of *Listeria monocytogenes* infection with trimethoprim-sulfamethoxazole: case report and review of the literature. *Rev Infect Dis* 1986;8:427.
TMP-SMX is an alternative drug in the penicillin-allergic patient.

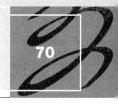

*I*nformation obtained by history and physical examination may provide clues to parasitic infections of the gastrointestinal tract. Diarrhea (especially in patients with AIDS; waterborne outbreak situation; nursery school/day care center workers; campers, backpacker, and hikers; suspected foodborne outbreak), bloating, weight loss, or unexplained eosinophilia in the context of a relevant epidemiologic and travel history requires that stool sample(s) be examined for ova and parasites (O & P).

Three discrete procedures usually are used for an O & P examination. The direct wet smear to visualize trophozoite motility; the concentration of stool to enrich the diagnostic stage of the parasite for microscopy; and the permanent stained smear to examine in-depth morphology of the parasite eggs or larval stages. Each of these procedures is designed for a specific purpose and forms an essential component of the total microscopic examination. Additionally, in some instances in which a particular pathogen is suspected (e.g., *Giardia lamblia*, *Cryptosporidium parvum*, and *Entamoeba histolytica/dispar*), commercially available immunodiagnostic kits may be used instead of or in addition to the routine light microscopy.

The number and frequency of fecal specimens to be collected varies with the diagnosis suspected. Most parasitology textbooks and laboratory manuals recommend the examination of at least three independently collected stool specimens to maximize the sensitivity of detection of intestinal O & P. Such recommendations are based on studies that have repeatedly shown improved rates of detection of diagnostic stages of parasites when multiple specimens were examined. This is because of the differential rates of expulsion of diagnostic stages of parasites in the feces. For example, roundworms such as *Ascaris*, hookworm, and *Trichuris* shed eggs more or less constantly and may be detected almost daily in stool. Other parasites, especially protozoa (*E. histolytica*, *E. dispar*) and the roundworm *Strongyloides stercoralis*, are passed out sporadically, often for only a few days at a time. In some helminth infections, particularly schistosomes, and those caused by *Diphyllobothrium* spp.and *Taenia* spp., eggs may be passed out in stool intermittently. In some instances purgation, usually with Fleet Phospho-Soda or Epsom salt, may increase the yield of some parasites, such as amoebae, *Giardia*, and *Strongyloides*, and it should be considered when their presence is strongly suspected clinically but specimens have been negative.

Many drugs and other substances can interfere with proper stool examination. Iron, bismuth, and mineral oil may interfere with the stool examination for 1 week or more; barium and dyes, iodine preparations, and antimicrobials may cause difficulty for as long as several weeks. Naturally passed stools are usually preferred for microscopic examination. Fecal specimens should be collected in a wide-mouthed container or carton. Urine is harmful to some parasites and must not contaminate the specimen. Stool samples should not be retrieved from the toilet water because water is destructive to some eggs and protozoa. Prompt examination or fixation in polyvinyl alcohol (PVA) fixative or 10% aqueous formalin is particularly important for soft or watery specimens. Formalin preserves eggs, cysts, and larvae for wet mount examination and for concentration. PVA-fixative preserves cysts and trophozoites for permanent staining. Specimens that cannot be examined or fixed quickly should be refrigerated at 4°C (39°F) and should not be frozen and thawed.

The healthcare professional may want to screen the sample before submitting it to the laboratory. Dark-colored stools may indicate bleeding high in the gastrointestinal tract, and fresh (bright red) blood most often is the result of bleeding at a lower level. In certain parasitic infections, for example *E. histolytica*, blood and mucus may be present in the stool. Consistency of the stool samples (formed, soft, or liquid) can also be a good indicator of the types or stages of parasites present. Generally, trophozoites (motile forms) of the intestinal protozoa are frequently detected in liquid specimens; both trophozoites and cysts might be found in a soft specimen. Protozoan cysts have commonly been discerned in formed specimens. Coccidian oocysts, microsporidian as well as helminth eggs may be found in any type of specimen. Mature proglottids of cestodes can sometimes be seen on or under the stool in the bottom of the collection container. Adult pinworms and *Ascaris* may occasionally be found on the surface or in the stool.

Microscopic examination is still the gold standard for making a diagnosis for most intestinal parasites. However, if a definitive identification of the parasite cannot be made, the stool specimen can be analyzed using molecular techniques such as polymerase chain reaction (PCR). PCR-generated fragments can be examined through restriction fragment length polymorphisms (RFLP) or DNA sequencing if further characterization is needed.

Following is a very brief overview of some of the conventional procedures used for determining some common parasites of temperate climates, in stool specimens.

 PROTOZOA

Multiple stool specimens are necessary in the diagnosis of intestinal amebiasis (*E. histolytica/dispar*). Specimens obtained by endoscopy with scraping of ulcers have a high yield. Biopsy material stained with paraaminosalicylic acid will demonstrate trophozoites. Wet preparations can identify amoebae with their linear motility. Permanent stains with trichrome or iron hematoxylin are used to identify *E. histolytica* by nuclear morphology and ingestion of red blood cells (RBCs). Concentration methods are superior to direct stool examination for the detection of cysts. Enzyme immunoassay (EIA) kits are now commercially available for the detection of fecal antigens for the diagnosis of intestinal amebiasis (e.g., *Entamoeba*: CELISA, Cellabs, Brookvale, NSW, Australia; ProSpecT, Remel, Lenexa, Kan, USA). Some of these assays use monoclonal antibodies that detect the galactose-inhibitable adherence protein in *E. histolytica*. Several EIA kits for antigen detection of both *E. histolytica* and *E. dispar* are also available (e.g., *E. histolytica* II, TechLab, Blacksburg, Va, USA). The only disadvantage of these tests is that the fresh and unpreserved stool specimens are needed to perform the assays.

Cyst excretion in *Giardia* infection varies from one specimen to another and is observer-dependent. Only about 80% of infections are detected, even when three daily specimens are examined. Cyst concentration techniques will improve overall yield. A recent study suggests that duodenal fluid obtained by aspiration is not superior to fecal specimens. Trophozoites also can be demonstrated in jejunal mucosal biopsy specimens. Detection of surface parasite antigen(s) via immunodiagnostic tools (e.g., direct flourescent antibody (DFA), EIAs, and rapid tests) are now considered to be the current tests of choice for diagnosis of giardiasis because they provide increased sensitivity over more commonly used microscopic techniques. For example, DFA assays use fluorescein isothiocyanate (FITC)-conjugated monoclonal antibody for the detection of *Giardia* cysts alone or in a combined kit for the simultaneous detection of *Giardia* cysts and *Cryptosporidium* oocysts (e.g., Merifluor, Meridian Bioscience, Inc., Cincinnati, Ohio, USA). Some commercial EIA kits are available also for the detection of *Giardia* antigen in fresh or refrigerated stool samples and in specimens preserved in formalin, MIF, or SAF fixatives (e.g., PARA-TECT™ Giardia Antigen 96, Medical Chemical Corporation, Torrance, Calif, USA).

Acid-fast staining methods, with or without stool concentration, are the most frequently used procedures in clinical laboratories for the diagnosis of *Cryptosporidium*. However, immunodetection of surface antigens of the parasite in fecal samples through monoclonal antibody-based DFA assays, EIAs, and rapid tests are now becoming more popular because they provide increased sensitivity over modified acid-fast staining techniques (e.g., Crypto CELISA, PARA-TECT™ *Cryptosporidium* 96). Acid-fast staining method also is useful in detecting the diagnostic stages of *Isospora belli* and *Cyclospora cayetanensis*. The spores of *Microsporidia* can be detected in the stool through staining with trichrome stains (Weber Green modified trichrome; Ryan Blue modified trichrome).

Rapid immunochromatographic procedures are available for the combined antigen detection of either *Cryptosporidium* and *Giardia*, or *Cryptosporidium*, *Giardia*, and *E. histolytica/dispar* (e.g., Triage, BioSite, San Diego, Calif, USA). This test offers the benefit of short test time (~20 min) and multiple results in one reaction device. The Meridian Merifluor DFA Kit for *Cryptosporidium/Giardia*, modified acid-fast stain for *Cryptosporidium* spp., or Wheatley's trichrome stain for *Giardia* spp. are used at the Centers for Disease Control and Prevention for routine identification of these parasites.

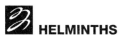 **HELMINTHS**

Microscopic identification of eggs in the stool is the most common method for diagnosing hookworm infection. Fixed stool samples are usually concentrated using the formalin-ethyl acetate sedimentation and the pellet is examined for hookworm eggs. However, the examination of the eggs cannot distinguish between *Necator americanus* and *Ancylostoma duodenale*, the two major species of hookworms. Larvae can be used to differentiate between *N. americanus* and *A. duodenale* by rearing filariform larvae in a fecal smear on a moist filter paper strip for 5 to 7 days (Harada-Mori Culture Method). Sometimes it may be necessary to distinguish between the rhabditiform larvae (L2) of hookworms and those of *Strongyloides stercoralis*.

To date, the definitive diagnosis of strongyloidiasis is accomplished by the detection of rhabditiform larvae (L2) in the stool. However, in the majority of uncomplicated cases of strongyloidiasis, the intestinal worm load is very low and larval output is minimal. In more than two-thirds of the cases, there are no more than 25 larvae per gram of stool. The examination of one stool sample has been shown to be negative in up to 70% of cases. Repeated examinations of stool specimens improve the chances of finding parasites in some studies; the diagnostic sensitivity increases to 50% with three stool examinations and can approach 100% if seven serial stool samples are examined. A number of techniques have been used to discern larvae in stool samples, including direct smear of feces in saline/Lugol's iodine stain, Baermann concentration, formalin-ethyl acetate concentration, Harada-Mori filter paper culture, and nutrient agar plate cultures. Concentrating the stool with formalin-ethyl acetate increases the yield, but dead individual larvae are more difficult to visualize at low magnification. The Baermann method and the Harada-Mori filter paper capitalize on the ability of *S. stercoralis* to enter a free-living cycle of development. They are much more sensitive than single stool smears but are rarely standard procedures in clinical parasitology laboratories. In the Harada-Mori technique, filter paper containing fresh fecal material is placed in a test tube with water that continuously soaks the filter paper by capillary action. Incubation at 30°C (86°F) provides conditions suitable for the development of larvae, which can migrate to either side of the filter paper. In the Baermann procedure, stool is placed on mesh screen and a coarse fabric in a funnel that is filled with warm water and connected to a clamped tubing. After an hour of incubation, larvae crawl out of the fecal suspension and migrate into the warm water, where they can be collected by centrifugation. In the agar culture method, stool sample is placed on a nutrient agar plate and incubated for at least 2 days. As the larvae crawl over the agar, they carry bacteria with them, thus creating visible tracks. Motile *S. stercoralis* larvae can also be seen with the aid of a dissecting microscope. However, this sensitive method for diagnosis of strongyloidiasis is not usually available on a routine basis in clinical microbiology laboratories.

Pinworm eggs (*Enterobius vermicularis*) also can be found, but less frequently, in the stool. Identification of eggs collected in the perianal area is the diagnostic method of choice. This should be done in the morning, before defecation and washing, by pressing transparent adhesive tape ("Scotch test," cellulose-tape slide test) on the perianal skin and then examining the tape placed on a slide. Alternatively, anal swabs or "Swube tubes" (a paddle coated with adhesive material) can be used. Similarly, microscopic identification of whipworm (*Trichuris trichiura*) eggs in feces is evidence of infection. Because eggs may be difficult to find in light infections, a concentration procedure is recommended. Because the severity of symptoms depends on the worm burden, quantification of the latter (e.g., with the Kato-Katz technique) can prove useful.

Identification of eggs and proglottids in feces by microscopy is diagnostic for many cestode infections, including taeniasis and diphyllobothriasis. Repeated examination and concentration techniques will increase the likelihood of detecting light infections. However identification of a specific species (i.e., *T. solium* or *T. saginata*) is not possible to do solely on the basis of microscopic examination of eggs, because all *Taenia* species produce eggs that are morphologically identical. Microscopic identification of mature/gravid proglottids or the examination of the scolex, will only determine the species of the infecting cestode.

Eggs can be present in the stool in infections with human blood flukes, *Schistosoma mansoni* and *S. japonicum*. The examination can be performed on a simple smear (1 to 2 mg of stool sample). Because eggs may be passed intermittently or in small amounts, their detection will be enhanced by repeated examinations and/or concentration procedures (such as the formalin-ethyl acetate technique). Additionally, for field surveys and investigational purposes, the egg output can be quantified by using the Kato-Katz technique (20 to 50 mg of fecal material) or the Ritchie technique.

In summary, more sensitive immunodiagnostic methods for organism detection in stool specimens are now commercially available for several protozoan parasites. However, stool analysis by microscopy is still the gold standard for diagnosis for most flatworms and round worms. (SLB)

Bibliography

Broussard JD. Optimal fecal assessment. *Clin Tech Small Anim Pract* 2003;18:218–230.
  This article reviews the plethora of diagnostic techniques available for fecal assessment. Indications, limitations, and issues of specimen handling for each technique are discussed. The optimal approach to the diagnosis of some common parasites, pathogens, abnormalities of flora, and metabolic conditions are covered.
DPDx Laboratory Identification of Parasites of Public Health Concern. Available at: http://www.dpd.cdc.gov/dpdx. Accessed November 5, 2004.
  An excellent Web site devoted to up-to-date information on the clinical manifestations, diagnosis, and treatment of a larger repertoire of parasites.
Garcia LS, Bruckner DA. *Diagnostic Medical Parasitology*. 2nd ed. Washington, DC: American Society of Microbiology; 1993431–455.
  An excellent compilation of diagnostic procedures have been presented in great detail. This book is a very good reference manual of diagnostic parasitology.
Heyworth MF. Parasitic diseases in immunocompromised hosts. Cryptosporidiosis, isosporiasis, and strongyloidiasis. *Gastroenterol Clin North Am* 1996;25:691–707.
  Important review dealing with parasitic infections in immunocompromised patients.
Katz DE, Taylor DN. Parasitic infections of the gastrointestinal tract. *Gastroenterol Clin North Am* 2001;30:797–815.
  This article updates recent advances in the body of knowledge of diagnosis and treatment of intestinal parasites. The article focus on the manifestations of disease in the immunocompetent adult host.
Liu LX, Weller PF. Strongyloidiasis and other intestinal nematode infections. *Infect Dis Clinic North Am* 1993;7:655–682.
  Continuing diagnostic and therapeutic challenges dealing with helminths have been discussed in this important review.
Long EG, Christie JD The diagnosis of old and new gastrointestinal parasites. *Clin Lab Med* 1995;15:307–331.
  A good overview of diagnostic methods for intestinal parasites.
Siddiqui AA, Berk SL. Diagnosis of *Strongyloides stercoralis* infection. *Clin Infect Dis* 2001;33:1040–1047.
  This review describes different methods of diagnosis (conventional and research) for strongyloidiasis (intestinal and disseminated). Also, the specificity limitations of the ELISA method for the detection of S. stercoralis are discussed at length.

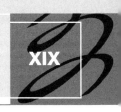

Antimicrobial, Antiviral, Antiparasitic, Antifungal Agents

XIX

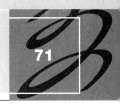
 $\mathcal{T}$here are at least five basic principles on which successful antimicrobial therapy must be based. These principles require knowledge of an antimicrobial's spectrum of activity, distribution and pharmacokinetics, toxicity, synergy and antagonism with other antimicrobials, and cost.

PRINCIPLE 1: SPECTRUM OF ACTIVITY

This principle is relevant to choosing an antimicrobial directed against a specific pathogen. First, the physician must determine the particular pathogen that is causing infection. Once the agent has been identified, an antimicrobial with particular activity against the organism causing disease can be chosen.

Identification of the most likely bacterium causing an infection is based on history, physical examination, epidemiology, and Gram's stain and culture of appropriate body fluids. For example, in a patient with pneumonia, several aspects of the history might be important. Whether the pneumonia is community or hospital acquired will provide a clue to the likely etiologic agent. Another clue to the identity of the organism causing pneumonia might be a patient history that includes having a sick parakeet, as psittacosis presents in a nonspecific manner. A history of a single shaking chill suggests the likelihood of a pneumococcal infection. Sputum that is foul smelling or has a fecal odor suggests an anaerobic component to the pneumonia. Physical examination, in addition to suggesting the focus of infection, may also be important in determining an etiologic agent. In a patient with cellulitis, for example, erysipelas seen on physical examination suggests group A β-hemolytic streptococcal infection. In a patient with gram-negative bacteremia, a black fluid-filled lesion suggesting ecthyma gangrenosum makes the diagnosis of *Pseudomonas* bacteremia most likely.

An increasing number of rapid laboratory tests are available for early, specific diagnosis; however, for bacterial infections, Gram's stain of the infected material is still extremely important in defining optimal antimicrobial therapy. In a patient with bacterial pneumonia, sputum Gram's stain is essential for optimal management. A patient who has empyema requires thoracentesis and Gram's stain of pleural fluid before antimicrobial therapy can be determined.

Once the physical examination and laboratory results, including Gram's stain, have been assessed, the physician makes the best possible determination about the likely bacterial pathogens causing infection. An antimicrobial with optimal activity against these pathogens must then be chosen. Narrow-spectrum antibiotics are preferred to prevent the emergence of resistance; however, the choice of narrow- versus broad-spectrum therapy will depend on the severity of illness, clinical clues to etiology, and issues of local hospital epidemiology.

Because host factors determine the potential severity of illness caused by an infection, an appraisal of the host's immune system and underlying diseases may help determine the most appropriate antibiotic.

PRINCIPLE 2: VOLUME OF DISTRIBUTION AND PHARMACOKINETICS

An antimicrobial may have excellent activity against a particular bacterium, but treatment will not be successful unless it reaches the site of infection in adequate concentrations.

For example, aminoglycosides alone are not usually chosen for gram-negative pneumonia because of concern about concentrations of aminoglycosides in bronchial washings. Nor would a first-generation cephalosporin be used for pneumococcal meningitis. Although the cephalosporin would have excellent activity against the pneumococcus, it does not enter the cerebrospinal fluid in adequate concentrations to be effective. Hence, in choosing an antimicrobial, it is necessary to know the specific pharmacokinetics of each and what antimicrobials can be expected to reach therapeutic levels in various body fluids.

Route of administration will be an important issue to obtain maximum efficacy. In most cases, the physician will choose between oral and parenteral therapy. Oral therapy usually will be chosen for mild infections and infections treated on an outpatient basis. Oral therapy will require assurance of patient compliance or assistance with compliance. The oral route will require that the patient does not have excessive nausea or vomiting. Oral absorption may be affected by meals or by concomitant medications. Some antibiotics can only be given by the parenteral route because of poor absorption. These include, for example, vancomycin, aminoglycosides, and amphotericin.

Intravenous antibiotics are given for life-threatening infections and for severe, chronic infections in some cases. For serious, chronic infections, intravenous therapy may be started in the hospital and continued at home or in an intermediate care facility. Continuous infusion or intermittent bolus infusion is still an area of controversy and one method may be better than another for specific types of infections and antibiotics.

 ## PRINCIPLE 3: ANTIMICROBIAL TOXICITY

The benefits of an antimicrobial must outweigh the risks. To make this assessment, the clinician must appreciate the side effects of each agent that is used and must then assess the benefits versus the risks of the drug in question. For example, in an elderly patient with *Klebsiella pneumoniae* pneumonia, a combination of cephalosporin and aminoglycoside may be chosen. This combination may have some nephrotoxic side effects (and the combination of cephalosporin and aminoglycoside likely causes increased nephrotoxicity compared with aminoglycoside alone), but in the case of a life-threatening infection such as *K. pneumoniae* pneumonia, this combination of antimicrobials would be the therapy of choice for many clinicians. In contrast, a patient with cystitis who is found to have *K. pneumoniae* in the urine would be treated with a very different regimen—one with a less toxic profile.

The toxicity of an antimicrobial must be assessed in regard to the specific patient. The likelihood of toxicity from an aminoglycoside is greater in an older patient with underlying renal disease than in a young adult. A patient who has had an episode of anaphylaxis to penicillin should not be treated with a cephalosporin.

 ## PRINCIPLE 4: ISSUES OF SYNERGY AND ANTAGONISM

When one antimicrobial enhances the other with more than just an additive effect, the interaction is called *synergy*. When an antimicrobial interferes with the activity of a second one, the effect is called *antagonism*. A bacteriostatic antimicrobial, for example, frequently slows the killing rate of a bactericidal antimicrobial.

Several examples of in vitro synergism have been shown to be important in the clinical setting. For example, the newer penicillins in combination with aminoglycosides are synergistic for *Pseudomonas aeruginosa*. In neutropenic patients with *Pseudomonas* bacteremia, the combination of a newer penicillin and an aminoglycoside is generally considered to be a combination of choice because of this synergistic relationship. There also have been some examples of clinical antagonism. For example, an early study on pneumococcal meningitis showed that the combination of penicillin and tetracycline was much less successful than penicillin alone in the treatment of this disease.

The use of more than one antimicrobial has become increasingly common in therapy, so the clinician must understand the potential synergistic and antagonistic relationships involved in combination antimicrobial therapy.

PRINCIPLE 5: COST OF ANTIMICROBIALS AND ANTIMICROBIAL ADMINISTRATION

In life-threatening infections, cost will not play a major role in choosing antimicrobial therapy; however, for mild infections, such as cystitis, or for antimicrobial prophylaxis, regimens may vary tenfold in cost. Therefore, the clinician must have some understanding of the cost of various antimicrobials.

OTHER ISSUES IN SELECTION

For some infections, bactericidal antimicrobials are mandatory. For example, in endocarditis, treatment with a bacteriostatic drug, such as erythromycin, has a higher failure rate than treatment with a bactericidal drug, such as penicillin. In this infection, a high level of inhibition is insufficient; for cure, adequate "killing" must be achieved. In some types of bacterial meningitis, a bactericidal drug also is recommended. For example, in gram-negative bacillary meningitis, a third-generation cephalosporin is preferred to chloramphenicol.

For some infections, the ability of antimicrobials to penetrate phagocytes may be necessary for cure. *Legionella pneumophila,* for example, can survive within phagocytic cells. Erythromycin, rifampin, and ciprofloxacin may penetrate alveolar macrophages and be curative in this infection. Some β-lactamase–stable cephalosporins have good in vitro activity against *Legionella* but are ineffective in treatment.

Because antimicrobials are often given intermittently, the ability of the offending agents to multiply between doses can present an important problem. Many antimicrobials produce an inhibitory effect on bacteria for a number of hours after exposure. With gram-positive cocci, this postantimicrobial effect is similar for all antimicrobial agents. However, for gram-negative bacilli, some antimicrobials, such as aminoglycosides and ciprofloxacin, have a postantimicrobial effect, whereas others, such as cephalosporins, may not. The clinical relevance of this phenomenon needs further evaluation.

The prevention of resistant organisms has become an increasing priority in establishing principles for antibiotic use. Antibiotics must be avoided in circumstances in which they are not necessary. This is particularly important in the management of upper respiratory infections that are not bacterial in origin. Similarly, not all cases of bronchitis, sinusitis, or pharyngitis require antibiotic therapy. (SLB)

Bibliography

Gonzales R, et al. Excessive antibiotic use for acute respiratory infections in the United States. *Clin Infect Dis* 2001;33:757.
Documents amount and cost of excess antibiotics used for upper respiratory infections, pharyngitis, and bronchitis. This has become a major issue in the emergence of antibiotic resistant organisms.

Gross PA. The potential for clinical guidelines to impact appropriate antimicrobial agent use. *Infect Dis Clin North Am* 1997;11:803.
Practice guidelines will become more important in antibiotic selection. These guidelines will require selection of narrow-spectrum antibiotics, when possible, with lowest possible toxicity.

Gupta K. Addressing antibiotic resistance. *Dis Mon* 2003;49:99.
Antibiotic recommendations may become dependent on the epidemiology of resistance in local areas. One example has become the role of trimethoprim-sulfa in community-acquired urinary tract infection.

Hessen MT, Kaye D. Principles of selection and use of antibacterial agents. *Infect Dis Clin North Am* 1995;9:531.
Includes basic principles of pharmacodynamics, monitoring of therapy, and reasons for treatment failure.

Medical Letter. The choice of antibacterial drugs. *Med Lett Drugs Ther* 2004;2:13.
Lists drugs of choice for common pathogens. Good consensus evaluation of new antimicrobial agents.

Moellering RC. Principles of anti-infective therapy. In: Mandell GL, Bennett JE, Dolin R, eds. *Principles and Practice of Infectious Diseases.* Vol 1. 5th ed. New York, NY: Churchill Livingstone; 2000:223.
Gives basic principles of therapy with emphasis on host factors as an important consideration.

Neu HC. General concepts on the chemotherapy of infectious diseases. *Med Clin North Am* 1987;71:1051.
Includes a discussion of bactericidal versus bacteriostatic drugs and intracellular versus extracellular location of bacteria, plus a brief description of the mechanism of action of each drug.

Rahal JJ Jr. Antibiotic combinations: the clinical relevance of synergy and antagonism. *Medicine (Baltimore)* 1978;57:179.
Reviews the relationship between in vitro testing and the clinical relevance of antimicrobial combinations.

Shlaes DM, et al. Society of Healthcare Epidemiology of America and Infectious Disease Society of America Joint Commission on the Prevention of Antimicrobial Resistance: guidelines for the prevention of antimicrobial resistance in hospitals. *Clin Infect Dis* 1997;25:584.
Antibiotic selection must take into account in prevention of the emergence of resistance. Narrow-spectrum antibiotics are preferred, but their selection will depend on local hospital epidemiology.

Skerret S, Statton C. New antibiotics in primary care. *Patient Care* 2004;7:17.
Update on the most recently approved antibiotics.

Thompson RL, Wright AJ. General principles of antimicrobial therapy. *Mayo Clin Proc* 1998;73:995.
Symposium on antibiotics and their selection. Stresses the importance of history and physical diagnosis in determining antibiotic therapy, but also the role of empirical therapy.

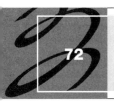

72   CHOOSING A FLUOROQUINOLONE

Fluoroquinolones (FQ) have emerged as important agents in the therapy/prevention of a wide number of infections. Reasons for this include (1) equal oral/parenteral bioavailability for many of these products; (2) ease of administration—typically b.i.d. or, more recently, q.d.; (3) numerous studies documenting use for many infections; (4) broad spectrum of activity; (5) relative safety; (6) excellent penetration into most body sites, including the prostate; and (7) intense marketing by pharmaceutical companies.

FQs have been available since the 1960s, when nalidixic acid (Negram®) was approved for uncomplicated lower urinary tract infections caused by susceptible organisms. Over the last 40 years, enhanced understanding of both the basic molecule and structure/activity relationships has allowed for targeted modifications resulting in decreased adverse reactions and variable spectra of activity. Major reviews of these have been published, and the interested reader is referred to them for further details. Related to this has been the production and rather rapid removal from the marketplace of several products demonstrated to have unacceptable toxicities, despite initial excitement in the community. These include trovafloxacin (Trovan®) and sparfloxacin (Zagam®). The former was associated with hepatotoxicity, whereas the latter was a cause for unacceptable phototoxicity.

MECHANISM OF ACTION

FQs work by binding with two target sites—DNA gyrase (topoisomerase II) and topoisomerase IV. Both are intimately involved with maintenance of DNA structure within a bacterium. FQs may have varying impact on one or the other. All FQs demonstrate concentration-dependent killing, indicating that pharmakinetics issues such as peak concentration to minimum inhibitory concentration (MIC) and area under the curve (AUC) to MIC may be best associated with clinical outcomes. Higher doses may have a favorable impact on this, and initial studies recently performed with levofloxacin (see below) indicate that higher doses for shortened durations of treatment may result in enhanced outcomes and perhaps also abort emergence of resistance.

The basic FQ molecule consists of what is called a bi-cyclic aromatic core; the presence of specific side chains (e.g., a ketone at the 4 position) is required for antibacterial activity. Substitution of the carbon at the 8 position has resulted in enhanced activity; the addition of halides at this site has been associated with increased phototoxicity. As a result of structural changes over time, FQs can be divided into four generations. First-generation FQs (e.g., nalidixic acid) have gram (−) activity generally only within the urinary tract. Second-generation agents, all of which have a fluoride on the molecule (e.g., ciprofloxacin) demonstrate enhanced gram (−) activity, capacity to be used in systemic infections, and modest (+) activity. Third-generation agents (e.g., levofloxacin) have enhanced gram (+) activity, especially against *Streptococcus pneumoniae,* and generally once-daily dosing. A category of fourth generation FQs has been used by some for agents with an enhanced anaerobic spectrum (e.g., trovafloxacin and, possibly, moxifloxacin).

 ADVERSE EFFECTS

Major adverse effects of FQs include gastrointestinal disturbance (nausea, vomiting, diarrhea) and CNS side effects (headache, dizziness). Most of these are not associated with discontinuation of the agent. Seizures are rare. All FQs have a demonstrated association with fetal cartilage disruption in animals, and currently are contraindicated in those younger than age 18. A human corollary may be tendinopathy, especially Achilles tendon rupture. This problem has been noted primarily in individuals with either renal dysfunction or corticosteroid use, and may occur within hours or up to several months after discontinuation of the product. Phototoxicity has been associated with selected products having a halide at the 8 position within the molecule (e.g., sparfloxacin). However potential for "rash" exists with all products. The potential for drug interactions exists with all FQs but is notably lower with newer agents. Prolongation of the QTc interval is rarely clinically important and is likely a class effect. Moxifloxacin and gatifloxacin contain recommendations in bold face to use carefully in patients at risk. This is probably related to blockade of potassium channel flux. Use of FQs in patients receiving class 1A antiarrhythmics and other agents capable of prolonging QTc should be undertaken gingerly. Drug interactions may occur with all products but are less likely with newer agents, such as levofloxacin, gatifloxacin, and moxifloxacin. All may bind with divalents, resulting in lack of gastrointestinal absorption. Newer products have limited interactions with warfarin, digoxin, phenytoin, theophylline, and cyclosporine. Gatifloxacin may have adverse effects on glucose metabolism.

Five major FQs—ciprofloxacin (Cipro®), levofloxacin (Levaquin®), gatifloxacin (Tequin®), gatifloxacin (Avelox®), and gemifloxacin (Factive®)—now exist and compete aggressively in the marketplace. Although there is much overlap among them, some differences are noteworthy and will be discussed further.

Table 72-1 presents selected differences among commonly used FQs. Ciprofloxacin is generally considered the FQ with the "best" activity against gram (−) bacilli, including Enterobacteriaceae and *P. aeruginosa*. Activity against other nonfermenting organisms such as *Stenotrophomonas* spp. and *Acinetobacter* spp. is variable. Over time, intense use of ciprofloxacin has been associated with increasing resistance best noted with *S. pneumoniae* and *P. aeruginosa*. In many institutions, only 50 to 60% of *P. aeruginosa*

TABLE 72-1   **Notable Issues With Selected Fluoroquinolones**

Feature	Ciprofloxacin	Levofloxacin	Gatifloxacin	Moxifloxacin
Dosing	b.i.d.	q.d.	q.d.	q.d.
Renal adjustment	Yes	Yes	Yes	No
Bone/joint infections	Yes	Maybe	Unknown	Unknown
Drug interactions	More	Less	Less	Less
Pneumococcal infection	No	Yes	Yes	Yes
"Atypical" coverage	Worse	Good	Good	Good
P. aeruginosa infection*	Best	OK	Unknown	Unknown
Anthrax	Preferred	Likely	Likely	Likely
QTc[†] prolongation	Less	Less	Bold print warning	Bold print warning
Tendinopathy	More	Less	Less	Less

*Check local sensitivity data.
[†]Likely a class effect. Check other agents concomitantly administered.

isolates, especially in critical care units, remain susceptible to this agent. Resistance has also been noted with *Salmonella* spp. It has more modest gram (+) activity against both *S. aureus* and *S. pneumoniae* than newer agents and requires b.i.d. dosing. Methicillin-resistant *S. aureus* is likely to be resistant to all FQs and they should not be used for management of this pathogen. Well-documented ciprofloxacin failures for pneumococcal pneumonia have been observed, and it should not be used for pneumococcal infections. Ciprofloxacin emerged as an agent of choice for management of cases of anthrax. Limited data exist for other FQs, but newer ones are likely to be effective. As with all newer FQs, oral bioavailability is excellent, and ciprofloxacin may be given orally for all indications as long as the patient reliably absorbs the product. Ciprofloxacin has been the best studied of FQs for management of bone and joint infections. Used as monotherapy, it is effective in osteomyelitis caused by susceptible Enterobacteriaceae, selected cases of *P. aeruginosa* and *S. aureus*. When combined with rifampin, it is a valuable regimen for management of osteomyelitis caused by sensitive staphylococci (generally not methicillin-resistant *S. aureus*) and has had success in infections associated with prostheses.

Levofloxacin, available both intravenously and orally, is the optical S-(−) isomer of ofloxacin and a "mainstay" FQ and has been heavily marketed and studied as a respiratory agent because of enhanced *S. pneumoniae* activity, including strains that are penicillin resistant, compared with earlier agents. It is also active against the atypical pathogens *Chlamydia pneumoniae*, *Mycoplasma pneumoniae*, and *Legionella* spp. while maintaining activity against *H. influenzae* and common Enterobacteriaceae. It thus provides excellent monotherapy against commonly encountered respiratory pathogens, can be given orally and once daily. Recent studies in community-acquired pneumonia (CAP) demonstrate that 5 days of treatment with 750 mg/day provides outcomes comparable to 10 days of therapy with 500 mg/day, with possibly higher likelihood of compliance and decreased adverse reactions. This agent also has been demonstrated to have efficacy for acute sinusitis and acute exacerbations of chronic bronchitis.

Gatifloxacin is available as both intravenous and oral product, and is marketed primarily as an agent for treatable respiratory illnesses, similar to those noted with levofloxacin. In vitro, it is approximately twice as active against *S. pneumoniae*, but the clinical implications of this are unknown.

Moxifloxacin is also marketed primarily as a "respiratory FQ" and is approximately twice as active against *S. pneumoniae* as gatifloxacin. It, like levofloxacin, has been approved for use against penicillin-resistant strains of *S. pneumoniae*, but clinical implications of its enhanced activity remain clinically unproven. It is the only FQ not requiring dosing adjustment for renal dysfunction.

Gemifloxacin, similar to moxifloxacin, has substantially enhanced activity against *S. pneumoniae* when compared with other FQs. It does not appear to have any major advantages or shortcomings compared with other agents and likely will be used as empiric therapy for lower respiratory infections.

 CONCLUSIONS

FQs are intensely marketed for many clinical indications. Overuse of these products has resulted in emergence of both gram (−) and gram (+) resistance. This has been best documented for *P. aeruginosa* (ciprofloxacin) and *S. pneumoniae* (ciprofloxacin). Methicillin-resistant *S. aureus* should generally be considered resistant to all FQs. Worsening resistance is likely to continue and may result in the loss of the entire class within several years. FQs should be selectively used when other agents are less valuable and when their spectrum of activity is suitable for the infection being treated. The author does not believe that they represent agents of choice for either sinusitis or acute exacerbation of chronic bronchitis, in which their activity against atypical organisms has limited clinical relevance. Their appropriate spectrum of activity for CAP makes levofloxacin, gatifloxacin, moxifloxacin, and gemifloxacin suitable for empiric monotherapy in noncritically ill patients and are thus recommended in guidelines.

FQs can generally be avoided in intra-abdominal infections. The author feels that other agents can often be used for skin/soft tissue infections, for which limited activity of FQs against *S. aureus* (and the emerging role of methicillin-resistant *S. aureus* in community-acquired skin/soft tissue infections) make these agents less desirable. FQs are excellent choices for prostatitis and acute urinary tract infections in nonpregnant adults, and selected agents are indicated also for some sexually transmitted diseases. However, progressive resistance of *Neisseria gonorrhoeae* may erode use for these infections. Ciprofloxacin (often with rifampin) has emerged as an excellent regimen for some patients with infections of bone and joint and may allow prolonged therapy of an infection historically treated parenterally. (RBB)

Bibliography

Ament PW. Predicting fluoroquinolone therapy outcomes: potential role of the AUC/MIC ratio. *Formulary* 1999;34:1033–1040.

The author, a pharmD, presents basic pharmacokinetic principles and how the AUC/MIC ratio may be a valid indicator of outcomes with FQ treatment. Both values can be calculated from either the literature or from the package insert. For gram (−) organisms, an AUC/MIC greater than 140, and for gram (+) pathogens an AUC/MIC greater than 30 (>30–55 for S. pneumoniae*) appears associated with better outcomes. Thus both pharmacokinetics of the individual FQ and activity against the offending organism may impact on outcome.*

Dunbar LM, et al. High-dose, short-course levofloxacin for community-acquired pneumonia: a new treatment paradigm. *Clin Infect Dis* 2003;37:752–760.

A multicenter, double-blinded, randomized study investigated the efficacy of levofloxacin 750 mg/day for 5 days versus the same agent administered for 10 days at 500 mg/day. Outcomes demonstrated at least equal efficacy with the shorter course of antibiotic. Less than 50% of persons in each group had microbiologic documentation of etiology of CAP. This study clinically justifies much prior nonhuman data concerning the concept of concentration-dependent killing. Other FQs are likely to have similar outcomes, but shorter courses of treatment with other agents, such as β-lactams, may not be associated with similar, good outcomes.

Khalig Y, Zhanel GG. Fluoroquinolone-associated tendonopathy: a critical review of the literature. *Clin Infect Dis* 2003;36:1404–1410.

A literature review revealed 98 cases of FQ-associated tendinopathy. Injury to the Achilles tendon was seen in about 90% of cases. Most (one-third) were associated with pefloxacin; ciprofloxacin was next most common. Most others were also incriminated, and it is felt to likely be a class effect. Renal dysfunction or use of corticosteroids were notable associated events. Mechanism is unknown; ischemia and direct collagen damage have been suggested.

Saravolatz LD, Leggett J. Gatifloxacin, gemifloxacin, and moxifloxacin: the role of 3 newer fluoroquinolones. *Clin Infect Dis* 2003;37:1210–1215.

The authors present an overview of in vitro and in vivo issues of these three newer FQs. The major advantage is enhanced pneumococcal activity of uncertain clinical importance. Gemifloxacin was associated with higher rates of nonphotosensitivity-related rash than other products. Use is likely to be for selected respiratory infections, but the authors correctly warn against overuse.

Sheld WM. Maintaining fluoroquinolone class efficacy: review of influencing factors. *Emerg Infect Dis* 2003;9:1–9

The author documents issues relating to the pressures resulting in FQ resistance. These are underdosing, overuse, and underappreciation of evolving resistance patterns. He depicts pharmacokinetic variances among products as they relate to different classes of bacteria. Using the most active agent in the highest dose is likely to lessen emergence of resistance and enhance clinical outcomes. As an example, ciprofloxacin is less active and, as a result, has poorer pharmacokinetics against S. pneumoniae and should not be used against this pathogen. Pharmokinetic tables for the varying FQs are presented.

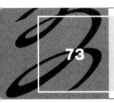

73 ANTIMICROBIAL-ASSOCIATED COLITIS

*G*astrointestinal side effects frequently complicate antimicrobial therapy. Of the adverse effects, diarrhea and an occasionally lethal pseudomembranous colitis have been the subject of numerous reports. Pseudomembranous colitis occurred in the preantimicrobial era, usually as a complication of an abdominal operation.

In 1977, based on studies in a hamster model, it was reported that clindamycin-associated colitis was caused by a toxin-producing organism, *Clostridium difficile*. Most cases of antimicrobial-associated diarrhea can be classified as *C. difficile*-associated or idiopathic. The role of other pathogens, such as *Candida albicans,* as a cause of antimicrobial-associated, *C. difficile*-negative disease requires more evidence.

Nearly all patients with *C. difficile* disease report use of an antimicrobial within the prior 6 weeks. Almost all antimicrobials have been implicated in cases of *C. difficile* disease; those most commonly involved are the cephalosporins, ampicillin or amoxicillin, and clindamycin. Most cases (total numbers) are associated with cephalosporin use, although the incidence rates are probably highest after use of clindamycin. Rarely, some antineoplastic drugs have been involved, such as fluorouracil and methotrexate. *C. difficile* should be considered as a cause of both community-acquired and nosocomial diarrhea; this organism is the most frequent cause of nosocomial diarrhea. In the hospital setting, numerous outbreaks of diarrhea as well as sporadic cases have been associated with *C. difficile*. The organism has been recovered from the hands of hospital personnel, and transmission by the hands appears to be an important mode of spread from patient to patient. In one study, use of vinyl gloves was associated with a fivefold decline in the incidence of *C. difficile* diarrhea.

C. difficile is an anaerobic gram-positive rod. Disease is localized to the colon. Pseudomembranes consisting of fibrin, mucus, epithelial cells, and leukocytes may be present, adhering to the underlying mucosa. Only 3% of healthy adults will be culture positive for *C. difficile*, in contrast to colonization rates of 50% in newborns. Colitis results from toxin production by the organism. Pathogenesis appears to involve four factors: (1) alteration in the intestinal flora secondary to antimicrobial therapy; (2) presence of *C. difficile*, usually from an exogenous source but sometimes in the patient's endogenous flora; (3) presence of an organism capable of producing toxins A and B; and (4) age-related susceptibility (the illness is uncommon in children, and older people are at increased risk).

The spectrum of disease ranges from asymptomatic to life threatening. The typical patient notes profuse watery diarrhea with abdominal pain 4 to 9 days after starting to take an antimicrobial. Diarrhea may begin after the antimicrobial has been discontinued. Fever and leukocytosis are often present. Fever and abdominal pain may occur without diarrhea. Fecal leukocytes are present in about half the patients, and the stool guaiac test result may be positive. A leukemoid reaction and hypoalbuminemia may occur. If the disease is untreated, complications include toxic megacolon, colonic perforation, and shock. The death rate may be 10% in elderly debilitated patients.

The diagnosis depends on demonstrating disease by endoscopy or *C. difficile* toxin by specific assay. Sigmoidoscopy is adequate in 67% of cases, but in about 33% of cases, disease involves only the right side of the colon. Computed tomography may suggest the diagnosis, demonstrating a characteristic thickening of the colon. A barium enema is best avoided because of the possibility of colonic perforation. Diagnosis is usually established by demonstrating the presence of toxin B by tissue culture assay. Endoscopy may be helpful when the result of the toxin assay for *C. difficile* is negative. Results of tissue culture assays for *C. difficile* toxin are positive in 95 to 100% of patients with antimicrobial-associated pseudomembranous colitis, 15 to 25% of patients with antimicrobial-associated diarrhea without confirmed pseudomembranous colitis, 2 to 8% of patients with antimicrobial exposure without diarrhea, and no healthy adults. False negatives occur in about 10% of patients. Stool culture for *C. difficile* is available but is used mainly for epidemiologic studies. Other available tests include a latex particle agglutination test, enzyme immunoassays, polymerase chain reaction, and a dot immunobinding assay. The latex agglutination test lacks the sensitivity (60%) of the tissue culture assay but has a specificity of 96%. One enzyme immunoassay had a sensitivity of 85%, in comparison with 94% for the tissue culture assay. The specificity of the enzyme immunoassay was excellent (98%). Further data are needed to define the role of the dot immunobinding assay and polymerase chain reaction in the diagnosis.

Therapy for antimicrobial-associated colitis consists of stopping the implicated antimicrobial and providing supportive care. If an antimicrobial is still needed to treat the underlying infection, an agent should be selected that is infrequently associated with this disease, such as a quinolone or an aminoglycoside. Although data are lacking, avoid use of a cephalosporin, ampicillin, or clindamycin. Oral vancomycin (125 mg four times daily) or metronidazole (500 mg three times daily) should be selected for patients with severe disease. Some patients with mild-to-moderate disease will respond if the implicated antimicrobial is discontinued and supportive therapy with fluids is provided. An advantage of metronidazole is its low cost. Treatment usually should be given for 7 to 10 days. Antidiarrheal agents must be avoided because they promote toxin retention in the colon. Corticosteroids are not indicated. Patients who are unable to take oral vancomycin should receive it by nasogastric tube. For patients who cannot take oral medications, parenteral metronidazole should be given along with oral vancomycin via a nasogastric tube or by a long tube. More data are needed on the optimal management of patients who cannot take oral medications. Most patients respond to oral vancomycin with defervescence within 24 hours and a reduction in diarrhea and abdominal cramps within 4 to 5 days. Response is poorer in patients with a toxic megacolon or other causes of an ileus.

Approximately 20% of patients will relapse within 4 weeks of completing therapy. Most relapses occur within 3 to 10 days after discontinuation of therapy. The frequency of relapse is the same whether vancomycin or metronidazole is used as initial therapy. Relapse does not depend on the duration of treatment, and repeated toxin assays are not indicated. Treatment of patients who relapse with oral vancomycin or metronidazole is usually effective. Bartlett has suggested two regimens for patients who have multiple relapses: (1) vancomycin plus rifampin for 10 to 14 days; or (2) vancomycin or metronidazole orally for 10 to 14 days followed by a 3-week course of cholestyramine, or cholestyramine plus lactobacilli, or vancomycin orally every other day. Other methods to restore the normal colon flora include administration of *Saccharomyces boulardii* orally for 1 month or *Lactobacillus* preparations.

Bibliography

Archibald LK, Banerjee SN, Jarvis WR. Secular trends in hospital-acquired *Clostridium difficile* disease in the United States, 1987–2001. *J Infect Dis* 2004;189:1585–1589.
Trends in Clostridium difficile *disease. Intensive care unit patients with prolonged stays are at higher risk.*

Bartlett JG. The 10 most common questions about *Clostridium difficile*-associated diarrhea/colitis. *Infect Dis Clin Pract* 1992;1:254.
Answers to questions regarding C. difficile *issues.*

Bartlett JG. *Clostridium difficile* infection: pathophysiology and diagnosis. *Semin Gastrointest Dis* 1997;8:12–21.
A review of diagnostic tests for the detection of C. difficile *toxins. Latex particle agglutination lacks sensitivity, and enzyme-linked immunosorbent assays and dot immunoblot assays may have a role in rapid diagnosis.*

Bartlett JG, et al. Antibiotic-associated pseudomembranous colitis due to toxin-producing clostridia. *N Engl J Med* 1978;298:531.
A toxin-producing clostridial species (C. difficile) *resistant to clindamycin is the likely cause of antimicrobial-associated pseudomembranous colitis.*

Climo MW, et al. Hospital-wide restriction of clindamycin: effect on the incidence of *Clostridium difficile*-associated diarrhea and cost. *Ann Intern Med* 1998;128:989–995.
Use of other antibiotics with anaerobic activity, such as cefotetan, ticarcillin-clavulanate, and imipenem-cilastatin, and a decreased use of clindamycin were associated with a decreased incidence of C. difficile *diarrhea.*

DiPersio JR, et al. Development of a rapid enzyme immunoassay for *Clostridium difficile* toxin A and its use in the diagnosis of *C. difficile*-associated disease. *J Clin Microbiol* 1991;29:2724.
A direct enzyme immunoassay test for C. difficile *toxin A had a sensitivity of 85% and specificity of 98%. Results were available in 2.5 hours, compared with 24 to 48 hours for the tissue culture assay for toxin.*

Do AN, et al. Risk factors for early recurrent *Clostridium difficile*-associated diarrhea. *Clin Infect Dis* 1998;26:954–959.
Relapse is more common than reinfection. Risk factors for relapse include a history of renal insufficiency and leukocytosis (cell count 5,000/mm³ or higher).

Fekety R. Guidelines for the diagnosis and management of *Clostridium difficile*-associated diarrhea and colitis. *Am J Gastroenterol* 1997;92:739–750.
Review. Unnecessary use of antibiotics should be avoided within the first 2 months after treatment of an episode of C. difficile *infection.*

Fekety R, et al. Recurrent *Clostridium difficile* diarrhea: characteristics of and risk factors for patients enrolled in a prospective, randomized, double-blinded trial. *Clin Infect Dis* 1997;24:324–333.
Factors associated with recurrent C. difficile *disease included (1) onset of initial disease in the spring, (2) prior episodes of* C. difficile *disease, (3) use of antibiotics for another infection during or shortly after the* C. difficile *episode, (4) female sex, and (5) certain strains of* C. difficile.

Fishman EK, et al. Pseudomembranous colitis: CT evaluation of 26 cases. *Radiology* 1991;180:57.
The computed tomographic findings are nonspecific and demonstrate an increase in bowel wall thickness with the "accordion sign."

George RH, Symonds JM, Dimock F. Identification of *Clostridium difficile* as a cause of pseudomembranous colitis. *Br Med J* 1978;1:695.
C. difficile *was isolated from the stools of patients with pseudomembranous colitis.*

Gerding DN, et al. *Infect Control Hosp Epidemiol* 1995;16:459–477.
A review of the diagnosis, epidemiology, infection control, and treatment of C. difficile *disease. Testing stools of asymptomatic patients for* C. difficile, *including testing for cure, is not indicated.*

Ho M, et al. Increased incidence of *Clostridium difficile*-associated diarrhea following decreased restriction of antibiotic use. *Clin Infect Dis* 1996;23(suppl 1):S102–S106.
C. difficile *disease increased after broad-spectrum antibiotics were removed from formulary restriction status.*

Hutin Y, et al. Prevalence of and risk factors for *Clostridium difficile* colonization at admission to an infectious diseases ward. *Clin Infect Dis* 1997;920–924.
Clostridium difficile was detected in the stools of 13% of patients on admission and was usually related to use of antibiotics in the prior month.

Jacobs J, et al. *Eur J Clin Microbiol Infect Dis* 1996;15:561–566.
In hospitalized patients with fewer than six stools per day, the prevalence of C. difficile is low (3%); in patients with more than six stools per day, the yield is 27%.

Johnson S, Gerding DN. *Clostridium difficile*-associated diarrhea. *Clin Infect Dis* 1998; 26:1027–1036.
Review. The pathogenesis of C. difficile colitis involves exogenous acquisition of the organism and antibiotic exposure.

Johnson S, et al. Prospective, controlled study of vinyl glove use to interrupt *Clostridium difficile* nosocomial transmission. *Am J Med* 1990;88:137.
Hand carriage of C. difficile by hospital personnel is an important means of spread of this organism. The use of vinyl gloves can reduce the incidence of disease.

Johnson S, et al. Treatment of asymptomatic *Clostridium difficile* carriers (fecal excretors) with vancomycin or metronidazole. *Ann Intern Med* 1992;117:297.
Asymptomatic excretion of C. difficile should not be treated.

Katz DA, Lynch ME, Littenberg B. Clinical prediction rules to optimize cytotoxin testing for *Clostridium difficile* in hospitalized patients with diarrhea. *Am J Med* 1996;100:487–495.
Patients without a history of antibiotic use within the past month and without either diarrhea (at least three watery stools) or abdominal pain are unlikely to have a positive result on C. difficile toxin assay.

Keighly MRB, et al. Randomized controlled trial of vancomycin for pseudomembranous colitis and postoperative diarrhea. *Br Med J* 1978;2:1667.
Oral vancomycin (125 mg every 6 hours) was effective for pseudomembranous colitis caused by toxigenic strains of C. difficile.

Kelly CP, LaMont JT. *Clostridium difficile* infection. *Annu Rev Med* 1998;49:375–390.
Review. Response usually occurs within 3 days after start of therapy.

Kreutzer EW, Milligan FD. Treatment of antibiotic-associated pseudomembranous colitis with cholestyramine resin. *Johns Hopkins Med J* 1978;143:67.
Cholestyramine (4 g three times daily), an anion-binding resin that may bind the toxin, was effective in 12 patients with pseudomembranous colitis.

Lemann F, et al. Arbitrary primed PCR rules out *Clostridium difficile* cross-infection among patients in a haematology unit. *J Hosp Infect* 1997;35:107–115.
Polymerase chain reaction can be helpful to type strains in the evaluation of an outbreak.

Manabe YC, et al. *Clostridium difficile* colitis: an efficient clinical approach to diagnosis. *Ann Intern Med* 1995;123:835–840.
Predictors of a positive C. difficile toxin assay included a positive fecal leukocyte test, semiformed stool, use of a cephalosporin, and onset of diarrhea 6 days after start of antibiotic therapy.

McFarland LV, et al. Nosocomial acquisition of *Clostridium difficile* infection. *N Engl J Med* 1989;320:204.
Fifty-nine percent of healthcare workers had a positive hand culture for C. difficile after contact with an infected patient.

Renshaw AA, Stelling JM, Doolittle MH. The lack of value of repeated *Clostridium difficile* cytotoxicity assays. *Arch Pathol Lab Med* 1996;120:49–52.
In only 1% of cases was a repeated C. difficile toxin assay useful if performed within a 7-day period.

Rifkin GD, et al. Antibiotic-induced colitis: implication of a toxin neutralized by *Clostridium sordellii* antitoxin. *Lancet* 1977;2:1103.
A clostridial toxin was isolated from two patients with pseudomembranous colitis. Oral vancomycin (500 mg every 6 hours) was given for 10 days, with resolution of the illness.

Salcedo J, et al. Intravenous immunoglobulin therapy for severe *Clostridium difficile* colitis. *Gut* 1997;41:366–370.
IV immunoglobulin may have a role in patients with C. difficile colitis who fail standard antibiotic therapy.

Stanley RJ, Melson GL, Tedesco FJ. The spectrum of radiographic findings in antibiotic-related pseudomembranous colitis. *Radiology* 1974;111:519.
Plaquelike mucosal lesions on barium enema are highly suggestive.
Tedesco FJ, Barton RW, Alpers DH. Clindamycin-associated colitis: a prospective study. *Ann Intern Med* 1974;81:429.
The authors noted a 21% incidence of diarrhea and a 10% incidence of pseudomembranous colitis in patients receiving clindamycin.
van den Berg RJ, et al. Characterization of toxin A-negative, toxin B-positive *Clostridium difficile* isolates from outbreaks in different countries by amplified fragment length polymorphism and PCR ribotyping. *J Clin Microbiol* 2004;42:1035–1041.
A discussion of worldwide strains that are toxin B positive and toxin A negative.

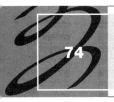

74 PERIOPERATIVE ANTIMICROBIAL PROPHYLAXIS

*I*nfections after surgical procedures are a major cause of morbidity and occasional mortality. Currently, surgical site infections (SSIs) represent up to 24% of all nosocomial infections, prolong hospital stay by 7 to 14 days, and cost in excess of $1 billion annually. It has been estimated that approximately 500,000 SSIs occur each year in the United States and result in more than 3,000 deaths.

The role of antibiotics is to reduce bacterial proliferation. When used prophylactically, these agents have been shown to decrease the likelihood of infection after selected types of surgery; however indiscriminate use may result in emergence of resistant pathogens, increased costs, adverse reactions, and a false sense of security. Some procedures are associated with a low risk of SSI, and the risks of perioperative antibiotics may outweigh the benefits.

Several general principles are important for prevention of SSIs. Asepsis and good surgical technique remain cornerstones for prevention of SSIs. Operating room cleanliness, adequate preoperative skin preparation, judicious shaving, level of activity in the operating room, and duration of preoperative hospitalization and surgical procedure are additional factors. The procedure itself mandates prophylactic antibiotics only if there is significant risk for postoperative site infection. Patient factors that may increase risk of SSI include poor nutrition, diabetes mellitus, old age, remote focus of infection, smoking, obesity, and immunosuppression. Once the need for prophylactic antibiotics has been determined, those which are most effective against the bacteria most commonly causing infection at the given surgical site should be chosen. The goal of antibiotic administration is to decrease intraoperative bacterial contamination to the point where it cannot overwhelm host defenses. Adequate levels of antibiotic at the operative site should be maintained for the entirety of the procedure.

 SURGICAL PROCEDURE CLASSIFICATION

Historically surgical procedures have been classified as (1) clean, (2) clean/contaminated, (3) contaminated, and (4) dirty/infected. Table 74-1 defines and gives examples of procedures within each class. In general, a major break in asepsis moves a procedure into the next higher class. Such a classification of procedures has been useful to help define anticipated postoperative infection rates. Clean operations are generally associated with infection rates lower than 2%. Clean/contaminated procedures performed without prophylaxis have

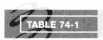

TABLE 74-1	Classification of Surgical Procedures	
Class	**Definition**	**Examples**
1. Clean	Nontraumatic, uninfected procedure without surgical procedural breaks; no entry of gastrointestinal, respiratory, or genitourinary tracts	Thyroidectomy, laminectomy, herniorrhaphy, breast surgery
2. Clean/contaminated	Entry of gastrointestinal, respiratory, or genitourinary tracts under controlled conditions without unusual contamination. Wounds may be mechanically drained	Appendectomy, hysterectomy, elective colorectal surgery, most elective biliary tract procedures
3/4. Contaminated/dirty	Surgery with overt spillage of gastrointestinal contents, open traumatic wounds, entry into infected biliary, gastrointestinal, or genitourinary tracts	Perforated diverticulitis, ruptured appendix, drainage of intra-abdominal abscess, repair of open compound fracture

historically been associated with wound infection rates above 8%, and often much higher. Factors within class 1 and 2 procedures, which are associated with a higher likelihood of infection, include abdominal surgery, surgery lasting longer than 2 hours, and more than three underlying diseases. The other classes are associated with infection rates above 30%; in these situations, the administration of antimicrobial agents should be considered therapeutic. Factored into this classification are additional clinical characteristics established by the Centers for Disease Control and Prevention as important in the likelihood of postoperative wound infection. These are an American Society of Anesthesiology (ASA) score of at least 3, duration of surgery beyond a "setpoint" for each surgical procedure, and class 3/4 surgery. Using the presence of these criteria (scored 0–3), the risk of infection increases from less than 2 to 13%. Thus, an individual with multiple comorbidities (ASA class 3 or greater) and anticipated prolonged surgery may benefit from antibiotic prophylaxis despite have "class 1" surgery.

Parenteral antimicrobials have been used for perioperative prophylaxis for several decades; however, only since the early 1980s have well-designed and controlled studies been performed that document efficacy in selected situations. Factors to be considered in prophylaxis include timing, duration, choice of agent, type of surgical procedure, and cost. Studies have shown that antimicrobial agents administered postoperatively (i.e., after contamination has occurred) or more than 2 hours preoperatively give no greater protection than placebo. In 2003, experts from the Medicare National Surgical Infection Prevention Project (NSIPP) recommended that the first antibiotic dose should start within 60 minutes of incision. With use of vancomycin or fluoroquinolones, infusion should be initiated within 120 minutes.. There is no consensus that infusion should be completed prior to incision. However, with use of a proximal tourniquet, the entire dose should be given before the tourniquet is inflated.

Most studies show that continuation of antibiotic prophylaxis after wound closure is not necessary. Adequate antibiotic concentrations should be maintained throughout the procedure, but the need for prolongation beyond this is unproven. Further use of antibiotics increases costs, encourages emergence of resistant organisms, and increases adverse reactions without additional benefits. No well-performed investigations have demonstrated enhanced efficacy with multiple-dose regimens, but for agents with short half-lives, redosing is indicated so that adequate concentrations are maintained during long procedures.

The agent chosen for prophylaxis should be safe and effective against most anticipated pathogens. To use agents most effectively, clinicians must have knowledge about likely postoperative pathogens in their institution. Of particular importance are data regarding the risk of methicillin-resistant *Staphylococcus aureus* (MRSA) or methicillin-resistant *Staphylococcus epidermidis* (MRSE), as the risk of these pathogens will require the increased use of vancomycin prophylactically (with its attendant risks of immediate complications and potential for emergence of vancomycin-resistant *Enterococcus faecium*). Alternatives to vancomycin exist and potentially include linezolid and daptomycin, but use of these agents for surgical prophylaxis is unproven and not currently recommended. There is no consensus regarding what percentage of MRSA (or MRSE) would require use of these agents. Additionally, no data demonstrate that such use decreases risk of MRSA or MRSE SSI.

Cefazolin remains the agent most commonly used and recommended for antibiotic perioperative prophylaxis. It can be used as a single preoperative 1-g dose for procedures lasting longer than 4 hours. For prolonged procedures a second dose may be given at about that time. Alternatively some experts recommend use of an extended half-life agent (e.g., cefotetan, ceftriaxone) when surgery is anticipated to extend beyond this length. Some authorities also recommend that antimicrobials used for treatment of established infections not be routinely used for prophylaxis. None of these agents is effective against MRSA or MRSE, however.

The role of prophylaxis for clean surgical procedures is controversial. With most of these, infection rates are extremely low, and large numbers of patients would have to receive antimicrobials to prevent small numbers of infections. However, when large numbers of patients have been studied, benefits have been shown for several apparently low-risk procedures (e.g., herniorrhaphy and some breast surgery). Patients with implantation of hardware or grafts and cardiac surgery patients should always receive prophylaxis. Additional clean procedures for which prophylaxis should be used include those lasting longer than 4 hours, in patients with coexistent distant infection, and those in insulin-dependent diabetics. The presence of these risks increases infection rates to almost 8%—approximately 300% more than in patients undergoing similar procedures without such risks.

Clean/contaminated surgical procedures benefit the most from antimicrobial prophylaxis, and, in general, perioperative antimicrobials represent the standard of care. Risks of infection from selected procedures may decline from more than 15% to well below 8%.

 SPECIFIC SURGICAL PROCEDURES

Biliary Tract Surgery

Cholelithiasis is associated with bactibilia in more than 50% of patients. Organisms most commonly identified are *Escherichia coli, Klebsiella* and *Proteus* spp., and *E. faecalis*. Risk factors for postoperative infection are age older than 70, cholelithiasis, jaundice, and positive bile cultures. In general, agents active against the common gram-negative enteric bacteria have proven effective. These include trimethoprim-sulfamethoxazole (TMP-SMX) and cefazolin. For high-risk patients, cefazolin 1 g is recommended. TMP-SMX is a reasonable alternative. Patients undergoing endoscopic retrograde cholangiopancreatography (ERCP) with risks for infection (age older than 70, common duct stones, obstruction, acute cholecystitis, and a nonfunctioning gallbladder) also benefit from prophylaxis.

Colorectal Surgery

Antimicrobial prophylaxis should always be used. Oral administration of antimicrobials, as well as cleansing enemas decreased postoperative wound infection rates when compared with controls of vigorous purgation alone; however, recent limitations on length of preoperative stay may impede the ability to perform satisfactory bowel cleansing. Oral neomycin plus erythromycin decreases wound infection rates from 43 to 9% when compared with controls. Similar results have been achieved with metronidazole and doxycycline. A standardized regimen for oral prophylaxis is given in Table 74-2.

The value of additional parenteral antimicrobials remains controversial. One study demonstrated that cefoxitin decreased infection rates from 18.3 to 6.6%. Many clinicians now add either a single preoperative dose of cefotetan or cefoxitin to a bowel preparation using nonabsorbable antimicrobials.

TABLE 74-2	Bowel Preparation for Elective Colorectal Operations
2 days prior to surgery	Low residue or liquid diet Magnesium citrate (30 mL of 50% solution at 10:00 AM, 2:00 PM, and 6:00 PM Fleet enema in evening until clear
1 day prior to surgery	Clear liquid diet Magnesium citrate × 2, or whole-gut lavage with polyethylene glycol electrolyte solution, 1 L/hr × 2–4 hr until clear (prior to use of oral antibiotics) Neomycin/erythromycin, 1 g each at 1:00 PM, 2:00 PM, and 11:00 PM
Day of surgery	Operate early AM Use appropriate parenteral antibiotic (generally cefoxitin or cefotetan) 30 minutes prior to initiation of surgery.

(Adapted from Nichols RL. Prophylaxis for surgical infections. In: Gorbach SL, Bartlett JG, Blacklow NR, eds. *Infectious Diseases.* 2nd ed. Philadelphia, Pa: WB Saunders and Co; 1998:470–480.)

Some practitioners have advocated the addition of specific anaerobic prophylaxis, such as parenteral metronidazole. A recent study suggests that the combination of oral and parenteral prophylaxis may result in lower postoperative infection rates.

When emergency colorectal operations must be performed on an unprepared bowel, the likelihood of fecal soilage is great. In this event, parenteral antimicrobial prophylaxis should be initiated. Cefoxitin or cefotetan are reasonable choices. Follow-up treatment depends on surgical findings. Gross spillage necessitates continuing antimicrobials for therapeutic reasons, but if no evidence of bowel perforation is noted, these agents can be discontinued.

A study of perioperative supplemental oxygen therapy in patients who underwent colorectal resection showed that patients who received supplemental oxygen during surgery and for 2 hours postoperatively had a 50% decrease in wound infection rate. This appears to be a practical and inexpensive method of decreasing the incidence of surgical wounds in this population.

Obstetric and Gynecologic Surgery

Vaginal hysterectomy benefits most from parenteral antimicrobial prophylaxis. Surgical wound infection rates decline from 20 to 40% down to 4 to 8% when prophylaxis is used. Cefotetan is currently recommended for both vaginal and abdominal hysterectomy, although cefazolin and cefoxitin are acceptable alternatives. Single-dose prophylaxis is sufficient. Metronidazole is an alternative, although it may be less effective when used as monotherapy than the cephalosporins. Cesarean sections are classified as low risk if they are done electively and are classified as high risk if rupture of membranes has occurred, if labor has started, or if done emergently. The same antibiotic choices as for hysterectomy apply. The antibiotic is generally not given until the umbilical cord is clamped to prevent masking any possible septic symptoms in the neonate.

The cost-benefit analyses of using cefazolin in both vaginal and abdominal hysterectomies demonstrate the importance of antimicrobial prophylaxis for both of these procedures. Costs were reduced by $1,777 and $716, respectively, and for vaginal and abdominal procedures, wound infection rates declined from 21.4 to 2.3% and 21.1 to 14.1%, respectively. The authors report that savings would be substantially higher if more expensive drugs or prolonged prophylaxis had been used. A single dose of cefazolin, 1 g intravenously, therefore, appears to be a prudent choice for antimicrobial prophylaxis in most obstetric and gynecologic operations.

Orthopedic Surgery (Total Hip and Knee Arthroplasty)

The recommended antibiotics for prophylaxis are cefazolin and cefuroxime. For patient with serious allergy or adverse reactions to ß-lactams, vancomycin or clindamycin is recommended. Several studies examining the duration of prophylaxis have found no benefit to prolonged antibiotic therapy. The NSIPP has recommended that antibiotic prophylaxis be discontinued within 24 hours from the completion of the surgery. There has been no evidence that continuing prophylaxis until all drains and catheters are removed will lower infection rates. In a recent meta-analysis, a single dose of a prophylactic antibiotic was as effective as multiple doses in hip fracture patients.

The need for antibiotic prophylaxis in patients undergoing dental procedures in the presence of prosthetic orthopedic devices is similarly controversial. Personal experience demonstrates that virtually all orthopedists strongly recommend use of antibiotics in these circumstances, but objective data to document need are lacking. Selected high-risk patients (defined as those with prolonged dental surgery or substantial underlying comorbidity) may benefit from short-course antimicrobials at the time of dental procedures. (RBB)

Bibliography

Abramowicz M, ed. Antimicrobial prophylaxis for surgery. *Treatment Guidelines from the Medical Letter* 2004;2:27–32.
The authors present a consensus of the antimicrobials of choice for surgical wound prophylaxis of numerous procedures. Cefazolin remains the drug of choice for many procedures.

Bratzler DW, Houck PM. Antimicrobial prophylaxis for surgery: An advisory statement from the National Surgical Infection Prevention Project. *Clin Infect Dis* 2004;38:1706–1715.
This advisory statement from experts representing the Medicare NSIPP provides general recommendations for antimicrobial prophylaxis and presents consensus statements regarding timing of first dose and appropriate duration of prophylactic therapy. Recommendations for prophylaxis are presented by type of surgery. It is an excellent single-source document for the areas covered.

Classen DC, et al. The timing of prophylactic administration of antibiotics and the risk of surgical wound infection. *N Engl J Med* 1992;326:281–286.
Approximately 2,800 patients were prospectively monitored to determine the relationship of postoperative wound infection to the timing of antimicrobial prophylaxis. Rates of infection were statistically higher when initiated either more than 2 hours preoperatively or postoperatively. The authors could not differentiate between groups that were given a first dose just prior to surgery or intraoperatively. This is a large clinical study that confirms many animal data.

Cruse PJE, Foord R. The epidemiology of wound infections: a 10-year prospective study of 62,939 wounds. *Surg Clin North Am* 1980;60:27–40.
The paper remains an excellent example of information that can be gathered with a great deal of leg work. The authors prospectively followed more than 60,000 surgical wounds over a 10-year period. The survey included telephone followup with patients at 28 days. There was a direct relationship between surgical wound class and risk of postoperative infection. The rate for clean procedures was 1.5% and 40% for class 4 procedures. Infection prolonged hospital stay by an average of 10 days. The authors conclude that wound infections can be decreased by using factors that include shortened hospital stay, preoperative hexachlorophene shower, minimal shaving, excellent surgical technique, and expeditious surgery.

DiPiro JT, et al. Single dose systemic antibiotic prophylaxis of surgical wound infections. *Am J Surg* 1986;152:552–559.
The authors critically evaluate the available literature on single-dose antimicrobial prophylaxis in surgery. Data are broken out by type of study and surgical procedure. Approximately 40 studies were identified, and in no instance was single-dose prophylaxis demonstrated to be inferior to a multiple-dose regimen.

Greif R, et al. Supplemental perioperative oxygen to reduce the incidence of surgical wound infection. *N Engl J Med* 2000;342:161–166.
The authors randomly assigned 500 patients to receive either 30% or 80% inspired oxygen during and after colorectal resection. The patients who received 80% oxygen had 50% fewer infections. Increased supplemental oxygen appears to be a practical method of decreasing postoperative wound infections.

Haley RW, et al. Identifying patients at high risk of surgical wound infection. *Am J Epidemiol* 1985;121:206–215.

Information concerning more than 59,000 surgical patients was used to establish risks for postoperative infections. Factors associated with postoperative infection included abdominal operation, surgical length longer than 2 hours, class 3 or 4 surgery, and more than three underlying diagnoses. The addition of factors other than surgical class identified at least twice as many infections.

Little JW. Patients with prosthetic joints: are they at risk when receiving invasive dental procedures? *Spec Care in Dentistry* 1997;17:153–161

The author, a dentist, presents existing data on the risks of prosthetic joint infection associated with invasive dental procedures. Little objective information exists that substantiates a valid risk. In this paper, the author also reviews statements for a variety of advisory boards which, in general, agree with his belief. Selected "high-risk" patients, which includes those undergoing prolonged dental surgery and those with substantial underlying comorbidities, may benefit from brief antibiotic prophylaxis.

Martin CE, and the French Study Group on Antimicrobial Prophylaxis in Surgery and the French Society of Anesthesia and Intensive Care. Antimicrobial prophylaxis in surgery: general concepts and clinical guidelines. *Infect Control Hosp Epidemiol* 1994;15:463–471.

The authors review basic principles of antibiotic prophylaxis in surgery and present recommendations for numerous specific procedures. They spend much time describing the ideal antibiotic, which of course does not exist. This manuscript remains an excellent resource for those interested in this topic.

Nichols RL, et al. Current practices of preoperative bowel preparation among North American colorectal surgeons. *Clin Infect Dis* 1997;24:609–619.

The authors sent questionnaires to more than 800 colorectal surgeons and received responses from 58%. All used some form of mechanical bowel preparation. Almost 90% also used antibiotics (the majority both oral and parenteral). The most common regimen was a combination of oral neomycin plus either metronidazole or erythromycin plus a parenteral antibiotic.

Platt R, et al. Perioperative antibiotic prophylaxis for herniorrhaphy and breast surgery. *N Engl J Med* 1990;322:153–160.

This important investigation validates the concept that patients with "clean" surgery, unassociated with implants or other major risks, may benefit from antimicrobial prophylaxis. In this study, ceforanide was used versus placebo in more than 1,200 patients undergoing herniorrhaphy or breast surgery. For both surgical procedures, patients who received antimicrobial prophylaxis were less likely to develop postoperative wound infection. It remains uncertain whether all clean surgical procedures would benefit similarly.

Southwell-Keely JP, et al. Antiobiotic prophylaxis in hip fracture surgery: a metaanalysis. *Clin Orthop* 2004;419:179–184.

The authors reviewed 15 randomized, controlled trials to determine the most effective prophylactic antibiotic regimen in hip fracture surgery. They determined that one dose of antibiotic yielded no better outcomes than multiple-dose regimens.

Ulualp K, Condon RE. Antibiotic prophylaxis for scheduled operative procedures. *Infect Dis Clin North Am* 1992;6:613–625.

A contemporary review that includes information on normal flora of various body areas and antimicrobial pharmacokinetics. Provides recommendations of specific antimicrobials for various types of procedures.

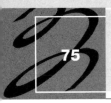

75 ANTIFUNGAL CHEMOTHERAPY

*F*ungi are an important cause of human infection. Some, such as *Histoplasma capsulatum, Blastomyces* spp., and *Coccidioides immitis* are indigenous to selected geographic areas, and are unlikely to be contracted by persons without habitation or travel histories. Others that include *Candida* spp., *Aspergillus/Mucor*, and *Cryptococcus neoformans* are more universally distributed and are seen primarily in patients with selected forms of immunosuppression or exposure to broad-spectrum antibiotics. No single agent provides coverage against all fungi, one of several reasons for targeted therapy whenever possible. Table 75-1 provides typical dosages for commonly used antifungals. Data on efficacy, safety, and dosing, as well as length of treatment, are much less well established than for most antibacterial agents. Reports of carefully controlled, prospective, and blinded studies are limited, and problems regarding the use of most of the antifungals are complicated further by difficulties with obtaining validated susceptibility testing and blood level determinations.

TABLE 75-1 **Dosages of Commonly Used Antifungal Agents**

Intravenous	Dosage	Common uses
Amphotericin B deoxycholate (IV)	0.3–1.5 mg/kg day	Most invasive fungal infections
Liposomal amphotericin B	3–5 mg/kg day	
Itraconazole	200–400 mg/day	Sporotrichosis, occasionally for pulmonary aspergillosis
Fluconazole	200–800 mg first dose, then 100–400 mg q 24 hr	Invasive *Candida* infections
Caspofungin acetate	70 mg/day (first day), then 50 mg/day	Invasive pulmonary aspergillosis
Voriconazole	6 mg/kg q12 hr × 2 doses. Then 4 mg/kg q 12 hr (dosing for *Candida* infections may be lower)	Invasive pulmonary aspergillosis
Oral		
Flucytosine	150 mg/kg day (four divided doses)	Adjunctive therapy of cryptococcal meningitis, *Candida* spp. urinary tract infections
Fluconazole	100–200 mg/day	See above
Voriconazole	400 mg q 12 hr × two doses, then 200 mg q 12 hr	See above
Itraconazole (capsules)	100–400 mg/day	See above
Itraconazole (liquid)	100 mg b.i.d.	
Amphotericin B (liquid)	100–500 mg q.i.d	Mucosal candidiasis

464

CLASSES OF ANTIFUNGAL DRUGS

Antifungal agents are grouped into several classes. *Polyenes* include amphotericin B, nystatin, and candicidin and are characterized by the presence of a hydrophilic region and four to seven double bonds. None are absorbed well after oral administration, and all are considered to be relatively toxic when parenterally administered. Additionally, all are poorly soluble in aqueous solvents. The mechanism of action, probably through binding to fungal ergosterol (a component of the fungal cell), allows for the formation of channels within the fungal cell membrane, with a resultant loss of vital elements. Lack of binding characterizes the occasionally resistant organism, such as *C. lusitaniae.*

Azoles (imidazoles and triazoles) include itraconazole, fluconazole, voriconazole, miconazole, terconazole, sulconazole, ketoconazole, and econazole. Within the United States, most use is of the first three agents. Imidazoles differ from triazoles by having two (rather than three) nitrogen atoms in the five-member azole ring. The triazole configuration increases tissue penetration, prolongs half-life, and enhances efficacy while decreasing toxicity. Unlike polyenes, which are active primarily against systemic mycoses, azoles are also effective against dermatophytes. The mechanism of action is through inhibition of intracellular cytochrome P-450, which is required for demethylation of the ergosterol precursor *lanosterol,* and is generally fungistatic.

Echinocandins represent the newest class of approved antifungals. Caspofungin acetate is the first of this class to be approved in the United States. All are likely to be available only parenterally. This class disrupts cell-wall synthesis through inhibition of 1,3 B-D- glucan synthase. *C. neoformans* lacks this enzyme and appears resistant to echinocandins. Human cells lack the cell wall, and thus echinocandins appear to be relatively nontoxic to humans.

 SPECIFIC DRUGS

Amphotericin B

Although the author feels that amphotericin B desoxycholate (Fungizone®) remains the standard for disseminated fungal infections, other agents that include fluconazole have emerged as agents of choice in selected infections (e.g., intensive care unit [ICU]-acquired candidemia). It is active against almost all pathogenic fungi, although occasional resistance and tolerance is encountered. The drug is poorly absorbed after oral administration and must be given intravenously for systemic infections. Its lack of absorption has made amphotericin B a useful component for bowel decontamination or candidal overgrowth syndromes in selected clinical situations. After parenteral administration, less than 5% is recovered in urine, and only 40% can be found in serum and other fluids. The remainder is presumably absorbed by cell membranes and is then slowly released over prolonged periods. The drug can be detected for more than 8 weeks after commonly used dosages. Blood levels of amphotericin B are typically below 2 μg/mL, an amount barely greater than the minimum inhibitory concentrations (MICs) of many of the fungi treated with this compound. The drug penetrates poorly into body fluids other than serum, and cerebrospinal fluid (CSF) levels have been demonstrated to be only about 2 to 3% of simultaneous serum levels. Nevertheless, occasional cures of central nervous system (CNS) infections, such as cryptococcal meningitis, have been effected with this drug.

Amphotericin B has poor solubility and is marketed with deoxycholate to ensure colloidal dispersion. It must be reconstituted with sterile water and then added to 5% dextrose in water (5% D/W) in an amount sufficient to provide a final concentration of 0.1 mg/mL. This formulation cannot be mixed with other solutions, and other compounds should not be admixed. It is no longer necessary to cover the bottle with a paper bag during administration. A 220-mm filter causes partial retention of the agent and should be avoided.

Amphotericin B is administered in doses of up to 1.5 mg/kg per day. An initial dose of 1 mg over 1 hour is recommended to ensure against possible anaphylaxis. If that dose is tolerated, the remainder of the prescribed dose is given over an additional 4 to 5 hours. Generally dosage modification for renal dysfunction is not needed. Although anecdotal reports of successful infusions lasting fewer than 4 to 6 hours have been published, occasionally severe adverse reactions, including cardiac arrest, have occurred with more rapid administration. Length of treatment depends on the disease. Under many circumstances, it may be necessary to render therapy for several months.

Relatively low doses of amphotericin B may be used in some cases of mucosal disease, such as stomatitis/esophagitis, as may occur in patients with AIDS. Dosage in these situations is generally 0.3 to 0.5 mg/kg, with total doses as low as 200 to 300 mg. Although azoles are generally preferred, some resistant cases may require therapy with amphotericin B desoxycholate.

Unusually, amphotericin B may be administered by alternative routes. As an example, selected cases of *Coccidioides immitis* meningitis may benefit from intrathecal therapy. Intra-articular regimens of less than 15 mg per dose have been used for selected fungal arthritides.

Adverse reactions to amphotericin B are common and may be severe. This compound should be administered by persons comfortable with its use. Extreme rigors, fever, and hypotension may be encountered, especially early in therapy, and may be life-threatening. Concurrent administration of hydrocortisone (25–50 mg) within the bottle may be beneficial. Also useful is premedication with agents, such as diphenhydramine or acetaminophen, 45 minutes prior to amphotericin infusion.

Nephrotoxicity is the most significant side effect of this agent and occurs in up to 80% of cases. Elevations of serum creatinine to 2 to 3 mg/dL are routinely noted and may necessitate interruption of treatment. Costs for amphotericin B-associated nephrotoxicity may have been underestimated. In a recent investigation, 30% of patients receiving this agent developed acute renal failure, with associated mortality of more than 50% in this population. Increased length of stay was 8 days. However, maintenance of adequate fluid and sodium loading are protective and should be part of the treatment strategy. Hypokalemia and hypomagnesemia are often noted, and may be exacerbated by other agents that may also cause this effect.

Anemia is routinely observed and is thought to be the result of either bone marrow suppression or inhibition of erythropoietin production. Thrombocytopenia or neutropenia rarely occurs; aplastic anemia has not been reported. Amphotericin B oral suspension (100 mg/mL) is episodically available, with use primarily targeted at HIV/AIDS patients with stomatitis/esophagitis. The recommended dose is 1 to 5 mL (100–500 mg) q.i.d. for a minimum of 2 weeks.

Liposomal Amphotericin B

Liposomes are phospholipid complexes that, when coupled with amphotericin B, allow better distribution of the product to fungi with decreased activity within human cells. This allows higher doses to be used with less human toxicity. Three liposomal amphotericin B products are available (amphotericin B lipid complex, Abelcet®; amphotericin B colloidal suspension, Amphotec®; and AmBisome, L-amB®) have decreased nephrotoxicity and at least equal efficacy of amphotericin B desoxycholate. Although they have varying pharmacokinetics, different clinical outcomes have not been proven. Dosing is generally 3 to 5 mg/kg. All lipid-based preparations appear associated with less renal dysfunction than amphotericin B desoxycholate, and this has been the driving force for utilization. Table 75-2 summarizes selected comparative data. All have the capacity to cause acute toxicity, but liposomal amphotericin B (AmBisome) may be the least likely to be so associated. Fortunately, many of the patients who receive the liposomal preparations will already be amphotericin B experienced and are less likely to have acute adverse reactions. The liposomal preparations also have been recommended for use in patients who have amphotericin B-associated nephrotoxicity.

Liposomal amphotericin B (AmBisome®) was shown to be associated with fewer breakthrough fungal infections compared with conventional amphotericin B in patients with fever and neutropenia, and was generally found to be safer. Higher cumulative doses also may be more safely administered. However, in the author's opinion, expense precludes their routine use. The availability of newer compounds, such as voriconazole and caspofungin acetate,

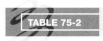

TABLE 75-2	Liposomal Amphotericin B Preparations		
Trade Name	Abelcet	Amphotec	AmBisome
FDA-approved indications	Invasive fungal infections refractory to amphotericin B	Invasive aspergillosis intolerant of full-dose amphotericin B, and treatment of aspergillosis when amphotericin B has failed	Empiric therapy for presumed fungal infection in patients with fever/neutropenia, cryptococcal meningitis in AIDS, diagnosis of *Aspergillus, Candida,* or *Cryptococcus* with failure of amphotericin B, visceral leishmaniasis, unacceptable toxicity with amphotericin B
Approval date (U.S.)	1995	1996	1997
Daily cost/ 100 mg*	$230	$186	$376

*Average wholesale price. Amphotericin B daily cost (1 mg/kg per day) = $33.20.

which are similarly priced to the lipid-based amphotericin B products, will likely result in decreased use of these agents.

Caspofungin Acetate

Caspofungin acetate (Cancidas®), the first of the echinocandins, represents a novel class of antifungal agent active against fungal cell wall. It acts by inhibiting beta (1.3)-D-glucan synthase, a critical component of fungal cell walls. It is active against virtually all *Candida* spp. and *Aspergillus* spp. However, *C. neoformans* and *Fusarium* spp. are likely resistant to this agent, as they lack this component of the cell wall. Caspofungin acetate is felt to be fungicidal against most *Candida* spp. Clinically it is effective for invasive aspergillosis, esophageal candidiasis, and invasive candidiasis. In studies of the latter condition, many strains were other than *C. albicans*. In this major investigation, fewer relapses were noted in patients receiving caspofungin acetate when compared with amphotericin B, with substantially less toxicity. Because of toxicities with the latter agent, some authors now consider caspofungin acetate a primary agent in the management of invasive candidiasis.

Dosing of caspofungin acetate is usually 70 mg/day for the first day, followed by 50 mg/day. No dosing adjustment is needed for renal insufficiency, but hemodialysis does not remove this agent. Although not an inhibitor of cytochrome P-450 hepatic enzyme systems, drug interactions are likely to occur with tacrolimus, cyclosporine, selected HIV medications (efavirenz, nelfinavir, and nevirapine), phenytoin, and rifampin. In these situations, a daily dose of caspofungin 70 mg has been recommended.

The possibility of synergy, by using agents with different modes of action is being explored, especially for the management of invasive aspergillosis. Future studies will be performed using an echinocandin plus either amphotericin B or an azole (with aspergillus activity) for the management of this disease.

Flucytosine

Flucytosine (Ancobon®) is a fluorinated pyrimidine related to fluorouracil, and is useful for selected candidal and cryptococcal infections. The mechanism of action is incompletely understood but is probably related to its conversion to fluorouracil within the fungal cell. It is well absorbed from the gastrointestinal tract and penetrates into most tissues. Most of the compound is excreted in active form in the urine, with levels averaging 200 to 500 μg/mL. Peak serum values are only 70 to 80 mg/day. Renal insufficiency (as may be seen with concurrent use of amphotericin B) may result in potentially toxic levels of flucytosine unless the dosage is regulated. The usual dosage of this drug is 150 mg/kg per day in four divided doses. The compound is supplied in either 250-mg or 500-mg tablets.

Flucytosine is relatively safe and usually well tolerated. Bone marrow depression may occur in the presence of renal dysfunction. The cause of this depression is not completely known but appears to be related to the metabolism of the parent compound to 5-fluorouracil. Suppression rarely occurs when blood levels of flucytosine are below 100 mg/mL. Presence of renal impairment necessitates dosage reduction. One method is to give a dose (37.5 mg/kg) at varying intervals depending on creatinine clearance; gfor example, every 6 hours at more than 40 mL/minute, every 12 hours at 20 to 40 mL/minute, and every 24 hours at 10 to 20 mL/minute. No nomogram is satisfactory for the anuric patient; however, blood levels can be measured by high-pressure liquid or gas chromatography. Flucytosine is cleared by hemodialysis or peritoneal dialysis, and a single dose of 37.5 mg/kg is recommended after each treatment. About 5% of individuals who receive this drug develop bone marrow depression, typically anemia or neutropenia. Nausea, diarrhea, and vomiting are occasionally seen but are infrequently severe and rarely necessitate discontinuation of therapy.

Use of flucytosine as monotherapy is indicated only in selected patients with candiduria, where rapid achievement of high levels may preclude emergence of resistance. It is most frequently used in combination with amphotericin B for serious cryptococcal infections. For cryptococcal meningitis in the HIV-negative patient, use of the two agents reduces the dose of amphotericin B (from 0.6 to 0.3 mg/kg) and the duration of therapy (from 10 to 6 weeks). In the presence of HIV, cryptococcal meningitis is not curable, and the addition of flucytosine may intensify anemia and other adverse reactions. However, some authorities recommend its use for the first 2 weeks of treatment. A recent publication used flucytosine plus fluconazole (vs. fluconazole alone) in AIDS patients with cryptococcal meningitis and demonstrated enhanced survivorship at 2 months (32% vs. 12%) and decreased headache at 1 month in those who received the combination. Other data suggest that the combination also may be useful for therapy of serious candidal infections. Flucytosine is not effective against infections caused by species of *Aspergillus* or *Mucor*.

Fluconazole

Fluconazole (Diflucan®) is available in both oral and intravenous formulations, and is the most utilized of the imidazoles. In vitro activity is present against most species of *Candida*, *C. neoformans*, *H. capsulatum*, *C. immitis*, and *Blastomyces* species. Activity against *Aspergillus* and *Mucor* is limited. Fluconazole is currently the major agent for management of infections caused by *C. albicans* and other "sensitive" *Candida* spp. It distributes well to tissues, and levels within inflamed meninges are 60 to 80% of those of serum. Clinically, fluconazole in doses of 100 to 200 mg daily has been successfully used for oropharyngeal and esophageal candidiasis. It is more effective than clotrimazole troches for the former and at least as effective as ketoconazole. A study using a daily 100-mg dose of fluconazole in AIDS patients demonstrated its superiority (endoscopically and clinically) over ketoconazole (200 mg daily) for therapy of *Candida* esophagitis.

Fluconazole at 200 mg/day orally is the agent of choice for maintenance therapy of cryptococcal meningitis in AIDS patients. Intravenous fluconazole is an important agent for the management of invasive candidal infections in seriously ill patients. Its ease of administration and excellent safety profile make it an appealing alternative to amphotericin B for disseminated candidal infections. At 400 mg/day, it appears to be as effective as amphotericin B for invasive *C. albicans* infections in nonneutropenic critically ill patients. Other species, including *C. tropicalis* and *C. parapsilosis*, also are generally susceptible. However, *C. krusei* is relatively resistant to fluconazole, *and C. glabrata* also may have enhanced resistance to this agent. Some clinicians have treated these with higher doses of fluconazole (e.g., 800–1200 mg/day); however, most prefer an alternative agent such as voriconazole. A loading dose double the daily dose should be administered to reach steady-state promptly.

Fluconazole inhibits cytochrome P-450 hepatic enzymes. Drug interactions resulting in higher levels of Coumadin, cyclosporin, and hydantoin, among others, have been observed. Rarely, other complications, such as hepatic failure, have been reported. This agent does not appear to impact on adrenal function or testosterone production—issues noted with selected earlier azoles. In patients receiving this agent, either for prolonged periods or repetitively (generally individuals treated for thrush with AIDS), failure may be noted related to resistance of *C. albicans* to this agent.

Voriconazole

Voriconazole (Vfend®) was approved by the Food and Drug Administration (FDA) in May 2002, initially for treatment of invasive aspergillosis and for treatment of several unusual organisms that include *Fusarium* and *Scedosporium* spp. It is available both orally and intravenously and is considered to have excellent oral bioavailability, in excess of 95%. Additionally, it distributes well to most tissues, including those in the central nervous system. Major advantages compared to fluconazole include activity against *Aspergillus* spp. and enhanced activatory against strains of *Candida* likely to be fluconazole resistant (e.g., *C. krusei* and *C. glabrata*). It has been demonstrated to be more effective and less toxic than amphotericin B desoxycholate in patients with invasive aspergillosis and also has been shown to be at least as effective as liposomal amphotericin B for empiric antifungal therapy in patients with neutropenia and persistent fever. In such situations, it has the additional advantage of oral administration, possibly for prolonged periods. Although active against "resistant" *Candida* spp., its value compared with other agents has not been proved.

Voriconazole has been associated with unique visual (retinal) adverse reactions seen in up to 30% of patients, generally within the first week. Individuals may complain of rapid onset of photophobia, color misperceptions, glare, or other conditions that generally last less than 30 minutes and are not associated with long-term complications. Other adverse reactions include rash and abnormalities of liver function. Voriconazole interacts with the cytochrome P-450 enzyme system and is potentially associated with numerous drug interactions. Examples of agents that should not be combined with voriconazole include rifampin and sirolimus. Agents requiring monitoring include warfarin, phenytoin, tacrolimus, and cyclosporine.

Voriconazole is very much a product in evolution. Its availability as an oral agent and the clinical experience against *Aspergillus* spp. make it a compelling choice for many persons with this infection. Clinical value for cryptococcal, coccidioidal, and histoplasmal infections is not proved. Its efficacy against *Candida* spp., especially those relatively resistant to fluconazole, is likely, but it is not yet clear whether it is a more effective product than its less expensive cousin.

Itraconazole

Itraconazole, available both intravenously and as capsules or oral suspension, is a triazole with potent in vitro activity against *Candida* spp., cryptococcus, *Aspergillus/Mucor*, and others, and is considered the agent of choice for lymphocutaneous sporotrichosis. Its major advantages clinically compared with fluconazole are that it has at least modest activity against *Aspergillus* spp. and has been proven effective for prophylactic use in febrile neutropenic patients, when consideration for infections with *Aspergillus* exists. When compared with amphotericin B for the latter indication, it was equally effective but with significantly decreased toxicity. Although favorable data for treatment of several forms of pulmonary aspergillosis exist, other agents that include amphotericin preparations, caspofungin acetate, and voriconazole are generally preferred, especially for severe infections. There do not appear to be defined benefits of this agent (compared to fluconazole) for infections associated with *Candida* spp. For oral administration, the solution is preferred to capsules because of enhanced gastrointestinal absorption and should be taken fasting. It has been approved for oral and esophageal candidiasis. The dosage is 100 to 200 mg/day; the solution should be vigorously swished for several seconds and swallowed.

An intravenous preparation of itraconazole is available, generally for individuals who cannot take the medication orally. Indications include patients with aspergillosis who are intolerant to amphotericin B. The typical dosage is 200 mg b.i.d. for 4 days followed by 200 mg daily.

Adverse effects are generally minor, although a case of fatal hepatitis has been reported. The recommended dosage of itraconazole ranges from 100 mg/day (superficial infections) to

400 mg/day (invasive aspergillosis). The duration of therapy is 3 days (vaginal candidiasis) to many months. As with other azoles, itraconazole interacts with the cytochrome P-450 system, and can lead to drug interactions with compounds that are metabolized through this system.

Ketoconazole

Ketoconazole is an oral preparation active in vitro against *Candida, Coccidioides, Blastomyces, Histoplasma,* and most dermatophytes. The usual daily dose is 200 to 400 mg. Use has generally been supplanted by other agents. It is extensively metabolized, and the dosage need not be altered in renal failure. Levels in the CSF and urine are low, and the drug should not be considered for use in infections at these sites. Oral administration of ketoconazole requires gastric acid for absorption, and this product must be given with food. In achlorhydric patients, administration with 8 ounces of Minute Maid orange juice, Coca Cola, Pepsi Cola, or Canada Dry ginger ale will improve absorption.

Ketoconazole has been successfully used for candidal infections involving mucous membranes, including esophagitis. It is inferior to fluconazole for esophageal candidiasis in AIDS patients, but its early use may prove less expensive initially. Outcomes with thrush in patients with HIV are similar between the two agents. It also has been reported useful for the management of coccidioidomycosis, histoplasmosis, and cryptococcal infection (nonmeningeal), sporotrichosis, and blastomycosis. Chronic relapsing forms of coccidioidomycosis and paracoccidioidomycosis appear to be stabilized with low doses of this agent given for up to 1 year. One study documents the efficacy and limited toxicity of high doses (up to 1,200 mg/day) in the management of CNS fungal infections.

Side effects of ketoconazole are minor, although hepatitis may occur and should be considered in patients on long-term, high-dose therapy. At least one fatal case of hepatitis caused by this drug has been reported in a patient who was receiving only 200 mg/day for 2 months. Additionally, it may depress synthesis of both testosterone and corticosteroids, which may result in oligospermia, gynecomastia, or abnormalities of menstruation. These side effects are associated more with higher daily dosage than with duration of therapy and are reversible on discontinuation of the drug.

Drug interactions are an important consideration with the use of ketoconazole. Agents that need to be used with caution with ketoconazole include (but are not limited to) H_2 antagonists, rifampin, terfenadine, cisapride, ddI, protease inhibitors, and cyclosporin.

Clotrimazole

Clotrimazole is a topical product useful in treating infections caused by both dermatophytes and *C. albicans.* It is available as a 1% ointment, a topical solution, a lozenge, and 100- and 500-mg vaginal tablets. Because of its broad spectrum of activity, it is often used when specific organism identification has not been accomplished. A controlled clinical trial has demonstrated the effectiveness of clotrimazole lozenges given five times daily in the treatment of chronic oral candidiasis; however, efficacy is less than that seen with fluconazole or ketoconazole.

Griseofulvin is an oral agent active only against dermatophytes. Therefore, diagnostic accuracy is necessary prior to beginning treatment. Griseofulvin is supplied as 125-mg, 250-mg, and 500-mg capsules or tablets, and peak blood levels of about 1 mg/mL are reached. The usual dose for adults is 500 mg twice daily, and therapy should be continued for more than 4 weeks, even if the infection clears before that time. For stubborn nail infections, therapy should be anticipated to last more than 3 months.

Side effects are minor and consist primarily of nausea, which may be noted in up to 15% of individuals. Occasionally, neuritis and mild confusion can be noted. Hematologic and hepatic dysfunction occurs rarely. Adverse drug interactions with warfarin can be seen.

Miscellaneous Agents

Terbinafine, a well-absorbed oral antifungal, is used in the United States primarily for the management of dermatophytes associated with onychomycoses. When administered in a dose of 250 mg/day for fingernail or toenail onychomycoses (6 weeks or 12 weeks, respectively), it is at least as effective as griseofulvin.

Supersaturated potassium iodide (SSKI) is used for the management of lymphocutaneous sporotrichosis. The drug is given orally, and treatment is initiated with a dose of 5 drops mixed in a liquid three times daily. The dose is increased by up to 4 drops/day to a maximum of 120 drops/day. If treatment is continued for several months, SSKI is effective and may preclude the need for harsher regimens. Toxicity is manifested by gastrointestinal upset or increased lacrimation or salivation. An acneiform rash may be noted at any stage of therapy and is generally not considered a reason to discontinue treatment. (RBB)

Bibliography

Hebrecht R, et al. Voriconazole versus amphotericin B for primary therapy of invasive aspergillosis. *New Engl J Med* 2002;347:408–415.
The authors conducted a randomized but unblinded study of these two agents in almost 300 patients with invasive aspergillosis. Almost all had hematologic malignancy or were bone marrow transplants patients. Use of voriconazole resulted in higher survival rates (70% vs. 58%) and fewer adverse reactions. Additionally, use of voriconazole allowed a substantial part of therapy to be oral.

Mora-Duarte J, et al. Comparison of caspofungin and amphotericin B for invasive candidiasis. *New Engl J Med* 2002;347:2020–2029.
The authors compared the two agents in patients with invasive candidiasis and performed a subset analysis in patients with proven candidemia. Caspofungin was noted to be at least as effective as amphotericin B and was associated with significantly less toxicity.

Ostrosky-Zeichner L, et al. Amphotericin B: time for a new "gold standard." *Clin Infect Dis* 2003;37:415–425.
The authors review the literature concerning the liposomal amphotericin B preparations, especially from controlled trials. They are of the opinion that liposomal preparations are generally at least the equivalent of amphotericin B desoxycholate and have a superior safety profile. Thus, they may now be "suitable replacements" for treatment of selected fungal infections. The authors do not directly address the substantial costs of these preparations, nor do they explore the potential value of other newer products (e.g., echinocandins or voriconazole) as alternatives for some individuals.

Singh RM, Perdue BE. Amphotericin B: a class review. *Formulary* 1998;33:424–447.
An excellent overview comparing the available formulations of amphotericin. Three liposomal forms have been FDA approved. All are substantially more expensive than amphotericin B deoxycholate, and it remains uncertain how much better they are clinically. It is very difficult to detect important differences among the three liposomal forms. One of them should probably be used for invasive disease associated with aspergillus. Although they are marketed as having advantages in patients with renal dysfunction associated with amphotericin B deoxycholate, the author has not found this problem to be significant when the original formulation is used carefully. All forms may be associated with acute toxicities and should be used with a loading dose and dose escalation.

Walsh TJ, et al. Amphotericin B lipid complex for invasive fungal infections: analysis of safety and efficacy in 556 cases. *Clin Infect Dis* 1998;26:1383–1396.
Patients who either clinically failed therapy with amphotericin B, had renal failure (drug induced or pretreatment), or acute amphotericin B toxicity were enrolled to receive amphotericin B lipid complex. Most patients were infected with either Aspergillus *or* Candida.*Approximately 60% demonstrated clinical response, including 40% with* Aspergillus. *Renal failure improved in those who entered the study with this condition. The authors correctly conclude that amphotericin B lipid complex is indicated for selected conditions.*

Walsh TJ, et al. Voriconazole compared with liposomal amphotericin B for empirical antifungal therapy in patients with neutropenia and persistent fever. *New Engl J Med* 2002;346;225–234.

The two products were compared in more than 800 patients with varying types of malignancies and chemotherapies who remained febrile more than 4 days with neutropenia despite broad-spectrum antibiotics, but without documented fungal infection at the time of enrollment. Although overall success was comparable between the two agents, voriconazole was associated with fewer breakthrough fungal infections, lower levels of toxicity, and allowed the switch to oral therapy in more than 20% of patients.

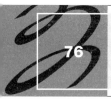

76 ANTIBIOTIC FAILURE

*A*ntibiotic failure can result from a variety of factors. An immunocompromised host is less likely to respond to appropriate antibiotics and may require combination therapy to achieve a satisfactory result. Febrile neutropenics, for example, might benefit from an aminoglycoside combined with a broad-spectrum penicillin agent. Patients with endocarditis also are often treated with combination therapy. Patients who have prosthetic-device infections often fail therapy, especially if retention of the prosthesis is maintained. Diabetics and patients with periphereal vascular disease often fail therapy as well. Some drug–drug interactions (iron and flouroquinolones) may impair the efficacy of an antibiotic. Some antibiotics may not be suited to treat certain infections in anatomic sites because they do not achieve significant levels in the affected tissues. For these reason, first-generation cephalosporins are not good choices for central nervous system infections. Likewise, aminoglycosides are ineffective antimicrobials when used as monotherapy for pulmonary infections. Individuals with hepatic or renal failure, or both, can be immunocompromised but can also be difficult to dose properly. Regimens that require multiple daily doses can be more difficult to take, leading to noncompliance.

Gastric acidity varies with age. There is a decline in gastric acidity such that gastric achlorhydria is found in 5.3% of people ages 20 to 29, in 16% of those ages 40 to 49, and in 35.4% of those older than age 60. The absorption of a number of antimicrobials through the oral route depends on their acid stability and the pH of gastric secretions. Decreased absorption can be a cause of lower serum and subsequently tissue levels of some antibiotics, which may lead to antibiotic failure. The absorption of intramuscularly administered antibiotics also may vary among patients, with lower levels being noted in some diabetic patients.

Renal function, likewise, varies with age. It is especially important to realize that calculated creatinine clearance may be significantly reduced in older patients, even though they may appear to have near-normal serum creatinine concentrations. Caution should be used when dosing certain antibiotics, such as penicillins or cephalosporins, to prevent the development of high serum levels that may produce severe neurotoxic reactions, such as myoclonus, seizures, or confusion. Other adverse reactions to the penicillins, such as reversible neutropenia, may be dose related and occur with increased frequency in older patients. Conversely, younger patients may require larger than expected doses of renally cleared antibiotics, such as vancomycin. Serum levels can be useful in managing these patients.

If an infection does not respond to antibiotic treatment alone, the patient should be evaluated for the presence of obstruction, necrotic tissue, hematoma, abscess, prosthetic devices, or venous thromboembolism. Computerized tomography, vascular studies, and nuclear scans might be helpful in determining the cause of fever. A trial of ibuprofen can be helpful in diagnosing tumor fever in cancer patients.

In an effort to help make the right choice of antibiotic intially, I have chosen to emphasize several key points to help understand how to choose the right antibiotic based on antimicrobial sensitivity tests.

 ## SPECIFIC TESTING MODALITIES

The National Committee for Clinical Laboratory Standards (NCCLS) publishes standards pertaining to various aspects of bacterial susceptibility testing. Generally speaking, most hospitals can perform susceptibility tests on aerobic bacteria. Usually, results are reported annually in an "antibiogram "for those antibiotics that are a part of the hospital's formulary. It is important to be familiar with your hospital's antibiogram, as it can be an invaluable tool to help guide empiric therapy pending formal suspectibility testing. For organisms not included in the NCCLS standards, consultation with an infectious disease specialist or reference lab is recommended for guidance in determining the need for susceptibility testing and in the interpretation of results.

The minimum inhibitory concentration (MIC), reported as micrograms per milliliter (μg/mL), is the lowest concentration of a specific antimicrobial agent that inhibits the test organism. Similarly, the minimal bactericidal concentration (MBC), also known as the minimal lethal concentration, is the lowest concentration of a specific antimicrobial agent that kills the test organism. The following definitions of *susceptible, intermediate,* and *resistant* are presented in one of the NCCLS documents (NCCLS. Performance Standards for Antimicrobial Susceptibility Testing. 8th Informational Supplement. NCCLS document M100-S8. Wayne, Pa: National Committee for Clinical Laboratory Standards; 1998).

1. Susceptible. The "susceptible" category implies that an infection due to the strain may be appropriately treated with the dosage of antimicrobial agent recommended for that type of infection and infecting species, unless otherwise contraindicated.
2. Intermediate. The "intermediate" category includes isolates with antimicrobial agent MICs that approach usually attainable blood and tissue levels and for which response rates may be lower than for susceptible isolates. The intermediate category implies clinical applicability in body sites where the drugs are physiologically concentrated (e.g., quinolones and β-lactams in urine) or when a high dosage of drug can be used (e.g., β-lactams). The intermediate category also includes a "buffer zone" that should prevent small, uncontrolled technical factors from causing major discrepancies in interpretations, especially for drugs with narrow pharmacotoxicity margins.
3. Resistant. Resistant strains are not inhibited by the usually achievable systemic concentrations of the agent with normal dosage schedules and/or that fall in the range in which specific microbial resistance mechanisms are likely (e.g., β-lactamases), and clinical efficacy has not been reliable in treatment studies

Anaerobes, fungi, and mycobacteria are not tested for routinely in most hospitals.

Disk Diffusion Testing

Perhaps the oldest, but still useful method is the disk diffusion test or Kirby-Bauer method. Disk susceptibility testing is based on the relationship between the concentration of drug necessary to prevent bacterial growth and the zone or area of growth inhibition around an antimicrobial-impregnated disk. Kirby-Bauer disk diffusion antibiotic suseptibility testing is performed by streaking a defined inoculum (compared with McFarland 0.5 OD standard) onto a large Mueller-Hinton agar plate. Then antibiotic-impregnated disks are placed onto the agar surface. As the bacteria grow (incubated at $35°C$ [$95°F$] for 18 hours), they are inhibited to varying degrees by the antibiotic diffusing from the disk. It has been determined that zones of inhibition of a certain diameter (varies for antibiotic and, to a lesser extent, bacterial species) correlate with sensitivity or resistance to the antibiotic tested. The diameter of the area around each disk that is free from visible bacterial growth is measured to the nearest millimeter. The zones of growth inhibition are compared with reference values, and the results are reported as "susceptible," "intermediately susceptible," or "resistant." The disk technique is an inexpensive, rapid, reproducible, and relatively simple means of evaluating antimicrobial susceptibility; however, standardized procedures must be followed. In addition, the disk diffusion test can be used only for microbes that grow rapidly on artificial media; thus, this technique is not reliable for evaluating the susceptibility of anaerobic and other fastidious bacteria. Interpretation of the organism as sensitive, intermediate, or resistant to the antibiotic depends on the zone diameter criteria for the particular organism–antibiotic combination. For example, for one of the *Enterobacteriaceae*, a zone diameter around an ampicillin disk of 17 mm or greater is considered susceptible, whereas for a *Staphylococcus* spp., the zone diameter for ampicillin must be 29 mm or larger to be considered susceptible.

Antibiotic Gradient Diffusion Testing/E test

The E test is an in vitro method for quantitative antimicrobial susceptibility testing whereby a preformed antimicrobial gradient from a plastic-coated strip diffuses into an agar medium inoculated with the test organism. The MIC is read directly from a scale on the top of the strip at a point where the ellipse of organism growth inhibition intercepts the strip. This commercially prepared strip creates a gradient of antibiotic concentration when placed on an agar plate inoculated with bacteria. After incubation, the intersection of the strip with the edge of the elliptic zone of inhibition is identified, and the MIC corresponds to the point where the bacterial growth crosses the numbered strip. In general, data from the E test have correlated very well with the results of broth or agar dilution susceptibility assays with only a few minor errors. The E test has greatly facilitated the ability of microbiology laboratories to determine MICs for *Streptococcus pneumoniae* and a variety of organisms, including fungi, and anaerobes.

β-Lactamase Assays

This method is used to detect β-lactamase production in *Haemophilus* spp., *Neisseria gonorrhoeae*, *Moraxella catarrhalis*, enterococci, and staphylococci. The current method used in the laboratory is the chromogenic cephalosporin (cefinase [nitrocefin] disk) test. The test organism is inoculated directly onto the filter paper disk impregnated with nitrocefin. If the organism produces β-lactamase, it will hydrolize the chromogenic cephalosporin, causing an electron shift that results in a colored product. β-Lactamases are enzymes capable of hydrolyzing the β-lactam ring of penicillins (penicillinases) or cephalosporins (cephalosporinases), thereby inactivating the drugs. Enterococcus fecalis produces a β-lactamase approximately 1% of the time. These strains are susceptible to ampicillin–sulbactam but not to ampicillin.

Dilution Susceptibility Tests

To determine the actual concentration of an antimicrobial required to inhibit bacterial growth, dilution tests must be performed. Dilution susceptibility testing methods are used to determine the minimal concentration of an antimicrobial agent required to inhibit or kill a microorganism. Antimicrobial agents are usually tested at (twofold) serial dilutions, and the lowest concentration that inhibits visible growth of an organism is the MIC. The concentration range used may vary with the drug, the organism tested, and the site of the infection. The method and principles of the microdilution method are essentially the same as the macrodilution method, except that the antimicrobial dilutions are in 0.1-mL volumes contained in wells of a microdilution tray (usually 96-well trays). One should keep in mind that the size of the bacterial inoculum, concentration of cations in the medium, and other technical factors can influence the outcome of the test.

Broth (or agar) containing twofold dilutions of a drug is inoculated with a standardized bacterial inoculum, and the cultures are incubated at 35°C (95°F) for 18 to 24 hours. In general, an organism is considered to be susceptible when the achievable peak serum concentration is at least fourfold greater than the measured MIC.

If a patient is immunocompromised or has an infection that is difficult to treat (endocarditis), or if tolerance is suspected, the lowest concentration of antimicrobial required to kill a bacterium can be determined. This value is referred to as the *minimum bactericidal concentration* (MBC). To determine the MBC, a broth dilution system is used. Tubes containing a broth medium, a standard bacterial inoculum, and varying concentrations of an antimicrobial are incubated for 18 to 20 hours. Aliquots of broth from tubes with no visible growth (the first of which corresponds to the MIC) are subcultured onto agar medium containing no drugs. Expressed in micrograms per milliliter, the MBC is the concentration of antimicrobial that kills at least 99.9% of the original bacterial inoculum. Measuring the MBC might reveal the phenomenon in which normally microbicidal drugs, such as penicillins and cephalosporins, inhibit the growth of a bacterium but do not kill it. *Tolerance* has been defined on the basis of the ratio of MBC to MIC, and it is said to be present when the ratio is greater than 16 or 32 (NCCLS. Methods for Determining Bactericidal Activity of Antimicrobial Agents. NCCLS document M26-T. Wayne, Pa: National Committee for Clinical Laboratory Standards; 1992.). The exact clinical significance of tolerance is controversial.

Often combination antimicrobial therapy is used for serious infections. In vitro assays (the two-dimensional broth dilution method and the time–kill curve method) have been developed to quantify the bactericidal activity of combinations of antimicrobials. These tests are technically difficult and labor-intensive, and they should be considered only in selected circumstances.

Serum Bactericidal Test

In the treatment of a patient with bacterial endocarditis or osteomyelitis, it is often important to know whether the prescribed dosages of antibiotics are achieving blood levels sufficiently high to kill the causative organism. This test can be difficult to interpret. It may be technically demanding for many labs and should be reserved for selected adults with serious infections that fail to respond to therapy. The NCCLS (NCCLS. Methodology for the Serum Bactericidal Test. NCCLS document M21-T. Wayne, Pa: National Committee for Clinical Laboratory Standards; 1992) published a tentative guideline in 1992 pertaining to the serum bactericidal test, but as with the guideline pertaining to the measurement of bactericidal activity, no approved standard has been published, and the test is rarely available in routine diagnostic laboratories.

The bacteriostatic level is the dilution of serum that inhibits visible bacteria growth; the bactericidal level is the serum dilution that kills 99.9% of the initial inoculum. The serum bactericidal test is an assay that quantifies the killing ability of serum from an antimicrobial-treated patient. The dose, the time the dose was given, and the time of collection must be recorded accurately. The pre-dose blood specimen is drawn immediately before administering the next dose of antibiotic in order to evaluate the trough (pre) level. Blood for the post-dose (peak) level should be drawn 1 hour after an intravenous infusion has been started, 1 hour after an intramuscular dose has been given, and 1 to 2 hours after an oral dose. Twofold dilutions of the serum are made with culture medium (Mueller-Hinton broth with pooled human serum), and the mixtures are inoculated with the patient's bacterial isolate. The serum bactericidal titer is defined as the highest dilution at which more than 99% of the bacterial inoculum is killed. If performed, this test is usually used in patients who are failing appropriate therapy for endocarditis. The test also has been used in granulocytopenic or immunosuppressed patients who have gram-negative bacteremia and in patients whose therapy has been changed from the parenteral to the oral route, including children with acute osteomyelitis and IV drug users with endocarditis. In general, a peak titer of 1:8 or 1:16 or more is considered desirable. In this author's opinion, these tests are too tedious to be of pratical value.

Antifungal Susceptibility Testing

Broth microdilution susceptibility tests of *Candida* spp. have now been standardized by the NCCLS. The establishment of a standardized broth reference method for antifungal susceptibility testing of yeasts has opened the door to a number of interesting and useful developments. The adaptation of the reference macrodilution method to a microdilution method has significantly increased the clinical utility of antifungal susceptibility testing, and both methods are now included in the NCCLS document M27-A. The publication of quality control limits for five antifungal agents, coupled with the establishment of interpretive MIC breakpoints for three agents, provides useful parameters to survey clinical isolates of *Candida* and other yeast species. Adaptations of the M27 microdilution method for testing molds also has proved feasible. These developments have made it possible for a number of recent studies designed to expand the capabilities of laboratories to perform antifungal susceptibility testing and to enhance our understanding of trends in antifungal susceptibility.

Molecular Methods

For some organisms it is becoming more possible to consider the use of molecular methods to detect reliably antimicrobial resistance as opposed to using conventional methods. For *Staphylococcus aureus,* current breakpoints used in both MIC and disk testing correlate well with presence of the *mecA* (MRSA) gene. On the contrary, for coagulase-negative staphylococci, the current NCCLS MIC breakpoint fails to detect nearly 16% of *mecA*-containing organisms.

Genotypic-based methods hold promise for the rapid and accurate detection or confirmation of antimicrobial resistance; however, phenotypic methods will continue to have an advantage when resistance to the same antimicrobial agent may be caused by several different mechanisms. The diversity of genetic mechanisms may exceed the capabilities of current molecular technology. Genotypic assays have the ability to detect resistance but not susceptibility. Although results can be obtained rapidly, many molecular methods are labor intensive, expensive, and lack standardization. Clinical studies will be required to validate the genotypic approach to detection of antimicrobial resistance. Molecular assays also are at risk for false-positive results because of contamination of specimens by other specimens that carry the DNA targeted for the assay, or carryover of amplified target DNA (amplicons) from a previous polymerase chain reaction (PCR) assay during sample preparation. Detection of certain genetic resistance loci in clinical specimens must be interpreted with caution, because organisms in normal flora may also harbor the same loci. All these factors must be taken into consideration when introducing a genotypic method in the clinical laboratory. Other considerations include cost, turnaround time, and assay performance.

Early diagnosis of *Mycobacterium tuberculosis* disease is crucial in initiating treatment and interrupting the train of transmission. The increasing incidence of multidrug-resistant tuberculosis (MDR-TB) worldwide has placed emphasis on the need for early detection of drug resistance, particularly to isoniazid and rifampicin. Molecular diagnostic techniques and automated culture systems have reduced turnaround times in the modern mycobacteriology laboratory, and the continuing evaluation and development of such techniques is increasing the use of molecular technology in developed nations. Simple phenotypic methods for the detection of resistance to first-line drugs and genotypic kit-form assays for detection of rifampicin resistance have been developed that have become key tools in the containment of MDR-TB.

Antiviral Susceptibility Testing

Assays that detect antiretroviral drug resistance in HIV recently have become available to clinicians. Phenotypic assays measure the drug susceptibility of the virus by determining the concentration of drug that inhibits viral replication in tissue culture. Genotypic assays determine the presence of mutations that are known to confer decreased drug susceptibility. Although each type of assay has specific advantages, limitations associated with these tests often complicate the interpretation of results. Several retrospective clinical trials have suggested that resistance testing may be useful in the assessment of the success of salvage antiretroviral therapy. Prospective, controlled trials have demonstrated that resistance testing improves short-term virologic response. Resistance testing is currently recommended to help guide the choice of new drugs for patients after treatment has failed and for pregnant women. Resistance testing also should be considered for treatment-naïve patients, to detect transmission of resistant virus.

Concordance between phenotypic and genotypic susceptibility testing for HIV was 81% for nucleoside reverse transcriptase inhibitors, 91% for nonnucleoside reverse transcriptase inhibitors, and 90% for protease inhibitors. Phenotypic and genotypic susceptibility appears to provide similar results. However, interpretation of genotypic results can be complicated, and both methods still require clinical validation.

Drug-resistant cytomegalovirus (CMV) should be considered when viral shedding persists after several weeks of therapy. The problem is most likely to arise in the setting of a severely immunosuppressed host with continuing or relapsing disease. Not all treatment failure can be attributed to drug resistance. The testing of CMV isolates for drug resistance in cell culture is time consuming and labor intensive. However, recent advances in understanding of the genetics of resistance have resulted in rapid genotypic assays for specific mutations in the viral UL97 phosphotransferase or UL54 DNA polymerase genes that can predict resistance and cross-resistance to specific drugs. This information may help in the selection of alternative therapy.

Extended-Spectrum β-Lactamase Detection

Extended-spectrum β-lactamase (ESBL)-producing strains of *Klebsiella* spp. may be difficult to detect in the laboratory. Isolates of these species with MICs of 2 μg/mL or greater for cefpodoxime, ceftazidime, or aztreonam should be considered as possible ESBL producers. Initially, such organisms may appear to be susceptible to cefoxitin, but this agent should not be used for these organisms. The most sensitive single method for detecting ESBL production at present is susceptibility testing with cefpodoxime using a MIC breakpoint of 2 μg/mL or greater or a disk breakpoint of 22 mm or less as an indicator of possible ESBL production. Both the E test and double-disk potentiation methods are also useful to detect ESBL producers. In these assays, an ESBL producer is detected by virtue of its enhanced sensitivity to a test antibiotic, such as ceftazidime, in the presence of a β-lactamase inhibitor, such as clavulanate. The MICs to these agents should decrease when testing is done with any of these agents along with clavulanic acid.

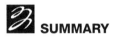 **SUMMARY**

Although the results of susceptibility assays are valuable in guiding antimicrobial therapy, they do not guarantee a response to treatment, and they cannot predict outcome. They should be viewed as an adjunct to—and not a substitute for—clinical judgement. Molecular methods will play an increasingly important role in this area. (JWM)

Bibliography

Barry AL, et al. Quality control limits for broth microdilution susceptibility tests of ten antifungal agents. *J Clin Microbiol* 2000;38:3457–3459.
   Broth microdilution susceptibility tests of Candida *spp. have now been standardized by the NCCLS.*
Ceri H, et al. The Calgary Biofilm Device: new technology for rapid determination of antibiotic susceptibilities of bacterial biofilms. *J Clin Microbiol* 1999;37:1771–1776.
   Minimal biofilm eradication concentrations, derived by using the Calgary Biofilm Device (CBD), demonstrated that for biofilms of the same organisms, 100 to 1,000 times the concentration of a certain antibiotic were often required for the antibiotic to be effective, whereas other antibiotics were found to be effective at the MICs. The CBD offers a new technology for the rational selection of antibiotics effective against microbial biofilms and for the screening of new effective antibiotic compounds.
Cormican MG, Marshall SA, Jones RN. Detection of extended-spectrum beta-lactamase (ESBL)-producing strains by Etest ESBL screen. *J Clin Microbiol* 1996;34:1880–1884.
   New testing approach to this difficult problem.
Chou S. Antiviral drug resistance in human cytomegalovirus. *Transpl Infect Dis* 1999;1:105–114.

Drug-resistant CMV should be considered when viral shedding persists after several weeks of therapy. The problem is most likely to arise in the setting of a severely immunosuppressed host with continuing or relapsing disease.

Dunne AL, et al. Comparison of genotyping and phenotyping methods for determining susceptibility of HIV-1 to antiretroviral drugs. *AIDS* 2001;15:1471–1475.

Phenotypic and genotypic susceptibility appears to provide similar results. However, interpretation of genotypic results can be complicated, and both methods still require clinical validation.

Ferraro MJ. Should we reevaluate antibiotic breakpoints? *Clin Infect Dis* 2001;33(suppl 3):S227–S229.

In the United States, the NCCLS has a mechanism in place to establish breakpoints initially and to review and publish updates on an annual basis. There should be a continued effort to coordinate both susceptibility testing methods and breakpoint determinations in various parts of the world.

Goessens WH, et al. Evaluation of the Vitek 2 system for susceptibility testing of Streptococcus pneumoniae isolates. *Eur J Clin Microbiol Infect Dis* 2000;19:618–622.

Vitek 2 (bioMerieux, France) is a new commercial system that allows rapid identification and rapid determination of the MIC of S. pneumoniae by monitoring the growth kinetics of the organisms in microwells. In conclusion, Vitek 2 shows good agreement with the reference method, as demonstrated by the low number of major errors, but it has a tendency to overestimate MICs, resulting in minor errors.

Hanna GJ, Caliendo AM. Testing for HIV-1 drug resistance. *Mol Diagn* 2001;6:253–263.

Resistance testing is currently recommended for patients who have virologic failure or no response to an antiretroviral regimen, and for pregnant women. Testing should also be considered in treatment-naive patients in areas of high prevalence of transmitted drug-resistant virus.

Hanna GJ, D'Aquila RT. Clinical use of genotypic and phenotypic drug resistance testing to monitor antiretroviral chemotherapy. *Clin Infect Dis* 2001;32:774–782.

Prospective, controlled trials have demonstrated that resistance testing improves short-term virologic response. Resistance testing is currently recommended to help guide the choice of new drugs for patients after treatment has failed and for pregnant women. Resistance testing also should be considered for treatment-naive patients, to detect transmission of resistant virus.

Kartsonis NA, D'Aquila RT. Clinical monitoring of HIV-1 infection in the ERA of antiretroviral resistance testing. *Infect Dis Clin North Am* 2000;14:879–899.

A practitioner's decision about when to initiate or change therapy in an HIV-infected patient should depend primarily on viral load results, and not on antiretroviral resistance test results. Moreover, resistance testing is no substitute for a thorough clinical and drug history.

King A. Recommendations for susceptibility tests on fastidious organisms and those requiring special handling. *J Antimicrob Chemother* 2001;48(suppl 1):77–80.

Fastidious organisms present problems in antimicrobial susceptibility testing related to particular cultural requirements or slow growth.

Louie M, Cockerill FR 3rd. Susceptibility testing. Phenotypic and genotypic tests for bacteria and mycobacteria. *Infect Dis Clin North Am* 2001;15:1205–1226.

Although results can be obtained rapidly, many molecular methods are labor intensive, expensive, and lack standardization. Clinical studies will be required to validate the genotypic approach to detection of antimicrobial resistance.

Olsson-Liljequist B, Nord CE. Methods for susceptibility testing of anaerobic bacteria. *Clin Infect Dis* 1994;18(suppl 4):S293–S296.

Susceptibility testing can be done by the dilution or diffusion methods, and the method chosen is dependent on the purpose of the assay. The agar dilution method is the NCCLS reference method and is well suited for surveillance studies. The broth microdilution method is recommended for routine susceptibility testing of anaerobes, but the E test, which has an antibiotic gradient and is used on agar plates, also seems to be useful for routine susceptibility testing of anaerobes.

Peterson LR, Shanholtzer CJ. Tests for bactericidal effects of antimicrobial agents: technical performance and clinical relevance. *Clin Microbiol Rev* 1992;5:420–432.

Bactericidal testing has been used for several decades as a guide for antimicrobial therapy of serious infections. In clinical laboratories, all bactericidal tests must be performed with rigorously standardized techniques and adequate controls, bearing in mind the limitations of the currently available test procedures.

Pfaller MA. Antifungal susceptibility testing: progress and future developments. *Braz J Infect Dis* 2000;4:55–60.

Incorporation of antifungal susceptibility testing methods into the clinical trials of new antifungal agents will facilitate the establishment of clinical correlates and further enhance the clinical utility of antifungal susceptibility testing.

Rosenblatt JE, Gustafson DR. Evaluation of the Etest for susceptibility testing of anaerobic bacteria. *Diagn Microbiol Infect Dis* 1995;22:279–284.

The E test is simple to perform and is a generally reliable method that is optimally read after 48 hours of incubation. It should be an acceptable alternative to the agar dilution standard, although results with certain organism-antimicrobial combinations should be read very conservatively because of the frequency of errors.

Sader HS, Pignatari AC. E test: a novel technique for antimicrobial susceptibility testing. *Rev Paul Med* 1994;112:635–638.

This report is based on the literature review of using the E test for susceptibility testing of the Xanthomonas maltophilia, S. pneumoniae, *and* S. viridans *group against eight different drugs.*

Wexler HM. Susceptibility testing of anaerobic bacteria—the state of the art. *Clin Infect Dis* 1993;16(suppl 4):S328–S333.

Demand for susceptibility testing of anaerobes has increased, but no consensus on procedure and interpretation has been achieved. The need for reliable methods for testing anaerobic bacteria extends from small hospital laboratories to large research centers.

Wilson JW, Bean P. A physician's primer to antiretroviral drug resistance testing. *AIDS Read* 2000;10:469–473, 476–478.

Genotypic assays identify specific "gene mutations" or nucleotide substitutions known to confer drug resistance, whereas phenotypic assays measure the amount of drug necessary to inhibit viral replication in vitro.

Woods GL. In vitro testing of antimicrobial agents. *Infect Dis Clin North Am* 1995;9:463–481.

With the exception of detecting high-level aminoglycoside resistance in enterococci as a means to predict synergism between these drugs and cell wall-active agents, the clinical relevance of assessing synergism is not well documented.

Woods GL, Witebsky FG. Susceptibility testing of Mycobacterium avium complex in clinical laboratories. Results of a questionnaire and proficiency test performance by participants in the College of American Pathologists Mycobacteriology E Survey. *Arch Pathol Lab Med* 1996;120:436–439.

Given the obvious interest in Mycobacterium avium *complex (MAC) susceptibility testing, standardized methodology that demonstrates interlaboratory reproducibility and, optimally, shows some correlation with clinical outcome is needed. Moreover, recommendations concerning indications for performing the test would be useful.*

Yao JD, et al. Comparison of E test and agar dilution for antimicrobial susceptibility testing of Stenotrophomonas (Xanthomonas) maltophilia. *J Clin Microbiol* 1995;33:1428–1430.

For most antimicrobial agents tested against S. maltophilia, *the E test is an acceptable alternative susceptibility test method.*

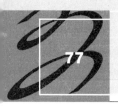

TREATMENT AND PREVENTION OF INFLUENZA

77

*I*nfluenza virus causes a common acute respiratory illness that may affect up to 20% of the population annually. Influenza-related illness is a major cause of loss of productivity. It accounts for more than 200,000 hospitalizations and is associated with about 20,000 deaths yearly in the United States. Although all age groups are susceptible to infection, those at the extremes of life or with chronic medical conditions are at greatest risk for complications and death.

VIRAL CHARACTERISTICS

Four influenza viruses, A, B, C, and D have been identified; only influenza viruses A and B are clinically relevant. All are members of the Orthomyxoviridae family. Influenza A virus infects several species of birds and other mammals, whereas influenza B virus only infects humans. However, transmission in people occurs only through direct person-to-person contact with aerosol droplets generated by sneezing or coughing.

Influenza viruses A and B are morphologically similar and possess two types of surface proteins: hemagglutinins (HA) and neuraminidases (NA). HAs represent binding sites for host respiratory tract cells. Once attached, the virus undergoes changes that permit replication. NA permits viral penetration and spread among these cells.

Influenza A viruses are divided into subclasses based on their HA and NA antigens. Generally, two influenza A subtypes circulate internationally; currently these are H1N1 and H3N2. Influenza vaccines are trivalent, containing these two subtypes as well as an influenza B strain.

The greatest indicator of virulence after infection has occurred is the level of preexisting host immunity. Thus *morbidity*, related to the acute infection, is highest in infants and children with naïve immune systems, but *mortality*, resulting from complications of influenza infection, is greatest among older persons, those with chronic medical conditions, and pregnant women. The introduction of new subtypes ("antigen shift") of influenza viruses leads to greater virulence among all ages. Because antibodies produced after exposure to influenza virus are anti-HA antibodies, HA mutations may render host antibodies inadequate in controlling subsequent influenza virus infection. Alternatively, "antigenic shift" represents a more profound phenomenon in which a novel influenza virus is formed that may be unaffected by preexisting immunity. Both influenza A and B may undergo antigenic shift, but only influenza A virus is capable of antigenic shift. Thus, only influenza A can cause pandemics such as those seen 1918, 1957, and 1977.

CLINICAL MANIFESTATIONS

Influenza A and B infection most commonly occur between December and May with similar, often severe, systemic manifestations and tracheobronchitis. After exposure, there is an asymptomatic incubation period lasting several days, followed by abrupt onset of fever, chills, cough, myalgias, headache, and malaise. Table 77-1 summarizes these. Fever usually resolves within 3 days, but cough and malaise may persist for weeks. High fevers, cervical lymph node enlargement, and croup are more common in children than in adults. Older

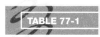

Symptom	Incidence
Sudden onset	75%
Headache	58%
Fever	51%
Cough	48%
Sore throat	46%
Myalgia	39%
Chills	37%

TABLE 77-1 Symptoms of Influenza Illness

patients may report atypically with minimal respiratory symptoms and high fever, lethargy, and confusion.

DIAGNOSIS

Influenza may be diagnosed clinically when appropriate symptoms are present during influenza season. In particular, individuals with two respiratory symptoms plus fever and myalgias, in the setting of an outbreak, likely have influenza. Alternatively, the presence of major rash or diarrhea likely represents other diagnoses. Infections that may appear similarly to viral influenza include respiratory syncytial virus (RSV) and adenovirus, among others.

If diagnosis of viral influenza is insecure, several methods for laboratory confirmation are available. Because treatment for influenza is effective only if started within 2 days of symptoms, enzyme-linked immunosorbent assays (ELISA) of nasopharyngeal secretions, which have an assay time of minutes, are most commonly used and can be used for both influenza A and B. However, cost-effectiveness analysis has demonstrated that for unvaccinated or high-risk ambulatory adults older than age 75 who report during influenza season, empiric treatment (without testing) is most cost effective. Those hospitalized with respiratory illness during influenza season should be tested, not only to guide therapy and provide diagnostic and prognostic information, but also to help control the spread of infection in the hospital. In nursing homes, residents with signs and symptoms of influenza should be tested for similar reasons, but also to determine if chemoprophylaxis of other residents is warranted. Viral culture and acute/chronic serologic testing also is available.

COMPLICATIONS

Primary viral pneumonia is most common in older adults or in persons with preexisting cardiac or pulmonary disease. It typically appears shortly after onset of influenza symptoms, with rapid progression of fever, tachypnea, tachycardia, hypoxia, and, occasionally, hypotension. Mortality is high and survivors may develop pulmonary fibrosis.

Secondary bacterial pneumonia also is more common among older persons and those with chronic pulmonary disease. Patients have typical influenza symptoms, often demonstrate modest clinical improvement, and then relapse with recurrence of fever, productive cough, and, occasionally, pleurisy. Bacteria most commonly associated with secondary pneumonia are *Streptococcus pneumoniae, Haemophilus influenzae, and Staphylococcus aureus.* This is one of the few instances when *S. aureus* should be clinically suspected as an etiology of community-acquired pneumonia. Methicillin-resistant *S. aureus* (MRSA) may be noted in this circumstance. Heart failure is a common complication of influenza infection in older adults with preexisting heart disease. Those with coronary heart disease also are at risk of myocardial infarction in the setting of primary viral pneumonia. Less commonly reported sequelae include myocarditis and pericarditis.

In children, croup may present with dry cough and stridor. Both influenza A and B may cause this complication, but the former is associated with more severe illness. Otitis media and seizures (resulting from high fever) also may complicate viral influenza in children. Encephalitis is noted uncommonly in both children and adults and typically occurs during the acute phase of illness with irritability, and confusion delirium. It has a high mortality rate.

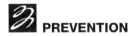

PREVENTION

Because influenza viral infection is spread by direct person-to-person contact with aerosol droplets generated by sneezing or coughing, its spread may be limited by practicing good "respiratory hygiene," such as sneezing/coughing into a tissue and then discarding it safely. Frequent hand washing with soap and water or with an alcohol-based hand cleaner also may reduce the number of individuals exposed to this virus.

Influenza vaccination is highly effective in preventing influenza illness and its complications and represents a standard of care. It should be administered prior to "flu season" and may prevent illness in 70 to 100% of healthy adults. Efficacy is lower in young children and in adults older than age 65 (30–60%). In nursing home populations, approximately 50% of those vaccinated may mount an adequate antibody response to the vaccine. However, it may still prove effective in preventing complications. In healthy working adults, vaccination reduces disease incidence, number of physician visits, and absenteeism. Despite the proven benefits of the vaccine, at least 33% of those older than age 65 and more than 50% of younger persons with indications for vaccination remain unvaccinated each year.

Healthcare providers represent an important group for vaccination consideration. In addition to decreasing absenteeism and hospitalizations, influenza vaccination of this population in chronic care facilities has been associated with decreased influenza-related morbidity and mortality among residents. However fewer than 50% of long-term care staff are vaccinated against influenza.

Currently, influenza vaccine is available in two forms: the intramuscular vaccine (Fluzone® and Fluvirin®) is trivalent, inactivated, prepared in eggs, and more commonly used. It currently contains three viral strains: influenza A subtypes H1N1 and H3N2, and one type B influenza strain. The annual determination of its exact components is made by the Food and Drug Administration (FDA), based on "best information" about strains most likely to be circulating. A single intramuscular dose is effective for most individuals. However; children younger than age 9 require two doses of vaccine if not vaccinated previously. The cost is less than $7 per dose.

An intranasal spray (FluMist®) represents a trivalent, live attenuated vaccine approved by the FDA in 2003 for use in healthy persons ages 5 to 49. Administration provides 96% protection in this group, and it may prove more acceptable for some individuals. At this time, it is not recommended for children younger than age 5, adults older than age 50, or persons with chronic medical conditions. It is also much more expensive than the intramuscular vaccine. Table 77-2 provides information regarding individuals at increased risk for influenza and its complications, and who should be vaccinated annually.

During the second half of 2004, the United States experienced an acute vaccine shortage that resulted in availability of only about 50% of the anticipated allotment of 100 million doses. As a result, the Centers for Disease Control and Prevention (CDC) Advisory Committee for Immunization Practices (ACIP) issued interim recommendations for vaccine use. These are summarized as follows:

Children ages 6 to 23 months
Adults age 75 and older
Individuals ages 2 to 74 with underlying chronic medical conditions
Females who will be pregnant during the influenza season
Nursing home residents
Children ages 6 months to 18 years on chronic aspirin therapy

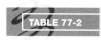

TABLE 77-2	Candidates for Annual Influenza Vaccine

Adults older than age 50
Children ages 6–24 months
Individuals older than 24 months with underlying chronic medical conditions
Children and teenagers who receive long-term aspirin therapy and may be at risk for developing Reye's syndrome
Nursing home residents
All healthcare workers including home care providers
Females who will be pregnant during influenza season and during second or third trimester if not vaccinated before conception.
Household contacts of children ages 2–6 months
Household members of persons in a high-risk group

Healthcare workers involved in direct patient care
Out-of-home caregivers and household contacts of children younger than age 6 months

Additionally, the CDC suggested that healthy adults ages 5 to 49 in the priority group above, who were not pregnant, receive the intranasal vaccine in lieu of the intramuscular form. The CDC also requested that all other individuals forego vaccination during the shortage. Future attempts to deal with this issue will include (1) inclusion of other companies to produce and distribute influenza vaccine in the United States, (2) development of novel technologies to produce and develop influenza vaccine in a more streamlined fashion, and (3) generation of data to prove that smaller doses of vaccine, perhaps administered intradermally, will provide adequate protection. This has recently been demonstrated in healthy individuals.

SIDE EFFECTS AND CONTRAINDICATIONS TO VACCINATION

Influenza vaccine is well tolerated and its side effects are usually minimal. With the intramuscular form, mild soreness at the injection site is the single most common reaction. The intranasal vaccine is associated with a mild upper respiratory illness in less than 15% of those who receive it. Because the viral strains are grown in chick embryos, an anaphylactic reaction to eggs is an absolute contraindication to the influenza vaccine. Inactivated influenza vaccine has been rarely associated with Guillain-Barré syndrome; thus the influenza vaccine should be avoided in individuals with a previous history of acute inflammatory polyneuropathy within 6 weeks of influenza vaccination. It also should be avoided in anyone with an acute febrile illness, children younger than age 6 months, and in pregnant women during the first trimester.

ANTIVIRAL CHEMOPROPHYLAXIS

Although vaccination is the preferred preventive strategy for influenza infection, use of antiviral agents in unvaccinated individuals or selected vaccinated groups at high risk of influenza during an outbreak is an alternative strategy (see Table 77-3). Amantadine (Symmetrel®), rimantadine (Flumadine®), and oseltamivir (Tamiflu®) represent antivirals approved for viral influenza prevention. Zanamivir (Relenza®) is available for treatment but not prevention, although it has been studied for this. Pharmacology of these agents is reviewed below (see "Treatment").

Amantadine and rimantadine are only effective in preventing influenza A infection. Their efficacy is comparable to that of the vaccine; preventing half of influenza infections and 70 to 90% of clinical disease. Oseltamivir has similar efficacy, but has the advantage of being active against both influenza A and B. For persons deemed candidates for influenza prevention but who cannot be vaccinated, antiviral chemoprophylaxis is begun at the

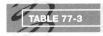

TABLE 77-3   Indications for Antiviral Chemoprophylaxis

High risk individuals vaccinated for the first time after influenza is circulating
Previously vaccinated older individuals exposed to an outbreak
Immune deficiency
Children younger than age 9 receiving the vaccine for the first time
Unvaccinated care providers of high risk individuals

onset of flu season and continues for 4 to 6 weeks during the season at risk. Those who have been vaccinated but are at high risk for influenza illness should be considered for prophylaxis during a period of presumed exposure. Chemoprophylaxis does allow for subclinical infection that induces an antibody response to current circulating influenza virus.

TREATMENT

Treatment of influenza includes specific antiviral therapy plus supportive measures. Four FDA-approved agents for the treatment of influenza exist and are summarized in Table 77-4. If administered within the first 48 hours of illness, they are effective in reducing the duration of symptoms by up to 2.5 days.

Amantadine and rimantadine are chemically related and possess activity against influenza A virus only. They are given orally, are well absorbed, and have relatively long half-lives that allow for once- or twice-daily administration. Because amantadine has a 50% higher peak plasma concentration, longer half-life in older adults, and is predominantly excreted in the kidneys, dose reduction is required in this population and in those with renal insufficiency.

Influenza viruses may develop resistance to these agents, which can be noted in up to 33% of persons. To reduce the emergence of resistant viruses, these drugs should be discontinued as soon as clinically warranted, typically after 3 to 5 days of treatment or within 24 to 48 hours after the disappearance of signs and symptoms.

Because amantadine (but not rimantadine) stimulates release of catecholamines, it may be associated with mild central nervous system side effects in 10% of those treated. These include jitters, insomnia, anxiety, and difficulty with concentration. Serious side effects that can include seizures and delirium are associated with high plasma drug concentrations. Both agents may cause nausea and vomiting.

The newer neuraminidase inhibitors, zanamivir and oseltamivir, were approved for treatment of both influenza A and influenza B. They possess a side-effect profile more favorable than the older agents, and influenza viruses are much less likely to develop drug resistance to them. Zanamivir is a powder given by aerosol inhalation by mouth; only 15% of the inhaled drug reaches the lungs. A significant amount of manual dexterity is required to administer this agent and it may not be appropriate for very frail

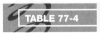

TABLE 77-4   Antiviral Drugs for Influenza

Antiviral drug	Approved ages	Daily Dose (children)	Daily dose (adults)	Daily dose (elderly)
Amantadine	≥ 1 yr.	5 mg/kg	200 mg	100 mg
Rimantadine	≥ 1 yr (prophylaxis) ≥ 18 yr. (treatment)	5 mg/kg	200 mg	100 mg
Zanamivir	≥ 7 yr	20 mg	20 mg	20 mg
Oseltamivir	≥ 18 yr.		150 mg	150 mg

older patients. It also can cause bronchospasm and a decline in respiratory function in patients with asthma or chronic obstructive pulmonary disease. Oseltamivir is a pill administered twice daily; dosage is reduced in patients with creatinine clearance less than 30 mL/min. It can rarely be associated with severe nausea or vomiting. Duration of therapy with either agent is 5 days. Resistance is much less likely than with amantadine and rimantadine.

Supportive treatment for influenza includes adequate hydration and rest during the acute illness and treatment of fever, headache, and myalgias in some individuals. Acetaminophen is a good agent for this. Aspirin should generally be avoided because of concern about inducing Reye's syndrome. Cough suppressants also may be used if this is particularly troublesome. (RBB)

Bibliography

Golden MP, Sajjad Z, Elgart L. Influenza and human immunodeficiency virus infection: absence of HIV progression after acute influenza infection. *Clin Infect Dis* 2001;32: 1366–1370.
A small number of patients with HIV were identified as having viral influenza during the 1998–1999 season. Most were infected with influenza A. None of this small number developed opportunistic infection or had unusual changes in the CD4 counts or viral load. The authors conclude that viral influenza had no important impact on their patients with HIV.

Gravenstein S, Davidson E. Current strategies for management of influenza in the elderly population. *Clin Infect Dis* 2002;35:729–737.
The authors present an excellent summary of strategies to deal with viral influenza in older patients. Vaccination represents the cornerstone of prevention and is the most cost-effective strategy. But other strategies include carefully chosen chemoprophylaxis, surveillance, and education.

The Medical Letter. Antiviral drugs for prophylaxis and treatment of influenza. 2004;46:85–87.
The writers provide a succinct overview of the four medications available for treatment and prophylaxis. They note that zanamivir is FDA-approved only for therapy, although they provide dosing for prevention as well. A "pearl" provided is that efficacy of the live-virus vaccine may be interfered with by use of antiviral medications. These should be discontinued at least 48 hours before use of Flumist[R] and not started for at least 14 days after live virus vaccination. The two neuraminidase inhibitors also may have activity against avian flu.

Interim influenza recommendations, 2004–2005 influenza season. *MMWR Morb Mortal Wkly Rep* 2004;53:1–2.
Because of the influenza vaccine shortage associated with contaminated batches of vaccine from a production plant in England, the CDC issued interim recommendations to provide vaccine to those most at need. The highest priority groups were identified, and persons at lower risk were implored not to ask for vaccine.

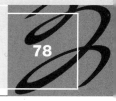
*A*IDS was first recognized in 1981 and its causative agent, now known as HIV type 1 (HIV-1), was identified in 1983. In the two decades since, the worldwide toll of AIDS-related morbidity and mortality has been devastating. Forty million people are living with HIV infection: 37 million adults and 2.5 million children younger than age 15. An estimated 5 million people acquired HIV infection in 2003, including 4.2 million adults and 700,000 children. AIDS caused the deaths of an estimated 3 million people in 2003, including 2.5 million adults and 500,000 children. UNAIDS has estimated that by 2010, 106 million children will have lost one or both parents, with 25 million of this group orphaned because of AIDS.

In the United States, the accumulated number of AIDS cases from the beginning of the epidemic through 2002 is estimated to be 886,575. The estimated number of deaths from AIDS is 501,669, including 496,354 adults and adolescents and 5,315 children younger than age 15.

Eighty-two percent of AIDS cases reported through 2002 in the United States occurred in males and 18% in females. Adult and adolescent AIDS cases totaled 877,275. Thirty-nine percent of these cases occurred in persons ages 39 to 44 and another 34% occurred in persons ages 25 to 34; 9,300 AIDS cases occurred in children younger than age 13. Among reported AIDS cases, 41% occurred in white (non-Hispanic) persons, 39% in black (non-Hispanic) persons, and 18% in Hispanics. The risk factors for acquiring AIDS in the reported cases include: male-to-male sexual transmission, 48%; injection drug use, 27.4% (19.6% in males and 7.7% in females); combined male-to-male sexual contact and injection drug use, 6.8%; heterosexual contact, 15.5% (5.8% in males and 9.7% in females); and other factors (hemophilia, blood transfusion, and perinatal transmission), 2.4%. The nationwide distribution of reported AIDS cases is uneven, with the highest rates reported in New York, California, Florida, Texas, and New Jersey.

The number of new AIDS diagnoses increased from 1990 through 1992, followed by a decline from 1993 through 1999. The annual number of deaths among persons with AIDS increased steadily until 1994, was constant during 1994 and 1995, declined significantly during 1996 and 1997, and was constant during 1998 and 1999. The declines in AIDS diagnoses and deaths since 1995 were caused primarily by the slower progression of HIV-associated immune deficiency among persons who used highly active antiretroviral therapy (HAART). Therefore, current trends in AIDS incidence and mortality indicate the success of the secondary prevention of severe disease and death in persons living with HIV, and not in behavior change that prevented the primary acquisition of HIV infection. HIV transmission continues to spread among men who have sex with men, intravenous drug users, and by heterosexual contact.

 ## SEXUAL TRANSMISSION

Sexual transmission accounts for 70% of cases of HIV infection in the United States, mostly male-to-male sexual contact, and 85% of cases in developing countries, mostly heterosexual contact. The probability of transmission ranges from 0.03 to 0.0003 per contact. The wide range is attributable to both the imprecision of the epidemiologic studies and the many cofactors that affect transmission, such as host susceptibility factors, host and virus infectiousness factors, the viral dose, and whether exposure is into the blood or onto mucus membranes. HIV infection and other sexually transmitted infections (STIs) are more easily transmitted from men to women than from women to men, with the male-to-female efficiency approximately four times greater than female-to-male transmission.

Among the host factors that affect the risk of sexual transmission, cervical ectopy has been shown in some but not all studies to increase the relative risk of HIV acquisition from 1.7 to 5.0. Lack of male circumcision is more consistently shown to affect transmission risk. Langerhans cells, abundantly present in the foreskin, may explain why the relative risk of transmission may be as high as eight times the risk in circumcised men. Certain host genetics, a mutation in the chemokine-receptor gene, explain how some sex workers and homosexual men remained uninfected despite repeated sexual contact with HIV-infected partners. Persons with homozygous mutation of the CKR5 gene appear to be resistant to infection. The prevalences of these mutations are inexplicably varied by race, with homozygosity found in 11% of whites but only 1.7% of blacks. Menstruation may increase the risk of acquiring HIV infection by 1.5 times. Bleeding during sexual intercourse appears to increase the odds of transmission by as much as 4.9 times. Finally, pregnancy itself has been found to increase the likelihood of viral presence in genital fluids.

STIs, especially ulcerative diseases such as chancroid, syphilis, and genital herpes simplex virus infection, raise the transmission risk by creating a portal of infection as well as a local accumulation of inflammatory cells that bind HIV infection. Transmission is also known to increase with noninfectious causes of genital tract inflammation, such as traumatic sexual intercourse and douching. Viral concentration in genital secretions may be the reason that infectiousness is increased in patients with late-stage disease and in primary HIV infection and decreased in patients on HAART. Furthermore, the various HIV subtypes or clades may differ in their tropism for Langerhans cells. Finally, HIV isolates from blood and genital secretions appear to differ phenotypically with respect to the efficiency of transmission.

Prevention of Sexual Transmission

Strategies to prevent sexual transmission of HIV infection include increasing the use of condoms and reducing unsafe sexual behavior, treatment of STIs, and increasing the use of antiretroviral therapy (ARV) to reduce the concentration of HIV in genital secretions. Behavioral interventions, for the most part, have focused on either heterosexual men, men who have sex with men, or intravenous drug users. Most studies of behavioral interventions to reduce unsafe sexual practices have methodologic weaknesses that prevent generally conclusive statements on effectiveness. An evidence-based review by Elwy and colleagues of interventions intended to prevent heterosexual transmission among men found a mixture of successful and unsuccessful programs. The successful interventions were carried out in the workplace, in the military, or in STI clinics. A variety of methods were used, including workplace counseling and HIV testing, a multiple-sector mass communication program in Thailand, and motivation and skills-building programs in STI clinics (only some of which were found to be effective).

For HIV infection, unlike other STIs, a number of carefully conducted studies using rigorous methods and measures have demonstrated that consistent latex condom use is a highly effective means of preventing HIV transmission. Epidemiologic studies conducted in real-life settings, in which one partner is infected with HIV and the other partner is not, demonstrate conclusively that the consistent use of latex condoms provides a high degree of protection. Another type of epidemiologic study involves examination of STI rates in populations rather than individuals. Such studies have demonstrated that when condom use increases within population groups, rates of STIs decline in these groups. Other studies have examined the relationship between condom use and the complications of STIs. For example, condom use has been associated with a decreased risk of cervical cancer, a human papillomavirus-associated disease. Although consistent use of HAART decreases viral concentrations in genital tract secretions and decreases transmission, instances of unsafe sexual practices among treated persons are a reminder that medical interventions must be coupled with behavioral interventions that promote safer sexual behavior.

Despite the evidence for the effectiveness of condoms in preventing the sexual transmission of HIV infection, recent doubts have been raised in the public media. An extensive review of available studies was conducted in June 2000 by a panel convened by National Institutes of Health (NIH), the Centers for Disease Control and Prevention (CDC), and the World Health Organization (WHO). The review concluded that condoms, when used correctly and consistently, are effective for preventing HIV infection in women and men and gonorrhea in men. The available data on other STIs, however, are less complete. In news items after the release of the review, there appear to have been a misunderstandings about the difference between "lack of evidence of effectiveness" and a "lack of effectiveness." Many reasons exist for the current lack of evidence. Studies to establish the effectiveness of condoms against specific STIs are difficult to conduct in an ethical and scientifically valid manner. Nonetheless, additional studies are currently under way. Until these or other studies providing additional reliable evidence can be completed, the effectiveness of condoms against some specific STIs will remain a matter of debate.

Because of the difficulties many women face negotiating the use of male condoms, the female condom is an important additional option to assist women in protecting themselves and their partners from both unwanted pregnancy and STIs. The female condom is a strong, soft, transparent polyurethane sheath inserted in the vagina before sexual intercourse, providing protection against both pregnancy and STI. It forms a barrier between the penis and the vagina, cervix and external genitalia. It is stronger than latex, causes no allergic reactions, and, unlike latex, may be used with both oil-based and water-based lubricants. It has no known side effects or risks. It can be inserted prior to intercourse, is not dependent on the male erection, and does not require immediate withdrawal after ejaculation.

 ## INJECTION DRUG USERS

Parenteral transmission, including drug injection, percutaneous occupational exposure, and receipt of infected blood, blood products, organs or tissues, is the most efficient way HIV is transmitted. The proportion of HIV/AIDS cases caused by exposure to infected blood other than illicit drug injection has declined dramatically since the mid-1980s when donor exclusion criteria were implemented, HIV diagnostic testing became available, and screening began of blood for transfusion.

Prevention of Injection Drug User Transmission

People who inject drugs should be regularly counseled to stop using and injecting drugs and should enter and complete substance abuse treatment. For those who cannot or will not stop injecting drugs, the following steps may be taken to reduce personal and public health risks. Never reuse or share syringes, water, or drug preparation equipment. Only use syringes obtained from a reliable source, such as pharmacies or needle exchange programs. Use a new, sterile syringe each time to prepare and inject drugs. If possible, use sterile water to prepare drugs; otherwise, use clean water from a reliable source, such as fresh tap water. Use a new or disinfected container ("cooker") and a new filter ("cotton") to prepare drugs. Clean the injection site with a new alcohol swab prior to injection. Safely dispose of syringes after one use.

 ## PERINATAL TRANSMISSION

Transmission of HIV from an infected mother can occur during pregnancy, during labor, or after delivery through breast milk. Most perinatal transmission occurs close to the time of or during childbirth. In the absence of any intervention, an estimated 15 to 30% of mothers with HIV infection will transmit the infection during pregnancy and delivery, and 10 to 20% through breast milk. HIV transmission from mother to child during pregnancy, labor, and delivery or by breast-feeding has accounted for 91% of all AIDS cases reported among

U.S. children. The past decade has witnessed a dramatic decline in mother-to-child HIV transmission (MTCT), as a result of intensive efforts to identify infected pregnant women to offer them ARV prophylaxis.

Before perinatal preventive treatments became available in the early 1990s an estimated 1,000 to 2,000 infants were born with HIV infection each year in the United States, with a high of 2,500 infants born in 1992. The number of HIV-infected infants born in 2000 is estimated to be 280 to 370. These declines reflect the widespread success of U.S. Public Health Service recommendations made for counseling and testing pregnant women for HIV, and for offering ARV therapy to infected women during pregnancy and delivery and for the infant after birth.

Prevention of Perinatal Transmission

The best ways to prevent infection in children are to prevent infection in women and to encourage early prenatal care, which includes HIV counseling and testing. In 1994, the Pediatric AIDS Clinical Trials Group Protocol 076 demonstrated that a three-part regimen of zidovudine could reduce MCTC by nearly 70%. The three-part regimen is oral zidovudine initiated at 14 to 34 weeks of gestation and continued throughout pregnancy, intravenous zidovudine during labor until delivery, and oral zidovudine for the first 6 weeks of the newborn's life. After release of the results of the study, zidovudine prophylaxis became a recommended standard of care, and in 1995 the U.S. Public Health Service recommended universal prenatal HIV counseling and voluntary testing. Since then, other studies have confirmed the effect of zidovudine, zidovudine plus lamivudine, and nevirapine in reducing MTCT. Today, even more aggressive ARV therapy is recommended to maximally suppress viral replication, both for the health of the mother as well as for the prevention of transmission to the child. Pregnancy is no longer considered to be a reason to defer HIV treatment.

Recommendations regarding the use of ARV therapy for pregnant women are subject to the unique considerations of the effect of changes in physiology that may affect dosing, the potential effect of the drugs on the woman, and the potential short- and long-term effects on the fetus and the newborn. Although data are uncertain, there may be an association of combination ARV on preterm birth. Pregnancy may increase the likelihood of ARV drug toxicity.

For HIV-infected pregnant women who have not received prior ARV therapy, the recommendations for initiation and choice of therapy are based on the same considerations used for persons who are not pregnant, and the risks and benefits must be considered and discussed. At the very least, the three-part zidovudine regimen should be recommended for all pregnant women. A combination of the three-part zidovudine regimen plus additional ARV drugs is recommended if the clinical status indicates a requirement for treatment or the HIV viral concentration is greater than 1,000 copies per milliliter. Women in the first trimester of pregnancy may consider delaying initiation of therapy until after 10 to 12 weeks' gestation.

HIV-infected pregnant women already receiving ARV therapy are recommended to continue it and to consider the three-part zidovudine regimen as part of the chemoprophylaxis. HIV-infected women in labor who have not had prior therapy have several options: the intrapartum and postpartum zidovudine components of the three-part regimen; zidovudine plus lamivudine during labor and for the newborn for 1 week; a single dose of nevirapine at the onset of labor and a single dose for the newborn at age 48 hours; and the two-dose nevirapine regimen combined with the intrapartum and postpartum zidovudine components of the three-part regimen. Infants born to HIV-infected mothers who have received no ARV should receive the postpartum component of the three-part zidovudine regimen. Some clinicians choose to administer zidovudine in combination with other ARV drugs to the newborns of mothers suspected of having zidovudine-resistant virus.

Cohort studies performed prior to the availability of plasma HIV RNA titer (viral load) testing and before the recommendation for HAART showed that cesarean delivery performed before the onset of labor or the rupture of membranes was associated with a reduction of MTCT rates of 55 to 80%, regardless of whether the pregnant woman received zidovudine. A randomized trial of mode of delivery found that elective cesarean delivery was associated with a 1.8% MTCT rate. Nonelective cesarean delivery performed after the onset of labor or the rupture of membranes was not associated with a decrease in transmission rate. The magnitude of benefit and the benefit-to-risk ratio of elective cesarean delivery for women who are taking HAART and who have fully suppressed viral replication are uncertain. The U.S. Public Health Service and the American College of Obstetrics and Gynecologists' Committee on Obstetric Practice have issued guidelines concerning the role of elective cesarean delivery for HIV-infected women with viral concentrations greater than 1,000 copies per milliliter.

 ## OCCUPATIONAL TRANSMISSION

Percutaneous needlestick exposure by a healthcare worker (HCW) to HIV-infected blood or body secretions is an uncommon cause of HIV transmission. Through December 2001, the Centers for Disease Control and Prevention reported 57 documented cases and an additional 138 "possible cases" of HIV seroconversion among HCWs after occupational exposure. Nevertheless, each needlestick exposure is an urgent health issue for both the exposed person and their physician in the workplace, the emergency department or the acute care setting. There are an estimated 380,000 needlestick injuries in U.S. hospitals each year and an unknown number of needlestick injuries in other healthcare settings.

The risk of infection after percutaneous needlestick exposure to HIV-infected blood is approximately 0.3% (95% confidence interval [CI], 0.2–0.5%). Retrospective studies indicate that the risk of transmission is increased when the needle was visibly contaminated with blood, when the needle had been inserted into a vein or artery, when the needlestick caused a deep injury, or when the source patient died within 2 months. A laboratory study indicates that more blood is transferred with deep injuries and injuries with hollow-bore needles rather than suture needles. The risk may be greater after exposure to source patients with high HIV viral load levels, but this is not proven. Transmission has been documented from source patients with undetectable viral load. The risk after mucous membrane exposure is about 0.09% (95% CI, 0.006–0.5%). The risk after exposure of nonintact skin and the risk after exposure to HIV-infected fluids other than blood or bloody fluids is far less and too low to be estimated. Transmission has not been documented after exposure to intact skin.

Prevention of Occupational Transmission

The rationale for postexposure prophylaxis (PEP) is based on uncertain but plausible assumptions about the pathogenesis of early HIV infection, the effect of prophylaxis on preventing infection, and the relative risks and benefits of various regimens. Animal studies demonstrate that tenofovir prevented simian immunodeficiency virus infection if given up to 24 hours after exposure, but resulted in incomplete protection if given 48 to 72 hours after exposure.

A case-control study of exposed HCWs found that zidovudine PEP reduced the transmission risk by 81% (95% CI, 43–94%). Nevertheless, 21 cases of the failure of PEP to prevent infection have been documented, including three cases of failure of triple-drug regimens. ARV resistance testing of source cases suggests that in some of these cases, the transmitted virus was found to have decreased susceptibility to zidovudine or other drugs used for PEP.

U.S. Public Health Service guidelines recommend that a basic 4-week regimen of two drugs (zidovudine and lamivudine, stavudine and lamivudine, or stavudine and didanosine) be started as soon as possible after most cases of HIV percutaneous exposure (Table 78-1). The recommendations for exposure through mucus membrane routes are similar. If the HIV status of the source patient is unknown, voluntary testing with a rapid HIV test can

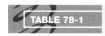

TABLE 78-1 Recommended HIV Postexposure Prophylaxis for Percutaneous Injuries

	Infection status of source				
Exposure type	HIV-positive class 1*	HIV-positive class 2*	Source of unknown HIV status[†]	Unknown source[§]	HIV-negative
Less severe[¶]	Recommend basic two-drug PEP	Recommend expanded three-drug PEP	Generally, no PEP warranted; however, consider basic two-drug PEP[‡] for source with HIV risk factors[††]	Generally, no PEP warranted; however, consider basic two-drug PEP[‡] in settings where exposure to HIV-infected persons is likely	No PEP warranted
More severe[§§]	Recommend expanded three-drug PEP	Recommend expanded three-drug PEP	Generally, no PEP warranted; however, consider basic two-drug PEP[‡] for source with HIV risk factors[††]	Generally, no PEP warranted; however, consider basic two-drug PEP[‡] in settings where exposure to HIV-infected persons is likely	No PEP warranted

*HIV Positive Class 1—asymptomatic HIV infection or known low viral load (e.g., < 1,500 RNA copies/mL). HIV Positive Class 2—symptomatic HIV infection, AIDS acute seroconversion, or known high viral load. If drug resistance is a concern, obtain expert consultation. Initiation of PEP should not be delayed pending expert consultation, and, because expert consultation cannot substitute for face-to-face counseling, resources should be available to provide immediate evaluation and follow-up care for all exposures.
[†] Source of unknown HIV status (e.g., deceased source person with no samples available for HIV testing).
[‡] The designation "consider PEP" indicates that PEP is optional and should be based on an individualized decision between the exposed person and the treating clinician.
[§] Unknown source (e.g., a needle from a sharps disposal container).
[¶] Less severe (e.g., solid needle and superficial injury)
[††] If PEP is offered and taken and the source is later determined to be HIV-negative, PEP should be discontinued.
[§§] More severe (e.g., large-bore hollow needle, deep puncture, visible blood on device, or needle used in patient's artery or vein).
(Source: Centers for Disease Control and Prevention. Available at: http://www.cdc.gov/mmwr/preview/mmwrhtml/rr5011a1.htm).

provide results in minutes to hours. If the source patient is determined to be HIV negative, prophylaxis should be discontinued.

The guidelines recommend an expanded 4-week regimen of three drugs for cases in which either the exposure is high risk or the source patient is determined to be HIV-Positive Class 2 (Table 78-1). Options for the third drug include the protease inhibitors indinavir and nelfinavir, the nonnucleoside inhibitor efavirenz, and the reverse transcriptase inhibitor abacavir. Adding a third drug increases the likelihood that adverse reactions will occur and therefore increases the likelihood that the prophylaxis course will not be completed. Treatment begun many days after exposure should be considered in the setting of high risk, as it may favorably affect the course of the acute retroviral syndrome in HCWs who seroconvert.

Exposed persons should be tested for HIV antibody status at the time of exposure to determine if infection is already present and periodically for 6 months to determine if seroconversion has occurred. HIV viral load testing is not recommended because of the high false-positive rate. Laboratory monitoring also should include complete blood count and renal and hepatic function testing at baseline and at 2 weeks. Additional clinical monitoring may be needed, depending upon the choice of ARV regimen used for prophylaxis. Postexposure care must also include evaluation of the risk of infection with hepatitis B virus and hepatitis C virus. (RBB)

Bibliography

Centers for Disease Control and Prevention. Updated U.S. Public Health Service guidelines for the management of occupational exposures to HBV, HCV, and HIV and recommendations for postexposure prophylaxis. *MMWR* 2001;50:1–42.

Gerberding JL. Occupational exposure to HIV in health care settings. *N Engl J Med* 2003;348:826–833.
Excellent in-depth reviews and recommendations for management. The authors stress the rapid initiation of ARV prophylactic regimens when indicated.

Centers for Disease Control and Prevention. Public Health Service Task Force. Recommendations for use of antiretroviral drugs in pregnant HIV-1-infected women for maternal health and interventions to reduce perinatal HIV-1 transmission in the United States. *MMWR* 2003; Available at: http://aidsinfo.nih.gov/guidelines/perinatal/PER_062304.pdf
This document provides the most recent recommendations for the management of HIV in pregnancy. At least zidovudine is indicated, and for patients who have been on an antiretroviral and then become pregnant, medications should be continued. Also includes recommendations for the role of elective cesarean delivery in preventing vertical transmission.

Elwy AR, et al. Effectiveness of interventions to prevent sexually transmitted infections and human immunodeficiency virus in heterosexual men: a systematic review. *Arch Intern Med* 2002;162:1818–1830.
An evidence-based review of interventions intended to prevent heterosexual transmission among men.

Marcus R, CDC Cooperative Needlestick Surveillance Group. Surveillance of health care workers exposed to blood from patients infected with the human immunodeficiency virus. *N Engl J Med* 1988;319:1118–1123.
Approximately 1,200 HCWs with blood exposures—more than 60% of them nurses—were followed. Most exposures resulted from needlestick injuries, and about a third were potentially preventable. The seroprevalence rate was 0.4%.

Royce RA, et al. Sexual transmission of HIV. *N Engl J Med* 1997;336:1072–1078.
An excellent review.

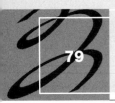

PRIMARY HIV INFECTION

79

*P*rimary HIV infection has often been referred to as mononucleosis-like syndrome. It should be considered in patients, either with or without obvious HIV exposure, who present with fever of an unknown cause. Early on the presumptive diagnosis can be based on a positive HIV-1 RNA level (usually more than 50,000 copies per milliliter) even in the absence of a positive enzyme-linked immunosorbent antibody assay (ELISA) and confirmatory Western blot antibody test for HIV. Early treatment may be beneficial.

Studies of persons with acute HIV-1 infection demonstrate selective infection by certain populations of HIV-1 variants. Transmitted viruses are typically macrophage-tropic but not T-cell–tropic. Glycoprotein 120, the viral-envelope protein, binds to the CD4 molecule on susceptible cells, but cell entry requires the presence of a coreceptor called CCR5. Such viruses recently have been renamed R5 viruses to reflect their coreceptor requirement, whereas T-cell–tropic viruses, which require CXCR4 for entry, are termed *X4 viruses*. Langerhans' cells are felt to be the earliest target of the virus and express CCR5 but not CXCR4, the coreceptor required for the entry of X4 viral isolates. After the initial rise in plasma viremia, often to levels in excess of 1 million RNA molecules per milliliter, there is a significant reduction from the peak viremia to a steady-state level of viral replication. There is a correlation between cytotoxic T-lymphocyte responses to the envelope protein and the reduction in plasma viral RNA. In contrast, neutralizing antibodies are not usually detectable until weeks to months after the reduction in replicating virus. Many of the symptoms of acute HIV-1 infection may reflect the immune response to the virus, and the symptoms usually resolve as the viral load in the plasma decreases. After the initial drop in viremia, a viral set-point is established. Persons with the highest viral loads will most likely have the most rapid rates of progression to the acquired immunodeficiency syndrome and death.

The signs and symptoms of acute HIV-1 infection usually appear within days to weeks after initial exposure. The acute illness may last from a few days to more than 10 weeks, but the duration is usually less than 14 days. The severity and the duration of the illness may have prognostic implications; severe and prolonged symptoms are correlated with rapid disease progression. Studies have show that perhaps between 50 to 90% of patients acutely infected with HIV experience symptoms of the acute retroviral syndrome. The most common findings of the syndrome, as illustrated in Table 79-1, are fever (80–90%), fatigue (70–90%), rash (40–80%), headache (32–70%), and lymphadenopathy (40–70%). The rash has a predilection for the upper thorax, face, and forehead and is usually recognized as an exanthem (macular or maculopapular oval or rounded lesions). Additional findings include pharyngitis, myalgia, nausea, vomiting, diarrhea, arthralgia, aseptic meningitis, retro-orbital pain, weight loss, depression, gastrointestinal distress, night sweats, and oral or genital ulcers. Symptoms usually develop within days to weeks after HIV exposure and last from a few days to several months, but usually fewer than 14 days. Often acute HIV infection may resemble infectious mononucleosis, influenza, severe streptococcal pharyngitis, viral hepatitis, toxoplasmosis, or even secondary syphilis. A high index of suspicion is required to make the diagnosis.

Laboratory studies performed during the initial infection may show lymphopenia and thrombocytopenia, but atypical lymphocytes are infrequent. The CD4+ cell count usually remains normal or decreases over several weeks. The ratio of CD4+ cells to CD8+ cells can be inverted. The recombinant ELISAs commonly used to diagnose established HIV-1 infection are usually negative in persons who present with acute infection. Serologic tests

TABLE 79-1	Signs and Symptoms of Primary HIV Infection

Findings	Frequency (%)
Fevers	>90%
Fatigue	>90%
Rash	>70%
Headache	32–70%
Lymphadenopathy	40–70%
Pharyngitis	50–70%
Myalgia, arthralgia	50–70%
Nausea, vomiting, or diarrhea	30–60%
Night sweats	50%
Oral ulcers	10–20%
Genital ulcers	5–15%
Thrombocytopenia	45%
Leukopenia	40%
Elevated hepatic enzymes	21%

first become positive approximately 22 to 27 days after acute infection in most patients. The detection of high-titer viral RNA or viral p24 antigen in a patient with a negative test for HIV-1 antibodies establishes the diagnosis of acute HIV-1 infection. The viral-RNA assay appears to be the more sensitive of the two tests, and it has been estimated to detect HIV-1 infection 3 to 5 days earlier than the p24 antigen test and 1 to 3 weeks earlier than standard serologic tests. Generally speaking, the levels of viral RNA will be higher than 50,000 molecules and may exceed 1 million molecules per milliliter. The quantitative plasma HIV-1 RNA level (viral load) by polymerase chain reaction (PCR) is 95 to 98% sensitive for HIV and becomes positive within 11 days of infection. Beware of false-positive HIV-1 RNA tests, which are usually less than 2,000 copies per milliliter. Subsequent documentation of seroconversion is essential to confirm the diagnosis of HIV-1 infection.

A blood sample should be obtained for both HIV-1 RNA testing and HIV ELISA when a patient at risk presents with the signs and symptoms of the syndrome along with a compatible history of exposure. HIV ELISA and HIV-1 RNA tests should be repeated 2 to 4 weeks after the resolution of symptoms in high-risk persons. If viral RNA quantitation is not available, a serum or plasma p24 antigen test may be used to detect viral infection before the appearance of HIV antibodies. If acute HIV infection is strongly suspected, but the HIV-1 RNA PCR test is negative or shows a low titer, the initial high level of viral RNA may have already subsided. The patient should be followed with HIV-1 antibody tests at 3 months, 6 months, and 1 year.

Early treatment is somewhat controversial but has been shown to restore important virus-specific cellular immune responses that appear to be involved in host responses that control viremia. Early treatment also may limit the extent of viral dissemination, restrict damage to the immune system, protect antigen-presenting cells, and reduce the chance of disease progression. Administration of potent antiretroviral therapy can result in a rapid and sustained decline in the viral load to below the limit of detection within 3 months. Some patients will rebound sooner than others if treatment is not continued. Furthermore, studies of CD4 and CD8 lymphocyte dynamics show restoration of the normal ratio, reflecting recovery of the immune system. Early institution of antiretroviral therapy has the advantage of keeping the viral load low by reducing replication and the appearance of resistant HIV phenotypes. It also may prevent immune depletion because of increased immune stimulation resulting from the strong antigenicity of HIV during primary infection. If acute HIV infection is not treated, the signs and symptoms disappear, along with the viremia. The person enters a prolonged stage of hidden viral replication during which the virus may not be culturable from the blood, and HIV-1 RNA levels may be low or undetectable. During the next 5 to 10 years, lymph node architecture is destroyed, certain CD4 and CD8 cell lines

TABLE 79-2	Useful Web Sites

Information	Address
Primary HIV links	http://www.thebody.com/treat/primary.html
Overview and images	http://health.allrefer.com/health/acute-hiv-infection-info.html
Postgraduate medicine	http://www.postgradmed.com/issues/1997/10_97/schacker.htm
Online resource	http://hivinsite.ucsf.edu/InSite.jsp?page=kb-03-01-11
Online text	http://hivmedicine.com/textbook/acuteinf.htm
Guidelines for HIV treatment	http://www.hivatis.org

are gradually depleted, and progression to symptomatic disease ultimately occurs. The new HIV treatment guidelines now recommend considering initiating treatment with an antiviral regimen when a patient's CD4+ T-cell count drops below 350 cells/mm^3 in asymptomatic individuals. The previous version of the guidelines advised physicians to consider therapy for patients with CD4+ T-cell levels below 500 cells/mm^3. The new guidelines also raise the bar for starting treatment in asymptomatic individuals based on the patient's viral load (plasma HIV RNA) level to more than 30,000 viral copies per milliliter, using the branched DNA test or more than 55,000 viral copies per milliliter using the reverse transcriptase polymerase chain reaction (RT-PCR) test—a substantial change from previous guidelines regarding when to initiate treatment, which were based on levels of HIV in the bloodstream of 10,000 copies per milliliter using the branched DNA test or 20,000 copies per milliliter using RT-PCR. The guidelines continue to recommend highly active antiretroviral therapy (HAART) for people with AIDS. The panel also recommends offering treatment to people who are diagnosed within 6 months of becoming HIV infected. Preliminary data suggest that treatment very early in the course of the infection may help preserve immune function and enable some patients to keep HIV in check, although the guidelines state that "on-going clinical trials are addressing the question of the long-term clinical benefit of potent treatment regimens" in acute infection. The current recommendation is to use, for an indefinite duration, combination antiretroviral therapy with at least three drugs to which the patient has never been exposed. One should stop all of the drugs if treatment is going to be discontinued.

The *Guidelines for the Use of Antiretroviral Agents in HIV-Infected Adults and Adolescents*, which are periodically updated to reflect new data about treatment of HIV infection, are available online at the HIV/AIDS Treatment Information Service (ATIS) Web site (http://www.hivatis.org). See Table 79-2 for other useful Web sites. (JWM)

Bibliography

Apoola A, et al. Primary HIV infection. *Int J STD AIDS* 2002;13:71–78.

Common symptoms are pyrexia, pharyngitis, malaise, lethargy, maculopapular rash, mucous membrane ulceration, lymphadenopathy, and headache. It can be reliably diagnosed by a positive virologic test in the absence of HIV-specific antibodies.

Colven R, et al. Retroviral rebound syndrome after cessation of suppressive antiretroviral therapy in three patients with chronic HIV infection. *Ann Intern Med* 2000;133:430–434.

A retroviral rebound syndrome similar to that seen in primary HIV syndrome can occur in patients with chronic HIV infection after cessation of suppressive antiretroviral therapy.

Corey L, Berrey MM. Antiretroviral therapy in primary HIV. *Adv Exp Med Biol* 1999;458:223–227.

Only clinical trials can define the relative benefit of initiating antiretrovirals during this stage of infection.

Kahn JO, Walker BD. Acute human immunodeficiency virus type 1 infection. *N Engl J Med* 1998;339:33–39.

Excellent, comprehensive review of the subject.

Kilby JM, et al. Recurrence of the acute HIV syndrome after interruption of antiretroviral therapy in a patient with chronic HIV infection: A case report. *Ann Intern Med* 2000;133:435–438.
Therapeutic interruption may be associated with profound viral rebound and recurrence of the acute HIV syndrome.

Kosel BW, Aweeka F. Drug interactions of antiretroviral agents. *AIDS Clin Rev* 2000;193–227.
Key points to remember when prescribing antiretroviral therapy are reviewed.

Nye F. Infectious mononucleosis: not always what it seems. *Hosp Med* 2001;62:388–389.

Perlmutter BL, et al. How to recognize and treat acute HIV syndrome. *Am Fam Physician* 1999;60:535–542, 545–546.
The diagnosis is based on a positive HIV-1 RNA level (more than 50,000 copies per milliliter) in the absence of a positive ELISA and confirmatory Western blot antibody test for HIV. Early diagnosis permits patient education as well as treatment that may delay disease progression.

Pilcher CD, et al. Diagnosing primary HIV infection. *Ann Intern Med* 2002;136:488–489; discussion 488–489.
Review of the different tests used to make the diagnosis.

Stephenson J. New HIV therapy guidelines. *JAMA* 2001; 285:1281.
Overview of the new guidelines.

Vanhems P, et al. Primary HIV-1 infection: diagnosis and prognostic impact. *AIDS Patient Care STDS* 1998;12:751–758.
Acute infection with HIV is symptomatic in approximately two-thirds to three-fourths of patients. Physicians should be aware of the broad clinical spectrum representative of primary HIV infection, which ranges from mild symptoms resembling classic mononucleosis infection to highly severe presentations. Progression to AIDS and to death has been associated with the severity of the acute HIV infection.

von Sydow M, et al. Antigen detection in primary HIV infection. *Br Med J (Clin Res Ed)* 1988;296:238–2340.
Serial blood samples were obtained from 21 homosexuals who had developed symptomatic primary infection with HIV after a median incubation time of 14 days.

Youle M. Is interruption of HIV therapy always harmful? *J Antimicrob Chemother* 2000;45:137–138.

Yu K, Daar ES. Primary HIV infection. Current trends in transmission, testing, and treatment. *Postgrad Med* 2000;107:114–116, 119–122.
Primary care physicians who recognize the signs and symptoms are in an ideal position to diagnose the disease at an early stage and to help stem the tide of new infections in the community.

TREATMENT OF *PNEUMOCYSTIS CARINII* PNEUMONIA IN AIDS

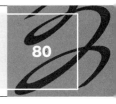

80

*P*atients with *Pneumocystis carinii* pneumonia (PCP) typically have a gradual onset of dyspnea accompanied by a nonproductive cough, weight loss, and fever. Physical findings are often unremarkable despite a strikingly abnormal radiograph. Sputum induction, monoclonal antibodies, and polymerase chain reaction (PCR) tests may be used to demonstrate the organism. Bronchoalveolar lavage usually will reveal the organism on Gomori silver stains.

Primary prophylaxis against *Pneumocystis* pneumonia in HIV-infected adults should be initiated when the CD4 count is less than 200 cells/μL or if there is a history of oropharyngeal candidiasis.

As approximately 40% of all HIV-infected patients with PCP have a second episode (usually within 18 months), a major goal is to prevent or delay subsequent episodes. In general, patients with CD4 cell counts of less than 200 cells/μL will have an 8.4% probability of acquiring PCP within 6 months, compared with a 0.5% probability in those whose CD4 cell counts were higher than 200. Patients who have already had a previous episode of PCP should receive lifelong secondary prophylaxis, unless sufficient reconstitution of the immune system has occurred as a result of HIV therapy. Primary or secondary prophylaxis should be discontinued in HIV-infected patients who have had a response to highly active antiretroviral therapy (HAART), as shown by an increase in the CD4+ cell count to more than 200 cells/mm^3 for a period of at least 3 months. It is important to restart prophylaxis if the CD4+ count falls to less than 200 cells/ mm^3.

Trimethoprim–sulfamethoxazole is most effective in treating severe PCP and in prevention of this disease. Corticosteroids recommended for HIV-infected patients with PCP who have hypoxemia (the partial pressure of arterial oxygen while the patient is breathing room air is under 70 mmHg or the alveolar–arterial gradient is above 35). They should be given

TABLE 80-1   **Treatment of PCP***

Drug	Dose	Side effects	Comments	Route
Trimethoprim-sulfamethoxazole	15–20 mg/kg of the TMP component divided q 6 hr	Rash, bone marrow toxicity, other	Drug of first choice	Intravenous or oral
Dapsone	100 mg per day. Usually with TMP	Hemolysis	Check for G6PD deficiency	Oral
Clindamycin and primaquine	600 mg t.i.d., and 30 mg per day	Diarrhea, bone marrow toxicity	Also rule out if the patient is G6PD deficient	Can be oral
Pentamidine	3–4 mg/kg IV q day	Parenteral has many side effects including hypoglycemia	Hyperglycemia may not become evident until several months after treatment is completed; diabetes has occurred as late as 150 days	IV
Atovaquone	750 mg suspension b.i.d.	Diarrhea	Give with food	Oral
Trimetrexate	45 mg/square meter of body surface IV q day	Bone marrow toxicity	Give with leucovorin	
Caspofungin			Experimental	

*Treat for 21 days total then begin suppression.

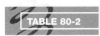

TABLE 80-2	Drugs for Prevention of PCP	
Drug	**Dose**	**Comments**
Trimethoprim-sulfamethoxazole	One double-or single-strength daily or one double-strength three times per week	Most effective medication but limited in some patients by side effects
Dapsone	Usually given as 100 mg daily.	A prior adverse reaction to TMP-SMX, however, means a risk of 33–38% for developing an adverse reaction to dapsone
Pentamidine	300 mg aerosol once per month	Pneumothoraces Extrapulmonary PCP is seen Risk of tuberculosis transmission Upper lobe PCP presentation
Atovaquone	1500 mg once daily	Newer formulation is better absorbed

prednisone at a dose of 40 mg twice daily for 5 days, then 40 mg daily on days 6 through 11, and then 20 mg daily on days 12 though 21. Because the clinical response may be delayed for as long as 5 days despite appropriate therapy, patients should be maintained on their initial regimen for 5 to 7 days before a determination of clinical failure and a change to an alternative drug are made. Prognosis is variable. Several studies have shown that patients with serum lactate dehydrogenase (LDH) levels less than 350 IU at the time of diagnosis have a better survival rate than those with higher serum LDH levels. Most survivors also show a decline in LDH levels by at least 7 days. Patients may be coinfected with other pathogens. Recovery of cytomegalovirus from bronchoscopy specimens, however, appears to have no significant impact on mortality when found in association with PCP.

Tables 80-1 and 80-2 list the medications useful in treating and preventing this disease. (JWM)

Bibliography

Abd AG, et al. Bilateral upper lobe Pneumocystis carinii pneumonia in a patient receiving inhaled pentamidine prophylaxis. *Chest* 1988;94:329–331.

Barber BA, et al. Clindamycin/primaquine as prophylaxis for Pneumocystis carinii pneumonia. *Clin Infect Dis* 1996;23:718–722.
Failure of clindamycin/primaquine (C/P) prophylaxis could be the result, at least in part, of underdosing (clindamycin, 300 mg/day; primaquine, 15 mg/day). C/P recipients had more nonspecific diarrhea than did trimethoprim-sulfamethoxazole (TMP-SMX) recipients (RR, 2.99; 95% CI, 1.61–5.55).

Blum RN, et al. Comparative trial of dapsone versus trimethoprim/sulfamethoxazole for primary prophylaxis of Pneumocystis carinii pneumonia. *J Acquir Immune Defic Syndr* 1992;5:341–347.
Development of toxicity to one drug does not invariably predict toxicity to the other.

Bucher HC, et al. Meta-analysis of prophylactic treatments against Pneumocystis carinii pneumonia and toxoplasma encephalitis in HIV-infected patients. *J Acquir Immune Defic Syndr Hum Retrovirol* 1997;15:104–114.

Casale L, et al. Decreased efficacy of inhaled pentamidine in the prevention of Pneumocystis carinii pneumonia among HIV-infected patients with severe immunodeficiency. *Chest* 1993;103:342–344.
Failure of inhaled pentamidine prophylaxis is seen almost exclusively among patients with CD4 lymphocyte counts below 60/mm³.

Castro M. Treatment and prophylaxis of Pneumocystis carinii pneumonia. *Semin Respir Infect* 1998;13:296–303.
Excellent review article

Caumes E, et al. A life-threatening adverse reaction during trimethoprim-sulfamethoxazole desensitization in a previously hypersensitive patient infected with human immunodeficiency virus. *Clin Infect Dis* 1996;23:1313–1314.

Cook DE, Kossey JL. Successful desensitization to dapsone for Pneumocystis carinii prophylaxis in an HIV-positive patient. *Ann Pharmacother* 1998;32:1302–1305.
> *This case suggests that utilization of a dapsone desensitization regimen may permit a viable treatment option in patients previously thought to be intolerant to the agent.*

Edelson PJ, et al. Dapsone, trimethoprim-sulfamethoxazole, and the acquired immunodeficiency syndrome. *Ann Intern Med* 1985;103:963.

Edelstein H, McCabe RE. Atypical presentations of Pneumocystis carinii pneumonia in patients receiving inhaled pentamidine prophylaxis. *Chest* 1990;98:1366–1369.
> *Clinicians who choose to use this effective and convenient mode of prophylaxis should be aware of the problems attendant to its use.*

Fulton B, et al. Trimetrexate. A review of its pharmacodynamic and pharmacokinetic properties and therapeutic potential in the treatment of Pneumocystis carinii pneumonia. *Drugs* 1995;49:563–576.
> *Trimetrexate is a folinic acid analogue structurally related to methotrexate, whose primary mechanism of action is believed to be inhibition of dihydrofolate reductase. Currently, trimetrexate should be considered as only as an alternative treatment option in immunocompromised patients with moderate to severe PCP who have not responded to or are intolerant of first-line therapy.*

Gluckstein D, Ruskin J. Rapid oral desensitization to trimethoprim-sulfamethoxazole (TMP-SMZ): use in prophylaxis for Pneumocystis carinii pneumonia in patients with AIDS who were previously intolerant to TMP-SMZ. *Clin Infect Dis* 1995;20:849–853.
> *These results indicate that most patients who are presumed to be TMP-SMZ–intolerant can be desensitized rapidly with oral TMP-SMZ and subsequently receive the drug for protracted periods as effective prophylaxis for PCP.*

Ioannidis JP, et al. A meta-analysis of the relative efficacy and toxicity of Pneumocystis carinii prophylactic regimens. *Arch Intern Med* 1996;156:177–188.

Kales CP, et al. Early predictors of in-hospital mortality for Pneumocystis carinii pneumonia in the acquired immunodeficiency syndrome. *Arch Intern Med* 1987;147:1413–1417.
> *One hundred forty-five patients were initially seen with PCP. Of the many features examined, several variables were identified early in the hospitalization for PCP that were associated with poor survival. These included multiple admissions, leukocytoses, elevated serum LDH levels, decreased arterial oxygen pressure (tension), decreased arterial carbon dioxide pressure (tension), and decreased serum albumin levels. Variables that were associated with increased survival included normal respiratory rates and normal findings on lung examination. Patients with multiple pulmonary infections displayed higher mortality rates than patients who had only PCP. Finally, our data did not suggest that the degree of immunosuppression affected in-hospital mortality for PCP.*

Leoung G, et al. A randomized, double-blind trial of TMP/SMX dose escalation vs. direct rechallenge in HIV+ persons at risk for PCP and with prior treatment-limiting rash or fever. 37th Interscience Conference on Antibiotics and Antimicrobial Chemotherapy, Toronto, Canada, 1997.
> *The results show that 75.3% (73/97) patients who underwent dose escalation compared with 57.4% (54/94) of patients directly rechallenged were able to continue TMP/SMX for 6 months Of note is that even without dose escalation, 57% of all patients with prior rash or fever were able to tolerate TMP/SMX after direct rechallenge. Although this offers hope that patients may be once again able to take TMP/SMX, it remains difficult to predict which patients will require desensitization and in whom it will ultimately be successful.*

MacGregor RR, et al. Efficacy and tolerance of intermittent versus daily cotrimoxazole for PCP prophylaxis in HIV-positive patients. *Am J Med* 1992;92:227–229.

Monk JP, Benfield P. Inhaled pentamidine. An overview of its pharmacological properties and a review of its therapeutic use in Pneumocystis carinii pneumonia. *Drugs* 1990;39:741–756.

Phair J, et al. The risk of Pneumocystis carinii pneumonia among men infected with human immunodeficiency virus type 1. Multicenter AIDS Cohort Study Group. *N Engl J Med* 1990;322:161–165.

We conclude that PCP is unlikely to develop in HIV-1-infected patients unless their CD4+ cells are depleted to 200/mm³ or below or the patients are symptomatic, and therefore that prophylaxis should be reserved for such patients.

Pretet S, et al. Long-term results of monthly inhaled pentamidine as primary prophylaxis of Pneumocystis carinii pneumonia in HIV-infected patients. *Am J Med* 1993;94:35–40.

Generally effective, but less so than TMP-SMX.

Ryan C, et al. Sulfa hypersensitivity in patients with HIV infection: onset, treatment, critical review of the literature. *WMJ* 1998;97:23–27.

Our findings indicate that the sulfa hypersensitivity reaction is more likely to develop in patients with advanced disease and that desensitization can restore tolerability to the drug in approximately two-thirds of those who attempt it.

Safrin S, et al. Comparison of three regimens for treatment of mild to moderate Pneumocystis carinii pneumonia in patients with AIDS. A double-blind, randomized trial of oral trimethoprim-sulfamethoxazole, dapsone-trimethoprim, and clindamycin-primaquine. ACTG 108 Study Group. *Ann Intern Med* 1996;124:792–802.

Differences in expected categories of toxicities associated with each regimen should guide the clinician in choosing first-line therapy, particularly for patients with baseline hepatic insufficiency or myelosuppression.

Sin DD, Shafran SD. Dapsone- and primaquine-induced methemoglobinemia in HIV-infected individuals. *J Acquir Immune Defic Syndr Hum Retrovirol* 1996;12:477–481.

Our study indicates that dapsone and primaquine alone or in combination can produce clinically significant methemoglobinemia in HIV-infected individuals, either in the setting of an overdose or when primaquine is instituted before dapsone has been cleared from the bloodstream.

Smego RA Jr, et al. A meta-analysis of salvage therapy for Pneumocystis carinii pneumonia. *Arch Intern Med* 2001;161:1529–1533.

The combination of clindamycin plus primaquine appears to be the most effective alternative treatment for patients with PCP who are unresponsive to conventional antipneumocystis agents.

The National Institutes of Health-University of California Expert Panel for Corticosteroids as Adjunctive Therapy for Pneumocystis Pneumonia. Consensus statement on the use of corticosteroids as adjunctive therapy for pneumocystis pneumonia in the acquired immunodeficiency syndrome. *N Engl J Med* 1990;323:1500–1504.

A consensus statement on adjunctive corticosteroid use in acute PCP concluded that corticosteroid treatment is beneficial and the risk of adverse reactions is low enough to recommend corticosteroids with anti-PCP therapy in patients with a partial pressure of oxygen (PaO₂) less than 70 mmHg, PAO₂–PaO₂ greater than 35 mmHg, or oxygen saturation less than 90% on room air, provided there are no specific contraindications (e.g., suspected tuberculosis or disseminated fungal infection; pp 293, 294). The consensus statement recommended the corticosteroid regimen of prednisone, or equivalent, 40 mg twice daily for 5 days, then 40 mg daily for 5 days, and then 20 mg daily until day 21 of therapy, based on the regimen used in one study (p 295). Corticosteroid treatment ideally should begin at the same time as anti-PCP therapy and no later than 72 hours after anti-PCP treatment has begun. Many clinicians use an alternative regimen of 40 mg of prednisone twice daily for 5 days, 40 mg daily for 5 days, and 20 mg daily for 5 days.

Thomas CF Jr, Limper AH. Pneumocystis pneumonia. *N Engl J Med* 2004;350:2487–2498.

Excellent, comprehensive review article.

Toma E, et al. Clindamycin with primaquine vs. trimethoprim-sulfamethoxazole therapy for mild and moderately severe Pneumocystis carinii pneumonia in patients with AIDS: a multicenter, double-blind, randomized trial (CTN 004). CTN-PCP Study Group. *Clin Infect Dis* 1998;27:524–5230.

This trial confirms that Cm/Prq is a reasonable alternative therapy for mild and moderately severe PCP.

Waskin H, et al. Risk factors for hypoglycemia associated with pentamidine therapy for Pneumocystis pneumonia. *JAMA* 1988;260:345–347.

This serious, potentially fatal reaction should be considered in all patients who are treated with pentamidine, particularly those receiving prolonged or recurrent therapy.
White A, et al. Clinical experience with atovaquone on a treatment investigational new drug protocol for Pneumocystis carinii pneumonia. *J Acquir Immune Defic Syndr Hum Retrovirol* 1995;9:280–285.
  The clinical experience of HIV+ patients treated with oral atovaquone for acute PCP under a Treatment Investigational New Drug (IND) protocol (mild or moderate PCP) and an Open-Label Study protocol (severe PCP) was evaluated.
Zaman MK, White DA. Serum lactate dehydrogenase levels and Pneumocystis carinii pneumonia. Diagnostic and prognostic significance. *Am Rev Respir Dis* 1988;137:796–800.
  The level of serum LDH has been reported to be useful as a marker of PCP in patients infected with HIV. Serial determinations of LDH during treatment for PCP showed that 27 of 36 (75%) of the survivors had gradual decreases of LDH, whereas 9 of 12 (75%) nonsurvivors had rising values during treatment.

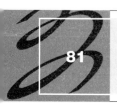

81 HIV-1 AND INFECTIONS OF THE CENTRAL NERVOUS SYSTEM

*T*here are many causes of neurologic disease in HIV-1–infected persons, including primary HIV infection-related syndromes and opportunistic infections. The high prevalence and variety of diseases affecting the CNS is a consequence of the direct involvement of the brain by HIV-1 as well as the profound immunosuppression that occurs with lymphocyte depletion.

MENINGITIS

A neurotropic retrovirus, HIV-1 appears to invade the central nervous system (CNS) during the primary infection. The virus has been isolated from the cerebrospinal fluid (CSF) of adults with acute HIV-1 infection and from those with AIDS. In addition, HIV-1 has been detected in a number of CNS cell populations, including endothelial cells, macrophages, and microglial cells. Because of the high prevalence of abnormal spinal fluid findings in this patient population, the results of the CSF analysis must be interpreted with caution. Patients are at risk to experience meningitis caused by a variety of microorganisms including fungi, parasites, and bacteria. In addition, lymphomatous meningitis can develop in these patients as a complication of a systemic lymphoma. HIV-1–infected patients also can present with syphilis as well.

  Cryptococcus neoformans, a fungus found in bird excreta and soil throughout the United States, is the most common cause of fungal meningitis in patients infected with HIV. *C. neoformans* has two varieties—*neoformans* and *gattii*. The species has four serotypes based on antigenic specificity of the capsular polysaccharide; these include serotypes A and D (*C. neoformans* var *neoformans*) and serotypes B and C (*C. neoformans* var *gattii*). The *C. neoformans* var *neoformans* is the most common variety in the United States and other temperate climates throughout the world and is found in aged pigeon droppings. *C. neoformans* var *gattii* develops in tropical and subtropical climates and is not associated with birds, but it grows in the litter around certain species of eucalyptus trees. Serotype A causes most cryptococcal infections in patients who are immunocompromised, including patients infected with HIV.

Cryptococcal meningitis is usually seen in HIV-1–infected patients whose CD4 cell counts are below 100. It may be the intial manifestation of AIDS. The most common symptoms of cryptococcal meningitis are headache, fever, and malaise. Diagnosis is made by the examination of the CSF, and the following are typical abnormalities: (1) normal or slightly elevated opening pressure; (2) lymphocytic pleocytosis (usually of less than 100 cells/mm^3); (3) elevated protein concentration; (4) decreased glucose concentration; and (5) positive cryptococcal antigen. Results of computed tomography (CT) and magnetic resonance imaging (MRI) are usually normal. Normal CSF findings do not rule out the disease, especially in patients with advanced disease. Spinal fluid cultures will reveal the presence of the fungus in virtually all patients, and blood cultures will be positive in 50 to 60% of cases. Fortunately, cryptococcal antigen is detectable in the CSF and serum in more than 90% of patients, typically at high titer (>1:1,024). Altered mentation (confusion, lethargy, obtundation), cranial nerve deficits, CSF cryptococcal antigen (CRAg) titers above 1:1024, and CSF white blood cell (WBC) counts below 20/mm^3 are risk factors associated with poor outcome. An India ink preparation commonly is used with CSF to identify the organism and to support a presumptive diagnosis, and up to 50% of patients with cryptococcal meningitis may have positive results.

Of note, because of defects in the mechanisms through which the polysaccharide is eliminated, cryptococcal antigen can remain detectable for extended periods. Serum and CSF CRAg titers often increase after initiation of antifungal treatment; however, the increased titers do not necessarily correlate with treatment failure. Titers of CRAg do not necessarily correlate with disease status.

Among patients with HIV infection and cryptococcal meningitis, induction therapy with amphotericin B (0.7 mg/kg per day) plus flucytosine (100 mg/kg per day for 2 weeks) followed by fluconazole (400 mg/day) for a minimum of 10 weeks is the treatment of choice. In view of the positive influence of flucytosine therapy on the mycologic outcome, its low degree of toxicity in a recent study, and data demonstrating its effectiveness in preventing relapses (regardless of the maintenance regimen), many experts believe that the addition of flucytosine to amphotericin B is warranted for induction therapy but there is some disagreement on this issue.

After 10 weeks of therapy, the fluconazole dosage may be reduced to 200 mg/day, depending on the patient's clinical status. An alternative regimen for AIDS-associated cryptococcal meningitis is amphotericin B (0.7–mg/kg per day) plus 5-flucytosine (100 mg/kg per day) for 6 to 10 weeks, followed by fluconazole maintenance therapy. Induction therapy beginning with an azole alone is generally discouraged. Lipid formulations of amphotericin B can be substituted for amphotericin B for patients whose renal function is impaired. Fluconazole (400–800 mg/d) plus flucytosine (100–150 mg/kg per day) for 6 weeks is an alternative to the use of amphotericin B, although toxicity with this regimen is high. Intrathecal or intraventricular amphotericin B may be used in refractory cases in which systemic administration of antifungal therapy has failed. Owing to its inherent toxicity and difficulty of administration, this therapy is recommended only in this salvage setting. Voriconazole has activity against *C. neoformans*, but its role in therapy remains undefined at this point. Caspofungin does not have any activity against this pathogen.

When the CSF culture is sterile, the patient is usually switched to maintenance fluconazole therapy (200 mg/day) indefinitely. Although somewhat less effective overall, itraconazole is a suitable alternative for patients unable to take fluconazole. Several treatment options exist for managing elevated intracranial pressure including intermittent CSF drainage by means of sequential lumbar punctures, insertion of a lumbar drain, or placement of a ventriculoperitoneal shunt. Medical approaches, such as the use of corticosteroids, acetazolamide, or mannitol, have not been definitively proven to be effective in the setting of cryptococcal meningitis but are occasionally used. Among patients with normal baseline opening pressure (<200 mm H$_2$O), a repeat lumbar puncture should be performed 2 weeks after initiation of therapy to exclude elevated pressure and to evaluate culture status. Repeat lumbar punctures may be considered after completion of therapy and at anytime there is clinical evidence to suggest relapse. CSF pleocytosis may persist for up to 6 months after successful treatment, and most patients should have normal CSF findings by 1 year after treatment. There are no established guidelines for the frequency or timing of surveillance lumbar punctures to evaluate for relapse.

For patients with elevated baseline opening pressure, lumbar drainage should remove enough CSF to reduce the opening pressure by 50%. Patients should initially undergo daily lumbar punctures to maintain CSF opening pressure in the normal range. When the CSF pressure is normal for several days, the procedure can be suspended. Occasionally patients who present with extremely high opening pressures (>400 mm H_2O) may require a lumbar drain, especially when frequent lumbar punctures are required to or fail to control symptoms. In cases in which repeated lumbar punctures or use of a lumbar drain fail to control elevated pressure symptoms, or when persistent or progressive neurologic deficits are present, a ventriculoperitoneal shunt is indicated. Owing to the intense fungal burden and large amount of replication in patients with HIV disease, adjunctive steroid therapy is not recommended for HIV-infected patients. Because there is a strong association between elevated intracranial pressure and early death, clinicians should monitor cerebrospinal fluid pressure even in the absence of symptoms and initiate aggressive management if the pressure is elevated.

United States Public Health Service (USPHS) guidelines have changed secondary prophylaxis recommendations for cryptococcosis to reflect data that reveal it is safe to discontinue secondary prophylaxis in patients who have had a sustained immunologic response on effective antiretroviral therapy. There have been two prospective case series of safely discontinuing secondary prophylaxis in patients with cryptococcal meningitis. In one study, six patients with disseminated cryptococcal disease, including one with a history of a brain abscess, discontinued antifungal prophylaxis after 1 year of prophylaxis and a sustained CD4 count >150 cells/mm³ (range 178–525) on antiretroviral treatment. One patient had both a positive CSF CRAg and serum CRAg at the time of enrollment. In another study, six patients, including three with serum CRAg titers higher than 1:8 discontinued antifungal prophylaxis after a median of 11 months of combination antiretroviral treatment with a CD4 count greater than 100 cells/mm³. None of the patients in either study has had a recurrence of cryptococcosis. Mussini and colleagues retrospectively evaluated 16 patients who had voluntarily discontinued antifungal therapy for cryptococcal meningitis versus 17 patients who continued antifungal therapy. The median CD4 T-cell count of the group who discontinued prophylaxis was 113 cells/mm³. None of the patients experienced a relapse of cryptococcosis after a median of 15 months.

For those patients who do not have a mass lesion, a lumbar puncture should be performed to send cultures for bacteria, mycobacteria, and fungi and a VDRL. Other useful tests to consider to help determine the etiology include a polymerase chain reaction (PCR) amplification for herpes simplex virus (HSV), varicella-zoster virus (VZV), cytomegalovirus (CMV), Epstein-Barr virus (EBV), and/or JC virus.

SPACE-OCCUPYING LESIONS IN THE BRAIN

HIV-1–infected patients frequently have abnormal findings on the neurologic examination and parenchymal lesions revealed by CT of the brain. Although a number of diseases can result in space-occupying lesions in the brain, the most common entities are toxoplasmosis and lymphoma. Pyogenic brain abscesses, cryptococcomas, tuberculomas, and Kaposi's sarcoma are rare causes of intracerebral masses in these patients.

A protozoan pathogen, *Toxoplasma gondii* is capable of causing single or multiple cerebral abscesses. The risk for cerebral disease approaches 10% among persons with HIV-1 infection who have serologic evidence of prior infection with *T. gondii*; indeed, toxoplasmosis has traditionally been the most common cause of intraparenchymal brain lesions in HIV-1–infected patients. The problem is usually seen in persons with CD4 cell counts below 100 mm³. Most patients with cerebral toxoplasmosis present with focal neurologic problems, such as aphasia, hemiparesis, and complete hemiplegia, that evolve during 1 to 2 weeks; headache, fever, seizures, and changes in mental status also occur. The head CT scan in patients with CNS toxoplasmosis usually shows ring enhancing lesions in 80 to 90% of patients. From 60 to 70% of patients have multiple lesions by CT or MRI. Lesions are most common in the frontal lobes, basal ganglia, and parietal lobes, and generally in cerebral white matter or subcortical gray matter. Although the test is not often required, MRI can detect lesions not visualized by CT; with MRI, multiple abscesses will be detected in more than 80% of patients. Patients with a solitary lesion are more likely (70%) to have lymphoma rather than toxoplamosis. *Toxoplasma* serologies are positive in more than 95% of patients with CNS infection, and up to 40% of HIV-positive patients with positive IgG anti-*Toxoplasma* antibodies develop active CNS toxoplasmosis within 2 years after the diagnosis of AIDS. A negative IgG titer is uncommon in a patient with reactivated toxoplasmosis and should prompt the clinician to consider another diagnosis, such as lymphoma. Analysis of the cerebrospinal fluid (CSF) in patients with toxoplasmic encephalitis (TE) usually reveals a normal glucose level, and protein levels are slightly elevated in more than half the patients. From 15 to 50% of patients show a mild mononuclear pleocytosis. Because the CSF changes are nondiagnostic, a lumbar puncture is not routinely indicated and carries a risk of herniation. Nevertheless, a PCR of the CSF to detect *T. gondii* DNA may prove to be a useful assay if fluid is obtained. PCR tests have high specificity but low sensitivity and should be considered only when standard diagnostic approaches are negative.

An acceptable approach to the HIV-1–infected patient with multiple ring-enhancing lesions is to give empiric antitoxoplasmal therapy to monitor the clinical response. Most patients with cerebral toxoplasmosis demonstrate an improvement in their systemic or neurologic symptoms within 2 weeks and a radiologic response within 3 weeks; of note, abnormalities on CT can persist for up to 6 months. The usual therapy is a combination of pyrimethamine (200 mg orally on the first day, then 75–100 mg daily), sulfadiazine (1–1.5 g orally every 6 hours), and folinic acid (10–15 mg daily) given for 4 to 6 weeks; clindamycin (600 mg intravenously or orally every 6 hours) can be used in patients intolerant of sulfadiazine. Sulfadiazine has good CNS penetration, but has many side effects, including neutropenia, nausea, vomiting, pyrimethamine diarrhea, rash, fever, interstitial nephritis, crystalluria, and nephrolithiasis that can result in acute renal failure. Pyrimethamine penetrates the CSF moderately well. Potentially limiting side effects include pancytopenia, headache, and gastrointestinal upset. To decrease the incidence of pancytopenia, 10 mg of folinic acid is administered orally with each dose of pyrimethamine. This addition does not negate the beneficial effect of pyrimethamine therapy, because *T. gondii* is unable to use folinic acid.

The high incidence of adverse reactions to sulfa drugs in patients with HIV disease, particularly neutropenia and rash, often leads to discontinuation of sulfadiazine, as up to 75% of patients treated with sulfadiazine and pyrimethamine develop a rash. When given with pyrimethamine and folinic acid, azithromycin, clarithromycin, doxycycline, and dapsone are among the other agents that have been shown to be effective in the therapy of CNS toxoplasmosis. Pyrimethamine and clindamycin, 450 to 600 mg orally or 600 to 1200 mg IV four times daily for the first 6 to 10 weeks, followed by a maintenance regimen of 300 mg orally four times daily is a suitable alternative regimen as prospective studies have demonstrated that clindamycin-pyrimethamine is as efficacious as sulfadiazine-pyrimethamine for acute treatment of TE. However, patients randomized to clindamycin-pyrimethamine treatment are almost twice as likely to relapse during maintenance therapy as those given sulfadiazine-pyrimethamine, although neither treatment was associated with a significant survival advantage. Atovaquone, a hydroxynaphthoquinone, can be used as salvage therapy in patients who cannot tolerate standard regimens or who have a relapse on such regimens. Small pilot studies have shown that 75 mg pyrimethamine daily plus 2 g clarithromycin daily and oral pyrimethamine at 75 mg per day plus azithromycin at 500 mg per day may be effective as well. Adjuvant therapy for patients with TE may include dexamethasone for abscesses associated with severe mass effect and phenytoin for infection-induced seizures.

A stereotactic or open brain biopsy is reserved for patients with single lesions that suggest lymphoma and for patients who fail to respond to antitoxoplasmal therapy within 7 to 14 days. The risks of brain biopsy and the frequency of CNS infection by *T. gondii* in HIV-infected patients suggest that clinically stable patients with one or more intracranial masses should be treated presumptively for TE. Guidelines from the American Academy of Neurology recommend that empiric treatment for toxoplasmosis should be instituted in all cases except (1) nonterminal cases with large lesions requiring open decompression and biopsy; (2) cases in which thallium[201] single photon-emission computed tomography ([201]T1 SPECT) or positron-emission tomography with ^{18}F-fluorodeoxyglucose([18]FDG-PET) suggest the presence of primary CNS lymphoma; or (3) cases in which a single intracranial mass is accompanied by negative serology for toxoplasmosis. The use of [201]T1 SPECT or [18]FDG-PET is considered optional, where available.

The outlook for patients with cerebral toxoplasmosis tends to be good, and many survive for extended periods. In contrast, the prognosis for patients with primary lymphoma is poor; most succumb within 2 to 4 months. Finally, because the discontinuation of antitoxoplasmal. therapy results in a recrudescence of the infection in up to 50% of treated patients, usually long-term (lifelong) suppressive therapy is indicated; pyrimethamine (25–50 mg daily) and folinic acid (5–10 mg daily) plus sulfadiazine (0.5–1.0 g four times daily) or clindamycin (300 mg four times daily) should be given. Secondary prophylaxis for toxoplasmosis may be discontinued in patients with a sustained increase in CD4+ counts (e.g., 6 months) to more than 200 cells/μL in response to highly active retroviral therapy (HAART) if they have completed their initial therapy and have no symptoms or signs of ongoing infection.

Primary lymphoma of the CNS, which has been associated with the EBV, is the lesion most frequently confused with toxoplasmosis. The estimated relative risk of non-Hodgkins lymphoma (NHL) associated with HIV infection is 100 times greater than in the general population. Usually the CD4+ lymphocyte count at diagnosis is less than 50/μL. Central nervous system lymphoma develops as single or multiple lesions in the deep regions of white matter, in the basal ganglia, and in the cerebellum. The clinical presentation is nonspecific, and approximately 50% of patients present with lethargy, confusion, and personality change. Symptoms alone do not reliably distinguish lymphoma from toxoplasmosis. Unfortunately, the anatomic location and CT appearance of toxoplasmosis and lymphoma are similar. Equally important, in up to 40% of patients, the malignancy is multicentric, and so the presence of more than one ring-enhancing lesion on CT does not exclude the possibility of a lymphoma; furthermore, 60 to 70% of patients with primary CNS lymphoma will have positive serologic tests for *T. gondii.*

Of note, in recent investigations, PCR for EBV DNA in CSF appears to be a very sensitive method for identifying patients with primary CNS lymphoma, and SPECT with thallium 201 has been reported as a novel method for accurately distinguishing toxoplasmosis from lymphoma, as discussed earlier. Some experts recommend that patients with CNS lesions typical for primary CNS lymphoma who are nonresponsive to antitoxoplasmosis treatment and who have positive CSF PCR results for EBV can be treated presumptively for the latter diagnosis, obviating the necessity for a biopsy. Studies have shown76% of patients treated with 4000 cGy of whole-brain radiation therapy showed evidence of significant clinical improvement, and 69% demonstrated complete or partial radiographic response. Most patients with CNS lymphoma treated with radiotherapy alone do have improvement in their neurologic symptoms but survival is short, with most individuals dying from complications of HIV disease. Survival is not improved by the addition of chemotherapy.

Less common opportunistic diseases that may cause an intracranial mass lesion include bacterial brain abscesses (including *Listeria monocytogenes* and *Bartonella* infections), candidiasis, nocardiosis, aspergillosis, coccidioidomycosis, histoplasmosis, cryptococcosis, cysticercosis, tuberculosis, syphilis, VZV infections, HSV infections, and Kaposi's sarcoma.

 ## ENCEPHALOPATHY

Patients infected with HIV-1 can present with changes in mental status because of meningitis or cerebral mass lesions. These patients can also experience a deterioration in cognitive function caused by intercurrent conditions, including viral encephalitis (CMV, HSV, herpes zoster virus, human herpesvirus 6) and metabolic encephalopathy (hypoxemia, drugs). Of note, PCR of the CSF for CMV DNA appears to be a rapid and sensitive technique for establishing a diagnosis of CMV encephalitis or ventriculoencephalitis, and PCR of the CSF has been used to monitor the response of AIDS patients with CMV disease to antiviral (ganciclovir) therapy. CMV encephalitis (CMVE) with dementia is well described neuropathologically as a multifocal, scattered micronodular encephalitis that resembles the HIV encephalitis-dementia syndrome. Patients with dementia caused by CMVE usually have a more acute onset and rapid progression than patients with HIV dementia (HIVD). Frequently reported symptoms include delirium and confusion, lethargy and somnolence, apathy and withdrawal, personality changes, and focal neurologic signs with cranial nerve involvement. The other major form of CMVE is that of a ventriculoencephalitis that characteristically occurs as a late and terminal event. Then onset of symptoms of the encephalitis may be rapid and associated with cranial nerve involvement and nystagmus. If an ependymitis is evident on imaging this is suggestive, but not necessarily diagnostic, for CMV infection. Similarly, CSF examination is nonspecific and cultures may be negative, even in pathologically proven CMV encephalitis. One should look for other signs of systemic CMV infection (retinal, gastrointestinal, or pulmonary) as well. Ganciclovir is the treatment of choice.

In patients with AIDS, the most common CNS infection caused by CMV is polyradiculopathy characterized by an ascending weakness in the lower extremities associated with a loss of deep tendon reflexes and a loss of bowel and bladder control. The syndrome frequently begins as low back pain with a radicular or perianal radiation, followed in a few weeks by a progressive flaccid paralysis. The CSF abnormalities are typically a pleocytosis with predominant polymorphonuclear leukocytosis and hypoglycorrhachia. Culture of CSF is usually negative, but antigen or DNA assays are sensitive methods of diagnosis. MRI may reveal enhancement of leptomeninges and clumping of lumbosacral roots.

HIV-infected persons also are at risk for the development of progressive multifocal leukoencephalopathy (PML) which is caused by JC virus, a polyoma virus that affects approximately 5% of patients with advanced HIV disease. It is characterized by an altered mental status, aphasia, ataxia, and hemiparesis, and, occasionally, seizures. Dementia, encephalopathy, and coma can occur with the more fulminant forms of the disease. CT studies in patients with PML characteristically reveal hypodense, nonenhancing lesions confined to the white matter. Traditionally, a brain biopsy has been required for definitive diagnosis; however, PCR of the CSF for JC virus DNA appears to be a useful assay. In many cases, there is progressive decline over the course of 4 to 5 months until death. There appears to be, however, a spectrum of disease possibly related to the degree of immune competence in HIV-infected persons. Stabilization of symptoms, either without treatment or in the setting of antiretroviral therapy, occurs in some patients with relatively high CD4 counts (>200), for whom PML is the CDC AIDS-defining illness. A controlled clinical trial showed no benefit of either IV or intrathecal araC when added to antiretroviral therapy; however, the topoisomerase inhibitor Topecan, which is active against both HIV and JC virus, is in pilot clinical trials for PML and may be more promising.

Also referred to as AIDS-related dementia and AIDS encephalopathy, the AIDS dementia complex is characterized by a progressive impairment in cognitive function that is accompanied by behavioral changes and motor abnormalities. Early in the course, patients with the AIDS dementia complex experience impairments in cognitive function, such as forgetfulness and an inability to concentrate, and personality changes, including apathy, withdrawal, and depression. As the condition progresses, the behavioral and motor abnormalities become more prominent and leg weakness, a loss of balance, and clumsiness of the arm and hands are common complaints. Late in the course, ataxia, psychiatric disturbances, mutism, paraplegia, incontinence, and myoclonus occur. CT scans reveal cortical atrophy and ventricular enlargement in most patients. Additionally, some patients have patchy or diffuse T_2-weighted abnormalities on MRI in the hemispheric white matter and, less commonly, the basal ganglia or thalamus. Most patients succumb within a few months after the onset of severe dementia. The severity of AIDS dementia complex parallels CSF levels of

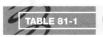
TABLE 81-1   **Useful Web Sites**

Web site	Address
Academy of Neurology Guidelines	http://www.aan.com/professionals/practice/pdfs/gl0079.pdf
Project Inform	http://www.projinf.org/fs/cryptoco.html
HIVpositive.com	http://www.hivpositive.com/index.html
Medline Plus	http://www.nlm.nih.gov/medlineplus/ency/article/000642.htm
CDC Toxoplasmosis Site	http://www.cdc.gov/ncidod/dpd/parasites/toxoplasmosis/

HIV-1 RNA. Among the nucleoside reverse transcriptase inhibitors, zidovudine, stavudine, and abacavir likely have the best penetration, and lamivudine penetrates to a lesser extent. Nevirapine, a nonnucleoside reverse transcriptase inhibitor, also has favorable penetration.

Table 81-1 presents useful Web sites. (JWM)

Bibliography

Aberg JA, et al. A pilot study of the discontinuation of antifungal therapy for disseminated cryptococcal disease in patients with acquired immunodeficiency syndrome, following immunologic response to antiretroviral therapy. *J Infect Dis* 2002;185:1179–1182.
Disseminated cryptococcal disease can be cured by prolonged antifungal therapy in some patients with AIDS who experience sustained CD4 lymphocyte increases while receiving HAART.

Aberg JA, et al. Clinical utility of monitoring serum cryptococcal antigen (sCRAg) titers in patients with AIDS-related cryptococcal disease. *HIV Clin Trials* 2000;1:1–6.
Although in the majority of patients the sCRAg titers appeared to decrease over time, we could not detect a significant correlation between sCRAg titer results of patients who had a clinical response to treatment and sCRAg titers in patients who experienced persistent disease, probable relapse, or definitive relapse of cryptococcal disease. We conclude that follow-up monitoring of the sCRAg titer is not useful in the management of patients with AIDS-related cryptococcal disease on treatment.

Aller AI, et al. Correlation of fluconazole MICs with clinical outcome in cryptococcal infection. *Antimicrob Agents Chemother* 2000;44:1544–1548.
It appears that the clinical outcome after fluconazole maintenance therapy may be better when the infecting C. neoformans strain is inhibited by lower concentrations of fluconazole for eradication (minimum inhibitory concentrations [MICs] <16 μg/mL) than when the patients are infected with strains that require higher fluconazole concentrations (MICs ≥16 μg/mL).

Andreoletti L, et al. Semiquantitative detection of JCV-DNA in peripheral blood leukocytes from HIV-1-infected patients with or without progressive multifocal leukoencephalopathy. *J Med Virol* 2002;66:1–7.
The predictive positive value of a positive JCV DNA PCR in peripheral blood cells for the diagnosis of PML in an HIV-infected patient was 16%, whereas the predictive negative value was 96%.

Antinori A, et al. Value of combined approach with thallium-201 single-photon emission computed tomography and Epstein-Barr virus DNA polymerase chain reaction in CSF for the diagnosis of AIDS-related primary CNS lymphoma. *J Clin Oncol* 1999;17:554–560.
Combined SPECT and EBV-DNA showed a very high diagnostic accuracy for AIDS-related primary CNS lymphoma (PCNSL). Because PCNSL likelihood is extremely high in patients with hyperactive lesions and positive EBV-DNA, brain biopsy could be avoided, and patients could promptly undergo radiotherapy or multimodal therapy. On the contrary, in patients showing hypoactive lesions with negative EBV-DNA, empiric anti-Toxoplasma therapy is indicated. In patients with discordant SPECT/PCR results, brain biopsy seems to be advisable.

Apisarnthanarak A, Powderly WG. Treatment of acute cryptococcal disease. *Expert Opin Pharmacother* 2001;2:1259–1268.
Currently, amphotericin B with or without flucytosine is regarded as the best initial therapy for patients with meningitis or more severe illness, although the azoles and other formulations of amphotericin B can be considered in other situations.

Choi SH, et al. The possible role of cerebrospinal fluid adenosine deaminase activity in the diagnosis of tuberculous meningitis in adults. *Clin Neurol Neurosurg* 2002;104:10–15.
Values higher than 15 U/L were not observed in any of the nontuberculous meningitis patients; therefore, adenosine deaminase (ADA) activity higher than 15 U/L could be a strong indication of tuberculous meningitis.

Cingolani A, et al. PCR detection of Toxoplasma gondii DNA in CSF for the differential diagnosis of AIDS-related focal brain lesions. *J Med Microbiol* 1996;45:472–476.
Six of 18 patients with toxoplasmic encephalitis, but none of the 70 patients with other disorders, were PCR positive (33.3% sensitivity and 100% specificity). Despite the

moderate sensitivity, the high specificity and positive predictive value (100%) make this assay a useful tool in the differential diagnosis of AIDS-related focal brain lesions as part of a series of CSF and neuroradiologic examinations.

Cinti SK, et al. Case report. Recurrence of increased intracranial pressure with antiretroviral therapy in an AIDS patient with cryptococcal meningitis. *Mycoses* 2001;44:497–501.

This is the first report of symptomatic elevated intracranial pressure occurring during HAART-related immune recovery in a patient with cryptococcal meningitis. Exacerbation of symptoms does not necessarily reflect mycologic failure that requires a change in antifungal therapy, but may relate to acutely increased intracranial pressure that will respond to simple measures, such as repeated lumbar punctures.

Dubois V, et al. Detection of JC virus DNA in the peripheral blood leukocytes of HIV-infected patients. *AIDS* 1996;10:353–358.

JCV DNA is detectable in the peripheral blood leukocytes (PBL) of 28.9% of HIV-infected persons, even in the early stages of infection. JCV is more seldomly amplified in HIV-negative immunocompromised patients. Further work is in progress to determine the prognostic value of the presence of JCV DNA in the blood of HIV-positive patients.

Dubois V, et al. Prevalence of JC virus viraemia in HIV-infected patients with or without neurological disorders: a prospective study. *J Neurovirol* 1998;4:539–544.

PML is a severe demyelinating disease, which is rapidly fatal and is caused by JCV infection, which especially occurs in HIV-infected patients. To investigate JCV pathophysiology and to evaluate the predictive value of JCV detection in blood, we looked for JCV DNA in leukocytes and plasma of 96 patients without any neurologic symptoms and 109 patients with neurologic diseases, among whom 19 were suffering from PML. JCV genome was detected in about 18% of all patients, i.e., 15.6% of patients with CNS disorders except PML, 13.5% of patients without neurologic symptoms, and significantly more often in PML patients (47.6%). Both leukocytes and plasma were tested; in plasma, JCV DNA was found in 36.1% of positive patients and in cells in 80.5%. Surprisingly in seven instances only the plasma contained JCV genome. One-year follow-up of these patients showed that the absence of JCV DNA in blood was associated with a very low probability of developing PML (negative predictive value = 0.99).

Eggers C, et al. Quantification of JC virus DNA in the cerebrospinal fluid of patients with human immunodeficiency virus-associated progressive multifocal leukoencephalopathy—a longitudinal study. *J Infect Dis* 1999;180:1690–1694.

Whereas an overall increase during progressive disease was confirmed, the virus burden was either constant or fluctuated irregularly during the intermediate stage of disease. This shows a variability of viral shedding during active disease that must be taken into account when the JCV load is measured by quantitative PCR for both the diagnosis of PML and monitoring under investigational treatment.

Feldmesser M, et al. Serum cryptococcal antigen in patients with AIDS. *Clin Infect Dis* 1996;23:827–830.

Ferrante P, et al. Comprehensive investigation of the presence of JC virus in AIDS patients with and without progressive multifocal leukoencephalopathy. *J Med Virol* 1997;52:235–242.

PML, a viral-induced demyelinating disease, is becoming relatively common, yet many diagnostic and pathogenetic aspects remain to be clarified. A study was undertaken in 64 AIDS patients suffering from various neurologic disorders, including PML (12 subjects), with the specific objective of searching for JCV DNA by nested PCR (n-PCR) in CSF, peripheral blood mononuclear cells (PBMCs), and urine collected from all patients. CSF examination, CD4 and CD8 counts, neurologic examinations, and neuroradiologic investigations were undertaken. JCV DNA was detected in 92% of CSF specimens in 75% of the PBMCs and urine samples from the PML patients, whereas among the non-PML patients JCV DNA was not detected in any CSF samples, but was found in 10% of PBMCs and in 39% of the urine specimens. BK virus (BKV) and JCV DNA viruria was observed simultaneously in 6% of the AIDS patients without PML. The routine CSF tests, including IgG oligoclonal bands, the Link, and Tourtellotte IgG indexes, did not show a typical pattern in PML cases. The data obtained clearly indicate that the detection of JCV DNA in CSF constitutes an efficient marker for PML diagnosis. The simultaneous presence of JCV DNA in the CSF, PBMCs, and urine samples from the

PML patients, who did not differ from controls with regard to their immunosuppressive status, suggests that JCV could be carried into the CNS by infected PBMCs.

Ferrante P, et al. PCR detection of JC virus DNA in brain tissue from patients with and without progressive multifocal leukoencephalopathy. *J Med Virol* 1995;47:219–225.
All 28 brain specimens from the patients with PML were positive for JCV DNA when tested by n-PCR and three of the latter were also positive for BKV DNA. These results were confirmed by an enzyme restriction analysis and a DNA hybridization assay. Interestingly, in this study, JCV DNA was also found in six brain tissue specimens from four subjects with diseases unrelated to PML or AIDS.

Gambarin K J, Hamill R.J. Management of increased intracranial pressure in cryptococcal meningitis. *Curr Infect Dis Rep* 2002;4:332–338.
Optimal therapy has not yet been firmly established, but the diagnostic evaluation and available treatment options are reviewed here, including frequent high-volume lumbar punctures, lumbar drains, ventriculoperitoneal shunting, and corticosteroids.

Garcia De Viedma D, et al. JC virus load in progressive multifocal leukoencephalopathy: analysis of the correlation between the viral burden in cerebrospinal fluid, patient survival, and the volume of neurological lesions. *Clin Infect Dis* 2002;34:1568–1575.
Virus load values of more than 4.68 log were associated with shorter patient survival time. No correlation was found between the virus load values and the global volume of brain tissue damaged. Our data suggest that factors other than the volume of neurologic lesions influence the shedding of JCV in the CSF.

Gasnault J, et al. Prolonged survival without neurological improvement in patients with AIDS-related progressive multifocal leukoencephalopathy on potent combined antiretroviral therapy. *J Neurovirol* 1999;5:421–429.
Their results demonstrate a benefit of combined antiretroviral therapy (CART) on survival of AIDS-related PML patients and suggest the need for an early, specific anti-JC virus treatment to limit the neurologic deterioration.

Giri JA, et al. Polyoma virus JC DNA detection by polymerase chain reaction in CSF of HIV infected patients with suspected progressive multifocal leukoencephalopathy. *Am Clin Lab* 2001;20:33–35.
Several studies had previously demonstrated the high sensitivity and specificity of JCV DNA detection in CSF by PCR. Many recent studies report a significant benefit of combined antiretroviral therapy on the survival of HIV patients without clear neurologic improvements. A negative correlation has been described between the concentration of JCV in the CSF and survival time in HIV-1 infected patients, and the level of immune depression may influence JCV replication. This suggests that a single CSF JCV viral load determination during the course of PML disease progression may be of prognostic value for managing HIV patients.

Heald AE, et al. Differentiation of central nervous system lesions in AIDS patients using positron emission tomography (PET). *Int J STD AIDS* 1996;7:337–346.
FDG-PET could accurately differentiate lymphoma from infections in 16 of 18 cases. Two cases of PML had high metabolic activity and could not be differentiated from lymphoma. FDG-PET shows great promise in differentiating lymphoma from infectious lesions in the CNS of patients with HIV infection.

Holland NR, et al. Cytomegalovirus encephalitis in acquired immunodeficiency syndrome (AIDS). *Neurology* 1994;44:507–514.
PCR of CSF samples identified CMV genome in 33% of cytomegalovirus encephalitis (CMVE) cases. CMVE was associated with periventricular enhancement on CTs and periventricular lesions with meningeal enhancement on MRI scans. CMVE should be particularly suspected in homosexual men presenting with subacute encephalopathy who have had AIDS for more than 1 year and have a history of systemic CMV infection. Other features supporting the diagnosis of CMVE include periventricular lesions, hyponatremia, and identification of CMV genome in CSF by PCR.

King MD, et al. Paradoxical recurrent meningitis following therapy of cryptococcal meningitis: an immune reconstitution syndrome after initiation of highly active antiretroviral therapy. *Int J STD AIDS* 2002;13:724–726.
Reported is a case of paradoxical recurrent meningitis in response to initiation of HAART in a patient receiving maintenance fluconazole for a previous diagnosis of cryptococcal meningitis.

Koralnik IJ, et al. JC virus DNA load in patients with and without progressive multifocal leukoencephalopathy. *Neurology* 1999;52:253–260.

The presence of JCV in the CSF is highly sensitive and specific for PML, and a high CSF JC viral load was associated with poor clinical outcome in patients receiving antiretroviral therapy. JCV quantification in the CSF constitutes a potentially important tool for monitoring clinical PML treatment trials.

Larsen RA. Treatment of cryptococcal meningitis. *N Engl J Med* 1997;337:1557; discussion 1557–1558.

Larsen RA, et al. Fluconazole combined with flucytosine for treatment of cryptococcal meningitis in patients with AIDS. *Clin Infect Dis* 1994;19:741–745.

In this pilot study of fluconazole combined with flucytosine, the rate of clinical success at 10 weeks was greater than that previously reported with regard to the use of fluconazole alone or amphotericin B alone.

Leenders AC, et al. Liposomal amphotericin B (AmBisome) compared with amphotericin B both followed by oral fluconazole in the treatment of AIDS-associated cryptococcal meningitis. *AIDS* 1997;11:1463–1471.

A 3-week course of 4 mg/kg AmBisome resulted in a significantly earlier CSF culture conversion than 0.7 mg/kg amphotericin B, had equal clinical efficacy, and was significantly less nephrotoxic when used for the treatment of primary episodes of AIDS-associated cryptococcal meningitis.

Liliang PC, et al. Use of ventriculoperitoneal shunts to treat uncontrollable intracranial hypertension in patients who have cryptococcal meningitis without hydrocephalus. *Clin Infect Dis* 2002;34:E64–E68.

Uncontrollable elevation of intracranial pressure associated with cryptococcal meningitis can be resolved by use of a ventriculoperitoneal (VP) shunt, even when imaging studies do not reveal hydrocephalus.

Low WK. Cryptococcal meningitis: implications for the otologist. *ORL J Otorhinolaryngol Relat Spec* 2002;64:35–37.

Cryptococcal meningitis can present to the otologist with hearing loss and vestibular dysfunction. Retrocochlear damage may result in cochlear implantation having a poor outcome.

Mamidi A, et al. Central nervous system infections in individuals with HIV-1 infection. *J Neurovirol* 2002;8:158–167.

We review the epidemiology, pathogenesis, clinical features, diagnosis, and management of five common CNS disorders in individuals with HIV-1 infection: TE, primary CNS lymphoma, cryptococcal meningitis, CMVE, and PML.

Martinez E, et al. Discontinuation of secondary prophylaxis for cryptococcal meningitis in HIV-infected patients responding to highly active antiretroviral therapy. *AIDS* 2000;4:2615–2617.

Matsiota-Bernard P, et al. JC virus detection in the cerebrospinal fluid of AIDS patients with progressive multifocal leucoencephalopathy and monitoring of the antiviral treatment by a PCR method. *J Med Microbiol* 1997;46:256–259.

The PCR method is useful for the detection of JCV in CSF samples and in the diagnosis of PML. However, the application of PCR for monitoring the effect of treatment remains to be established.

Menichetti F, et al. High-dose fluconazole therapy for cryptococcal meningitis in patients with AIDS. *Clin Infect Dis* 1996;22:838–840.

Fluconazole (800–1,000 mg IV) was administered to 14 consecutive patients with AIDS and cryptococcal meningitis. At 10 weeks the rate of clinical success was 54.5%. At the end of treatment, eight (72.7%) of 11 patients responded to fluconazole. The median time to the first negative CSF culture was 33.5 days (95% confidence interval [CI], 18.3–67.3); the median time for patients with initial CSF cryptococcal antigen titers of 1:1,024 or more was 66 days compared with 18 days for patients with initial CSF cryptococcal antigen titers of less than 1:1,024 (P = .06). The median time to the first negative CSF culture for patients with an isolate for which the MIC was 4 μg/mL was 56 days compared with 16 days for patients with an isolate for which the MIC was less than 4 μg/mL (P = .11). High-dose fluconazole might be an effective and well-tolerated therapeutic option for patients with AIDS and acute cryptococcal meningitis.

Nelson MR, et al. The role of azoles in the treatment and prophylaxis of cryptococcal disease in HIV infection. *AIDS* 1994;8:651–654.

Fluconazole is an effective treatment for cryptococcal meningitis. For prophylaxis after meningitis, a dose of 400 mg fluconazole is the preferred treatment; lower doses are associated with a higher relapse rate.

Newton PN, et al. A randomized, double-blind, placebo-controlled trial of acetazolamide for the treatment of elevated intracranial pressure in cryptococcal meningitis. *Clin Infect Dis* 2002;35:769–772.

The trial was terminated prematurely because patients who received acetazolamide developed significantly lower venous bicarbonate levels and higher chloride levels and had more frequent serious adverse events than did subjects who received placebo.

Nwokolo NC, et al. Cessation of secondary prophylaxis in patients with cryptococcosis. *AIDS* 2001;15:1438–1439.

The authors report their experience of the cessation of secondary antifungal prophylaxis in patients responding to highly active antiretroviral therapy.

Powderly WG. Editorial response: management of cryptococcal meningitis–have we answered all the questions? *Clin Infect Dis* 1996;22:329–330.

Powderly WG. Recent advances in the management of cryptococcal meningitis in patients with AIDS. *Clin Infect Dis* 1996;22(suppl 2):S119–S123.

The drug of choice for maintenance therapy is fluconazole (200 mg/day). A recent trial showed that fluconazole was superior to itraconazole (200 mg/day) as suppressive therapy.

Powderly WG, et al. A controlled trial of fluconazole or amphotericin B to prevent relapse of cryptococcal meningitis in patients with the acquired immunodeficiency syndrome. The NIAID AIDS Clinical Trials Group and Mycoses Study Group. *N Engl J Med* 1992;326:793–798.

Fluconazole taken by mouth is superior to weekly intravenous therapy with amphotericin B to prevent relapse in patients with AIDS-associated cryptococcal meningitis after primary treatment with amphotericin B.

Robinson PA, et al. Early mycological treatment failure in AIDS-associated cryptococcal meningitis. *Clin Infect Dis* 1999;28:82–92.

Multivariate analyses identified that titer of cryptococcal antigen in CSF, serum albumin level, and CD4 cell count, together with dose of amphotericin B, had the strongest joint association with failure to achieve negative CSF cultures by day 14. Among patients with similar CSF cryptococcal antigen titers, CD4 cell counts, and serum albumin levels, the odds of failure at week 10 for those without negative CSF cultures by day 14 was five times that for those with negative CSF cultures by day 14 (odds ratio, 5.0; 95% CI, 2.2–10.9). Prognosis is dismal for patients with AIDS-related cryptococcal meningitis.

Rollot F, et al. Discontinuation of secondary prophylaxis against cryptococcosis in patients with AIDS receiving highly active antiretroviral therapy. *AIDS* 2001;15:1448–1449.

Saag MS, et al. A comparison of itraconazole versus fluconazole as maintenance therapy for AIDS-associated cryptococcal meningitis. National Institute of Allergy and Infectious Diseases Mycoses Study Group. *Clin Infect Dis* 1999;28:291–296.

The factor best associated with relapse was the patient having not received flucytosine during the initial 2 weeks of primary treatment for cryptococcal disease (relative risk = 5.88; 95% CI, 1.27–27.14; P = .04). Fluconazole remains the treatment of choice for maintenance therapy for AIDS-associated cryptococcal disease. Flucytosine may contribute to the prevention of relapse if used during the first 2 weeks of primary therapy.

Saag MS, et al. Practice guidelines for the management of cryptococcal disease. Infectious Diseases Society of America. *Clin Infect Dis* 2000;30:710–718.

Among patients with HIV infection and cryptococcal meningitis, induction therapy with amphotericin B (0.7–1 mg/kg per day) plus flucytosine (100 mg/kg per day for 2 weeks) followed by fluconazole (400 mg/day) for a minimum of 10 weeks is the treatment of choice. After 10 weeks of therapy, the fluconazole dosage may be reduced to 200 mg/day, depending on the patient's clinical status. Fluconazole should be continued for life. An alternative regimen for AIDS-associated cryptococcal meningitis is amphotericin B (0.7–1 mg/kg per day) plus 5-flucytosine (100 mg/kg per day) for 6 to 10 weeks, followed by fluconazole maintenance therapy. Induction therapy beginning with an azole alone is generally discouraged. Lipid formulations of amphotericin B can be substituted for amphotericin B for patients whose renal function is impaired. Fluconazole (400–800 mg/ day) plus flucytosine (100–150 mg/kg per day) for 6 weeks is an alternative to the use of amphotericin B, although toxicity with this regimen is high.

Sheng WH, et al. Successful discontinuation of fluconazole as secondary prophylaxis for cryptococcosis in AIDS patients responding to highly active antiretroviral therapy. *Int J STD AIDS* 2002;13:702–705.

No relapse of cryptococcosis was detected in these patients after a median observation duration of 9 months (range, 5.5–4.1 months, mean, 14.6 months) after discontinuation.

Skiest DJ. Focal neurological disease in patients with acquired immunodeficiency syndrome. *Clin Infect Dis* 2002;34:103–115.

The combination of PCR and neuroimaging techniques may obviate the need for brain biopsy in selected cases. However, stereotactic brain biopsy, which is associated with relatively low morbidity rates, remains the reference standard for diagnosis. Highly active antiretroviral therapy has improved the prognosis of several focal CNS processes, most notably toxoplasmosis, PML, and CMV encephalitis.

Skiest DJ, et al. SPECT thallium-201 combined with Toxoplasma serology for the presumptive diagnosis of focal central nervous system mass lesions in patients with AIDS. *J Infect* 2000;40:274–281.

In a series of HIV-infected patients, Tl-201 SPECT was able to accurately differentiate primary brain lymphoma from other causes of focal CNS lesions in most patients; however, both false-positive and false-negative results occurred. By combining Tl-201 SPECT with serum Toxoplasma IgG, diagnostic accuracy was improved.

Straus DJ. Human immunodeficiency virus-associated lymphomas. *Med Clin North Am* 1997;81:495–510.

The important features of the HIV-associated CNS lymphomas are also described.

Vago L, et al. JCV-DNA and BKV-DNA in the CNS tissue and CSF of AIDS patients and normal subjects. Study of 41 cases and review of the literature. *J Acquir Immune Defic Syndr Hum Retrovirol* 1996;12:139–146.

Their data demonstrates that JCV-DNA and, rarely, BKV-DNA can be detected in the CNS of immunocompromised patients with and without PML and in the CNS of HIV-negative subjects. However, only HIV-positive patients with clinically evident PML and JCV-DNA in the brain have PCR-detectable JCV-DNA in their CSF.

van der Horst CM, et al. Treatment of cryptococcal meningitis associated with the acquired immunodeficiency syndrome. National Institute of Allergy and Infectious Diseases Mycoses Study Group and AIDS Clinical Trials Group. *N Engl J Med* 1997;337: 15–21.

Although consolidation therapy with fluconazole is associated with a higher rate of CSF sterilization, itraconazole may be a suitable alternative for patients unable to take fluconazole.

Witt MD, et al. Identification of patients with acute AIDS-associated cryptococcal meningitis who can be effectively treated with fluconazole: the role of antifungal susceptibility testing. *Clin Infect Dis* 1996;22:322–328.

Logistic regression modeling revealed that a negative blood culture, a low MIC of fluconazole (per the microtiter method), and treatment with flucytosine were factors independently associated with successful treatment.

Wright D, et al. Central nervous system opportunistic infections. *Neuroimaging Clin North Am* 1997;7:513–525.

The neuroimaging features, when coupled with the clinical and laboratory findings, often suggest the correct diagnosis and enable the physician to initiate therapy.

Yiannoutsos CT, et al. Relation of JC virus DNA in the cerebrospinal fluid to survival in acquired immunodeficiency syndrome patients with biopsy-proven progressive multifocal leukoencephalopathy. *Ann Neurol* 1999;45:816–821.

The detection and semiquantitation of JCV DNA in CSF is prognostic of survival and is a marker of the course of PML. CSF samples from 15 AIDS patients with biopsy-proven PML were analyzed by semiquantitative PCR. A low JCV burden was predictive of longer survival compared with a high JCV burden (median survival from entry, 24 [2–63] vs. 7.6 [4–17] weeks). Further analyses indicated a possible threshold of 50 to 100 copies/µL separating high- and moderate-risk cases. Patients with a JCV load below this level survived longer than those with a JCV load above it.

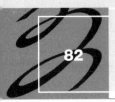

82   FEVER IN THE HIV-INFECTED PATIENT

*W*hen an HIV-infected patient has a fever for more than 4 weeks without an obvious cause, the condition can be defined as fever of unknown origin (FUO). An infectious etiology is overwhelmingly the most common cause of FUO in HIV-infected patients in contrast to other types of patients with FUO. When the CD4 cell count is below 200/mm^3, the clinician should resist the temptation to attribute the fever to the HIV infection itself; prophylactic trimethoprim-sulfamethoxazole (TMP-SMX) reduces, but does not eliminate, the possibility of *Pneumocystis carinii* pneumonia (PCP) and invasive toxoplasmosis. Respiratory symptoms may be more subtle than one would expect in these cases of PCP, and a high index of suspicion is needed to make the diagnosis. A fever without associated symptoms can be the exclusive presentation of PCP, toxoplasmosis, invasive cryptococcal disease, tuberculosis, or lymphoma.

A single etiology was determined in the majority of patients in a recent large retrospective analysis, but up to 20% may have multiple etiologies. Regional variations in the prevalence of these infections account for the differences noted between series reported from Europe compared with the United States. Tuberculosis and leishmaniasis are much more commonly reported from France and Spain than from the United States as causes of FUO. Chaga's disease is a possibility for patients from endemic areas. Even within the United States, differences in the prevalence of endemic fungi such as histoplasmosis vary widely according to geography. For the IV drug addict with HIV infection, more fevers are caused by bacterial infections (pneumonia, soft-tissue infections, bacteremia, endocarditis, septic arthritis, osteomyelitis, tuberculosis) as compared with other risk groups (Table 82-1).

When fever develops in an HIV-infected patient with a CD4 cell count above 200/mm^3, diagnostic considerations would include bacterial infections, drug abuse-related disorders, tuberculosis, and other disorders more so than traditional opportunistic infections. Neutropenia is a risk factor for bacteremia in the HIV-infected patient, and the possibility of endocarditis should be considered in patients with a history of drug abuse. It is essential that the physician assessing a febrile, HIV-infected patient with a CD4 cell count above 200/mm^3 perform a careful and thorough examination, and if no obvious clues to the source of the

TABLE 82-1   **Major Causes of Fever by Location***

GI tract	Pulmonary	Esophagus	Eye	Skin
CMV	PCP	HSV	CMV	Bacillary
Isospora	TB	MAC·	Toxoplasmosis	Angiomatosis
Cyclospora	Histoplasmosis	CMV		Kaposi's sarcoma
Microspòridia	Pneumococcus	Candida		
Salmonella	Lymphoma			
Lymphoma				

*See Chapter 81 as well.
TB, Tuberculosis; HSV, Herpes simplex virus.

fever are revealed by the medical history and physical examination, arrange for a complete blood count (CBC), blood cultures, urinalysis, evaluation of liver enzymes, and chest roentgenography. However, it is important to appreciate that chest roentgenogram findings may be negative in a patient who has PCP, and analysis of induced sputum with stains and cultures can be helpful to establish the diagnosis of PCP. If these tests are negative, a bronchoalveolar lavage should be considered.

For the patient with a CD4 cell count below 200/mm^3, there must be more concern for opportunistic infections. Numerous investigations have identified rather characteristic CD4 cell counts for specific opportunistic infections (PCP, <200 mm^3; toxoplasmosis, <100/mm^3; histoplasmosis, <100/mm^3; *Mycobacterium avium* complex [MAC] infection, <50/mm^3; and cytomegalovirus [CMV] infection, <50/mm^3). Febrile AIDS patients who present a particular diagnostic challenge include the following: patients with tuberculosis or PCP who have either no respiratory symptoms or normal chest roentgenography findings; those with central nervous system toxoplasmosis in the absence of neurologic manifestations; patients with symptoms of invasive MAC infection weeks to months before detection of the organism on blood cultures; patients with disseminated histoplasmosis and no pulmonary symptoms or chest roentgenography abnormalities; and patients receiving numerous medications, any one of which has the potential to cause fever. CMV infection may result in pneumonia, colitis, and meningoencephalitis rather than as retinitis in some patients.

Drugs may also cause fever, and the list of medications capable of producing drug-related fever is extensive and includes such compounds as antimicrobials (trimethoprim-sulfamethoxazole [TMP-SMX], clindamycin, amphotericin B, dapsone), antimycobacterials (isoniazid, rifampin), antineoplastic agents (bleomycin, methotrexate), and antiepileptics (phenytoin, carbamazepine). Protease inhibitors also may cause diarrhea and kidney stones. Pentamidine and nucleoside analogues may cause pancreatitis as well. Nucleoside analogues (especially combinations of ddi/d4t) also may cause a lactic acidosis syndrome that might be confused with sepsis.

If the initial history and physical examination (including a dilated ophthalmologic study), chest roentgenogram, routine blood cultures, serum liver chemistries, and studies of induced sputa fail to explain the patient's febrile state, additional diagnostic studies include an assay for serum cryptococcal antigen; lysis–centrifugation blood cultures (to isolate *Bartonella henselae, Histoplasma capsulatum,* MAC); sinus roentgenography; a gallium 67 scan; and a serum lactate dehydrogenase determination (a significantly elevated concentration is suggestive of PCP, tuberculosis, toxoplasmosis, disseminated histoplasmosis, or lymphoma). A negative gallium scan would help exclude PCP. Persistent unexplained fever would suggest the need for computed tomography of the chest (pathologic adenopathy would suggest tuberculosis or lymphoma), abdomen (to detect MAC infection, tuberculosis, CMV colitis, hepatic abscess, splenic abscess, infectious cholangitis, visceral Kaposi's sarcoma, and non-Hodgkin's lymphoma), and brain (to detect toxoplasmosis in the patient without neurologic manifestations); analysis of the cerebrospinal fluid (to identify evidence of tuberculosis, cryptococcosis, or lymphoma); and, if the epidemiologic history is appropriate, a test for *Histoplasma* antigen in urine and serum. On occasion, biopsy for peritoneal masses or abnormal retroperitoneal lymph nodes, guided by computed tomography, will establish the cause of fever.

If the above studies are negative and the patient is anemic or losing weight, a bone marrow aspiration and biopsy should be considered. Alternatively, if there is no contraindication, and particularly if the patient demonstrates abnormal liver enzymes, splenomegaly, or peripheral lymphadenopathy, the more sensitive liver biopsy might be undertaken. These procedures have the potential to assist in the diagnosis of MAC infection, tuberculosis, cryptococcosis, histoplasmosis, and lymphoma. Disseminated MAC infection is the single most common cause of HIV-associated FUO in the United States, and empiric therapy against this pathogen might be useful after obtaining blood cultures for this organism. (JWM)

Bibliography

Armstrong WS, et al. Human immunodeficiency virus-associated fever of unknown origin: a study of 70 patients in the United States and review. *Clin Infect Dis* 1999;28:341–345.

The most common diagnoses were disseminated Mycobacterium avium *complex infection (DMAC, 31%), PCP (13%), CMV infection (11%), disseminated histoplasmosis (7%), and lymphoma (7%). In this U.S. series, FUO occurs most often in the late stage of HIV infection, individual cases often have multiple etiologies, and DMAC is the most common diagnosis.*

Barbado FJ, et al. Fever of unknown origin: classic and associated with human immunodeficiency virus infection. a comparative study. *J Med* 2001;32:152–162.

The authors concluded that predominance of Mycobacteria *and absence of collagen diseases make FUO associated with HIV a different form of FUO. No differences were found in approach and time to diagnosis.*

Chariyalertsak S, et al. Case-control study of risk factors for Penicillium marneffei infection in human immunodeficiency virus-infected patients in northern Thailand. *Clin Infect Dis* 1997;24:1080–1086.

The author's data suggest that recent exposure to a potential environmental reservoir of organisms in the soil may be associated with disseminated P. marneffei *infections among patients with AIDS in Northern Thailand.*

Francisci D, et al. The pp65 antigenaemia test as a predictor of cytomegalovirus-induced end-organ disease in patients with AIDS. *AIDS* 1997;11:1341–1345.

The negative predictive value (NPV) of the test was 92%, and the positive predictive value (PPV) was 45.8%. This test could be used as an alternative to polymerase chain reaction in order to select patients at higher risk of CMV disease who can be treated with preemptive anti-CMV therapy.

Lambertucci JR, et al. Fever of undetermined origin in patients with the acquired immunodeficiency syndrome in Brazil: report on 55 cases. *Rev Inst Med Trop Sao Paulo* 1999;41:27–32.

The medical records of patients with AIDS admitted to a general hospital in Brazil from 1989 to 1997 were reviewed retrospectively with the aim at defining the frequency and etiology of FUO in HIV-infected patients of a tropical country and to evaluate the usefulness of the main diagnostic procedures.

Lozano F, et al. Impact of highly active antiretroviral therapy on fever of unknown origin in HIV-infected patients. *Eur J Clin Microbiol Infect Dis* 2002;21:137–139.

The study findings suggest that the use of highly active antiretroviral therapy (HAART) has reduced the frequency of fever of unknown origin in HIV-infected patients, but the etiology of the condition remains mostly unchanged.

Mayo J, et al. Fever of unknown origin in the HIV-infected patient: new scenario for an old problem. *Scand J Infect Dis* 1997;29:327–336.

Some HIV-infected patients with FUO remain undiagnosed after a thorough investigation; these individuals should be managed conservatively. Symptomatic treatment is the best option for terminally ill patients in whom benefit from a detailed investigation of the cause of fever is not expected.

Mayo J, et al. Fever of unknown origin in the setting of HIV infection: guidelines for a rational approach. *AIDS Patient Care STDS* 1998;12:373–378.

In this overview the authors stress, from a practical point of view, some points to be considered in the evaluation of the HIV-infected patient who presents with fever of unknown origin, as well as the usefulness and yield of several diagnostic procedures.

Miller RF, et al. Pyrexia of undetermined origin in patients with human immunodeficiency virus infection and AIDS. *Int J STD AIDS* 1996;7:170–175.

Unexplained fever in this patient group should not be ascribed to HIV infection itself and should be vigorously investigated to find a cause.

Rodriguez JN, et al. [Usefulness of bone marrow examination in patients with advanced HIV infection]. *Rev Clin Esp* 1996;196:213–216.

In the authors' experience, the investigation of bone marrow specimen was of little help to clarify the possible etiology of cytopenia and febrile syndromes of unknown origin in patients with advanced HIV infection.

Roger PM, et al. Liver biopsy is not useful in the diagnosis of mycobacterial infections in patients who are infected with human immunodeficiency virus. *Clin Infect Dis* 1996;23:1302–1304.

Liver biopsy (LB) has been advocated for the detection of mycobacterial infections in patients infected with HIV. Noninvasive studies are preferable to LB for the diagnosis of mycobacterial infections in HIV-infected patients.

Sartori AM, et al. Follow-up of 18 patients with human immunodeficiency virus infection and chronic Chagas' disease, with reactivation of Chagas' disease causing cardiac disease in three patients. *Clin Infect Dis* 1998;26:177–179.

A series of 18 patients with chronic Chagas' disease and HIV infection were followed up for 2 to 66 months (median, 15.5 months). Specific antitrypanosomal treatment with benznidazole was effective in reducing the level of parasitemia and improving the clinical condition in three of the four patients treated.

Sepkowitz KA. FUO and AIDS. *Curr Clin Top Infect Dis* 1999;19:1–15.

Sirisanthana T, Supparatpinyo K. Epidemiology and management of penicilliosis in human immunodeficiency virus-infected patients. *Int J Infect Dis* 1998; 3:48–53.

Penicillium marneffei is a dimorphic fungus that can cause systemic mycosis in humans. It is endemic in Southeast Asia, the Guangxi province of China, Hong Kong, and Taiwan. The patients usually present with fever, anemia, weight loss, skin lesions, generalized lymphadenopathy, and hepatomegaly. The skin lesions are most commonly papules with central necrotic umbilication. The average number of CD4+ T lymphocytes at presentation is 64 cells/mm^3. The fungus is usually sensitive to amphotericin B, itraconazole, and ketoconazole.

Supparatpinyo K, et al. Penicillium marneffei infection in patients infected with human immunodeficiency virus. *Clin Infect Dis* 1992;14:871–874.

For 11 of these 21 patients, the presumptive diagnosis of P. marneffei infection could be made by microscopic examination of Wright's-stained bone marrow aspirate and/or touch smears of skin specimens obtained by biopsy several days before the results of culture were available.

Whitely W, et al. Pyrexia of undetermined origin in the era of HAART. *Sex Transm Infect* 2000;76:484–488.

General review of the subject.

PREVENTION OF OPPORTUNISTIC INFECTION IN THE HIV-INFECTED PATIENT

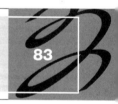

83

rimary prophylaxis in the HIV-positive patient is designed to prevent initial infection. *Secondary prophylaxis* is offered to prevent recurrence or reactivation of an established infection. Physicians should use prophylaxis for those disorders associated with substantial morbidity or mortality. Traditionally we have initiated prophylaxis based on the CD4 cell count, as researchers have identified the ranges within which most opportunistic infections are manifested. Before primary prophylaxis is initiated, one must exclude active disease. Traditionally, this is accomplished through a combination of medical history, physical examination, laboratory tests, and chest roentgenography (Table 83-1).

HIV-infected adults and adolescents, including pregnant women and those on highly active antiretroviral therapy (HAART), should receive primary chemoprophylaxis against *Pneumocystis carinii* pneumonia (PCP) if they have a CD4+ T-lymphocyte count of less than 200/μL or a history of oropharyngeal candidiasis. Persons who have a CD4+ T-lymphocyte percentage of less than 14% or a history of an AIDS-defining illness but do not otherwise qualify, should also be considered for prophylaxis. Trimethoprim-sulfamethoxazole (TMP-SMZ) is the recommended prophylactic agent. One double-strength tablet daily is the preferred regimen. However, 1 single-strength tablet daily is also effective and might

TABLE 83-1 Prevention of Opportunistic Illness

Opportunistic illness	Criteria for initiating primary prophylaxis	Criteria for discontinuing primary prophylaxis	Criteria for restarting primary prophylaxis	Criteria for initiating secondary prophylaxis	Criteria for discontinuing secondary prophylaxis	Criteria for restarting secondary prophylaxis
PCP[i]	CD4+ <200 cells/μL or oropharyngeal candidiasis	CD4+ >200 cells/μL for ≥3 months	CD4+ <200 cells/μL	Prior PEP	CD4+ >200 cells/μL for ≥3 months	CD4+ <200 cells/μL
Toxoplasmosis[ii]	IgG antibody to toxoplasma and CD4+ <100 cells/μL	CD4+ >200 cells/μL for ≥3 months	CD4+ <100–200 cells/μL	Prior toxoplasmic encephalitis	CD4+ >200 cells/μL sustained (e.g., ≥6 months) and Completed initial therapy and Asymptomatic for TE	CD4+ <200 cells/μL
Disseminated MAC[iii]	CD4+ <50 cells/μL	CD4+ >100 cells/μL for ≥3 months	CD4+ <50–100 cells/μL	Documented disseminated disease	CD4+ >100 cells/μL sustained (e.g., ≥6 months) and Completed 12 months of MAC therapy and Asymptomatic for MAC	CD4+ <100 cells/μL
Cryptococcosis[vi]	None	Not applicable	Not applicable	Documented disease	CD4+ >100–200 cells/μL sustained (e.g., ≥6 months) and Completed initial therapy and Asymptomatic for cryptococcosis	CD4+ <100–200 cells/μL

Pathogen					
Histoplasmosis[v]	None	Not applicable	Not applicable	Documented disease	No criteria recommended for stopping	Not applicable
Coccidioido-mycosis[vi]	None	Not applicable	Not applicable	Documented disease	No criteria recommended for stopping	Not applicable
Cytomegalo-virus[vii] retinitis	None	Not applicable	Not applicable	Documented end-organ disease	CD4+ >100–150 cells/µL sustained (e.g., ≥6 months) and No evidence of active disease Regular ophthalmic examination	CD4+ <100–150 cells/µL

[i] Chemoprophylaxis for PCP should be administered to pregnant women as is done for other adults and adolescents.

[ii] They should be advised not to eat raw or undercooked meat, particularly undercooked lamb, beef, pork, or venison. If the patient owns a cat, the litter box should be changed daily, preferably by an HIV-negative, nonpregnant person; alternatively, the patient should wash his or her hands thoroughly after changing the litter box. TMP-SMZ can be administered to pregnant women for prophylaxis against TE as described for PCP.

[iii] Organisms of MAC are common in environmental sources, such as food and water, but there are no specific recommendations regarding avoidance of exposure. Chemoprophylaxis for MAC disease should be administered to pregnant women as is done for other adults and adolescents. However, because of general concerns about administering drugs during the first trimester of pregnancy, some providers may choose to withhold prophylaxis during the first trimester. Azithromycin is the drug of choice. For secondary prophylaxis (chronic maintenance therapy), azithromycin plus ethambutol is the preferred drug treatment.

[iv] No evidence exists that exposure to pigeon droppings is associated with an increased risk for acquiring cryptococcosis. Prophylaxis with fluconazole or itraconazole should not be initiated during pregnancy.

[v] Patients whose CD4+ T-lymphocyte counts are less than 200 cells/µL should try to avoid activities known to be associated with increased risk (e.g., creating dust when working with surface soil; cleaning chicken coops that are heavily contaminated with droppings; disturbing soil beneath bird-roosting sites; cleaning, remodeling, or demolishing old buildings; and exploring caves). Because of the embryotoxicity and teratogenicity of itraconazole in animal systems, primary prophylaxis against histoplasmosis should not be offered during pregnancy.

[vi] Although HIV-infected persons living in or visiting areas in which coccidioidomycosis is endemic cannot completely avoid exposure to *Coccidioides immitis*, they should, when possible, avoid activities associated with increased risk. The potential teratogenicity of fluconazole and itraconazole should be considered when assessing the therapeutic options for HIV-infected women who become pregnant while receiving chronic maintenance therapy for coccidioidomycosis.

[vii] Indications for prophylaxis are the same for pregnant women as for nonpregnant women. The choice of agents to be used in pregnancy should be individualized after consultation with experts.

(Adapted from http://www.cdc.gov/mmwr/preview/mmwrhtml/rr5108a1.htmd).

be tolerated better than 1 double-strength tablet daily. Of note, 1 double-strength tablet three times weekly is also effective. TMP-SMX has the potential to decrease the development of other diseases, such as cerebral toxoplasmosis, isosporiosis, salmonellosis, and infections caused by *Nocardia* spp., *Listeria* spp., and *Haemophilus influenzae*. Patients who have experienced adverse events, including fever and rash, might better tolerate reintroduction of the drug with a gradual increase in dose (i.e., desensitization), according to published regimens or reintroduction of TMP-SMZ at a reduced dose or frequency. It is estimated that less than 70% of patients can tolerate such reinstitution of therapy. It has been shown that TMP-SMX can precipitate headache, nausea, vomiting, fever, pruritus, rash, and hematologic and hepatic toxicity, and this medication can produce drug–drug interactions with oral anticoagulants, phenytoin, glipizide, and methotrexate. If TMP-SMZ cannot be tolerated, prophylactic regimens that can be recommended as alternatives include dapsone, dapsone plus pyrimethamine plus leucovorin, aerosolized pentamidine administered by the Respirgard II^{TM} nebulizer, and atovaquone.

For patients seropositive for *Toxoplasma gondii* who cannot tolerate TMP-SMZ, recommended alternatives for prophylaxis against both PCP and toxoplasmosis include dapsone plus pyrimethamine or atovaquone with or without pyrimethamine. Oral clindamycin and primaquine *cannot* be recommended as prophylaxis. Adverse reactions noted with dapsone include rash and bone marrow suppression. Dapsone cannot be used in patients with glucose-6-phosphate dehydrogenase deficiency. A screening test should be ordered before initiating prophylaxis with this medication. Pyrimethamine can cause neutropenia and thrombocytopenia. Aerosolized pentamidine should be administered only to those patients who cannot tolerate the alternative prophylactic agents, as it is a less effective form of prophylaxis, particularly for patients with CD4 cell counts below 100/mm^3. It also does not offer protection against invasive toxoplasmosis and has been associated with the development of extrapulmonary *P. carinii* infection. Aerosolized pentamidine has induced cough, bronchospasm, pneumothorax, pancreatitis, hypoglycemia, and nephrotoxicity. Prophylactic failure with aerosolized pentamidine has resulted in atypical PCP (cysts, blebs, pneumothoraces). A risk of tuberculosis (TB) transmission is possible as well if the patient is coinfected with TB.

Primary and secondary *Pneumocystis* prophylaxis should be discontinued for adult and adolescent patients who have responded to HAART with an increase in CD4+ T-lymphocyte counts to more than 200 cells/μL for 3 months or longer. In observational and randomized studies supporting this recommendation, the majority of patients were taking antiretroviral regimens that included a protease inhibitor (PI), and the majority had a CD4+ T-lymphocyte cell count of more than 200 cells/μL for 3 months or longer before discontinuing PCP prophylaxis. The median CD4+ T-lymphocyte count at the time prophylaxis was discontinued was more than 300 cells/μL, and certain patients had a sustained suppression of HIV plasma ribonucleic acid (RNA) levels below detection limits of the assay used. Median follow-up ranged from 6 to 16 months. Discontinuing primary prophylaxis among these patients is recommended because, apparently, prophylaxis adds limited disease prevention (i.e., for PCP, toxoplasmosis, or bacterial infections) and because discontinuing drugs reduces pill burden, potential for drug toxicity, drug interactions, selection of drug-resistant pathogens, and cost. Prophylaxis should be reintroduced if the CD4+ T-lymphocyte count decreases to less than 200 cells/μL.

HIV-infected persons should be tested for immunoglobulin G (IgG) antibody to *Toxoplasma* soon after the diagnosis of HIV infection to detect latent infection with *T. gondii*. All HIV-infected persons, including those who lack IgG antibody to *Toxoplasma*, should be counseled regarding sources of toxoplasmic infection. They should be advised not to eat raw or undercooked meat, including undercooked lamb, beef, pork, or venison. Specifically, lamb, beef, and pork should be cooked until it is no longer pink inside. HIV-infected persons should wash their hands after contact with raw meat and after gardening or other contact with soil; in addition, they should wash fruits and vegetables well before eating them raw. If the patient owns a cat, the litter box should be changed daily, preferably by an HIV-negative, nonpregnant person; alternatively, patients should wash their hands thoroughly after changing the litter box. Patients should be encouraged to keep their cats inside and not to adopt or handle stray cats. Cats should be fed only canned or dried commercial food or well-cooked table food, not raw or undercooked meats. Patients need not be advised to part with their cats or to have their cats tested for toxoplasmosis.

Toxoplasma-seropositive patients who have a CD4+ T-lymphocyte count of less than 100/μL should be given prophylaxis against toxoplasmic encephalitis (TE). Apparently, the double-strength tablet daily dose of TMP-SMZ recommended as the preferred regimen for PCP prophylaxis is effective against TE as well and is therefore recommended. If patients cannot tolerate TMP-SMZ, the recommended alternative is dapsone-pyrimethamine, which is also effective against PCP. Atovaquone with or without pyrimethamine also can be considered. Prophylactic monotherapy with dapsone, pyrimethamine, azithromycin, or clarithromycin cannot be recommended. *Toxoplasma*-seronegative persons who are not taking a PCP prophylactic regimen known to be active against TE should be retested for IgG antibody to *Toxoplasma* when their CD4+ T-lymphocyte counts decline to less than 100/μL to determine whether they have seroconverted and are therefore at risk for TE. Prophylaxis against TE should be discontinued among adult and adolescent patients who have responded to HAART with an increase in CD4+ T-lymphocyte counts to more than 200 cells/μL for 3 months or longer. Prophylaxis should be reintroduced if the CD4+ T lymphocyte count decreases to less than 100 to 200 cells/μL.

Patients who have completed initial therapy for TE should be administered lifelong suppressive therapy unless immune reconstitution occurs as a consequence of HAART. The combination of pyrimethamine plus sulfadiazine plus leucovorin is highly effective for this purpose. A commonly used regimen for patients who cannot tolerate sulfa drugs is pyrimethamine plus clindamycin; however, apparently, only the combination of pyrimethamine plus sulfadiazine provides protection against PCP as well. Patients receiving secondary prophylaxis (i.e., chronic maintenance therapy) for TE are, apparently, at low risk for recurrence of TE when they have successfully completed initial therapy for TE, remain asymptomatic with regard to signs and symptoms of TE, and have a sustained increase in their CD4+ T-lymphocyte counts of more than 200 cells/μL after HAART (e.g., ≥6 months). Discontinuing chronic maintenance therapy among such patients is a reasonable consideration. Some specialists would obtain a magnetic resonance image of the brain as part of their evaluation to determine whether discontinuing therapy is appropriate. Secondary prophylaxis should be reintroduced if the CD4+ T-lymphocyte count decreases to less than 200 cells/μL.

Adults and adolescents who have HIV infection should receive chemoprophylaxis against disseminated MAC disease if they have a CD4+ T-lymphocyte count of less than 50 cells/μL. Three FDA-approved prophylactic regimens are currently available: azithromycin (1,200 mg orally every week), clarithromycin (500 mg orally twice a day), and rifabutin (300 mg orally every day). The combination of clarithromycin and rifabutin is no more effective than clarithromycin alone for chemoprophylaxis and is associated with a higher rate of adverse effects than either drug alone; this combination should not be used. The combination of azithromycin with rifabutin is more effective than azithromycin alone; however, the additional cost, increased occurrence of adverse effects, potential for drug interactions, and absence of a difference in survival when compared with azithromycin alone do not warrant a routine recommendation for this regimen. Azithromycin is probably the preferred prophylaxis; it is administered once a week, shares with clarithromycin the ability to prevent respiratory infections, is unsurpassed in efficacy by any other regimen, appears to be safe in pregnancy, and does not appear to have a potential for drug–drug interactions, which is a characteristic of clarithromycin. Clarithromycin has the potential to cause drug interactions with theophylline, carbamazepine, digoxin, ritonavir, cisapride, felodipine, fluconazole, warfarin, ergotamine, terfenadine, astemizole, and buspirone. Rifabutin is an effective prophylactic agent and is not associated with the development of resistant organisms. Rifabutin has caused rash, myalgias, arthralgia, nausea, headache, uveitis, thrombocytopenia, and hepatitis. A major concern with rifabutin is the potential for drug–drug interactions, such as with fluconazole, phenytoin, methadone, warfarin, oral contraceptives, dapsone, clarithromycin, phenytoin, saquinavir, indinavir, nelfinavir, ritonavir, zidovudine, beta blockers, and oral hypoglycemics.

If clarithromycin or azithromycin cannot be tolerated, rifabutin is an alternative prophylactic agent for MAC disease, although rifabutin-associated drug interactions make this agent difficult to use. Before prophylaxis is initiated, disseminated MAC disease should be ruled out by clinical assessment, which might include obtaining a blood culture for MAC if warranted. Because treatment with rifabutin could result in rifampin resistance among persons who have active TB, active TB should also be excluded before rifabutin is used for prophylaxis. Primary MAC prophylaxis should be discontinued among adult and adolescent patients who have responded to HAART with an increase in CD4+ T-lymphocyte counts to more than 100 cells/μL for 3 months or longer. Primary prophylaxis should be reintroduced if the CD4+ T-lymphocyte count decreases to less than 50 to 100 cells/μL.

Patients are at low risk for recurrence of MAC when they have completed a course of 12 months or more of treatment for MAC, remain asymptomatic with respect to MAC signs and symptoms, and have a sustained increase (e.g., $\geq$6 months) in their CD4+ T-lymphocyte counts to more than 100 cells/μL after HAART. It appears that discontinuing chronic maintenance therapy among such patients is reasonable. Some specialists recommend obtaining a blood culture for MAC, even for asymptomatic patients, before discontinuing therapy to substantiate that disease is no longer active. Secondary prophylaxis should be reintroduced if the CD4+ T-lymphocyte count decreases to less than 100 cells/μL. Rifabutin or clarithromycin, when taken for MAC prophylaxis, have been found to protect against cryptosporidiosis.

When HIV infection is first recognized, the patient should receive a tuberculin skin test (TST) by administration of intermediate-strength (5-TU) purified protein derivative (PPD) by the Mantoux method. Routine evaluation for anergy is not recommended. All HIV-infected persons who have a positive TST result ($\geq$5 mm of induration) should undergo chest radiography and clinical evaluation to rule out active TB. All HIV-infected persons, regardless of age, who have a positive TST result but have no evidence of active TB and no history of treatment for active or latent TB should be treated for latent TB infection. Options include isoniazid daily or twice weekly (BII) for 9 months; 4 months of therapy daily with either rifampin or rifabutin; or 2 months of therapy with either rifampin and pyrazinamide or rifabutin and pyrazinamide. Reports exist of fatal and severe liver injury associated with treatment of latent TB infection among HIV-uninfected persons treated with the 2-month regimen of daily rifampin and pyrazinamide; therefore, using regimens that do not contain pyrazinamide among HIV-infected persons whose completion of treatment can be ensured is prudent. Because HIV-infected persons are at risk for peripheral neuropathy, those receiving isoniazid should also receive pyridoxine. Decisions to use a regimen containing either rifampin or rifabutin should be made after carefully considering potential drug interactions, including those related to PIs and nonnucleoside reverse transcriptase inhibitors (NNRTIs). Directly observed therapy (DOT) should be used with intermittent dosing regimens and when otherwise operationally feasible. HIV-infected persons who are close contacts of persons who have infectious TB should be treated for latent TB infection, regardless of their TST results, age, or prior courses of treatment, after a diagnosis of active TB has been excluded. For persons exposed to isoniazid- or rifampin-resistant TB, decisions to use chemoprophylactic antimycobacterial agents other than isoniazid alone, rifampin or rifabutin alone, rifampin plus pyrazinamide, or rifabutin plus pyrazinamide should be based on the relative risk for exposure to resistant organisms and should be made in consultation with public health authorities. Although the reliability of TST might diminish as the CD4+ T-lymphocyte count declines, annual repeat testing should be considered for HIV-infected persons who are TST negative on initial evaluation and who belong to populations in which a substantial risk for exposure to *M. tuberculosis* exists. Clinicians should consider repeating TST for persons whose initial skin test was negative and whose immune function has improved in response to HAART (i.e., those whose CD4+ T-lymphocyte count has increased to >200 cells/μL). Administering bacille Calmette-Guérin (BCG) vaccine to HIV-infected persons is contraindicated because of its potential to cause disseminated disease. Chronic suppressive therapy for a patient who has successfully completed a recommended regimen of treatment for TB is unnecessary.

HIV specialists recommend that antifungal prophylaxis not be used routinely to prevent cryptococcosis because of the relative infrequency of cryptococcal disease, lack of survival benefits associated with prophylaxis, possibility of drug interactions, potential antifungal drug resistance, and cost. Apparently, adult and adolescent patients are at low risk for recurrence of cryptococcosis when they have successfully completed a course of initial therapy for cryptococcosis, remain asymptomatic with regard to signs and symptoms of cryptococcosis, and have a sustained increase (e.g., ≥6 months) in their CD4+ T-lymphocyte counts to more than 100 to 200 cells/μL after HAART. Discontinuing chronic maintenance therapy among such patients is a reasonable consideration, although recurrences can occur. Some HIV specialists would perform a lumbar puncture to determine if the cerebrospinal fluid (CSF) is culture negative before stopping therapy, even if patients have been asymptomatic; other specialists do not believe this is necessary. Maintenance therapy should be reinitiated if the CD4+ T-lymphocyte count decreases to 100 to 200 cells/μL.

Primary prophylaxis with oral ganciclovir can be considered for HIV-infected adults and adolescents who are CMV-seropositive and who have a CD4+ T-lymphocyte count of less than 50 cells/μL; however, this is not usually recommended. Maintenance therapy can be discontinued safely among adult and adolescent patients with CMV retinitis whose CD4+ T-lymphocyte counts have indicated a sustained (e.g., ≥6 months) increase to more than 100 to 150 cells/μL in response to HAART. Such decisions should be made in consultation with an ophthalmologist and should take into account such factors as magnitude and duration of CD4+ T-lymphocyte increase, anatomic location of the retinal lesion, vision in the contralateral eye, and the feasibility of regular ophthalmologic monitoring. All patients who have had anti-CMV maintenance therapy discontinued should continue to undergo regular ophthalmologic monitoring for early detection of CMV relapse as well as for immune reconstitution uveitis. CMV viral load or other markers of CMV infection (e.g., antigenemia or viral deoxyribonucleic acid [DNA] tests) are not well standardized; their role in predicting relapse remains to be defined. Relapse of CMV retinitis occurs among patients whose anti-CMV maintenance therapies have been discontinued and whose CD4+ T lymphocyte counts have decreased to less than 50 cells/μL. Therefore, reinstitution of secondary prophylaxis should occur when the CD4+ T-lymphocyte count has decreased to less than 100 to 150 cells/μL. Relapse has been reported among patients whose CD4+ T-lymphocyte counts are more than 100 cells/μL, but such reports are rare.

After a complete history of previous cervical disease has been obtained, HIV-infected women should have a pelvic examination and a Papanicolaou (Pap) smear. In accordance with the recommendation of the Agency for Health Care Policy and Research, the Pap smear should be obtained twice during the first year after diagnosis of HIV infection and, if the results are normal, annually thereafter.

Adults and adolescents who have a CD4+ T-lymphocyte count of 200 cells/μL or higher should be given a single dose of 23-valent polysaccharide pneumococcal vaccine if they have not received this vaccine during the previous 5 years. Immunization should also be considered for patients with CD4+ T-lymphocyte counts of less than 200 cells/μL, although clinical evidence has not confirmed efficacy. Revaccination can be considered for patients who were initially immunized when their CD4+ T-lymphocyte counts were less than 200 cells/μL and whose CD4+ counts have increased to more than 200 cells/μL in response to HAART. The duration of the protective effect of primary pneumococcal vaccination is unknown. Periodic revaccination can be considered; an interval of 5 years has been recommended for persons not infected with HIV and might be appropriate for persons infected with HIV. However, no evidence confirms clinical benefit from revaccination. Incidence of *H. influenzae* type B (Hib) infection among adults is low. Therefore, Hib vaccine is not usually recommended for adult use. An annual influenza vaccination is recommended for all patients. Hepatitis B vaccine should be given where appropriate. (JWM)

Current recommendations for prevention can be found on the Web:

http://www.cdc.gov/mmwr/preview/mmwrhtml/rr5108a1.htmd
http://www.hivatis.org

Bibliography

Aberg JA, et al. Localized osteomyelitis due to Mycobacterium avium complex in patients with human immunodeficiency virus receiving highly active antiretroviral therapy. *Clin Infect Dis* 2002;35:E8–E13.
Described three patients who developed atypical manifestations of Mycobacterium avium *complex (MAC) infection longer than 10 months (range, 3–16 months) after attaining sustained CD4(+) T-cell counts of more than 100 cells/μL while receiving antiretroviral therapy and not receiving MAC prophylaxis.*

Deayton JR. Changing trends in cytomegalovirus disease in HIV-infected patients. *Herpes* 2001;8:37–40.

Many individuals have been able to discontinue maintenance therapy for CMV with a low risk of disease recurrence to date.

DiRienzo AG, et al. Efficacy of trimethoprim-sulfamethoxazole for the prevention of bacterial infections in a randomized prophylaxis trial of patients with advanced HIV infection. *AIDS Res Hum Retroviruses* 2002;18:89–94.

In patients with advanced HIV infection not taking highly active antiretroviral therapy, the treatment strategy that initiates prophylaxis with trimethoprim-sulfamethoxazole *(TMP-SMZ) is superior to those initiating with Aerosol Pentamidine (AP) or Dapsone (DAP) for preventing any bacterial infection, with most of the advantage manifested through infectious diarrhea, sinusitis/otitis media, and pneumonia.*

Furrer H, Cohort Study tS t. Management of opportunistic infection prophylaxis in the highly active antiretroviral therapy era. *Curr Infect Dis Rep* 2002;4:161–174.

Incidence of opportunistic infections (OIs) has declined and survival after an OI has improved. Achieving a CD4 count of 200 cells/L after 6 months of antiretroviral therapy (ART) is a valuable marker for low risk of OI afterward.

Kaplan JE, et al. Viral load as an independent risk factor for opportunistic infections in HIV-infected adults and adolescents. *AIDS* 2001;15:1831–1836.

Viral load is an independent risk factor for OI and should be considered in special situations, such as in decisions to discontinue primary or secondary OI prophylaxis after CD4 lymphocyte counts have increased in response to ART.

Kaplan JE, et al. Guidelines for preventing opportunistic infections among HIV-infected persons—2002. Recommendations of the U.S. Public Health Service and the Infectious Diseases Society of America. *MMWR Recomm Rep* 2002;51:1–27, 29–46.

Major changes since the last edition of the guidelines include (1) updated recommendations for discontinuing primary and secondary OI prophylaxis among persons whose CD4+ T-lymphocyte counts have increased in response to antiretroviral therapy; (2) emphasis on screening all HIV-infected persons for infection with hepatitis C virus; (3) new information regarding transmission of human herpesvirus 8 infection; (4) new information regarding drug interactions, chiefly related to rifamycins and antiretroviral drugs; and (5) revised recommendations for immunizing HIV-infected adults and adolescents and HIV-exposed or -infected children.

Petrosillo N, et al. Nosocomial bloodstream infections among human immunodeficiency virus-infected patients: incidence and risk factors. *Clin Infect Dis* 2002;34:677–685.

Nosocomial blood stream infections (NBSIs) continue to occur frequently and remain severe and life-threatening manifestations.

Pierce AB, Hoy JF. Is the recommendation for pneumococcal vaccination of HIV patients evidence based? *J Clin Virol* 2001;22:255–261.

It may be more cost effective to concentrate efforts on strategies to improve adherence to ARV therapy, as this has unequivocally been shown to be associated with a reduction in the incidence of pneumococcal disease.

Sax PE. Opportunistic infections in HIV disease: down but not out. *Infect Dis Clin North Am* 2001;15:433–455.

Despite the significant improvement in patient survival and reduction in the incidence of HIV-related opportunistic infections with the introduction of potent, combination antiretroviral therapy, these infections remain a significant challenge in the management of HIV-infected patients.

Trikalinos TA, Ioannidis JP. Discontinuation of Pneumocystis carinii prophylaxis in patients infected with human immunodeficiency virus: a meta-analysis and decision analysis. *Clin Infect Dis* 2001;33:1901–1909.

The authors performed a meta-analysis and a decision analysis on the discontinuation of prophylaxis for PCP in patients infected with HIV who had adequate immune recovery while receiving highly active antiretroviral therapy. Discontinuation of PCP prophylaxis in patients with adequate immune recovery is a useful strategy that should be widely considered.

Zeller V, et al. Discontinuation of secondary prophylaxis against disseminated Mycobacterium avium complex infection and toxoplasmic encephalitis. *Clin Infect Dis* 2002;34: 662–667.
Patients were followed up for a median of 29 months after discontinuation of secondary prophylaxis; no relapses occurred in patients with a history of TE, and three relapses occurred in patients with a history of disseminated MAC infection (incidence, four relapses per 100 person-years).

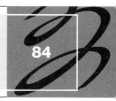

ANTIRETROVIRAL THERAPY   84

*T*his is an exciting subject, but it is time sensitive. The reader is encouraged to attend conferences, read the latest journals, and carefully surf the Internet to obtain the latest information.

 ## VIRAL LIFECYCLE

It begins with binding of the gp120 component of the viral envelope to the CD4 cell surface molecule and a 7-transmembrane cellular coreceptor for the virus. Next, fusion of the viral lipid envelope to the cellular membrane occurs through the fusion domain of gp41, another component of the envelope gp160 protein. The viral core will then enter the cell and the viral RNA is reverse transcribed into double-stranded DNA in the cytoplasm by the reverse transcriptase (RT) enzyme. Double-stranded HIV DNA has to be transported to the nucleus. At this point it is inserted into chromosomal DNA of the target cell. Transcription and translation will follow. It is important to note that the protease activity is necessary for processing of the core (gag) polyprotein and the gag/pol precursor polyprotein before production of infectious virions can occur.

Combination therapy targeting different steps in the above lifecycle appears to be necessary to impede the virus lifecycle efficiently. Highly active antiretroviral therapy (HAART) has dramatically changed the natural history of this infection.

INDIVIDUAL AGENTS AND CLASSES OF ANTIRETROVIRALS

Nucleoside reverse transcriptase inhibitors (NRTIs) compete with natural deoxynucleotide triphosphates at the RT active site for incorporation into DNA. When incorporated, NRTIs act as DNA chain terminators because they lack the 3′ hydroxyl moiety necessary for chain elongation. See Table 84-1 for characteristics of the individual inhibitors. Cross-resistance occurs within this family of drugs.

Nonnucleoside reverse transcriptase inhibitors (NNRTIs) bind to RT at a site that is distinct from the substrate binding site. NNRTIs do not require phosphorylation to become active, and they do not act as competitive inhibitors of RT or as DNA chain terminators. As before, cross-resistance occurs within this family of inhibitors but not with the NRTI medications. See Table 84-2 for characteristics of this family of drugs.

TABLE 84-1 Nucleoside Reverse Transcriptase Inhibitors

Drug	Usual dose	Metabolism	Side effects	Other
Abacavir (Ziagen)	300 mg b.i.d. Available in Trizivir too	No food restrictions No dose adjustment in renal insufficiency	In approximately 5% of patients, abacavir causes a hypersensitivity reaction that can be life-threatening	Mutations at codon 184, 65, and 151 are important
Didanosine (Videx, ddi)	400 mg q.d. (capsule or tablets) 200 mg b.i.d. (tablets) 250 mg b.i.d (buffered powder)	Should be taken on an empty stomach, 1 hour before or 2 hours after a meal Adjust for renal insufficiency	Diarrhea, neuropathy, pancreatitis	Reduce didanosine dose to 250 mg q.d. when used with tenofovir Mutations at 184, 151 appear to be important
Emtricitabine (Emtriva)	200 mg q.d. Hepatitis B?	No food restrictions. Adjust for renal insufficiency	Rare overall. The most common adverse effects noted in clinical trials of emtricitabine with other antiviral agents were headache, diarrhea, nausea, and rash	HIV isolates with resistance to emtricitabine by virtue of a mutation at RT codon 184 have been shown to be cross-resistant to lamivudine and zalcitabine, but retained sensitivity to abacavir, didanosine, stavudine, tenofovir, and zidovudine
Lamivudine (Epivir, 3TC)	150 mg b.i.d 300 mg q.d. Also in Trizivir Lamivudine is active against hepatitis B virus	No food restrictions Adjust for renal insufficiency	Rare	Mutation at codon 184 may reverse resistance associated with thymidine analogues.
Stavudine (Zerit, d4T)	40 mg b.i.d (immediate release) 100 mg q.d. (extended release)	No food restrictions Adjust for renal insufficiency	Peripheral neuropathy Lactic acidosis	Mutations at codons 41, 151 215 are important
Zidovudine (Retrovir, azidothymidine, AZT)	300 mg b.i.d Also in Trizivir	No food restrictions Adjust for renal insufficiency	Anemia. Loss of appetite, nausea, vomiting, malaise, headache, weakness and dizziness	Perinatal transmission is reduced by AZT
Tenofovir (Viread)	300 mg q.d.	No food restrictions Adjust for renal insufficiency	Not as toxic as adefovir but some cases of renal impairment associated with the use of tenofovir, including cases of acute renal failure and Fanconi syndrome have been reported	Adenosine nucleotide analogue Avoid coadministration of Reyataz or consider ritonavir-boosted atazanavir Interacts with Videx K65R mutation appears to be important

(Adapted from http://hivinsite.ucsf.edu/InSite.jsp?page=md-rr-18).

Drug	Usual dose	Metabolism	Side effects	Other
Delavirdine (Rescriptor)	400 mg t.i.d.	No food restrictions No dose adjustment is necessary in renal insufficiency Delavirdine inhibits metabolism by cytochrome P450 3A (CYP3A)	The most common symptomatic side effect of delavirdine is rash, usually occurring within 1–3 weeks of treatment Rash is not usually severe	Several drug interactions
Efavirenz (Sustiva)	600 mg q.d.	Efavirenz should be taken on an empty stomach, at bedtime No dose adjustment is necessary in renal insufficiency Efavirenz interacts with the cytochrome P450 3A (CYP3A) enzyme system	Often a sense of an altered mental state, which usually resolves within the first month of treatment Sleep disturbances Rash is also common but is seldom serious and usually resolves after 2–3 weeks without discontinuation of therapy	Increases in methadone dose should be considered when efavirenz therapy is initiated
Nevirapine (Viramune)	200 mg q.d. for 14 days, then 200 mg b.i.d. Likelihood of rash is reduced by the recommended initiation of nevirapine at half treatment dose, with increase to full dose if no rash is present after 2 weeks	No food restrictions No dose adjustment is necessary in renal insufficiency Cytochrome P450 3A (CYP3A) inducer	Rash often occurs in the first 6 weeks of treatment Women tend to be at higher risk than men for developing nevirapine-associated rash Symptomatic liver toxicity occurs in 4% of patients Transaminases should be monitored closely, especially during the first 18 weeks of treatment Patients with higher CD4 counts (>250 cells/μ in women, and >400 cells/μ in men) at initiation of nevirapine therapy, particularly women, are at greater risk for acute symptomatic hepatic events, including death, especially in the first 6 weeks of therapy Patients with chronic hepatitis B or C infection appear to be at higher risk for later hepatic events	Increases in methadone dose should be considered when nevirapine therapy is initiated A perinatal regimen of nevirapine (single oral dose to the mother at onset of labor, followed by a single oral dose to the newborn) showed a dramatic reduction, comparable or superior to an oral zidovudine regimen, in mother-to-child transmission of HIV HIV resistant to NNRTIs was detected in the blood of participating mothers 6 weeks after the single dose of nevirapine Nevirapine-resistant virus was also detected in infants for whom the regimen did not prevent HIV transmission

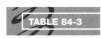

TABLE 84-3	**Combination Antiretroviral Medications**	
Combination	**Individual agents**	**Dose**
Combivir	AZT plus Epivir	One b.i.d.
Trizivir	AZT plus Epivir plus Abacavir	One b.i.d.
Truvada	Emtricitabine* and Tenofovir	Once daily
Epzicom	Abacavir plus Epivir	Once daily

*Emtriva is an NRTI for the treatment of HIV infection in adults. The drug works by inhibiting RT, the enzyme that copies HIV RNA into new viral DNA.

Table 84-3 provides information about combination antiretrovirals. Compliance is increased by the use of these medications.

HIV-1 protease cleaves the gag precursor polyprotein into the p24 and p17 virion components necessary for viral infectivity. These potent agents also demonstrate cross-resistance as well. Tables 84-4 and 84-5 illustrate their individual characteristics.

Entry inhibition is a newer approach to targeting the virus lifecycle. Fusion inhibitors offer a promising approach to antiretroviral therapy. The HIV-1 fusion inhibitor *enfuvirtide* (Fuzeon) binds to a protein on HIV's surface called gp41. Once it does this, HIV cannot successfully bind with the surface of T cells, thus preventing the virus from infecting healthy cells.

TOXICITY OF HAART

Toxicities such as gastrointestinal disturbances and rash are common in all the main classes of drugs (NRTIs, NNRTIs, and protease inhibitors (PIs), whereas other toxicities are more specific for each of the individual classes or agents. Please see Tables 84-1 through 84-4 for more details.

In addition to inhibiting viral RT, NRTIs also inhibit cellular DNA polymerase γ, which is involved in mitochondrial DNA replication. Inhibition of DNA polymerase γ results in several different toxicities. These include myopathy, peripheral neuropathy, bone marrow toxicity, pancreatitis, and hepatic steatosis with lactic acidosis. Abnormal lipid metabolism has occasionally been observed in patients who are taking PI-sparing regimens. The mechanism responsible for this association has been postulated to be mitochondrial toxicity of NRTIs as well.

Rash and Stevens-Johnson syndrome may occur with use of any of the NNRTIs and abacavir. Abacavir should never be given as a rechallenge.

Of note, there are several class-specific adverse effects are associated with the use of protease inhibitors. Triglyceride and cholesterol levels may become elevated, and significant insulin resistance, hyperglycemia, and even frank diabetes mellitus may occur. Peripheral fat wasting and central fat accumulation, as well as "buffalo humps" similar to Cushing's disease, may occur. It appears that there is a homology between HIV protease and two proteins, cytoplasmic retinoic acid-binding protein type 1, and low-density lipoprotein-receptor–related proteins that regulate lipid metabolism.

Caution must be taken when using other drugs that are metabolized by the cytochrome P450 pathway in conjunction with NNRTIs or PIs. Several of these drugs, including rifampin, rifabutin, and methadone are commonly used in patients with HIV infection.

IMMUNE RECONSTITUTION

In many cases of successful HAART, slow increases in CD4+ T-cell numbers follow the sharp increase that occurs within the first few weeks of therapy. This slow increase is largely the result of appearance of naïve cells. Partial normalization of perturbed T-cell receptor $V\beta$

TABLE 84-4   Older Protease Inhibitors

Drug	Usual dose	Metabolism	Side effects	Other
Indinavir (Crixivan)	Single PI 800 mg q 8 hr Boosted Indinavir 800 mg+ ritonavir 100–200 mg b.i.d.*	Take on an empty stomach or with a light snack, but not within 1 hour before or 2 hours after a full meal unless it is boosted by ritonavir Drink an extra 1.5 L per day to reduce the risk of nephrolithiasis No dose adjustment is necessary in renal insufficiency Metabolized by CYP3A4. Drug interactions	Kidney stones Asymptomatic hyperbilirubinemia	The tablet and powder formulations of didanosine should not be taken at the same time as indinavir because the buffer in these formulations may interfere with indinavir absorption M46I, V82A, I84V mutations are important
Nelfinavir (Viracept)	1250 mg b.i.d. 750 mg t.i.d.	Take with a meal No dose adjustment is necessary in renal insufficiency An inhibitor of cytochrome P450 3A (CYP3A)	Diarrhea is commonly reported	The D30N mutation does not appear to be associated with resistance to other drugs, unlike the 90M mutation, which is less commonly selected by nelfinavir, but it confers or contributes to resistance to all other protease inhibitors
Saquinavir (Fortovase [sgc], Invirase [hgcl]	Single PI 1200 mg t.i.d. (soft gel capsules) 600 mg t.i.d. (hard gel capsules)* Saquinavir (hgc or sgc) 1,000 mg b.i.d. Saquinavir (hgc or sgc) 1,600 mg q.d. + ritonavir 100 mg q.d.	This drug should be taken with or after a meal No adjustment in renal insufficiency Cytochrome P450 3A4 isoenzyme metabolized Drug interactions Saquinavir should not be used as the sole protease inhibitor in regimens containing efavirenz, but the addition of ritonavir may boost saquinavir to therapeutic levels in combination with efavirenz	Well tolerated, some gastrointestinal distress with the pill burden	The soft-gel capsules allow better absorption and improved potency However, fully active levels of saquinavir may be attained by combining either formulation with ritonavir Resistance mutations (G48V, L90M) selected by saquinavir frequently confer or contribute to resistance against other protease inhibitors.

sgc, Soft gel capsules; hgc, Hard gel capsules.

TABLE 84-5 Newer Protease Inhibitors

Drug	Usual dose	Metabolism	Side effects	Other
Fosamprenavir (Lexiva)	**Boosted** Fosamprenavir 700 mg b.i.d.+ ritonavir 100 mg b.i.d. Fosamprenavir 700 mg b.i.d.+ ritonavir 100 mg b.i.d. Coadministration of fosamprenavir with lopinavir/ritonavir causes reductions in levels of both amprenavir and lopinavir; it appears that this adverse interaction cannot be overcome by increasing ritonavir levels. Avoid this combination **Single PI:**1400 mg b.i.d.	No food restrictions No adjustments for renal impairment Cytochrome P450 3A4 (CYP3A4) metabolized Coadministration of fosamprenavir with efavirenz has been shown to decrease amprenavir levels, but boosting with sufficient doses of ritonavir may maintain therapeutic amprenavir levels in the presence of efavirenz	Rash, nausea, and diarrhea Fosamprenavir appears to induce fewer gastrointestinal adverse effects than amprenavir. Laboratory abnormalities include hyperlipidemia and possible increases in transaminase levels	Prodrug of amprenavir Only the twice-daily boosted regimen is approved in PI-experienced patients Mutations selected by fosamprenavir are also characteristic of amprenavir resistance, and include I50V, I54L/M, V32I, I47V, and M46I. These mutations do not appear to confer significant cross-resistance to other protease inhibitors. It appears that resistance to fosamprenavir may develop more readily during treatment with unboosted fosamprenavir than during treatment containing ritonavir-boosted fosamprenavir

Atazanavir (Reyataz)	400 mg q.d.	Take with food	Symptomatic side effects may include jaundice (in approximately 10% of individuals), nausea, and diarrhea	Pharmacologic boosting of atazanavir is recommended when coadministered with certain interacting medications, including tenofovir, efavirenz, and nevirapine
	Atazanavir 300 mg q.d. + ritonavir 100 mg q.d. if boosted	Higher gastric ph may decrease absorption	Isolated hyperbilirubinemia	Administer didanosine tablets on an empty stomach and 2 hours before or 1 hour after food or atazanavir.
	PI experienced patients and those with potential drug level-lowering interactions need to be boosted	No adjustment for renal impairment	Elevations of AST and ALT may occur	Novel I50L mutation
		Atazanavir is a substrate of the cytochrome P450 3A4 isoenzyme and may alter serum concentrations of other drugs metabolized by this pathway	More lipid friendly than other PIs	Efavirenz and rifampin both decrease lopinavir levels significantly
				If five or more mutations are present at baseline, the probability of failure increases
Lopinavir + ritonavir (Kaletra)	400/100 mg BID	Take with food	Diarrhea and nausea	
Each capsule contains 133.3 mg lopinavir + 33.3 mg ritonavir		No adjustments for renal impairment	Elevated cholesterol and triglyceride levels	
		A potent inhibitor of cytochrome P450 3A (CYP3A) and CYP2D6, as well as an inducer of other hepatic enzymes	Liver toxicity is possible	
		Many drug interactions		

repertoires during HAART suggested that some of these cells might be thymically derived and that qualitative as well as quantitative immune reconstitution might be possible. This translates into the ability to discontinue suppressive or preventive therapy for opportunistic infections in many patients with HIV infection.

The flip side of this immune reconstitution is an inflammatory syndrome occurring days to months after the start of HAART, which can at times be confusing to the clinician and hazardous to the patient. This syndrome can be elicited by infectious and noninfectious antigens. This phenomenon can occur in two different settings, depending on whether antiretroviral therapy (ART) was started in a patient treated for ongoing opportunistic infection or in a clinically stable patient with or without requiring primary prophylaxis. Microbiologically, the possible pathogenic pathways involve recognition of antigens associated with ongoing infection or recognition of persisting antigens associated with past (nonreplicating) infection. The interval between the start of ART and the onset of IRS ranges from less than 1 week to several months, but the majority of events occur within the first 8 weeks. In terms of management, specific antimicrobial therapy, nonsteroidal anti-inflammatory drugs, and/or steroids should be considered on a case by case basis. See Table 84-6 for more details.

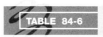 **TABLE 84-6** **Reconstitution Syndromes**

Syndromes	Comments	Onset	Management
MAC	Lymphadenitis, fever, abnormal CXR	Usually within the first 8 wks, but it can take several months in some cases.	In terms of management, specific antimicrobial therapy, nonsteroidal anti-inflammatory drugs, IVIG, thalidomide or steroids can be used on a case by case basis
CMV	Vitreitis, cystoid macular edema, uveitis		
HZV	Localized zoster		
TB	Abnormal CXR, mediastinal and peripheral adenopathy		
Cryptococcal	Worsening headache, CSF pleocytosis, palsy, hearing loss, abscess, mediastinitis, lymphadenitis		
Pneumocystis jirovecii	Pneumonitis		
Hepatitis B and C viruses	Hepatitis		

CXR, Chest X-ray; CMV, Cytomegalovirus; HZV, Herpes zoster virus; TB, Tuberculosis; CSF, Cerebrospinal fluid.

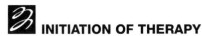

INITIATION OF THERAPY

Decisions regarding initiation or changes in antiretroviral therapy should be guided by monitoring the laboratory parameters of plasma HIV RNA (viral load) and CD4+ T-cell count in addition to the patient's general overall condition. A patient's willingness to comply with these regimens also should be factored into these decisions. Studies have shown that more than 95% adherence to a regimen was associated with an 81% incidence of virologic success.

There is strong evidence for treating patients with less than 200 CD4+ T cells/mm³, but the optimal time to initiate antiretroviral therapy among asymptomatic patients with CD4+ T-cell counts higher than 200 cells/mm³ is disputed. Regarding CD4+ T-cell count monitoring, the Multicenter AIDS Cohort Study (MACS) demonstrated that the 3-year risk for progression to AIDS was 38.5% among patients with 201 to 350 CD4+ T cells/mm³, compared with 14.3% for patients with CD4+ T cell counts higher than 350 cells/mm³. However, the short-term risk for progression also was related to the level of plasma HIV RNA, and the risk was relatively low for those persons with less than 20,000 copies/mL. An evaluation of 231 persons with CD4+ T-cell counts of 201 to 350 cells/mm³ demonstrated that the 3-year risk for progression to AIDS was 4.1% for the 74 patients with HIV RNA less than 20,000; 36.4% for those 53 patients with HIV RNA 20,001 to 55,000 copies/mL; and 64.4% for those 104 patients with HIV RNA greater than 55,000 copies/mL.

For persons with more than 200 CD4+ T cells/mm³, the decision to offer therapy must balance the desire of the patient for treatment, consideration of the prognosis for disease-free survival as determined by baseline CD4+ T-cell count and viral load levels, and assessment of the potential toxicity that might result from initiating antiretroviral therapy. The decision to initiate antiretroviral therapy should be guided by monitoring the laboratory parameters

 Recommendations to Begin Therapy

Category of disease	CD4 count (mm³)	Plasma RNA level	Comments
Symptomatic Disease or AIDS	Any value	Any value	Treat
Asymptomatic, AIDS	<200	Any value	Treat
Asymptomatic	>200 but <350	Any value	Offer treatment*
Asymptomatic	>350	>100,000	Offer or monitor CD4 closely†
Asymptomatic	>350	<100,000	Defer therapy‡

*Clinical benefit has been demonstrated in controlled trials only for patients with CD4+ T cells <200/mm³; however, the majority of clinicians would offer therapy at a CD4+ T-cell threshold <50/mm³. A recent evaluation of data from MACS of 231 persons with CD4+ T-cell counts >200 and <350 cells/mm³ demonstrated that of 40 (17%) persons with plasma HIV RNA <10,000 copies/mL, none progressed to AIDS by 3 years. Of 28 individuals (29%) with plasma viremia of 10,000–20,000 copies/mL, 4% and 11% progressed to AIDS at 2 and 3 years, respectively. Plasma HIV RNA was calculated as reverse-transcriptase polymerase chain reaction values from measured bDNA values. (Source: Phair JP, et al. Virologic and immunologic values allowing safe deferral of antiretroviral therapy. *AIDS* 2002;16:2455–2459).
†Some experienced clinicians recommend initiating therapy, recognizing that the 3-year risk for untreated patients to develop AIDS is >30%; in the absence of increased levels of Plasma HIV RNA, other clinicians recommend deferring therapy and monitoring the CD4+ T cell count and level of plasma HIV RNA more frequently; clinical outcome data after initiating therapy are lacking.
‡Many experienced clinicians recommend deferring therapy and monitoring the CD4+ T-cell count, recognizing that the 3-year risk for untreated patients to experience AIDS is <15%.
(Adapted from http://aidsinfo.nih.gov/guidelines/adult/AA_032304.html).

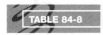

Type of Web site	URL
HIV drug interactions	http://www.hiv-druginteractions.org/
HIV drug interactions	http://www.projinf.org/fs/drugin.html
HIV consultation site	http://www.ucsf.edu/hivcntr/index.html
HIV medications overview	http://www.aidsmeds.com/List.htm
HIV medications drug chart	http://www.aidsmeds.com/lessons/DrugChart.htm
HIV information	http://www.hopkins-aids.edu/
NIH HIV information site	http://aidsinfo.nih.gov/
General antibiotic guide	http://www.hopkins-abxguide.org/
HIV therapy overview	http://home.mdconsult.com/das/journal/view/39539684-2/N/12327987?ja=281464&PAGE=1.html&sid=287154850&source=
Epzicom	http://www.epzicom.com/
Truvada	http://www.gilead.com/wt/sec/truvada
Fuzeon	http://www.fuzeon.com/

TABLE 84-8 Useful HIV Therapy Web Sites

that best predict the rate of disease progression (plasma viremia) and that reflect the degree of damage that has been sustained by the immune system (CD4 count), as well as the overall health of the patient. See Table 84-7 for more details.

CD4+ T-cell counts should be measured initially at the time of diagnosis, and then repeated every 3 to 4 months to evaluate the continuing effectiveness of therapy. When deciding on therapy initiation, the CD4+ T-lymphocyte count and plasma HIV RNA measurement should be performed twice to ensure accuracy and consistency of measurement. Plasma HIV RNA levels also should be measured initially and again at 2 to 8 weeks after initiation of antiretroviral therapy. This second measurement allows the clinician to evaluate the regimen's effectiveness. One should expect a decrease ($\sim$1.0 log$_{10}$) in viral load by 2 to 8 weeks. For the majority of patients, one should see a decrease below detectable levels (usually <50 RNA copies/mL) by 16 to 24 weeks. Factors that may preclude this from happening include a lack of patient adherence, malabsorption, or drug interactions. If HIV RNA remains detectable in plasma after 16 to 24 weeks of therapy, the plasma HIV RNA test should be repeated to confirm the result and a change in therapy should be considered. Plasma HIV RNA levels should not be measured during or within the 4 weeks after successful treatment of any intercurrent infection.

Table 84-8 lists several useful Web sites for review. (RBB)

Bibliography

Acosta EP, Gerber JG. Position paper on therapeutic drug monitoring of antiretroviral agents. *AIDS Res Hum Retroviruses* 2002;18:825–834.
This position paper offers guidelines to aid clinicians who choose to incorporate therapeutic drug monitoring (TDM) into the routine care of their patients.
Badri SM, et al. How does expert advice impact genotypic resistance testing in clinical practice? *Clin Infect Dis* 2003;37:708–713.
Consideration should be given to enlisting expert assistance in the interpretation of genotypic resistance testing (GRT) results in routine clinical practice.
Buckingham SJ, et al. Immune reconstitution inflammatory syndrome in HIV-infected patients with mycobacterial infections starting highly active anti-retroviral therapy. *Clin Radiol* 2004;59:505–513.
These cases illustrate the diverse chest radiographic appearances of immune reconstitution inflammatory syndrome (IRIS) occurring after HAART in patients with

mycobacterial and HIV coinfection. Significant mediastinal lymphadenopathy occurred in three of these five patients (with associated tracheal narrowing in two patients); four patients developed pulmonary infiltrates and one had an effusion. The cases further highlight that the onset of IRIS may be delayed for several months after HAART is started.

French MA, et al. Immune restoration disease after antiretroviral therapy. *AIDS* 2004; 18:1615–1627.
Review article.

Havlir DV. Strategic approaches to antiretroviral treatment. *Top HIV Med* 2003;11:145–149.
A useful clinical framework for decision making in antiretroviral treatment is to consider treatment options and goals at four decision points: initial therapy, early treatment failure, late treatment failure with high CD4+ cell count, and late treatment failure with low CD4+ cell count. This article summarizes a presentation given by Diane V. Havlir, MD, at the March 2003 International AIDS Society-USA course in Los Angeles.

Hirsch HH, et al. Immune reconstitution in HIV-infected patients. *Clin Infect Dis* 2004; 38:1159–1166.
State of the art review article.

Hirsch MS, et al. Antiretroviral drug resistance testing in adults infected with human immunodeficiency virus type 1: 2003 recommendations of an International AIDS Society-USA Panel. *Clin Infect Dis* 2003;37:113–128.
Resistance testing is recommended in cases of acute or recent HIV infection, for certain patients who have been infected as long as 2 years or more prior to initiating therapy, in cases of antiretroviral failure, and during pregnancy. Limitations of resistance testing remain, and more study is needed to refine optimal use and interpretation.

Johnson SC, et al. Recurrences of cytomegalovirus retinitis in a human immunodeficiency virus-infected patient, despite potent antiretroviral therapy and apparent immune reconstitution. *Clin Infect Dis* 2001;32:815–819.
The clinical significance of this case and of other recently reported cases is discussed.

Kaplan JE, et al. When to begin highly active antiretroviral therapy? Evidence supporting initiation of therapy at CD4+ lymphocyte counts <350 cells/μL. *Clin Infect Dis* 2003; 37:951–958.
The increased hazard associated with CD4+ cell counts of 200 to 349 cells/μL was modest but supports initiation of HAART at CD4+ cell counts less than 350 cells/μL, particularly in patients with high virus loads.

Kuritzkes DR. Management of patients with virologic and metabolic failure. *AIDS Read* 2003;13(6 suppl):S17–S22.
A difficult topic is addressed in this review.

Lori F, Lisziewicz J. Structured treatment interruptions for the management of HIV infection. *JAMA* 2001;286:2981–2987.
Results from randomized, controlled trials and more definitive means of gauging the status of the patient's immune system must be available before this treatment method is extended beyond the research setting.

Lori F, et al. Immune reconstitution and control of HIV. *HIV Clin Trials* 2004;5:170–182.

McGowan JP, Shah SS. Prevention of perinatal HIV transmission during pregnancy. *J Antimicrob Chemother* 2000;46:657–668.
Transmission of the human immunodeficiency virus (HIV) from mother to child can occur in utero, during labor, or after delivery from breastfeeding. The majority of infants are infected during delivery. Maternal HIV-1 plasma viral load at delivery is the most important predictor of vertical transmission. The impact of recent advances in the management of HIV infection in pregnancy is discussed with regard to their feasibility in resource-poor countries.

Mofenson LM, Munderi P. Safety of antiretroviral prophylaxis of perinatal transmission for HIV-infected pregnant women and their infants. *J Acquir Immune Defic Syndr* 2002;30:200–215.
This article focuses on a review of what is known about safety of antiretroviral regimens used to interrupt mother-to-child transmission for women and their children.

Ogedegbe AE, et al. Hyperlactataemia syndromes associated with HIV therapy. *Lancet Infect Dis* 2003;3:329–337.

This article reviews the current published work on these issues, identifies areas of controversy, and addresses directions for future research.

Rakhmanina NY, et al. Therapeutic drug monitoring of antiretroviral therapy. *AIDS Patient Care STDS* 2004;18:7–14.

A number of clinical trials have demonstrated that drug serum concentrations are an important factor in response to therapy for HIV, but whether TDM will become a tool for the routine management of HIV infection remains to be determined.

Schambelan M, et al. Management of metabolic complications associated with antiretroviral therapy for HIV-1 infection: recommendations of an International AIDS Society-USA panel. *J Acquir Immune Defic Syndr* 2002;31:257–275.

Review article.

Sharland M, et al. PENTA guidelines for the use of antiretroviral therapy in paediatric HIV infection. Pediatric European Network for Treatment of AIDS. *HIV Med* 2002;3:215–226.

These guidelines are aimed at assisting pediatricians in Europe with ART prescribing. They provide a more cautious approach to starting therapy than current pediatric U.S. guidelines.

Shelburne SA 3rd, Hamill RJ. The immune reconstitution inflammatory syndrome. *AIDS Rev* 2003;5:67–79.

Review article.

Temesgen Z, et al. Initial antiretroviral therapy in chronically-infected HIV-positive adults. *Expert Opin Pharmacother* 2004;5:595–612.

This article reviews the factors that should be considered in the selection of an initial antiretroviral regimen and presents the currently available evidence regarding the status of individual antiretroviral agents and treatment strategies relative to these factors.

Thorne C, Newell ML. Prevention of mother-to-child transmission of HIV infection. *Curr Opin Infect Dis* 2004;17:247–252.

Yeni PG, et al. Treatment for adult HIV infection: 2004 recommendations of the International AIDS Society-USA Panel. *JAMA* 2004;292:251–265.

Comprehensive review of this subject. Several excellent tables.

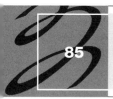

85 DRUG INTERACTIONS IN PATIENTS WITH HUMAN IMMUNODEFICIENCY SYNDROME

The expanding arsenal of antiretrovirals includes nucleoside reverse transcriptase inhibitors (NRTs), protease inhibitors (PIs), nonnucleoside reverse transcriptase inhibitors (NNRTIs), and fusion inhibitors, with a lot more in the pipeline. In addition to these virus-specific drugs, patients with HIV/AIDS often require additional agents to prevent or treat opportunistic infections; counteract wasting, depression, or anxiety; treat neoplasia; or ameliorate the metabolic side effects of select antiretrovirals. Thus medications for hyperlipidemia, diabetes mellitus, hypertension, lipodystrophy, and osteopenia also are often used. Factor into the equation the extended life expectancy of a patient on highly active antiretroviral therapy (HAART), the resultant aging of the HIV-positive population, the increased popularity of alternative medications, and the marketing of combined antiretroviral medications (Combivir®, Truvada®, Epzicom®, Trizivir®), and it becomes instantly obvious why many patients are on polypharmacy. Incidence of drug interactions in patients taking few agents has been estimated at about 5%. With polypharmacy, this can be expected to at least quadruple. The clinician must be acutely aware of the potential for drug and food interactions, some of which may be life threatening. The following discussion focuses on mechanisms for drug interactions and depicts many of the most common. It is not meant to be inclusive. With the large number of drugs that patients frequently ingest, and with the introduction of new antiretrovirals, it is likely that interactions heretofore unknown will be uncovered.

Mechanisms for drug/drug and drug/food interactions are multiple and involve two basic concepts. *Pharmacodynamic* interactions occur when the interplay of substances affects toxicity or antiretroviral activity. Examples include the simultaneous use of several nephrotoxic agents or the use of products that compete for binding to the same site and thus prove antagonistic (e.g., zidovudine plus stavudine). Table 85-1 lists some of the relevant drugs that share toxicities. In *pharmacokinetic* interactions, the blood level of the therapeutic agent is affected. This may be because of altered gastrointestinal absorption, modified protein binding and transport, inhibited or induced hepatic metabolism, or impaired renal filtration or excretion.

Many of the complex and life-threatening interactions associated with HIV-related agents are to the result of altered hepatic metabolism. The cytochrome P-450 system is susceptible to both induction and inhibition. Different drugs affect different cytochrome gene "families" and "subfamilies." CYP3 is responsible for the metabolism of many HIV medications. Our inability to easily determine plasma levels of antiretroviral drugs increases the dangers of altered metabolism and polypharmacy. Alternatively, improved understanding of the cytochrome system enables the exploitation of selected drug interactions for the patient's benefit. As an example, coadministration of ritonavir and a second protease inhibitor can inhibit CYP3 metabolism, producing a "boosting" effect on the second PI. The resultant increase in drug concentration and prolongation of drug half-life enables the patient to reduce pill burden and simplify dosing schedules.

 ## NUCLEOSIDE REVERSE TRANSCRIPTASE INHIBITORS

Table 85-2 summarizes major interactions for products within this category. NRTIs are prodrugs that are converted to the active state by intracellular phosphorylation. These drugs generally have more limited interactions. Knowledge of each drug's profile and toxicity, however, is essential for both efficacy and safety.

Didanosine (DDI) is unstable in gastric acid and is, therefore, manufactured either with buffers or in an enteric-coated/delayed-release form. The pharmacokinetics of DDI in its chewable/dispersible tablet and oral solution forms is susceptible to changes in gastric pH. Acidic medications (e.g., indinavir) may decrease the bioavailability of DDI, whereas those that require acid for absorption (e.g., ketoconazole, itraconazole) should not be coadministered. The buffering agents in the nonenteric-coated forms of DDI also may interfere with absorption of tetracycline and fluoroquinolones. Other NRTI pharmacokinetic interactions include inhibition of intracellular phosphorylation of zidovudine by ribavirin. Tenofovir and emtricitabine are eliminated by both glomerular filtration and active tubular secretion; other compounds that undergo active secretion (acyclovir, ganciclovir) may cause variations in drug levels. The combination of DDI and tenofovir has the potential to increase the levels of the former to potentially toxic levels; the mechanism for this is unclear.

Pharmacodynamic interactions include the potential for stavudine, DDI, and zalcitabine to cause peripheral neuropathy (along with isoniazid and linezolid) and pancreatitis (along with pentamidine, ritonavir, and lopinavir). Similarly, zidovudine and other commonly used AIDS medications (sulfa drugs, dapsone, ganciclovir, pyrimethamine, interferons, flucytosine) may cause additive myelosuppression.

 ## PROTEASE INHIBITORS

PIs are included in many highly active regimens for the management of HIV/AIDS. They are metabolized by the cytochrome P450 isoenzyme CYP3A and, to varying degrees, act as inhibitors of this enzyme. If drug combinations are not scrutinized for other agents primarily

TABLE 85-1 HIV-Related Drugs With Overlapping Toxicities

Bone marrow suppression	Peripheral neuropathy	Pancreatitis	Nephro-toxicity	Hepato-toxicity	Rash	Diarrhea	Ocular effects
Amphotericin B	Didanosine	Co-trimoxazole	Acyclovir (IV, high dose)	Azithromycin	Abacavir	Atovaquone	Didanosine
Cidofovir	Isoniazid	Lamivudine	Adefovir	Clarithromycin	Amprenavir	Clindamycin	Ethambutol
Co-trimoxazole	Linezolid	(children)	Aminoglycosides	Delavirdine	Atovaquone	Didanosine	Linezolid
Cytotoxic	Stavudine	Pentamidine	Amphotericin B	Efavirenz	Clarithromycin	Lopinavir/Ritonavir	Rifabutin
Chemotherapy	Zalcitabine	Ritonavir	Cidofovir	Fluconazole	Co-trimoxazole	Nelfinavir	Voriconazole
Dapsone		Stavudine	Foscarnet	Isoniazid	Dapsone	Ritonavir	
Flucytosine		Zalcitabine	Indinavir	Itraconazole	Delavirdine	Tenofovir	
Ganciclovir			Pentamidine	Ketoconazole	Efavirenz		
Hydroxyurea			Tenofovir	Neviparine	Fosamprenavir		
Interferon-α				(NRTIs)	Neviparine		
Linezolid				PIs	Sulfadiazine		
Peginterferon-α				Rifabutin	Voriconazole		
Primaquine				Rifampin			
Pyrimethamine				Voriconazole			
Ribavirin							
Rifabutin							
Sulfadiazine							
Trimetrexate							
Valganciclovir							
Zidovudine							

(Adapted from Table 23: HIV-Related Drugs with Overlapping Toxicities, in Guidelines for the Use of Antiretroviral Agents in HIV-1 Infected Adults and Adolescents in the U.S. Department of Health and Human Services database at http://aidsinfo.nih.gov/drugs/.)

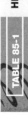

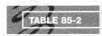

| **TABLE 85-2** | **Major Interactions With Nucleoside Reverse Transcriptase Inhibitors** |

Agent	Interacting drug	Result
Zidovudine (AZT)	Probenecid, fluconazole, atovaquone, methadone	↑ levels of zidovudine
	Rifampin, nelfinavir, ritonavir, ribavirin	ribavirin inhibits phosphorylation of AZT
DDI, buffered preparation	Itraconazole, ketoconazole, indinavir, delavirdine, fluoroquinolones, tetracycline, atazanavir, amprenavir, ritonavir	↓ absorption of interacting drug
Didanosine, buffered and enteric coated	Ganciclovir, allopurinol, tenofovir, cidofovir, probenecid	↑ levels of didanosine, possible shared elimination pathways
	Methadone	↓ levels of didanosine
	ribavirin	↑ risk of mitochondrial toxicity
Zalcitabine (ddC)	DDI antacids	Cross-resistance ↓ absorption of zalcitabine
Stavudine (d4T)	Zidovudine	Competitive inhibition of intracellular phosphorylation of stavudine
Lamivudine (3TC)	TMP/SMX	↓ levels of lamivudine
	DDI, ddC	Cross-resistance
Abacavir (ABC)	Methadone	↑ levels of methadone
Tenofovir (TDF)	Atazanivir, lopinavir/ritonavir	↓ levels of atazanivir and lopinovir/ritonavir, ↑ tenofovir
	Acyclovir, ganciclovir	Shared active renal tubular secretion, variable results
Emtricitabine (FTC)	No reported interactions	

(Adapted from Table 21: Drug Interactions Between Antiretrovirals and other Drugs: PIs, NNRTIs, and NRTIs, in Guidelines for the Use of Antiretroviral Agents in HIV-1 Infected Adults and Adolescents in the U.S. Department of Health and Human Services database at http://aidsinfo.nih.gov/drugs/.)

metabolized by this system, the effects of increased drug levels can be severe and life threatening. Agents to avoid with all PIs include astemizole (Hismanal®), cisapride (Propulsid®), pimozide (Orap®), bepridil (Vascor®), and terfenadine (Seldane®, no longer available in the United States); increased levels of these drugs can cause cardiac dysrhythmias. Others to use with extreme caution include the antiarrhythmics amiodarone, disopyramide, and quinine (cardiac toxicity), the antidepressants bupropion and nefazodone, and the ergot alkaloids (neurotoxicity), benzodiazepines (prolonged sedation), the HMG-CoA reductase inhibitors simvastatin and lovastatin (myopathy, rhabdomyolysis), and the PDE5 inhibitors (hypotension, visual changes, priapism). In addition to these medications that should be avoided with all PIs, Table 85-3 depicts several drug-specific interactions. Less drastic elevations of drug levels may be seen with many other drugs, such as the serotonin-reuptake inhibitors and tricyclic antidepressants, requiring a patient-by-patient search for new or augmented drug side effects. Similarly, other medications can alter the concentration of PIs. Rifampin, rifabutin, phenytoin, carbamazepine, phenobarbital, dexamethasone, and St. John's wort, for example, induce CYP, enhancing PI clearance and thereby lowering the antiretroviral concentrations to potentially subtherapeutic levels.

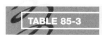

TABLE 85-3	**Major Interactions With Protease Inhibitors***	

Drug	Interacting agent	Result
Ritonavir (Norvir)	Oral contraceptives, theophylline, methadone	↓ levels of interacting drug
	Rifabutin, clarithromycin, atorvastatin, oral antifungals, sedatives, anticonvulsants, selected antiarrhythmics	↑ levels of interacting drug
	Rifampin	↓ levels of ritonavir
Indinavir (Crixivan)	Carbamazepine	↑ levels of interacting drug
	Clarithromycin, atorvastatin, trimethoprim	levels of interacting drug
	DDI	↓ indinavir absorption
	Rifampin, grapefruit juice, vitamin C	↓ levels of indinavir
	Ritonavir, rifabutin, oral antifungals	↑ levels of indinavir
Nelfinavir (Viracept)	Oral contraceptives	↓ levels of interacting drug
	Rifabutin, atorvastatin	levels of interacting drug
	Rifampin, rifabutin, anticonvulsants	↓ levels of nelfinavir
Saquinavir (Fortovase, Invirase)	Pravastatin	↑ levels of interacting drug
	Clarithromycin, atorvastatin	↑ levels of interacting drug
	Rifampin, rifabutin, anticonvulsants, dexamethasone, garlic	↓ levels of saquinavir
	Ritonavir, oral antifungals, grapefruit juice	↑ levels of saquinavir
Lopinavir	Oral contraceptives, methadone, phenytoin	↓ levels of interacting drug
	Select antiarrhythmics, carbamazepine, atorvastatin, rifabutin, oral antifungals, clarithromycin	↑ levels of interacting drug
	Rifampin	↓ levels of lopinavir
	Anticonvulsants	↓ levels of interacting drug
Amprenavir and fosamprenavir	Rifabutin, oral contraceptives, atorvastatin	↓ levels of interacting drug
	Rifampin, oral contraceptives	↓ levels of amprenavir and fosamprenavir
	Delavirdine	Varying results
Atazanavir	Calcium channel blockers, Rifabutin, atorvastatin, clarithromycin, oral contraceptives	↑ levels of interacting drug
	Proton-pump inhibitors, antacids, buffered, medications	↓ levels of atazanavir (↓ absorption)

*Avoid with all protease inhibitors: astemizole, cisapride, terfenadine, pimozide, ergotamines, midazolam and triazolam (require a monitored situation), St. Johns wort. Sildenafil, vardenafil and tadalafil levels may be dangerously increased.
(Adapted from Table 20: Drugs That Should Not Be Used With PI or NNRTI Antiretrovirals and Table 21: Drug Interactions Between Antiretrovirals and other Drugs: PIs, NNRTIs, and NRTIs, in Guidelines for the Use of Antiretroviral Agents in HIV-1 Infected Adults and Adolescents in the U.S. Department of Health and Human Services database at http://aidsinfo.nih.gov/drugs/.)

Of the older medications, ritonavir is the most potent CYP inhibitor, indinavir and nelfinavir are comparable inhibitors, and saquinavir is the least potent inhibitor and thus carries the least risk of drug interactions. Low-dose ritonavir is often used to boost levels of other PIs. These pairings allow for lower doses of the coadministered PI and a less demanding medication schedule but may have a larger impact on CYP450 enzymes and a higher potential for adverse drug reactions. Ritonavir and nelfinavir also increase the activity of the enzyme glucuronosyltransferase, which reduces serum estrogen concentrations and renders oral contraceptives less reliable. Alternatively, hormonal contraceptives have been shown to decrease levels of amprenavir to subtherapeutic levels.

The desire for PIs with fewer side effects (hyperlipidemia, diabetes, redistribution of body fat, etc.) and fewer drug interactions has led to the development of more of these agents. Newer medications, however, are still metabolized by the CYP system and have most of the same warnings and contraindications of the older ones. Fosamprenavir, the prodrug of amprenavir, has improved bioavailability; both of these PIs are sulfonamides and should be used with caution in patients with known sulfa allergies. Atazanavir does not appear to cause the typical increase in cholesterol or triglycerides but has been found to cause PR interval prolongation. Patients on calcium-channel antagonists or beta-blockers and patients with atrioventricular conduction abnormalities may require electrocardiogram monitoring. When atazanavir is administered with clarithromycin, the dose of the latter should be reduced by 50% to prevent toxic levels of clarithromycin and possible QTc prolongation.

NONNUCLEOSIDE REVERSE TRANSCRIPTASE INHIBITORS

Similar to the PIs, NNRTs are metabolized by the cytochrome P-450 system. However, whereas delavirdine is a potent CYP isoenzyme inhibitor, nevirapine is an inducer, and efavirenz may function as either. Agents of this class, therefore, have varying effects on coadministered drugs. For example, plasma concentrations of PIs frequently increase with

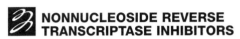

TABLE 85-4	**Interactions With Nonnucleoside Reverse Transcriptase Inhibitors**

Agent	Interacting drug	Effect
Nevirapine (Viramune)	Oral contraceptives, indinavir, saquinavir, methadone	↓ levels of interacting drug
	Rifampin, Rifabutin	↓ levels of nevirapine
	Ketoconazole, itraconazole, clarithromycin, erythromycin	↑ levels of interacting drug
Delavirdine (Rescriptor)	Indinavir, saquinavir, erythromycin, simvastatin, atorvastatin, sildenafil	↑ levels of interacting drug
	Rifampin	↓ levels of delavirdine
	Ketoconazole, itraconazole, clarithromycin, erythromycin, ritonavir	↑ levels of delavirdine
Efavirenz (Sustiva)	Oral contraceptives	↑↓ levels of interacting drug
	Rifabutin, clarithromycin, methadone	↓ levels of interacting drug
	Rifampin	↓ levels of efavirenz
	Ritonavir	↑↓ levels of efavirenz and interacting drug

(Adapted from Table 20: Drugs That Should Not Be Used With PI or NNRTI Antiretrovirals and Table 21: Drug Interactions Between Antiretrovirals and other Drugs: PIs, NNRTIs, and NRTIs, in Guidelines for the Use of Antiretroviral Agents in HIV-1 Infected Adults and Adolescents in the U.S. Department of Health and Human Services database at http://aidsinfo.nih.gov/drugs/.)

coadministration of delavirdine but decrease with nevirapine. When PIs are combined with efavirenz, the results are variable. Studies have demonstrated that plasma concentrations of ritonavir increase, but levels of amprenavir, indinavir, lopinavir, nelfinavir, and saquinavir decrease. Ketoconazole and voriconazole increase NNRT concentrations to potentially toxic levels, whereas their own concentrations are diminished and potentially ineffective.

In general, astemizole, terfenadine, cisapride, midazolam, triazolam, rifampin, ergot alkaloids, and St. John's wort should not be combined with NNRTs. Many other agents that should be used with caution include rifabutin, clarithromycin, oral contraceptives, anticonvulsants (carbamazepine, phenobarbital, phenytoin), anticoagulants, methadone. Interactions with most agents are complex and incompletely studied. Table 85-4 lists many of the known relevant interactions.

Delavirdine requires an acidic pH for absorption; antacids and buffered preparations of didanosine should be separated from delavirdine by at least 1 hour, and long-term coadministration with H_2-blockers or proton-pump inhibitors is not recommended.

 FUSION INHIBITORS

Enfuvirtide (Fuzeon®) is the first approved fusion inhibitor. No drug interactions with other antiretrovirals or with other medications have been identified to date that warrant dose modification. (RBB)

Bibliography

Dasgupta A, Okhuysen PC. Pharmacokinetic and other drug interactions in patients with AIDS. *Ther Drug Monit* 2001;23:591–605.

A readable review of the most relevant drug interactions that occur during treatment of HIV-infected patients. In addition to sections on antiretrovirals, the article also provides information on other commonly used medications, including antimycobacterias, antifungals, medications used for treating CNS disease and chemical dependency, and herbal supplements/medications.

McDonald CK, Gerber JG. Avoiding drug interactions with antiretroviral agents (parts 1 and 2). *J Respir Dis* 1998;19:24–25, 103–113.

A two-part review of drug interactions in HIV-infected patients. An older source, but it reviews relevant pharmacokinetic principles and the basics of drug metabolism as they pertain to HIV medications.

Murphy RL. Reviving protease inhibitors: new data and more options. *JAIDS* 2003;33:S43–S52.

A review of currently used PIs, common PI toxicities, boosted PIs, a synopsis of the studies that have investigated the use of these PI combinations, and a summary of promising new PIs.

Web sites providing information on antiretroviral drug interactions: http://hivinsite.ucsf.edu

AIDS info is a service of the U.S. Department of Health and Human Services. The database provides HIV/AIDS drug fact sheets describing each drug's use, pharmacology, and side effects and includes both approved and investigational HIV/AIDS drugs. Information is provided in English and Spanish and with the option of a technical or nontechnical version. http://www.medscape.com/px/hivscheduler

HIV InSite is a project of the UCSF Center for HIV Information. A database of the Food and Drug Administration (FDA)-approved antiretroviral drugs allows one to search for interactions by the antiretroviral drug, the interacting drug, or the interacting drug class. On the home page, click on "Medical." Then, in the left-hand column, under the subheading of "Antiretroviral Management," click on "Drug Interactions Database." http://aidsinfo.nih.gov/drugs/

Medscape requires free registration for viewing. The interactive program allows selection of a multidrug regimen, for which it provides potential interactions and generates the optimal daily schedule for the multidrug regimen. It focuses on drugs commonly

used in patients with HIV; the list is therefore limited. http://www.fda.gov/medwatch/
how.htm
*MedWatch is a resource provided by the FDA for obtaining drug safety informa-
tion and archiving adverse events. Forms are available for both clinicians and con-
sumers to report suspected serious adverse events, product problems, or medication
errors associated with the use of an FDA-regulated drug, biologic, device, or dietary
supplement.*

ROLE OF HIV RESISTANCE TESTING   86

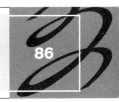

*R*esistance is usually due to changes in viral genes, called mutations. These mechanisms vary depending on drug class: chain termination for nucleoside reverse transcription
inhibitors (NRTIs)—impairing analogue incorporation or analogue removal, the latter being a classic thymidine-associated mutations (TAMs) mechanism; impaired binding to active
pocket for nonnucleoside reverse transcriptase inhibitors (NNRTIs); changing the shape of
the enzyme for protease inhibitors (PIs); or changing the gp41 protein sequence for fusion
inhibitors.

The term *primary* is used to indicate mutations that reduce drug susceptibility by
themselves, whereas the term *secondary* is used to indicate mutations that reduce drug
susceptibility or improve the replicative fitness of isolates with a primary mutation. Primary
(major) mutations interfere with the ability of the drug to bind to the target enzyme and may
confer measurable phenotypic drug resistance by themselves. Secondary (minor) mutations
function to improve the activity of an altered enzyme or enhance the fitness of a mutant virus.
Their phenotypic effect is usually dependent on the presence of other mutations. Mutations
are designated in a shorthand format using single-letter abbreviations for the amino acids en-
coded by a particular triplet of nucleotides (a codon). The normal, or wild-type (WT), amino
acid present at a particular location in a protein is given, followed by the location (amino acid
position, or codon number), followed by the new amino acid that has replaced the WT amino
acid. Because HIV mutates easily and reproduces very rapidly, a person may have many
different HIV strains in his or her body. These changes are the result of the inability of HIV-
1RT to *proofread* nucleotide sequences during replication. Replication is not really all that
efficient, and this feature is exacerbated by others, such as the high rate of HIV-1 replication
in vivo and by recombination. As a result, *quasispecies* evolve in individuals after primary
infection and can lead to drug resistance. The main problem in the clinical setting is that a
mutant selected for by a failing regimen may have some degree of cross-resistance to other
drugs in the same class that have not yet been prescribed to that patient. The development
of cross-resistance may lead to a reduced virologic or immunologic response to subsequent
regimens. Unfortunately it appears that resistant virus strains also can be transmitted between individuals. In the United States, it is estimated that about 10% of new infections are
with HIV strains harboring resistance to at least one of the three major classes of anti-HIV
drugs.

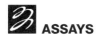 **ASSAYS**

The HIV *genotype* refers to the actual DNA sequence of the virus; the *phenotype* reflects the physical traits or behavior expressed by the genotype. Current commercially available genotypic and phenotypic assays both test HIV-1. Both genotype and phenotype testing methods require the use of polymerase chain reaction (PCR) technology to amplify the HIV-1 genes of interest (protease [PR] and reverse transcriptase [RT]) from patients' plasma samples. Genotypic tests look for genetic mutations that have been linked to drug resistance. Phenotypic tests assess which drugs can stop HIV growing in a lab setting. To accurately measure drug resistance, people should be on anti-HIV drugs and have a viral load of over 1,000 copies. Otherwise, the results may not be accurate or the test cannot be performed. *Genotypic resistance* testing refers to identifying mutations that have clinical resistance and is currently the most common method used. *Phenotypic testing* would be a closer match to traditional resistance testing in that one looks at how a virus grows in a certain concentration of drug. In that respect it more closely resembles disk diffusion testing for bacteria than does genotypic testing. Phenotypic testing would be similar to identifying a high minimum inhibitory concentration (MIC) to oxacillin to identify an organism as methicillin-resistant *Staphylococcus aureus* (MRSA), whereas genotypic testing would be more similar to identifying the mec or MRSA gene itself.

As a consequence of the very short half-life of HIV-1 in plasma, only actively replicating virus can be isolated from this source; thus the sequence of plasma virus represents the quasispecies most recently selected by antiretroviral drug therapy. After extraction, the contiguous protease and RT genes are reverse transcribed to cDNA and then amplified using PCR to generate sufficient DNA for genotypic or phenotypic testing. Genotypic testing detects the presence of mutations in a patient's virus population by identifying codon changes that differ from the standard, or "wild-type," genetic sequence of HIV. Phenotypic tests provide information about the relative amount of antiretroviral drug required to suppress replication of the patient virus, compared with the amount of drug needed to suppress replication of a laboratory strain of virus ("wild-type"). However, the results of both genotypic and phenotypic tests are complex and require expert interpretation if they are to be used successfully to help guide physicians in their use of antiretroviral therapy. One must remember that failure is more complex than just the genotype mutations that are present. Noncompliance, malabsorption, and drug interactions all play a role in a patient's lack of response.

Genotypic Assays

HIV genotypic assays detect specific mutations or nucleotide substitutions in the gag-pol region of the HIV-1 genome. This region encodes for the RT and protease enzymes, the targets of current antiretroviral drugs. Specific gene sequences are compared with that of a reference (wild-type) virus, and mutations associated with decreased susceptibility to specific antiretroviral drugs are identified.

HIV genotyping has historically been the more commonly used technology for drug resistance testing and generally used a two-step procedure: a PCR step to amplify a specific region of the HIV genome, and a specific mutation detection methodology that distinguishes each type of genotyping assay. The three most prevalent mutation detection methodologies are DNA sequencing, gene chip arrays, and the line probe assay (see Table 86-1).

Phenotypic Assays

Drug susceptibility testing involves culturing a fixed inoculum of HIV in the presence of serial dilutions of an inhibitory drug. Phenotypic assays use recombinant virus composed of a patient's virus PR and RT genes, which are inserted into a standard reference strain of virus. Like genotypic tests, current phenotypic assays also use PCR to amplify the gag-pol region of HIV-1. These assays, however, create a recombinant virus by introducing the RT gene, the protease gene, or both obtained from a clinical HIV isolate into a WT laboratory clone from which the corresponding gene(s) have been deleted. The recombinant virus is then

TABLE 86-1	Genotypic Methodologies
Gene sequence	A machine reads the gene sequence of the protease and RT genes.
Line probe assay, or LiPA	LiPA uses a specific probe to detect resistant mutations. There is a probe for each of the mutations known to lead to drug resistance. It can detect mutations that make up as little as 2–5% of the total virus population.
Gene chip	A third method, called GeneChip, uses a chip that has many markers built onto it. A blood sample is put onto the chip and it is passed through a scanner. The results are compiled by a computer which shows any mutations in the genes.

tested in vitro for the amount of each particular drug needed to inhibit virus replication by 50% (50% inhibitory concentration, IC_{50}), relative to the amount of drug needed to inhibit a reference strain of virus. This recombinant virus contains an indicator gene and is used in vitro to infect host cells in culture. Results are reported in the form of the fold change in drug susceptibility relative to a reference strain of HIV-1. An increase in IC_{50}, increase in resistance, and decrease in susceptibility are each different ways of expressing the fact that more drug is needed to inhibit the patient's virus in vitro relative to the reference virus. These assays are not designed to determine the amount of drug required to inhibit virus replication in vivo, but rather to compare the drug concentration required to inhibit a fixed inoculum of the isolated virus with the concentration required to inhibit the same inoculum of WT virus.

Pros and Cons of the Tests

A genotype test is cheaper and much faster than a phenotypic test but still costs $300 to $600. Results usually return within a week. A major problem with genotypic testing is that it will miss unknown gene mutations. A mutation that does not cause resistance by itself could lead to resistance when combined with other mutations. A phenotypic test usually requires a blood sample from someone with a viral load over 1,000. It can detect mutations that make up 10 to 20% of the total viral load. A drawback compared to genotypic testing is the higher cost at $800 to $1,000 per test. Also, the results may take 4 to 6 weeks to return.

Drugs are not usually tested in combinations. Because there are so many possible combinations of drugs, this would be very expensive and time-consuming. Some genotypic methods (line-probe assay or chip-based) interrogate only a limited subset of the positions in which resistance mutations may occur; these limited tests may be less appropriate for clinical use as an adjunct to managing the use of various antiretroviral combinations.

 SPECIFIC MUTATIONS BY DRUG

HIV Protease Mutations

The HIV protease enzyme is responsible for the posttranslational processing of the viral gag- and gag-pol-encoded polyproteins to yield the structural proteins and enzymes of the virus. Resistance is mediated by either a mutation in the substrate cleft or other types of mutations. Protease inhibitor (PI) resistance usually develops gradually from the accumulation of multiple primary and secondary mutations. Most primary mutations, by themselves, cause a two- to fivefold reduction in susceptibility to one or more PIs. However, this level of resistance is often insufficient to interfere with the antiviral activity of these drugs. Higher levels of resistance are resulting from the accumulation of additional primary and secondary mutations are often required for clinically significant reductions in drug susceptibility.

Saquinavir (SQV)

L90M and G48V are considered the key signature mutations developing with saquinavir therapy.

Indinavir (IDV)

Although V82A is often considered the key signature mutation developing with indinavir therapy, mutations M46I, I84V, and L90M also are often seen. Patients failing indinavir are often resistant to nelfinavir.

Nelfinavir (NFV)

D30N, and to a lesser degree L90M, are the key signature mutations developing with nelfinavir therapy. Since D30N does not result in cross-resistance to other PIs and is the most common mutation in patients failing nelfinavir, using nelfinavir as a first PI may preserve the other drugs of this class in later regimens.

Amprenavir (APV)

Although I50V is considered the key signature mutation developing with amprenavir therapy, other pathways to resistance are seen. Mutations at position 54, as well as those at 32, 46, 47, and 84, have a substantial effect on amprenavir. If a patient has developed only the I50V mutation as a result of amprenavir failure, susceptibility to other PIs should be preserved. Lopinavir susceptibility is reduced by the I50V mutation but in isolation it may not preclude use of the drug. Patients who have failed other PIs may often show various degrees of reduced susceptibility to amprenavir.

Lopinavir (LPV)

Mutations at positions 10, 20, 24, 32, 36, 46, 47, 48, 50, 53, 54, 63, 71, 73, 77, 82, 84, 90, and 93 may all contribute to some degree to lopinavir resistance. Data clearly suggest, however, that because of boosting, the combination of lopinavir/ritonavir can inhibit PI-resistant virus, resulting in clinical utility.

 NUCLEOSIDE REVERSE TRANSCRIPTION INHIBITORS

AZT

The most common mutations associated with drug resistance include M41L, D67N, K70R, L210W, T215Y/F, and K219 Q/E. Recently, mutations associated with resistance to either AZT or d4T have become known as TAMs, nucleoside analog mutations (NAMs), and/or nucleotide excision mutations (NEMs), as it is increasingly evident that both thymidine analogs can select for the same resistance-conferring mutations in RT and that these same mutations can confer a degree of resistance to either drug.

At least two NRTI mutations (L74V and M184V) and two NNRTI mutations (L100I and Y181C) partially reverse AZT resistance mediated by classic pathway mutations. AZT does not appear to select for the K65R mutation.

Didanosine

L74V is the most common mutation during didanosine (ddI) monotherapy and causes between two- and eightfold ddI resistance depending on the genetic context in which it develops. K65R causes three- to fivefold resistance to ddI but occurs rarely in clinical settings. M184V confers two- to fivefold ddI resistance and occurs in about 10% of patients receiving ddI. Finally, multinucleoside resistance through Q151M or the b3-b4 insertion develops in about 10% of patients receiving NRTI combinations.

D4T

The spectrum of mutations responsible for d4T resistance is not well characterized, but increasing evidence points to a role for the same mutations associated with resistance to AZT, that is, TAMs (also known as NEMs). The notion that AZT and d4T are cross-resistant is strengthened by the observation that the most common mutations in patients receiving d4T include the AZT-resistance mutations M41L and T215Y. Other potential mechanisms of cross-resistance between d4T and other drugs include multinucleoside resistance mediated by Q151M and the b3-b4 insertion.

3TC

M184V is the most common mutation causing 3TC resistance. Isolates with M184V are nearly 1,000-fold resistant to 3TC. In addition to causing high-level resistance to 3TC and low-level resistance to ddI, dideoxycytidine (ddC), and abacavir, M184V can hypersensitize HIV-1 isolates to AZT, adefovir, and tenofovir.

Abacavir

Q151M and its associated multinucleoside resistance mutations confer abacavir (ABC) resistance. The common RT mutation, M184V, which reduces ABC susceptibility twofold, has little or no effect by itself on virologic response to ABC. In previously untreated patients, ABC is the most potent NRTI virologically. Unfortunately, patients whose virus isolates contain multiple TAMs and 184V will have little benefit from ABC salvage therapy.

Tenofovir

Mutations associated with tenofovir (TDF) resistance include K65R, T69N/S/A/ins (high-level, multi-NRTI resistance), and Q151M (multi-NTRI resistance). In addition, the NEMs M41L, D67N, L210W, T215/F/Y, and K219Q/E/N can contribute to TDF resistance.

See Table 86-2 for more details regarding this class.

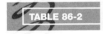 **TABLE 86-2**   **NRTI Resistance**

Resistance mutations	Blocks incorporation	Excision increased	Comments
TAMS	No	Yes	Thymidine analog mutations (41, 67, 70, 210, 215, 219). These can accumulate
MI84V	Yes	No	Blocks 3TC and others
K65R*	Yes	No	Rare with AZT. Common with 3TC, ddI, and ABC
Q151M	Discrimination results from a selective decrease of the catalytic rate constant k_{pol} The binding affinities of the triphosphate analogues for RT remain unchanged.		Q151M, by itself, causes intermediate levels of resistance to AZT, ddI, ddC, d4T, and ABC When occurring together with V75I, F77L, and F116Y, it causes high-level resistance to each of these NRTIs and low-level resistance to 3TC and TDF.

*Although important in selecting this mutation, the net effect on tenofovir itself may be essentially neutral because the decreased incorporation is balanced out by the decreased excision.

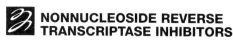

NONNUCLEOSIDE REVERSE TRANSCRIPTASE INHIBITORS

Isolates carrying single resistance mutations (K103N, V106A, Y181C, Y188C) have a 200-fold or greater increase in IC_{50} to nevirapine compared to WT isolates. Isolates carrying the V106A or Y188C mutations may remain susceptible to other NNRTIs (delavirdine, efavirenz). Isolates carrying the Y181C mutation are resistant to delavirdine but susceptible to efavirenz.

Isolates carrying the L100I or K103N mutations have a 20- to 30-fold increase in IC_{90} to efavirenz compared to WT isolates. The combination of K103N with either L100I, V108I, or P225H leads to an increase in IC_{90} of 100-fold or greater.

In contradistinction with other NNRTIs, the emergence of high-level resistance to efavirenz may require the accumulation of multiple mutations within the same viral genome. In this way, the barrier to resistance may be somewhat higher.

SPECIFIC RESISTANCE POSITIONS

PI Resistance Positions

Position: 84
I84V causes phenotypic and clinical resistance to SQV, RTV, IDV, NVF, and APV and contributes to LPV/r resistance.

Position: 54
Mutations at position 54 (generally I54V, less commonly I54T/L/M) contribute to resistance to each of the six approved PI and have been commonly reported during therapy with IDV, RTV, APV, SQV, and LPV/r. I54T/L/M is more common in amprenavir-treated patients.

Position: 46
Mutations at position 46 contribute to resistance to each of the PI except SQV and have been reported during therapy with IDV, RTV, APV, NFV, and LPV/r.

NRTI Positions

Mutation: K65R
K65R confers intermediate levels of resistance to ddI, ABC, and 3TC, but occurs rarely in vivo. The combination of K65R and M184V causes complete resistance to 3TC and greatly affects ddI and ABC. If a triple nucleoside regimen of TDF, ABC, and 3TC are used together, the K65R/M184 combination will cause what essentially amounts to having a patient on monotherapy with TDF. Interestingly, AZT-containing regimens rarely have K65R mutations. Perhaps the combination of Trivir and TDF might be more effective for this reason, but this is not proven at this time.

Mutation: M41L
M41L is associated with resistance to AZT and d4T, and to a lesser extent, ABC, ddI, ddC, and TDF, particularly when present with T215Y or F.

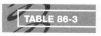 **TABLE 86-3** Useful Industry Web Sites

http://www.virco.be/
http://www.labcorp.com/
http://www.phenosense.com/
http://www.trugene.com/index.cfm
http://www.innogenetics.com/site/diagnostics.html

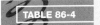

TABLE 86-4	Online Resources
Los Alamos HIV sequence database	http://hiv-web.lanl.gov
The International AIDS Society-USA	http://www.iasusa.org
Stanford HIV RT and protease sequence database	http://hivdb.stanford.edu
HIV ResistanceWEB.	http://www.hivresistanceweb.com
HIV InSite Knowledge Base Chapter April 2004	http://hivinsite.ucsf.edu/InSite?page=kb-03-02-06& doc=kb-03-02-07

Mutation: K70R

K70R is associated with AZT and d4T resistance, particularly when present with T215Y or F.

Mutation: Q151M

This mutation develops in about 5% of patients who receive dual NRTI therapy with ddI in combination with AZT or d4T.

NNRTI Positions

Mutation: K103N

K103N is currently the most clinically important NNRTI resistance mutation because it causes 20- to 50-fold resistance to each of the available NNRTI.

Mutation: Y181C/I

Y181C/I causes greater than 30-fold resistance to NVP and DLV and two- to threefold resistance to EFV. Nonetheless, NVP-treated patients with isolates containing Y181C generally have only transient virologic responses to EFV-containing salvage regimens.

Please see Tables 86-3 and 86-4 for more information concerning online resources. (JWM)

Bibliography

Barbour JD, et al. Evolution of phenotypic drug susceptibility and viral replication capacity during long-term virologic failure of protease inhibitor therapy in human immunodeficiency virus-infected adults. *J Virol* 2002;76:11104–11112.
Authors conclude that HIV may be constrained in its ability to become both highly resistant and highly fit and that this may contribute to the continued partial suppression of plasma HIV RNA levels that is observed in some patients with drug-resistant viremia.
Betts BJ, et al. Algorithm specification interface for human immunodeficiency virus type 1 genotypic interpretation. *J Clin Microbiol* 2003;41:2792–2794.
Despite the low number of patients and the short follow-up period, this study suggests that during failing therapy with analogue nucleosides, a phenotypic analysis could be performed in spite of an HIV genotypic sensitivity pattern.
Boyer PL, et al. Selective excision of AZTMP by drug-resistant human immunodeficiency virus reverse transcriptase. *J Virol* 2001;75:4832–4842.
Two distinct mechanisms can be envisioned for resistance of human immunodeficiency virus type 1 (HIV-1) RT to nucleoside analogs: one in which the mutations interfere with the ability of HIV-1 RT to incorporate the analog and the other in which the mutations enhance the excision of the analog after it has been incorporated.
Hanna GJ, D'Aquila RT. Clinical use of genotypic and phenotypic drug resistance testing to monitor antiretroviral chemotherapy. *Clin Infect Dis* 2001;32:774–782.
Prospective, controlled trials have demonstrated that resistance testing improves short-term virologic response. Resistance testing is currently recommended to help guide the choice of new drugs for patients after treatment has failed and for pregnant women.

Resistance testing should also be considered for treatment-naive patients, to detect transmission of resistant virus.

Hirsch MS, et al. Antiretroviral drug resistance testing in adults infected with human immunodeficiency virus type 1: 2003 recommendations of an International AIDS Society-USA Panel. *Clin Infect Dis* 2003;37:113–128.

Properly used resistance testing can improve virologic outcome among HIV-infected individuals. Resistance testing is recommended in cases of acute or recent HIV infection, for certain patients who have been infected as long as 2 years or more prior to initiating therapy, in cases of antiretroviral failure, and during pregnancy.

Hirsch MS, et al. Questions to and answers from the International AIDS Society-USA Resistance Testing Guidelines Panel. *Top HIV Med* 2003;11:150–4.

Concordance between phenotypic and genotypic susceptibility testing was 81% for NRTIs, 91% for NNRTIs, and 90% for PIs. Complete concordance between phenotype and genotype for all 14 drugs evaluated was observed in three (17%) patient samples. Phenotypic and genotypic susceptibility appear to provide similar results. However, interpretation of genotypic results can be complicated, and both methods still require clinical validation.

Shafer RW. Genotypic testing for human immunodeficiency virus type 1 drug resistance. *Clin Microbiol Rev* 2002;15:247–277.

Excellent summary. This review describes the genetic mechanisms of HIV-1 drug resistance and summarizes published data linking individual RT and protease mutations to in vitro and in vivo resistance to the currently available HIV drugs.

White KL, et al. Molecular mechanisms of resistance to human immunodeficiency virus type 1 with reverse transcriptase mutations K65R and K65R+M184V and their effects on enzyme function and viral replication capacity. *Antimicrob Agents Chemother* 2002;46:3437–3446.

HIV-1 RT resistance mutations K65R and M184V result in changes in susceptibility to several nucleoside and nucleotide RT inhibitors. K65R-containing viruses showed decreases in susceptibility to TDF, ddI, ABC, and (−)-beta-D-dioxolane guanosine (DXG—the active metabolite of amdoxovir), but appeared to be fully susceptible to zidovudine and stavudine in vitro. Viruses containing the K65R and M184V mutations showed further decreases in susceptibility to ddI and ABC but increased susceptibility to TDF compared to the susceptibilities of viruses with the K65R mutation.

Youree BE, et al. Antiretroviral resistance testing for clinical management. How does expert advice impact genotypic resistance testing in clinical practice? *AIDS Rev* 2002;4:3–12.

Consideration should be given to enlisting expert assistance in the interpretation of genotypic resistance testing results in routine clinical practice.

Pages followed by f indicate figures; pages followed by t indicate tables.